IMMUNOLOGY
A Short Course

To
Lisa, Jonathan, and Jennifer
R.C.

To
Ilene, Caroline, Alex, and Pearl
G.S.

IMMUNOLOGY
A Short Course

SEVENTH EDITION

Richard Coico
SUNY Downstate College of Medicine, Brooklyn, New York

Geoffrey Sunshine
Heath Effects Institute, and Tufts University School of Medicine, Boston, Massachusetts

WILEY Blackwell

This edition first published 2015 © 2015 by John Wiley & Sons Ltd

Registered office: John Wiley & Sons, Ltd, The Atrium, Southern Gate, Chichester, West Sussex, PO19 8SQ, UK

Editorial offices: 9600 Garsington Road, Oxford, OX4 2DQ, UK
The Atrium, Southern Gate, Chichester, West Sussex, PO19 8SQ, UK
111 River Street, Hoboken, NJ 07030-5774, USA

For details of our global editorial offices, for customer services, and for information about how to apply for permission to reuse the copyright material in this book, please see our website at www.wiley.com/wiley-blackwell.

Library of Congress Cataloging-in-Publication Data

Coico, Richard, author.
  Immunology : a short course / Richard Coico, Geoffrey Sunshine. – Seventh
edition.
     p. ; cm.
  Includes bibliographical references and index.
  ISBN 978-1-118-39691-9 (pbk.)
  I. Sunshine, Geoffrey, author. II. Title.
  [DNLM: 1. Allergy and Immunology. 2. Immune System Diseases. 3. Immune
System Processes. 4. Immunity. QW 504]
  QR181
  616.07′9–dc23

                                                    2014023101

A catalogue record for this book is available from the British Library.

Wiley also publishes its books in a variety of electronic formats. Some content that appears in print may not be available in electronic books.

Cover image: Russell Kightley

Set in 10/12 pt Times by Toppan Best-set Premedia Limited
Printed and bound in Singapore by Markono Print Media Pte Ltd

1 2015

CONTENTS IN BRIEF

CONTENTS

ABOUT THE AUTHORS

Richard Coico is Professor of Cell Biology and Medicine and Vice Dean for Scientific Affairs at SUNY Downstate College of Medicine in New York. His major research interest concerns the study of the physiologic role of IgD—a B-cell membrane immunoglobulin co-expressed with IgM. Another area of research concerns computational approaches to the identification of candidate vaccines for several hemorrhagic viruses, including Ebola and Lassa Fever viruses. He serves on several editorial boards including *Current Protocols in Immunology*.

Geoffrey Sunshine is a Senior Scientist at the Health Effects Institute in Boston, Massachusetts, which funds research worldwide on the health effects of air pollution. He is also a lecturer in the Tufts School of Medicine immunology course. For several years, he has directed a course in immunology for graduate dental students at Tufts University School of Dental Medicine and previously directed a course for veterinary students at Tufts University School of Veterinary Medicine. He was also a member of the Sackler School of Graduate Biomedical Sciences at Tufts University, doing research on antigen presentation and teaching immunology to medical graduate and undergraduate students.

CONTRIBUTORS

Philip L. Cohen
Temple University School of Medicine
Philadelphia, Pennsylvania

Susan R.S. Gottesman
Department of Pathology
SUNY Downstate College of Medicine
Brooklyn, New York

PREFACE AND ACKNOWLEDGMENTS

As with our previous editions, the seventh edition of *Immunology: A Short Course* is intended to provide the reader with a clear and concise overview of our current understanding of the physiology of the immune system as well as the pathophysiology associated with various immune-mediated diseases. Although our knowledge of how the immune system develops and functions and the ways in which these physiological phenomena can fail or be compromised and thereby cause disease has significantly expanded since the previous edition, we have preserved our commitment to the motto *less is more*, the guiding light of this series. We are still committed to teaching our students and presenting to our readers only the information that we consider absolutely essential. To reflect this new knowledge, we have updated and rewritten every chapter in the sixth edition to incorporate new findings or to remove information that no longer reflects current thinking. We have also provided new multiple choice questions and answers at the end of each chapter so that the reader can evaluate his or her understanding. We have also made one other pivotal change as compared with earlier editions: At its most basic level, and since the first edition of the book, we have introduced the subject of immune response by highlighting the fact that it can be split into two arms: the innate response and the adaptive immune response. The past decade has witnessed the delineation of innate immunity in ways that have revolutionized our understanding of host–pathogen interactions and their impact on defense mechanisms in infectious diseases. Because of this growth in knowledge, we have added a new chapter on the subject of innate immunity (Chapter 2).

Other advances since the sixth edition include an explosion of targeted therapies for diseases ranging from cancer to Crohn's disease. For many years the path toward this goal was principally pharmacologic in nature. Now, with the advent of hybridoma technology to generate monoclonal antibodies and their use in translational studies in humans, we have entered an era in which we are witnessing the potential for these antibodies to treat many different diseases including inflammatory and autoinflammatory disorders and cancer. Indeed, many antibody therapies are now approved for clinical use by the U.S. Food and Drug Administration. Similarly, the growth in our knowledge of cytokines, together with the successful development of soluble cytokine

receptors (antagonists), cytokine analogs, and anti-cytokine or anti-cytokine receptor antibodies has yielded many opportunities for therapeutic exploitation of this knowledge. The seventh edition highlights some of these important therapeutic successes and possibilities for success. We have also woven discussion of these therapies into chapters that deal with basic immune mechanisms. Our goal is to inspire the reader to consider how advances in the field of immunology have generated clinical and translational fruits that have improved health both through the prevention of infectious diseases using vaccines and by treating diseases with a variety of immune-based biological *magic bullets*, a term first coined by Paul Ehrlich more than 100 years ago.

Our goal is to provide a basic understanding of the immune system. For the reader who would like a more in-depth knowledge of clinical conditions, we refer in the text at several places to clinical cases in a companion book *Immunology: Clinical Case Studies and Disease Pathophysiology*, edited by Warren Strober (NIAID/NIH) and Susan Gottesman (SUNY-Downstate) (ISBN: 9780471326595, see http://bit.ly/ICCSDPsg). We are confident that the synergy created by the material in the seventh edition of *Immunology: A Short Course* and the linked clinical cases will be a true asset to students of medicine and other health professions.

We are very grateful to Dr. Philip Cohen (Temple University School of Medicine), who updated Chapter 13 on the subject of "Tolerance and Autoimmunity." We would also like to thank Dr. Susan Gottesman (SUNY-Downstate), who updated Chapter 18, "Immunodeficiency Disorders and Neoplasias of the Lymphoid System." We also offer our profuse thanks to Dr. Gottesman for reviewing and providing comments on drafts of every chapter, as well as writing many of the multiple choice questions and answers that are found on the accompanying website.

Richard Coico would like acknowledge the loving, enduring support of his wife, Lisa, during the writing of this book. "Her encouragement and inspiration is second to none with two possible exceptions, namely, our children, Jonathan and Jennifer. Jonathan, a talented writer himself, and Jennifer, an emerging public health advocate, are each blessed with patience and bright inquisitive minds"—the ideal mix of attributes for children and students alike. Finally, once again, he would like to thank his mentor, Dr. G. Jeanette Thorbecke, who greatly influenced his commitment and passion to the field of immunology. Special thanks also go to co-workers, including secretaries, office assistants, and other staff members who helped with the preparation of the manuscript.

Geoffrey Sunshine would like to thank his companion lecturers in the Tufts University School of Medicine immunology course, Peter Brodeur and Arthur Rabson. They provided enormous help in addressing the key questions of what is important to teach students who know little or no immunology and how best to present this information. Peter also gave many constructive suggestions during the prepara-

tion of the current edition. In addition, Geoffrey would like to thank his wife, Ilene, for her continued support and understanding during the writing, and his daughter, Caroline, for her help in revising the Glossary.

The authors also wish to express their appreciation to our copyeditor, William Krol; Stephanie Sakson, at Toppan Best-set Premedia; and to Martin Davies, Karen Moore, Elizabeth Norton, and Sam French of John Wiley and Sons, who helped to publish the seventh edition.

Richard Coico
Geoffrey Sunshine

HOW TO USE YOUR TEXTBOOK

FEATURES CONTAINED WITHIN YOUR TEXTBOOK

Standard **icons** are used throughout this book to denote different immunological molecules

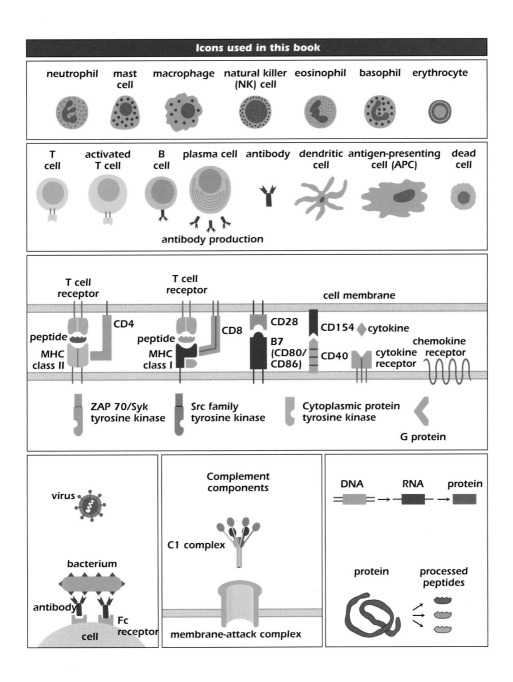

Your textbook is full of **photographs, illustrations, and tables**.

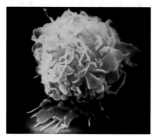

Figure 2.2. A PMN (surrounded by erythrocytes) with trilobed nucleus and cytoplasmic granules (×950). (Reproduced with permission from Olana and Walker, *Infect Med* 19: 318 [2007].)

arms of the immune system beginning with elements of the innate immune system followed by the adaptive immune system. But it is important to underscore the interrelationship of these two arms of our immune system. Clearly, they are interrelated developmentally due to their common hematopoietic precursor, the pluripotential stem cell. A classic example of their functional interrelationship is illustrated by the roles played by innate immune cells involved in *antigen presentation*. These so-called *antigen-presenting cells* (APCs) do just what their name implies: they present antigens (e.g., pieces of phagocytized bacteria) to T cells within the adaptive immune system. As will be discussed in great detail in subsequent chapters, T cells must interact with APCs that display antigens for which they are specific in order for the T cells to be activated to generate antigen-specific responses. Thus, while the title of this section implies that the cells described below are principally involved in innate immune responses, it is important to recognize their important role in adaptive immune responses (Chapter 3) at this early stage of study of the immune system.

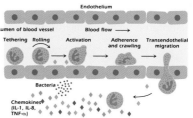

Figure 2.3. Scanning electron micrograph of macrophage with ruffled membrane and surface covered with microvilli (×5200). (Reproduced with permission from *J Clin Invest* 117 [2007].)

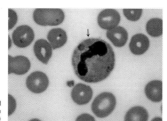

TABLE 2.2. Acute Phase Proteins

Protein	Immune System Function
C-reactive protein	• Binds to phosphocholine expressed on the surface of dead or dying cells and some types of bacteria • Opsonin
Serum amyloid P component	Opsonin
Serum amyloid A	• Recruitment of immune cells to inflammatory sites • Induction of enzymes that degrade extracellular matrix
Complement factors	• Opsonization, lysis, and clumping of target cells • Chemotaxis
Mannan-binding lectin	Mannan-binding lectin pathway of complement activation
Fibrinogen (α β globulin), prothrombin, factor VIII, von Willebrand factor	• Coagulation factors • Trapping invading microbes in blood clots. • Some cause chemotaxis
Plasminogen	Degradation of blood clots
Alpha 2-macroglobulin	• Inhibitor of coagulation by inhibiting thrombin. • Inhibitor of fibrinolysis by inhibiting plasmin
Ferritin	Binding iron, inhibiting microbe iron uptake
Hepcidin	Stimulates the internalization of ferroportin, preventing release of iron bound by ferritin within intestinal enterocytes and macrophages
Ceruloplasmin	Oxidizes iron, facilitating for ferritin, inhibiting microbe iron uptake
Haptoglobin	Binds hemoglobin, inhibiting microbe iron uptake
Orosomucoid (Alpha-1-acid glycoprotein, AGP)	Steroid carrier
Alpha 1-antitrypsin, Alpha alpha 1-antichymotrypsin	Serpin, downregulates inflammation

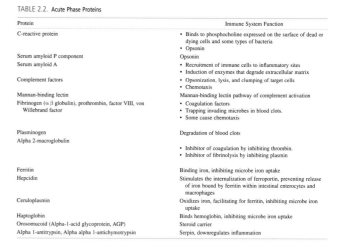

Figure 2.11. Leukocyte adhesion to endothelium leads to their adhesion, activation, and extravasation from the blood to tissue where they are needed to help destroy (e.g., phagocytize) pathogens such as bacteria that initiate this response.

Self-assessment review questions help you test yourself after each chapter.

REVIEW QUESTIONS

For each question, choose the ONE BEST answer or completion.

1. Which of the following applies uniquely with respect to B cells found in secondary lymphoid organs?
   A) present as precursor B cells
   B) express only IgM
   C) terminally differentiate into plasma cells
   D) undergo proliferation

2. The germinal centers found in the cortical region of lymph nodes and the peripheral region of splenic periarteriolar lymphatic tissue
   A) support the development of immature B and T cells
   B) function in the removal of damaged erythrocytes from the circulation
   C) act as the major source of stem cells and thus help maintain hematopoiesis
   D) provide an infrastructure that on antigenic stimulation contains large populations of B lymphocytes and plasma cells
   E) are the sites of natural killer T (NKT)-cell differentiation

3. Which of the following sequence correctly describes lymphocyte migration from lymph nodes to blood?
   A) postcapillary venules, efferent lymphatic vessels, thoracic duct, vena cava, heart
   B) postcapillary venules, afferent lymphatic vessels, thoracic duct, vena cava, heart
   C) postcapillary venules, efferent lymphatic vessels, vena cava, thoracic duct, heart
   D) postcapillary venules, afferent lymphatic vessels, vena cava, thoracic duct, heart

4. Clonal expansion of which of the following cells occurs following their direct interaction with the antigen for which they are specific?
   A) macrophages
   B) basophils
   C) B cells
   D) T cells
   E) mast cells

The case icon indicates that you can find a correlated clinical case in *Immunology: Clinical Case Studies and Disease Pathophysiology*, edited by Warren Strober (NIAID/NIH) and Susan Gottesman (SUNY-Downstate) (ISBN: 9780471326595; see http://bit.ly/ICCSDPsg).

The anytime, anywhere textbook

Wiley E-Text

For the first time, your textbook comes with free access to a **Wiley E-Text: Powered by VitalSource** version—a digital, interactive version of this textbook that you own as soon as you download it.

Your **Wiley E-Text** allows you to:

Search: Save time by finding terms and topics instantly in your book, your notes, even your whole library (once you've downloaded more textbooks).

Note and Highlight: Color code, highlight, and make digital notes right in the text so you can find them quickly and easily.

Organize: Keep books, notes, and class materials organized in folders inside the application.

Share: Exchange notes and highlights with friends, classmates, and study groups.

Upgrade: Your textbook can be transferred when you need to change or upgrade computers.

Link: Link directly from the page of your interactive textbook to all of the material contained on the companion website.

The **Wiley E-Text** version will also allow you to copy and paste any photograph or illustration into assignments, presentations, and your own notes.

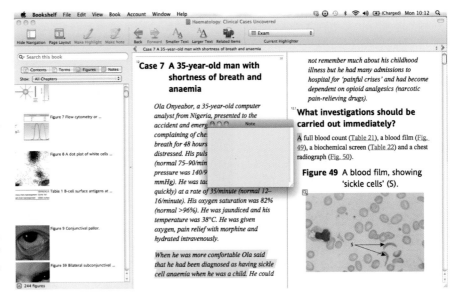

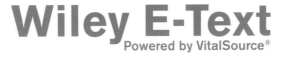

***To access your** Wiley E-Text:*

- Find the redemption code on the inside front cover of this book and carefully scratch away the top coating of the label. Visit **www.vitalsource.com/software/ bookshelf/downloads** to download the Bookshelf application to your computer, laptop, tablet, or mobile device.
- If you have purchased this title as an e-book, access to your **Wiley E-Text** is available with proof of purchase within 90 days. Visit **http://support.wiley.com** to request a redemption code via the "Live Chat" or "Ask A Question" tabs.
- Open the Bookshelf application on your computer and register for an account.
- Follow the registration process and enter your redemption code to download your digital book.
- For full access instructions, visit **www.wileyimmunology.com/coico**.

The VitalSource Bookshelf can now be used to view your Wiley E-Text **on iOS, Android, and Kindle Fire!**

- **For iOS:** Visit the app store to download the VitalSource Bookshelf: **http://bit.ly/17ib3XS**.
- **For Android and Kindle Fire:** Visit the Google Play Market to download the VitalSource Bookshelf: **http://bit.ly/ BSAAGP**.

You can now sign in with the email address and password you used when you created your VitalSource Bookshelf Account.

Full E-Text support for mobile devices is available at: **http://support.vitalsource.com**.

CourseSmart

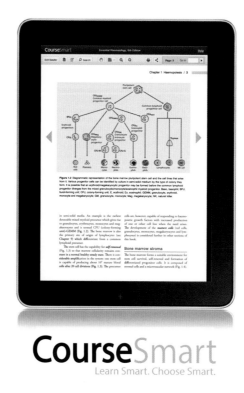

CourseSmart gives you instant access (via computer or mobile device) to this Wiley-Blackwell e-book and its extra electronic functionality, at 40% off the recommended retail print price. See all the benefits at **www.coursesmart.com/students**.

Instructors ... receive your own digital desk copies!

CourseSmart also offers instructors an immediate, efficient, and environmentally friendly way to review this textbook for your course. For more information visit **www.coursesmart.com/instructors**.

With **CourseSmart**, you can create lecture notes quickly with copy and paste, and share pages and notes with your students. Access your **CourseSmart** digital textbook from your computer or mobile device instantly for evaluation, class preparation, and as a teaching tool in the classroom.

Simply sign in at **http://instructors.coursesmart.com/bookshelf** to download your Bookshelf and get started. To request your desk copy, hit "Request Online Copy" on your search results or book product page.

We hope you enjoy using your new textbook. Good luck with your studies!

ABOUT THE COMPANION WEBSITE

Don't forget to visit the companion website for this book:

 www.wileyimmunology.com/coico

There you will find valuable material designed to enhance your learning, including:

- Multiple choice questions
- Sample cases to give you a flavor of those to be found in the companion volume, *Immunology: Clinical Case Studies and Disease Pathophysiology* by Warren Strober and Susan Gottesman
- Flashcards
- Downloadable figures

Scan this QR code to visit the companion website:

OVERVIEW OF THE IMMUNE SYSTEM

INTRODUCTION

Anyone who has had the good fortune to hear an orchestra brilliantly perform a symphony composed by one of the great masters knows that each of the carefully tuned musical instruments contributes to the collective, harmonious sound produced by the musicians. In many ways, the normally tuned immune system continuously plays an orchestrated symphony to maintain homeostasis in the context of host defenses. However, as William Shakespeare noted, "Untune that string, and, hark, what discord follows!" (*Troilus and Cressida*). Similarly, an untuned immune system can cause discord, which manifests as autoimmunity, cancer, or chronic inflammation. Fortunately for most of us, our immune system is steadfastly vigilant in regard to tuning (regulating) itself to ensure that its cellular components behave and interact symbiotically to generate protective immune responses that ensure good health. In many ways the immune system can be described in anthropomorphic terms: Its memory allows it to remember and recognize pathogens years or decades after initial exposure; it can distinguish between the body's own cells and those of another organism; and it makes decisions about how to respond to particular pathogens—including whether or not to respond at all, as will be discussed in Chapters 2 and 3.

In his penetrating essays, scientist–author Lewis Thomas, discussing symbiosis and parasitism, described the forces that would drive all living matter into one huge ball of protoplasm were it not for regulatory and recognition mechanisms that allow us to distinguish self from nonself.

The origins of these mechanisms go far back in evolutionary history, and many, in fact, originated as markers for allowing cells to recognize and interact with each other to set up symbiotic households. Genetically related sponge colonies that are placed close to each other, for example, will tend to grow toward each other and fuse into one large colony. Unrelated colonies, however, will react in a different way, destroying cells that come in contact with each other and leaving a zone of rejection between the colonies.

In the plant kingdom, similar types of recognition occur. In self-pollinating species, a pollen grain landing on the stigma of a genetically related flower will send a pollen tubule down the style to the ovary for fertilization. A pollen grain from a genetically distinct plant either will not germinate or the pollen tubule, once formed, will disintegrate in the style. The opposite occurs in cross-pollinating species: self-marked pollen grains disintegrate, whereas nonself grains germinate and fertilize.

The nature of these primitive recognition mechanisms has not been completely worked out, but almost certainly it involves cell-surface molecules that are able to specifically bind and adhere to other molecules on opposing cell surfaces. This simple method of molecular recognition has evolved over time into the very complex immune system that retains, as its essential feature, the ability of a protein molecule to recognize and bind specifically to a particular shaped structure on another molecule. Such molecular recognition is the underlying principle involved in the discrimination between self and nonself during an immune response. It is the purpose of this book to describe how the fully

Immunology: A Short Course, Seventh Edition. Richard Coico and Geoffrey Sunshine.
© 2015 John Wiley & Sons, Ltd. Published 2015 by John Wiley & Sons, Ltd.
Companion Website: www.wileyimmunology.com/coico

mature immune system—which has evolved from this simple beginning—makes use of this principle of recognition in increasingly complex and sophisticated ways.

Perhaps the greatest catalyst for progress in this and many other biomedical areas has been the advent of molecular biologic techniques. It is important to acknowledge, however, that certain technological advances in the field of molecular biology were made possible by earlier progress in the field of immunology. For example, the importance of immunologic methods (Chapter 6) used to purify proteins as well as identify specific cDNA clones cannot be understated. These advances were greatly facilitated by the pioneering studies of Köhler and Milstein (1975), who developed a method for producing monoclonal antibodies. Their achievement was rewarded with the Nobel Prize in Medicine. It revolutionized research efforts in virtually all areas of biomedical science. Some monoclonal antibodies produced against so-called tumor-specific antigens have now been approved by the US Food and Drug Administration for use in patients to treat certain malignancies. Monoclonal antibody technology is, perhaps, an excellent example of how the science of immunology has transformed not only the field of medicine but also fields ranging from agriculture to the food science industry.

Given the rapid advances occurring in immunology and the many other biomedical sciences and, perhaps most important, the sequencing of the human genome, every contemporary biomedical science textbook runs a considerable risk of being outdated before it appears in print. Nevertheless, we take solace from the observation that new formulations generally build on and expand the old rather than replacing or negating them completely. Let's begin, therefore, with an overview of innate and adaptive immunity (also called *acquired immunity*) which continue to serve as a conceptual compass that orients our fundamental understanding of host defense mechanisms.

INNATE AND ADAPTIVE IMMUNITY

The Latin term *immunis*, meaning "exempt," gave rise to the English word *immunity*, which refers to all the mechanisms used by the body as protection against environmental agents that are foreign to the body. These agents may be microorganisms or their products, foods, chemicals, drugs, pollen, or animal hair and dander.

Innate Immunity

Innate immunity is conferred by all those elements with which an individual is born and that are always present and available at very short notice to protect the individual from challenges by foreign invaders. The major properties of the innate immune system are discussed in Chapter 2. Table 1.1 summarizes and compares some of the features of the innate and adaptive immune systems. Elements of the innate system

TABLE 1.1. Major Properties of the Innate and Adaptive Immune Systems

Property	Innate	Adaptive
Characteristics	Antigen nonspecific	Antigen specific
	Rapid response (minutes to hours)	Slow response (days)
	No memory	Memory
Immune components	Natural barriers (e.g., skin, mucous membranes)	Lymphocytes
	Phagocytes and natural killer cells	Antigen recognition molecules (B and T cell receptors)
	Soluble mediators (e.g., complement)	Secreted molecules (e.g., antibody)
	Pattern recognition molecules	

include body surfaces and internal components, such as the skin, the mucous membranes, and the cough reflex, which present effective barriers to environmental agents. Chemical influences, such as pH and secreted fatty acids, constitute effective barriers against invasion by many microorganisms. Another noncellular element of the innate immune system is the complement system. As in the previous editions of this book, we cover the subject of complement in Chapter 14.

Numerous other components are also features of innate immunity: fever, interferons (Chapter 12), other substances released by leukocytes, and pattern-recognition molecules (*innate receptors*), which can bind to various microorganisms (e.g., Toll-like receptors or TLRs; Chapter 2), as well as serum proteins such as β-lysin, the enzyme lysozyme, polyamines, and the kinins, among others. All of these elements either affect pathogenic invaders directly or enhance the effectiveness of host reactions to them. Other internal elements of innate immunity include phagocytic cells such as granulocytes, macrophages, and microglial cells of the central nervous system, which participate in the destruction and elimination of foreign material that has penetrated the physical and chemical barriers.

Adaptive Immunity

We introduce the subject of adaptive immunity in Chapter 3. Later chapters provide more details about the cellular and molecular features of this arm of the immune system. Adaptive immunity came into play relatively late, in evolutionary terms, and is present only in vertebrates. Although an individual is born with the capacity to mount immune responses to foreign substances, the number of B and T cells available for mounting such responses must be expanded before one is said to be immune to that substance. This is achieved by activation of lymphocytes bearing antigen-specific receptors following their contact with the antigen. Antigenic stimulation of B cells and T cells together with antigen-presenting cells (APCs) initiates a chain of events that leads to proliferation of activated cells together with a program of differentiation events that generate the B- or T-effector cells responsible for the humoral or cell-mediated responses, respectively. These events take time to unfold (days to weeks). Fortunately, the cellular and noncellular components of the innate system are rapidly mobilized (minutes to hours) to eliminate or neutralize the foreign substance. One way to think about this host defense strategy is to consider this as a one-two punch launched initially by innate cells and noncellular elements of the immune system that are always available to quickly remove or cordon off the invader, followed by a round of defense that calls into play cells of the adaptive immune system (B and T cells) that are programmed to react with the foreign substance by virtue of their antigen-specific receptors. Moreover, the clonal expansion of these cells—a process first explained by the clonal selection theory discussed in the section below—gives rise to an arsenal of antigen-specific cells available for rapid responses to the same antigen in the future, a phenomenon referred to as *memory responses*. By this process, the individual acquires the immunity to withstand and resist a subsequent attack by, or exposure to, the same offending agent.

The discovery of adaptive immunity predates many of the concepts of modern medicine. It has been recognized for centuries that people who did not die from such life-threatening diseases as bubonic plague and smallpox were subsequently more resistant to the disease than were people who had never been exposed to it. The rediscovery of adaptive immunity is credited to the English physician Edward Jenner, who, in the late eighteenth century, experimentally induced immunity to smallpox. If Jenner performed his experiment today, his medical license would be revoked, and he would be the defendant in a sensational malpractice lawsuit: He inoculated a young boy with pus from a lesion of a dairy maid who had cowpox, a relatively benign disease that is related to smallpox. He then deliberately exposed the boy to smallpox. This exposure failed to cause disease! Because of the protective effect of inoculation with cowpox (vaccinia, from the Latin word *vacca*, meaning "cow"), the process of inducing adaptive immunity has been termed *vaccination*.

The concept of vaccination or immunization was expanded by Louis Pasteur and Paul Ehrlich almost 100 years after Jenner's experiment. By 1900, it had become apparent that immunity could be induced against not only microorganisms but also their products. We now know that immunity can be induced against innumerable natural and synthetic compounds, including metals, chemicals of relatively low molecular weight, carbohydrates, proteins, and nucleotides.

The compound to which the adaptive immune response is induced is termed an *antigen*, a term initially coined due to the ability of these compounds to cause antibody responses to be generated. Of course, we now know that antigens can generate antibody-mediated and T-cell–mediated responses.

CLONAL SELECTION THEORY

A turning point in immunology came in the 1950s with the introduction of a Darwinian view of the cellular basis of specificity in the immune response. This was the now universally accepted clonal selection theory proposed and developed by Jerne and Burnet (both Nobel Prize winners) and by Talmage. The clonal selection theory had a truly revolutionary effect on the field of immunology. It dramatically changed our approach to studying the immune system and stimulated research carried out during the last half of the twentieth century. This work ultimately provided us with knowledge regarding the molecular machinery associated with activation and regulation of cellular elements of the immune system. The essential postulates of this theory are summarized below.

As we have discussed earlier, the specificity of the immune response is based on the ability of B and T lymphocytes to recognize particular foreign molecules (antigens) and respond to them in order to eliminate them. The process of clonal expansion of these cells is highly efficient, but there is always the rare chance that errors or mutations will occur, resulting in the generation of cells bearing receptors that bind poorly or not at all to the antigen, or, in a worse-case scenario, cells that have autoreactivity. Under normal conditions, nonfunctional cells may survive or be aborted with no deleterious consequences to the individual. In contrast, the rare self-reactive cells are clonally deleted or suppressed by other regulatory cells of the immune system charged with this role among others. If such a mechanism were absent, autoimmune responses might occur routinely. It is noteworthy that during the early stages of development, lymphocytes with receptors that bind to self-antigens are also produced, but fortunately they are also eliminated or functionally inactivated. This process gives rise to the initial repertoire of mature lymphocytes that are programmed to generate antigen-specific responses with a relatively minute population functionally benign, albeit potentially autoreactive cells (Figure 1.1). The circumstances and predisposing genetic conditions that may lead to the latter phenomenon are discussed in Chapter 13.

As we have already stated, the immune system is capable of recognizing innumerable foreign substance serving as antigens. How is a response to any one antigen accomplished? In addition to the now-proven postulate that self-reactive clones of lymphocytes are functionally inactivated or aborted, the clonal selection theory proposed the following:

- T and B lymphocytes of a myriad of specificities exist before there is any contact with the foreign antigen.
- Lymphocytes participating in an immune response express antigen-specific receptors on their surface membranes. As a consequence of antigen binding to the lymphocyte, the cell is activated and releases various products. In the case of B lymphocytes, these receptors, so-called *B-cell receptors* (BCRs), are the

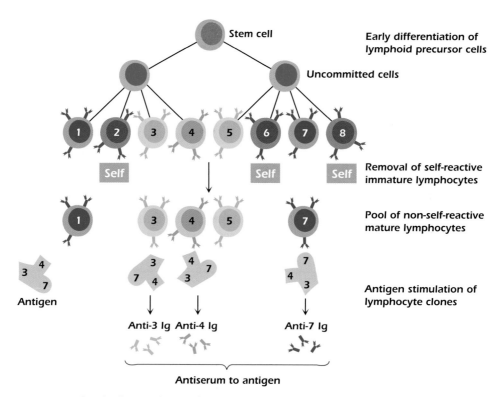

Figure 1.1. Clonal selection theory of B cells leading to antibody formation.

very molecules that subsequently get secreted as antibodies following B-cell activation.

- T cells have receptors denoted as T-cell receptors (TCRs). Unlike the B-cell products, the T-cell products are not the same as their surface receptors but are other protein molecules, called **cytokines**, that participate in elimination of the antigen by regulating the many cells needed to mount an effective immune response.
- Each lymphocyte carries on its surface receptor molecules of only a single specificity as demonstrated in Figure 1.1 for B cells and also holds true for T cells.

These postulates describe the existence of a large repertoire of possible specificities formed by cellular multiplication and differentiation before there is any contact with the foreign substance to which the response is to be made. The introduction of the foreign antigen then selects from among all the available specificities those with specificity for the antigen, enabling binding to occur. The scheme shown in Figure 1.1 for B cells also applies to T cells; however, T cells have receptors that are not antibodies and secrete molecules other than antibodies.

The remaining postulates of the clonal selection theory account for this process of selection by the antigen from among all the available cells in the repertoire.

- Immunocompetent lymphocytes combine with the foreign antigen, or a portion of it termed the epitope or antigenic determinant, by virtue of their surface recep-

tors. They are stimulated under appropriate conditions to proliferate and differentiate into clones of cells with the corresponding epitope-specific receptors.

- With B-cell clones, this will lead to the synthesis of antibodies having the same specificity. In most cases, the antigen stimulating the response is complex and contains many different epitopes, each capable of activating a clone of epitope-specific B cells. Hence, collectively, the clonally secreted antibodies constitute what is often referred to as polyclonal antiserum, which is capable of interacting with the multiple epitopes expressed by the antigen.
- T cells are similarly selected by appropriate epitopes or portions thereof. Each selected T cell will be activated to divide and produce clones of the same specificity. Thus the clonal response to the antigen will be amplified, the cells will release various cytokines, and subsequent exposure to the same antigen will now result in the activation of many cells or clones of that specificity. Instead of synthesizing and releasing antibodies like the B cells, the T cells synthesize and release cytokines. These cytokines, which are soluble mediators, exert their effect on other cells to grow or become activated facilitating elimination of the antigen. Several distinct regions of an antigen (epitopes) can be recognized: Several different clones of B cells will be stimulated to produce antibody, whose sum total is an antigen-specific antiserum that is made up of antibodies of differing specificity (Figure 1.1); all the T-cell clones that recog-

nize various epitopes on the same antigen will be activated to perform their function.

A final postulate was added to account for the ability to recognize self-antigens without making a response:

- Circulating self-antigens that reach the developing lymphoid system before some undesignated maturational step will serve to shut off those cells that recognize it specifically, and no subsequent immune response will be induced.

ACTIVE, PASSIVE, AND ADOPTIVE IMMUNIZATION

Adaptive immunity is induced by immunization, which can be achieved in several ways:

- *Active immunization* refers to immunization of an individual by administration of an antigen.
- *Passive immunization* refers to immunization through the transfer of specific antibody from an immunized individual to a nonimmunized individual.
- *Adoptive immunization* refers to the transfer of immunity by the transfer of immune cells.

Major Characteristics of the Adaptive Immune Response

The adaptive immune response has several generalized features that characterize it and distinguish it from other physiologic systems, such as circulation, respiration, and reproduction. These features are as follows:

- *Specificity* is the ability to discriminate among different molecular entities and to respond only to those uniquely required, rather than making a random, undifferentiated response.
- *Adaptiveness* is the ability to respond to previously unseen molecules that may in fact never have naturally existed before on earth.
- *Discrimination between self and nonself* is a cardinal feature of the specificity of the immune response; it is the ability to recognize and respond to molecules that are foreign (nonself) and to avoid making a response to those molecules that are self. This distinction, and the recognition of antigen, is conferred by specialized cells (lymphocytes) that bear on their surface antigen-specific receptors.
- *Memory*, a property shared with the nervous system, is the ability to recall previous contact with a foreign molecule and respond to it in a learned manner, that is, with a more rapid and larger response. Another term often used to describe immunologic memory is ***anamnestic response***.

When you reach the end of this book, you should understand the cellular and molecular bases of these features of the immune response.

Cells Involved in the Adaptive Immune Response

For many years, immunology remained an empirical subject in which the effects of injecting various substances into hosts were studied primarily in terms of the products elicited. Most progress came in the form of more quantitative methods for detecting these products of the immune response. A major change in emphasis came in the 1950s with the recognition that lymphocytes were the major cellular players in the immune response, and the field of cellular immunology came to life.

A convenient way to define the cell types involved in adaptive immunity is to divide the host defense mechanisms into two categories, namely B-cell and T-cell responses, respectively. While this is an oversimplified definition, it is, by and large, the functional outcome of adaptive immune responses. Thus, defining the cells involved begins with a short list, namely, B and T cells. These cells are derived from a common lymphoid precursor cell but differentiate along different developmental lines, as discussed in detail in Chapters 8–10. In short, B cells develop and mature in the bone marrow whereas T-cell precursors emerge from the bone marrow and undergo critical maturation steps in the thymus.

Antigen-presenting cells (APCs), such as macrophages and dendritic cells, constitute the third cell type that participates in the adaptive immune response. Although these cells do not have antigen-specific receptors as do the lymphocytes, they process and present antigen to the antigen-specific receptors expressed by T cells. The APCs express a variety of cell-surface molecules that facilitate their ability to interact with T cells. Among these are the major histocompatibility complex (MHC) molecules as discussed in Chapter 9. MHC molecules are encoded by a set of polymorphic genes expressed within a population. While we now understand that their physiologic role is concerned with T-cell–APC interactions, in clinical settings, MHC molecules determine the success or failure of organ and tissue transplantation. In fact, this observation facilitated their discovery and the current terminology (major *histocompatibility* complex) used to define these molecules. Physiologically, APCs process protein antigens intracellularly, resulting in the constellation of peptides that noncovalently bind to MHC molecules and ultimately get displayed on the cell surface.

Other cell types, such as neutrophils and mast cells, also participate in adaptive immune responses. In fact, they participate in both innate and adaptive immunity. While these cells have no specific antigen recognition properties and can be activated by a variety of substances, they are an integral part of the network of cells that participate in host defenses and often display potent immunoregulatory properties.

HUMORAL AND CELLULAR IMMUNITY

Adaptive immune responses have historically been divided into two separate arms of defense, namely, B-cell–mediated or humoral immune responses, and T-cell–mediated or cellular responses. Today, while we recognize that B and T cells have very distinct yet complementary molecular and functional roles within our immune system, we understand that the two arms are fundamentally interconnected at many levels. "Experiments of nature," a term coined by Robert A. Good in the 1950s when describing the immune status of humans with a congenital mutation associated with an athymic phenotype, have provided significant insights related to the interdependence of these two arms of the immune system. Athymic mice that fail to develop thymic tissue (a similar phenomenon in humans is called **DiGeorge Syndrome**), results in a profound T-cell deficiency with accompanying abnormalities in B-cell function. The molecular explanation for the latter is now well understood. Without T-cell help, B cells are unable to generate normal antibody responses and, in particular, to undergo immunoglobulin class switching (see Chapters 8 and 10). The help normally provided by T cells is delivered in several ways, including their synthesis and secretion of a variety of cytokines that regulate many events in B-cells required for proliferation and differentiation (see Chapter 12).

Humoral Immunity

B cells are initially activated to secrete antibodies after the binding of antigens to antigen-specific membrane immunoglobulin (Ig) molecules (B-cell receptors [BCRs]), which are expressed by these cells. It has been estimated that each B cell expresses approximately 100,000 BCRs of exactly the same specificity. Once ligated, the B cell receives signals to begin making the secreted form of this immunoglobulin, a process that initiates the full-blown antibody response whose purpose is to eliminate the antigen from the host. Antibodies are a heterogeneous mixture of serum globulins, all of which share the ability to bind individually to specific antigens. All serum globulins with antibody activity are referred to as immunoglobulins (see Chapter 5). These molecules have common structural features, which enable them to do two things: (1) recognize and bind specifically to a unique structural entity on an antigen (namely, the epitope), and (2) perform a common biologic function after combining with the antigen. Immunoglobulin molecules consist of two identical light (L) chains and two identical heavy (H) chains, linked by disulfide bridges. The resultant structure is shown in Figure 1.2. The portion of the molecule that binds antigen consists of an area composed of the amino-terminal regions of both H and L chains. Thus each immunoglobulin molecule is symmetric and is capable of binding two identical epitopes present on the same antigen molecule or on different molecules. In addition to differences in the antigen-binding portion of different immunoglobulin molecules, there are other differences, the most important of which are those in the H chains. There are five major classes of H chains (termed γ, μ, α, ε, and δ). On the basis of differences in their H chains, immunoglobulin molecules are divided into five major classes—IgG, IgM, IgA, IgE, and IgD—each of which has several unique biologic properties. For example, IgG is the only class of immunoglobulin that crosses the placenta, conferring the mother's immunity on the fetus, and IgA is the major antibody found in secretions such as tears and saliva. It is important to remember that antibodies in all five classes may possess precisely the same specificity against an antigen (antigen-combining regions), while at the same time having different functional (biologic effector) properties. The binding between antigen and antibody is not covalent but depends on many relatively weak forces, such as hydrogen bonds, van der Waals forces, and hydrophobic interactions. Since these forces are weak, successful binding between antigen and antibody depends on a very close fit over a sizable area, much like the contacts between a lock and a key.

Besides the help provided by T cells in the generation of antibody responses, noncellular components of the innate immune system collectively termed the **complement system**, play a key role in the functional activity of antibodies when they interact with antigen (Chapter 14). The reaction between antigen and antibody serves to activate this system, which consists of a series of serum enzymes, the end result of which is lysis of the target in the case of microbes such as bacteria or enhanced phagocytosis (ingestion of the antigen) by phagocytic cells. The activation of complement also results in the recruitment of highly phagocytic polymorphonuclear (PMN) cells or neutrophils, which are active in innate immunity.

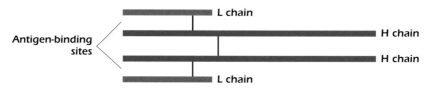

Figure 1.2. Typical antibody molecule composed of two heavy (H) and two light (L) chains. Antigen-binding sites are noted.

CELL-MEDIATED IMMUNITY

In contrast to humoral immune responses that are mediated by antibody, cell-mediated responses are T-cell mediated. However, this is an oversimplified definition since the effector cell responsible for the elimination of a foreign antigen such as a pathogenic microbe can be an activated T cell expressing a pathogen-specific TCR or it can be a phagocytic cell that gets activated by innate receptors that they express and the cytokines produced by activated T cells (Figure 1.3). Unlike B cells, which produce soluble antibody that circulates to bind its specific antigens, each T cell, bearing approximately 100,000 identical antigen receptors (TCRs) circulates directly to the site of antigen expressed on APCs and interacts with these cells in a cognate (cell-to-cell) fashion (Chapter 11). As will be discussed in later chapters of this book, activated T cells do release soluble mediators such as cytokines but these are not antigen specific.

There are several phenotypically distinct subpopulations of T cells, each of which may have the same specificity for an antigenic determinant (epitope), although each subpopulation may perform different functions. This is somewhat analogous to the different classes of immunoglobulin molecules, which may have identical specificity but different biologic functions. Several major subsets of T cells exist: helper T cells (T_H cells), which express molecules called CD4, and cytotoxic T cells (T_C cells), which express CD8 molecules on their surface. Another population of T cells that possesses suppressor activity is the T regulatory cell (Treg cells).

The functions ascribed to the various subsets of T cells include the following:

- ***B-cell help.*** T_H cells cooperate with B cells to enhance the production of antibodies. Such T cells function by releasing cytokines, which provide various activation signals for the B cells. As mentioned earlier, cytokines are soluble substances, or mediators that can regulate proliferation and differentiation of B cells, among other functions. Additional information about cytokines is presented in Chapter 12.
- ***Inflammatory effects.*** On activation, certain T_H cells releases cytokines that induce the migration and activation of monocytes and macrophages, leading to inflammatory reactions (Chapter 17).
- ***Cytotoxic effects.*** T_C cells become cytotoxic killer cells that, on contact with their target cell, are able to deliver a lethal hit, leading to the death of the latter. These T cells are termed ***T cytotoxic*** (T_C) cells. In contrast with T_H cells, they express molecules called CD8 on their membranes and are, therefore, CD8$^+$ cells.
- ***Regulatory effects.*** Helper T cells can be further subdivided into different functional subsets that are commonly defined by the cytokines they release. As you will learn in subsequent chapters, these subsets (e.g., T_H1, T_H2) have distinct regulatory properties that are mediated by the cytokines they release (Chapter 12). T_H1 cells can negatively cross-regulate T_{H2} cells and vice versa. Another population of regulatory T cells, the Treg cells, co-expresses CD4 and a molecule called CD25 (CD25 is part of a cytokine receptor known as the interleukin-2 receptor α chain; Chapter 12). The regulatory activity of these CD4$^+$/CD25$^+$cells and their role in actively suppressing autoimmunity are discussed in Chapter 13.
- ***Cytokine effects.*** Cytokine produced by each of the T-cell subsets (principally T_H cells) exert numerous effects on many cells, lymphoid and nonlymphoid. Thus directly or indirectly T cells communicate and collaborate with many cell types.

For many years, immunologists have recognized that cells activated by antigen manifest a variety of effector phenomena. It is only in the past few decades that they began to appreciate the complexity of events that take place in activation by antigen and communication with other cells. We know today that just mere contact of the TCR with antigen is not sufficient to activate the cell. In fact, at least two signals must be delivered to the antigen-specific T cell for activation to occur: Signal 1 involves the binding of the TCR to antigen, which must be presented in the appropriate manner by APCs. Signal 2 involves co-stimulators that include certain cytokines such as interleukin-1 (IL-1), IL-4, and IL-6 (Chapter 12) as well as cell-surface molecules expressed on APCs, such as CD40 and CD86 (Chapter 11). The term ***co-stimulator*** has been broadened to include stimuli such as microbial products (infectious nonself) and damaged tissue (Matzinger's "danger hypothesis") that will enhance signal 1 when that signal is relatively weak.

Once T cells are optimally signaled for activation, a series of events takes place and the activated cell synthesizes and releases cytokines. In turn, these cytokines come in

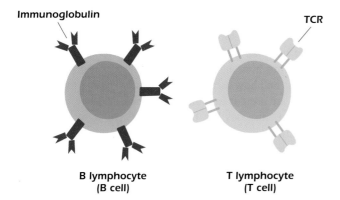

Immunoglobulin　　　　　　　　　**TCR**

B lymphocyte　　　**T lymphocyte**
(B cell)　　　　　　**(T cell)**

Figure 1.3. Antigen receptors expressed as transmembrane molecules on B and T lymphocytes.

contact with appropriate cell surface receptors on different cells and exert their effect on these cells.

Although the humoral and cellular arms of the immune response have been considered as separate and distinct components, it is important to understand that the response to any particular pathogen may involve a complex interaction between them, as well as the components of innate immunity. All this with the purpose of ensuring a maximal survival advantage for the host by eliminating the antigen and, as we shall see, by protecting the host from mounting an immune response against self.

GENERATION OF DIVERSITY IN THE IMMUNE RESPONSE

The most recent tidal surge in immunologic research represents a triumph of the marriage of molecular biology and immunology. While cellular immunology had delineated the cellular basis for the existence of a large and diverse repertoire of responses, as well as the nature of the exquisite specificity that could be achieved, arguments abounded on the exact genetic mechanisms that enabled all these specificities to become part of the repertoire in every individual of the species.

Briefly, the arguments were as follows:

- By various calculations, the number of antigenic specificities toward which an immune response can be generated could range upward of 10^6–10^7.
- If every specific response, in the form of either antibodies or T-cell receptors, were to be encoded by a single gene, did this mean that more than 10^7 genes (one for each specific antibody) would be required in every individual? How was this massive amount of DNA carried intact from individual to individual?

The pioneering studies of Tonegawa (a Nobel laureate) and Leder, using molecular biologic techniques, finally addressed these issues by describing a unique genetic mechanism by which B-cell immunologic receptors (BCRs) of enormous diversity could be produced with a modest amount of DNA reserved for this purpose.

The technique evolved by nature was one of genetic recombination in which a protein could be encoded by a DNA molecule composed of a set of recombined minigenes that made up a complete gene. Given small sets of these minigenes, which could be randomly combined to make the complete gene, it was possible to produce an enormous repertoire of specificities from a limited number of gene fragments. This is discussed in detail in Chapter 7.

Although this mechanism was first elucidated to explain the enormous diversity of antibodies that are not only released by B cells but that, in fact, constitute the antigen- or epitope-specific receptors on B cells (BCRs), it was subsequently established that the same mechanisms operate in generating diversity of the antigen-specific T-cell receptor (TCR). Mechanisms operating in generating diversity of B-cell receptors and antibodies are discussed in Chapter 7. Those operating in generating diversity of TCR are discussed in Chapter 10. Suffice it to say at this point that various techniques of molecular biology, that permit genes not only to be analyzed but also to be moved around at will from one cell to another, have continued to provide impetus to the onrushing tide of progress in the field of immunology.

BENEFITS OF IMMUNOLOGY

While we have thus far discussed the theoretical aspects of immunology, its practical applications are of paramount importance for survival and must be part of the education of students.

The field of immunology has been in the public limelight since the successful use of polio vaccines in the mid-twentieth century. More recently, the spectacular transplantation of the human heart and other major organs, such as the liver, has been the focus of much publicity. Public interest in immunology was intensified by the potential application of the immune response to the detection and management of cancer. In the 1980s, the general public became familiar with some aspects of immunology because of the alarming spread of acquired immune deficiency syndrome (AIDS).

The innate and adaptive immune systems play an integral role in the prevention of and recovery from infectious diseases and are, without question, essential to the survival of the individual. Metchnikoff was the first to propose in the 1800s that phagocytic cells formed the first line of defense against infection and that the inflammatory response could actually serve a protective function for the host. Indeed, innate immune responses are responsible for the detection and rapid destruction of most infectious agents that are encountered in the daily lives of most individuals. We now know that innate immune responses operate in concert with adaptive immune responses to generate antigen-specific effector mechanisms that lead to the death and elimination of the invading pathogen. Chapter 21 presents information concerning how our immune systems respond to microorganisms and how methods developed to exploit these mechanisms are used as immunoprophylaxis. Vaccination against infectious diseases has been an effective form of prophylaxis. Immunoprophylaxis against the virus that causes poliomyelitis has significantly reduced the incidence of this dreadful disease. Indeed, the previously widespread disease, smallpox, has been eliminated from the face of the earth. The last documented case of natural transmission of smallpox virus was in 1972. Unfortunately, the threat of biologic weapons has prompted new concerns regarding the reemergence of certain infectious diseases, including smallpox. Fortunately, public health vaccination initiatives can be applied to prevent or significantly curtail the threat of weaponized microbiological agents.

Recent developments in immunology also hold the promise of immunoprophylaxis against malaria and several other parasitic diseases that plague many parts of the world and affect billions of people. Vaccination against diseases in domestic animals promises to increase the production of meat in developing countries, while vaccination against various substances that play roles in the reproductive processes in mammals offers the possibility of long-term contraception in humans and companion animals such as cats and dogs.

DAMAGING EFFECTS OF THE IMMUNE RESPONSE

The enormous survival value of the immune response is self-evident. Adaptive immunity directed against a foreign material has as its ultimate goal the elimination of the invading substance. In the process, some tissue damage may occur as the result of the accumulation of components with nonspecific effects. This damage is generally temporary. As soon as the invader is eliminated, the situation at that site reverts to normal.

There are instances in which the power of the immune response, although directed against foreign substances—some innocuous such as some medications, inhaled pollen particles, or substances deposited by insect bites—produces a response that may result in severe pathologic consequences and even death. These responses are known collectively as *hypersensitivity reactions* or *allergic reactions*. An understanding of the basic mechanisms underlying these disease processes has been fundamental in their treatment and control and, in addition, has contributed much to our knowledge of the normal immune response. The latter is true because both utilize essentially identical mechanisms; however, in hypersensitivity, these mechanisms are misdirected or out of control (see Chapters 15–17).

Given the complexity of the immune response and its potential for inducing damage, it is self-evident that it must operate under carefully regulated conditions, as does any other physiologic system. These controls are multiple and include feedback inhibition by soluble products as well as cell–cell interactions of many types, which may either heighten or reduce the response. The net result is to maintain a state of homeostasis so that when the system is perturbed by a foreign invader enough response is generated to control the invader, and then the system returns to equilibrium; in other words, the immune response is shut down. However, its memory of that particular invader is retained so that a more rapid and heightened response will occur should the invader return. Disturbances in these regulatory mechanisms

may be caused by conditions such as congenital defects, hormonal imbalance, or infection, any of which can have disastrous consequences. AIDS may serve as a timely example: It is associated with an infection of T lymphocytes that participate in regulating the immune response. As a result of infection with the human immunodeficiency virus (HIV), which causes AIDS, there is a decrease in occurrence and function of one vital subpopulation of T cells, which leads to immunologic deficiency and renders the patient powerless to resist infections by microorganisms that are normally benign. An important form of regulation concerns the prevention of immune responses against self-antigens. As discussed in Chapter 13, this regulation may be defective, thus causing an immune response against self to be mounted. This type of immune response is termed *autoimmunity* and is the cause of diseases such as some forms of arthritis, thyroiditis, and diabetes, which are very difficult to treat.

THE FUTURE OF IMMUNOLOGY

For the student, a peek into the world of the future of immunology suggests many exciting areas in which the application of molecular and computational techniques promises significant dividends. To cite just a few examples, let us focus on vaccine development and control of the immune response. In the former, rather than the laborious, empirical search for an attenuated virus or bacterium for use in immunization, it is now possible to use pathogen-specific protein sequence data and sophisticated computational methods (bioinformatics) to identify candidate immunogenic peptides that can be tested as vaccines. Alternatively, DNA vaccines involving the injection of DNA vectors that encode immunizing proteins may revolutionize vaccination protocols in the not-too-distant future. The identification of various genes and the proteins or portions thereof (peptides) that they are encoding makes it possible to design vaccines against a wide spectrum of biologically important compounds. Another area of great promise is the characterization and synthesis of cytokines that enhance and control the activation of various cells associated with the immune response as well as with other functions of the body. Techniques of gene isolation, clonal reproduction, the polymerase chain reaction, and biosynthesis have contributed to rapid progress. Powerful and important modulators have been synthesized by the methods of recombinant DNA technology and are being tested for their therapeutic efficacy in a variety of diseases, including many different cancers. In some cases, cytokine research efforts have already moved from the bench to the bedside with the development of therapeutic agents used to treat patients. Finally, and probably one of the most exciting areas, is the technology to genetically engineer cells and even whole animals, such as mice, that lack one or more specific traits (gene knockout) or that carry a specific trait (transgenic). These and other immune-based experimental systems are the subject of Chapter 6. They allow the immunologist to study the effects of such traits on the immune system and on the body as a whole with the aim of understanding the intricate regulation, expression, and function of the immune response, and with the ultimate aim of controlling the trait to the benefit of the individual. Thus our burgeoning understanding of the functioning of the immune system, combined with the recently acquired ability to alter and manipulate its components, carries enormous implications for the future of humankind.

THE SHORT COURSE BEGINS HERE

This brief overview of the immune system is intended to orient the reader about the complex yet fascinating subject of immunology. In the remaining chapters we provide a more detailed account of the workings of the immune system, beginning with its cellular components, followed by a description of the structure of the reactants and the general methodology for measuring their reactions. This is followed by chapters describing the formation and activation of the cellular and molecular components of the immune apparatus required to generate a response. A discussion of the control mechanisms that regulate the scope and intensity of immune responses completes the description of the basic nature of immunity. Included in this section of the book is a chapter on cytokines (Chapter 12), the soluble mediators that regulate immune responses and play a significant role in hematopoiesis. Next are chapters that deal with the great variety of diseases involving immunologic components. These vary from ineffective or absent immune responses (immunodeficiency) to those produced by aberrant immune responses (hypersensitivity) to responses to self-antigens (autoimmunity). This is followed by chapters that describe the role of the immune response in transplantation and discuss antitumor reactions. Chapter 21 focuses on the spectrum of microorganisms that challenge the immune system and how immune responses are mounted in a vigilant, orchestrated fashion to protect the host from infectious diseases. Included is a discussion of immunoprophylaxis using vaccines that protect us from variety of pathogenic organisms. Without question, the successful use of vaccines helped revolutionize the field of medicine in the twentieth century. What lies

ahead in the twenty-first century are research efforts related to the development of crucial new vaccines to protect humankind from naturally occurring pathogenic viruses and microorganisms that have just begun to plague us (most notably HIV), have been engineered as potential biologic weapons, or have yet to be identified.

With the enormous scope of the subject and the extraordinary richness of detail available, we have made every effort to adhere to fundamental elements and basic concepts required to achieve an integrated, if not extensive, understanding of the immune response. If the reader's interest has been aroused, many current books, articles, and reviews, and growing numbers of educational Internet sites, including the one that supports this textbook (see the preface), are available to flesh out the details on the scaffolding provided by this book.

REFERENCES AND BIBLIOGRAPHY

Amsen D, Backer RA, Helbig C. (2013) Decisions on the road to memory. *Adv Exp Med Biol* 785: 107.

Birnbaum ME, Dong S, Garcia KC. (2012) Diversity-oriented approaches for interrogating T-cell receptor repertoire, ligand recognition, and function. *Immunol Rev* 250(1): 82.

Blom B, Spits H. (2006) Development of human lymphoid cells. *Ann Rev Immunol* 24: 287.

Boehm T, Bleul CC. (2007) The evolutionary history of lymphoid organs. *Nature Immunol* 8: 131.

Brownlie RJ, Zamoyska R. (2013) T cell receptor signalling networks: branched, diversified and bounded. *Nat Rev Immunol* 13(4): 257.

Carroll MC, Isenman DE. (2012) Regulation of humoral immunity by complement. *Immunity* 37(2): 199.

Köhler G, Milstein C. (1975) Continuous cultures of fused cells secreting antibody of predefined specificity. *Nature* 256(5517): 495.

Matzinger P. (1994) Tolerance, danger and the extended family. *Ann Rev Immunol* 12: 991.

Ohkura N, Kitagawa Y, Sakaguchi S. (2013) Development and maintenance of regulatory T cells. *Immunity* 38(3): 414.

Pieper K, Grimbacher B, Eibel H. (2013) B-cell biology and development. *J Allergy Clin Immunol* 131(4): 959.

Shevach EM. (2002) CD4+, CD25+ suppressor T cells: More questions than answers. *Nature Rev Immunol* 2: 389.

Swanson CL, Pelanda R, Torres RM. (2013) Division of labor during primary humoral immunity. *Immunol Res* 55(1–3): 277.

2

INNATE IMMUNITY

INTRODUCTION

Every living organism is confronted by continual intrusions from its environment. Our immune systems are equipped with a network of mechanisms to safeguard us from infectious microorganisms that would otherwise take advantage of our bodies for their own survival. In short, the immune system has evolved as a surveillance system poised to initiate and maintain protective responses against virtually any harmful foreign element we might encounter. These defenses range from physical and chemical barriers—elements of innate immunity—to highly sophisticated systems that constitute the adaptive immune system. Here, we describe the principle elements of innate immunity, which is a primordial immune defense system that is present from birth. The major role of this host defense system is to provide a rapid, first line of defense against pathogens. We will discuss the participating organs, cells, and molecular components of innate immunity and their physiological roles that, in many cases, include dynamic interactions with elements of the adaptive immune system. Thus, innate immune responses are important not only because they are an independent arm of the immune system but also because they profoundly influence the nature of adaptive immune responses.

PHYSICAL AND CHEMICAL BARRIERS OF INNATE IMMUNITY

Most organisms and foreign substances cannot penetrate intact skin but can enter the body if the skin is damaged.

Some microorganisms can enter through sebaceous glands and hair follicles. However, the acid pH of sweat and sebaceous secretions and the presence of various *fatty acids and hydrolytic enzymes* (e.g., *lysozymes*) all have some antimicrobial effects, therefore minimizing the importance of this route of infection. In addition, soluble proteins, including the *interferons* (see Chapter 12) and certain members of the *complement system* (see Chapter 14) found in the serum, contribute to nonspecific immunity. Interferons are a group of proteins made by cells in response to viral infection, which essentially induces a generalized antiviral state in surrounding cells. Activation of complement components in response to certain microorganisms results in a controlled enzymatic cascade, which targets the membrane of pathogenic organisms and leads to their destruction. An important innate immune mechanism involved in the protection of many areas of the body, including the respiratory and gastrointestinal tracts, involves the simple fact that surfaces in these areas are covered with mucous. In these areas, the mucous membrane barrier traps microorganisms, which are then swept away by ciliated epithelial cells toward the external openings. The hairs in the nostrils and the cough reflex are also helpful in preventing organisms from infecting the respiratory tract. The elimination of microorganisms from the respiratory tract is aided by pulmonary or alveolar macrophages, which, as we shall see later, are phagocytic cells able to engulf and destroy some microorganisms. Similarly, phagocytic cells called *microglial cells* provide innate immune defense within the central nervous system. Microorganisms that have penetrated the mucous membrane

Immunology: A Short Course, Seventh Edition. Richard Coico and Geoffrey Sunshine.
© 2015 John Wiley & Sons, Ltd. Published 2015 by John Wiley & Sons, Ltd.
Companion Website: www.wileyimmunology.com/coico

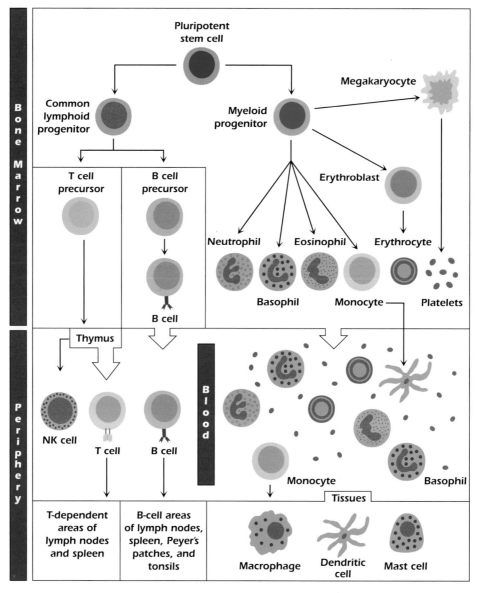

Figure 2.1. Developmental pathways of various hematopoietic cells from pluripotential bone marrow stem cells.

barrier can be phagocytized by macrophages or otherwise transported to lymph nodes, where many are destroyed. The environment of the gastrointestinal tract is made hostile to many microorganisms by other innate mechanisms, including the hydrolytic enzymes in saliva, the low pH of the stomach, and the proteolytic enzymes and bile in the small intestine. The low pH of the vagina serves a similar function.

Origin, Differentiation, and Characterization of Cells of the Innate Immune System

Once an invading microorganism has penetrated the various physical and chemical barriers, the next line of defense

consists of various specialized cells whose purpose is to destroy the invader. These include the ***polymorphonuclear leukocytes*** (white blood cells containing a segmented lobular nucleus and include eosinophils, basophils, and neutrophils), ***monocytes***, and ***macrophages***, each of which is derived from hematopoietic precursor cells. The developmental pathways of each of the hematopoietic cells are shown in Figure 2.1. Cells of the innate immune system derive from myeloid precursors whereas cells associated with the adaptive immune system are derived from common lymphoid precursors.

The immune system has evolved to exploit virtually each of the hematopoietic cell populations. As we have already pointed out, it is convenient to discuss the major

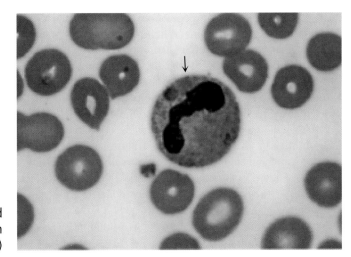

Figure 2.2. A PMN (surrounded by erythrocytes) with trilobed nucleus and cytoplasmic granules (×950). (Reproduced with permission from Olana and Walker, *Infect Med* 19: 318 [2007].)

arms of the immune system beginning with elements of the innate immune system followed by the adaptive immune system. But it is important to underscore the interrelationship of these two arms of our immune system. Clearly, they are interrelated developmentally due to their common hematopoietic precursor, the pluripotential stem cell. A classic example of their functional interrelationship is illustrated by the roles played by innate immune cells involved in *antigen presentation*. These so-called *antigen-presenting cells* (APCs) do just what their name implies: they present antigens (e.g., pieces of phagocytized bacteria) to T cells within the adaptive immune system. As will be discussed in great detail in subsequent chapters, T cells must interact with APCs that display antigens for which they are specific in order for the T cells to be activated to generate antigen-specific responses. Thus, while the title of this section implies that the cells described below are principally involved in innate immune responses, it is important to recognize their important role in adaptive immune responses (Chapter 3) at this early stage of study of the immune system.

Polymorphonuclear Leukocytes. Polymorphonuclear (PMN) leukocytes are a population of cells also referred to as ***granulocytes***. These include the basophils, eosinophils, and neutrophils. Granulocytes are short-lived phagocytic cells that contain the enzyme-rich lysosomes, which can facilitate destruction of infectious microorganisms (Figure 2.2). They also produce peroxide, superoxide radicals, and nitric oxide, which are toxic to many microorganisms. Some lysosomes also contain bactericidal proteins, such as lactoferrin. PMN leukocytes play a major role in protection against infection. Defects in PMN cell function are accompanied by chronic or recurrent infection.

Macrophages. Macrophages are phagocytes derived from blood ***monocytes*** (Figure 2.3). The monocyte itself is a small, spherical cell with few projections, abundant cyto-

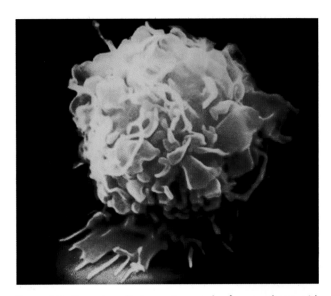

Figure 2.3. Scanning electron micrograph of macrophage with ruffled membrane and surface covered with microvilli (×5200). (Reproduced with permission from *J Clin Invest* 117 [2007].)

plasm, little endoplasmic reticulum, and many granules. Following migration of monocytes from the blood to various tissues, they undergo further differentiation into a variety of histologic forms, all of which play a role in phagocytosis, including the following:

- ***Kupffer cells***, in the liver; large cells with many cytoplasmic projections
- ***Alveolar macrophages***, in the lung
- ***Splenic macrophages***, in the red pulp
- ***Peritoneal macrophages***, free-floating in peritoneal fluid
- ***Microglial cells***, in the central nervous tissue

Each of these macrophage populations constitutes part of the cellular members of the *reticuloendothelial system* (RES), which is widely distributed throughout the body. The major function of the RES is to phagocytize microorganisms and foreign substances that are in the bloodstream and in various tissues. The RES also functions in the destruction of aged and imperfect cells, such as erythrocytes.

Although associated with diverse names and locations, many of these cells share common features, such as the ability to bind and engulf particulate materials and antigens. Because of their location along capillaries, these cells are most likely to make first contact with invading pathogens and antigens and, as we shall see later, play a large part in the success of innate as well as adaptive immunity (also called *acquired immunity*).

In general, cells of the macrophage series have two major functions. One, as their name ("large eater") implies, is to engulf and, with the aid of all the degradative enzymes in their lysosomal granules, break down trapped materials into simple amino acids, sugars, and other substances for excretion or reuse. Thus these cells play a key role in the removal of bacteria and parasites from the body. As noted above and discussed in detail in later chapters, the second major function of the macrophages is to take up antigens, process them by denaturation or partial digestion, and present them, on their surfaces, to antigen-specific T cells (i.e., the process of antigen presentation).

Dendritic Cells.   Dendritic cells (DCs) are critically important members of the innate immune system due to their highly efficient APC properties that enable them to trigger adaptive immune responses carried out by T cells (see Chapter 10). Like other innate immune cells, they recognize and phagocytize pathogens and other antigens but their ability to present antigens to T cells far exceeds that of other APCs. They are found as migrating dendritic cells in the blood, nonmigratory *follicular dendritic cells* (fDCs) in primary and secondary follicles of the B cell areas of lymph nodes and spleen (see Chapter 3), *interdigitating cells* of the thymus, and *Langerhans cells* in the skin. Another type of dendritic cell is the *plasmacystoid DC* (pDC). Unlike other DC subpopulations that are derived from myeloid precursor cells, pDCs are derived from lymphoid precursors. Like all DCs, pDCs display antigen-presenting function, but they are distinguished by their ability to produce large amounts of alpha/beta interferons (IFN-α/β) in response to viral and bacterial stimuli (see Chapter 12).

Natural Killer Cells.   Altered features of the membranes of abnormal cells, such as those found on virus-infected or cancer cells, are recognized by natural killer (NK) cells, which are cytotoxic. NK cells probably play a role in the early stages of viral infection or tumorogenesis, before the large numbers of activated cytotoxic T

lymphocytes are generated. Histologically, NK cells are large granular lymphocytes. The intracellular granules contain preformed biologically potent molecules that are released when NK cells make contact with target cells. Some of these molecules cause the formation of pores in the membrane of the target cell, leading to its lysis. Other molecules enter the target cell and cause apoptosis (programmed cell death) of the target cell by enhanced fragmentation of its nuclear DNA. Hence, they are able to lyse certain virus-infected cells and tumor cells without prior stimulation.

Unlike cytotoxic T lymphocytes, which recognize target cells in an antigen-specific fashion due to their expression of T cell receptors (TCRs), NK cells lack antigen-specific receptors. How, then, do they seek and destroy their targets? They do this by using a mechanism involving cell–cell contact, which allows them to determine whether a potential target cell has lost a particular self-antigen, namely, major histocompatibility complex (MHC) class I. MHC class I is expressed on virtually all nucleated cells. NK cells express receptors called *killer-cell inhibitory receptors* (KIR), which bind to MHC class I molecules expressed on normal cells. When ligated, KIRs inhibit downstream events that would otherwise cause the NK cell to be activated, causing degranulation and destruction of the target cells. Virus-infected or transformed (tumor) cells have significantly reduced numbers of MHC class I molecules on their surfaces. Thus, when such cells encounter NK cells, they fail to effectively engage KIRs and therefore become susceptible to NK cell-mediated cytotoxicity (Figure 2.4).

Natural Killer T Cells.   Recognized more than a decade ago, natural killer T (NKT) cells differentiate from thymic precursors through signals emanating from cortical thymocytes during TCR engagement. Like other T cells, these cells express TCRs, although with restricted variability. Their semi-invariant TCRs recognize a mammalian

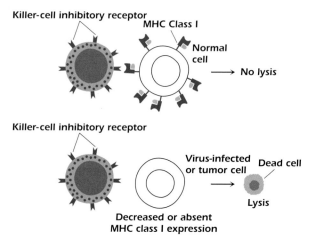

Figure 2.4. NK-cell inhibitory receptors and killing.

glycosphingolipid (isoglobotrihexosylceramide), as well as microbial α-glycuronylceramides found in the cell wall of Gram-negative, lipopolysaccharide (LPS)-negative bacteria. NKT cells are unique in terms of their functional status because they fall somewhere between the innate and the adaptive immune systems. Following activation, they secrete several regulatory cytokines, including interleukin-4 (IL-4) and interferon-γ and kill target cells via Fas–Fas ligand interactions that cause apoptosis (Chapter 12). NKT cells also regulate a range of immunopathological conditions, but the mechanisms and the ligands involved remain unknown.

Innate Lymphoid Cells. Innate lymphoid cells (ILCs) constitute a heterogeneous family of innate immune cells that have been shown to aid in protective immunity at the acute phase of infections, tissue remodeling, anatomical containment of commensals microorganisms (e.g., microbiota that inhabit our gastrointestinal tract in a symbiotic relationship in which one species is benefited while the other is unaffected), wound healing, and in maintaining the epithelial integrity at mucosal sites. ILCs have also been associated with pathophysiological conditions, such as airway and gut inflammation. ILCs, which include a population called ***lymphoid tissue-inducer*** (LTi) cells, share a lymphoid morphology, are dependent on the interleukin-2 receptor γ (IL-2Rγ) chain (discussed in Chapter 12) for their development but lack the rearranged antigen receptors or markers that are expressed on cells of myeloid origin or cells of the adaptive immune system discussed in Chapter 3. Subsets of ILCs express cell-surface molecules that were previously thought to be restricted to NK cells. However, NK cells are distinct from the more recently discovered ILCs and can be divided into ILC subsets that are highly diverse with respect to their capacity of producing cytokines. This diversity matches that of T cells, and this has led to the hypotheses that ILCs act in early stages of the immune response against infectious microorganisms when the adaptive response is not yet operational.

From this brief outline, it can be seen that each of these cellular components of the innate immune system has diverse roles that serve the host's initial attempt to eliminate foreign substances and pathogens to the generation of antigen-specific adaptive immune responses that ultimately give rise to long-term immunity. Finally, as producers of an array of cytokines, soluble mediators of immune responses (see Chapter 12), these cells influence the functional properties of many other cell types within the immune system. For example, they can enhance the phagocytic activity of macrophages to increase their killing of pathogens, as well as the cytotoxic effects of NK cells. Thus, innate immune cells are pivotal players in strategies employed by the immune system to ensure protection of the host against infectious microorganisms. They are also called into play whenever physical barriers of defense are compromised (e.g., skin

wounds). In either case, mobilization of innate immune cells following injury or infection generates a physiologic response known as ***inflammation***. This is discussed in more detail in the section that follows.

PATTERN RECOGNITION: THE HALLMARK OF INNATE IMMUNE RESPONSES

Now that we have outlined the origins and major characteristics of innate immune cells, we will discuss the sophisticated yet elegantly simple ways in which these cells initiate their host defense roles: ***pattern recognition***. The underlying host defense mechanism associated with this arm of the immune system is the ability of innate cells and specific soluble mediators they produce to recognize and respond to evolutionarily conserved microbial structures termed ***pathogen-associated molecular patterns*** (PAMPs). Detection of PAMPs by innate immune cells occurs via soluble and cell-associated germline-encoded ***pattern recognition receptors*** (PRRs). It is important to note that this feature of innate immune recognition of pathogens differs markedly from recognition mechanisms associated with the adaptive immune system as illustrated in Figure 2.5. As will be discussed in subsequent chapters, B and T lymphocytes (also called B and T cells, respectively) express somatically generated antigen-specific receptors. Thus, these receptors are not germline encoded but rather the translational products of multiple genes that are pieced together by gene rearrangement that occurs during their development. Many PRRs are highly expressed on DCs—highly efficient APCs—where they can be located on the cell surface, in endocytic compartments, or the cytoplasm. Upon recognition of foreign antigen, particularly in the presence of PAMPs, DCs help to initiate an adaptive immune responses by B cells (which produce antigen-specific antibody) and T cells (which express antigen-specific T cell receptors). Adaptive responses take days to weeks to develop but last considerably longer (years) than innate responses, which are very rapid (minutes to hours) and last less time (days or weeks). In addition, in contrast with adaptive immune responses that ultimately result in the generation of clonally expanded, highly antigen-specific memory B and T cells, activated innate immune cells do not expand or generate memory cells.

Pattern Recognition Receptors

Most microorganisms encountered daily in the life of a healthy individual are detected and destroyed within minutes to hours by innate defense mechanisms. Mechanistically, innate immunity is carried out by nonspecific physical and chemical barriers (e.g., the skin, acid pH or the stomach), cellular barriers (e.g., phagocytes), and molecular pattern-based reactions. This section describes the latter mechanism, which is used by a phylogenetically diverse set of

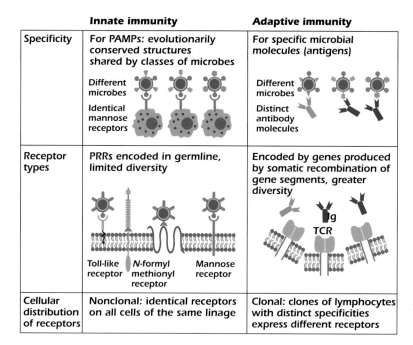

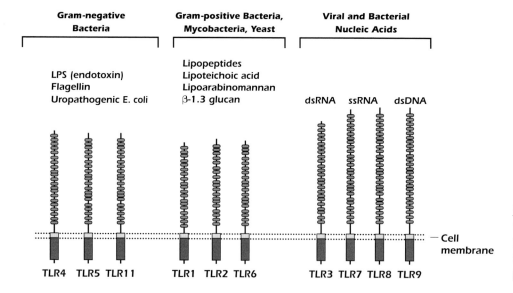

Figure 2.5. Comparison of specificity and cellular distribution of receptors used in innate and adaptive immunity.

Figure 2.6. Pattern-recognition receptors called TLRs binding to molecules with specific pattern motifs expressed by various pathogens.

species (fish, fruit flies, mammals) to enable host defense systems to detect the presence of foreign antigens that may do harm: the pattern recognition receptors (PRRs). Based on their molecular structure, PRRs can be divided into multiple families, including Toll-like receptors (TLRs), C-type lectin receptors (CLRs), NOD-like receptors (NLRs), and RIG-I-like receptors (RLRs).

Toll-like Receptors.   A major class of pattern recognition receptors is the **Toll-like receptors** (TLRs). The Toll gene family was originally discovered for its contribution to

dorsoventral patterning in *Drosophila melanogaster* embryos. Later, studies showed that Toll genes encode proteins that play a critical role in the fly's innate immune response to microbial infection. Further investigation then confirmed the existence of homologous proteins in mammals (TLRs) that can activate phagocytes and DCs to respond to pathogens. TLRs make up a large family of receptors and each recognizes specific microbial molecular patterns (Figure 2.6). Activation of cells expressing TLRs following receptor ligation also facilitates initiation of adaptive immune responses due to the production of proinflammatory cytokines by these activated cells. This phenomenon illustrates, yet again, the important functional and coordinated relationship that exists between the innate and adaptive immune systems.

TLRs are expressed as membrane-bound or cytoplasmic receptors that recognize a remarkably large number of PAMPs expressed by viral, bacterial, fungal and parasitic pathogen. TLR1, TLR2, TLR4, TLR5, and TLR6 are primarily expressed on the plasma membrane where they sense specific molecules on the surface of microbes. In contrast, TLR3, TLR7, TLR8, and TLR9 traffic from the endoplasmic reticulum to endolysosomal compartments where they recognize RNA and DNA. TLRs initiate signaling pathways through interactions with adaptor proteins, including MyD88 and Toll/interleukin-1 receptor domain-containing adaptor inducing IFN-β (TRIF). Adaptor proteins function as flexible molecular scaffolds that mediate protein–protein and protein–lipid interactions in signal transduction pathways. When specific TLRs interact with adaptor proteins, signal transduction pathways are activated resulting in generation of mitogen-associated protein kinases (MAPKs), nuclear factor kappaB (NF-κB), and transcription of interferon regulatory factor (IRF)-responsive genes.

C-Type Lectin Receptors.
C-type lectin receptors (CLRs), which are membrane-bound receptors, comprise a large family of receptors that bind to carbohydrates in a calcium-dependent manner (by definition, all lectins bind to carbohydrates). They are involved in fungal recognition and the modulation of the innate immune response.

f-Met-Leu-Phe Receptors.
A group of receptors specific for formylated peptides such as N-formylmethionine (fMet), are expressed at high levels on the membranes of polymorphonuclear and mononuclear phagocytes. fMet is specifically used for initiation of protein synthesis in bacteria. It is not used in cytosolic protein synthesis of eukaryotes. Synthetic formylated peptides have been shown to be chemotactic for phagocytes, leading to the concept of formylated peptides as PAMPs.

NOD-Like Receptors.
NOD-like receptors (NLRs) constitute a family of intracellular PRRs. The primary role of these cytoplasmic receptors is to recognize cytoplasmic PAMPs and/or the endogenous danger signal, thereby inducing immune responses. NLRs are characterized by a tripartite-domain organization with a conserved nucleotide-binding oligomerization domain (NOD) and leucine-rich repeats (LRRs). Certain NLRs can assemble into a multiprotein complex called the *inflammasome*, which activates an enzyme called *caspase-1* that can cleave immature forms of certain cytokines, such as IL-1 into active, mature cytokines (Figure 2.7). As the name implies, generation of inflammasomes is associated with inflammatory responses

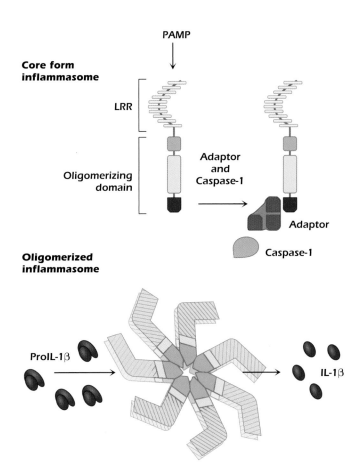

Figure 2.7. Binding of pathogen-associated molecular patterns (PAMPs) to the core form of an inflammasome. Binding of PAMPs to leucine-rich repeats (LRRs) on cytoplasmic inflammasomes causes the core form to bind to an adaptor protein and caspase-1. This is followed by oligomerization of the inflammasome, which enables it to catalyze the conversion of inactive IL-1 β to active IL-1β.

triggered by microbial pathogens. Inflammation will be discussed later in this chapter. In this capacity, inflammasomes meaningfully contribute to the healthy resolution of infections. However, activation of inflammasomes also contributes to cytokine-driven inflammation central to the pathology of autoimmune and autoinflammatory diseases. Consequently, inflammasomes are now major drug targets for autoimmune and chronic inflammatory diseases. Moreover, recent studies have described the genetic association of mutations in NLR genes with several chronic inflammatory barrier diseases, such as Crohn's disease and asthma, and with rare autoinflammatory syndromes including familial cold urticaria, Muckle–Wells syndrome, and Blau syndrome.

RIG-I-Like Receptors.
RIG-I-like receptors (RLRs) constitute a family of three cytoplasmic RNA helicases that are critical for host antiviral responses. They sense

double-stranded RNA, a replication intermediate for RNA viruses, leading to production of type I interferons (interferon-α and interferon-β) in infected cells.

COMPLEMENT

Another major soluble element of the innate immune system is the complement system. Complement will be discussed in detail in Chapter 14. Briefly, it is made up of approximately 25 proteins, most of which are produced in the liver. They work together to assist or "complement" the action of antibodies in destroying bacteria. Complement also helps to rid the host of antibody-coated antigens (so-called *opsonized* antigens). Certain complement proteins that cause blood vessels to become dilated and then leaky contribute to the redness, warmth, swelling, pain, and loss of function that characterize inflammatory responses.

Complement proteins circulate in the blood in an inactive form. Each component takes its turn in a precise chain of steps known as the ***complement cascade*** (Figure 2.8). The end products are molecular cylinders called the ***membrane attack complex*** (MAC), which are inserted into the cell walls that surround the invading bacteria. This results in the development of puncture holes causing fluids to flow in and out of the bacteria. Consequently, the bacterial cell walls swell, burst (lysis), and the bacteria are killed. There are three complement activation pathways as discussed in detail in Chapter 14. When the first protein in the complement series (C1q) is activated by an antibody that has been made in response to a microbe (e.g., bacteria), this initiates the chain of events resulting in the generation of MAC that causes lysis of the microbe. This is known as the ***classical***

activation pathway and is part of complement's participation in the adaptive immune response. However, the ***alternative activation pathway*** involves direct binding of certain complement components, such as C3, to the surfaces of pathogens without the participation of antibody. This binding triggers a conformational change in the protein that initiates the downstream cascade leading to the generation of MAC followed by lysis of the microbe. Finally, the ***lectin activation pathway*** involves other complement components such as C2 and C4, which are lectins that also bind directly, in this case to mannan moieties expressed on pathogens. As with the other two pathways, this results in activation of other complement components leading to MAC production and lysis of the pathogen.

Other components of the complement system by directly binding to bacteria make bacteria more susceptible to phagocytosis by innate immune cells. Phagocytic cells express complement receptors, and when they encounter complement-coated bacteria (also referred to as opsonized bacteria), this greatly facilitates their binding to and phagocytosis of the bacteria. Complement components generated during the complement cascade can beckon other immune cells (phagocytes and other leukocytes) to the area where invading bacteria are present. Thus, complement plays a role in locally mobilizing host defense mechanisms. Finally, like all biologically complex systems involving activation of proteins with the ability to promote potentially harmful consequences to the host (e.g., inflammation), the complement system is endowed with regulatory proteins that help to terminate the process. Table 2.1 summarizes the functional properties of the proteins involved in the complement cascade. These will be discussed further in Chapter 14.

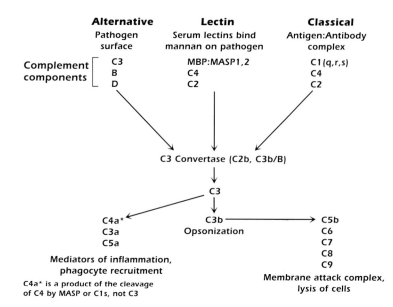

Figure 2.8. The three complement activation pathways: classical, alternative, and lectin.

Intracellular and Extracellular Killing of Microorganisms

Another hallmark of innate immunity is the ability of certain innate immune cells to sample their environment by engulfing macroparticles (*endocytosis*) or individual cells (*phagocytosis*). Endocytosis is the process whereby macromolecules present in extracellular tissue fluid are ingested by cells. This can occur either by pinocytosis, which involves non-specific membrane invagination, or by receptor-mediated endocytosis, a process involving the selective binding of macromolecules to specific membrane receptors. In both cases, ingestion of the foreign macromolecules generates

endocytic vesicles filled with the foreign material, which then fuse with acidic compartments called endosomes. Edosomes then fuse with lysosomes containing degradative enzymes (e.g., nucleases, lipases, proteases) to reduce the ingested macromolecules to small breakdown products, including nucleotides, sugars, and peptides (Figure 2.9).

Phagocytosis. Phagocytosis is the ingestion by individual cells of invading foreign particles, such as bacteria. It is a critical protective mechanism of the immune system. Many microorganisms release substances that attract phagocytic cells. Phagocytosis may be enhanced by a variety of factors that make the foreign particle an easier target. These factors, collectively referred to as *opsonins* (the Greek word meaning "prepare food for"), consist of antibodies and various serum components of complement (see Chapter 14). After ingestion, the foreign particle is entrapped in a phagocytic vacuole (phagosome), which fuses with lysosomes, forming the phagolysosome. The latter release their powerful enzymes, which digest the particle.

Phagocytes can also damage invading pathogens through the generation of toxic products in a process known as the ***respiratory burst***. Production of these toxic metabolites is induced during phagocytosis of pathogens such as bacteria and catalyzed by a set of interrelated enzyme pathways. The most important of these are nitric oxide (inducible nitric oxidase synthase), hydrogen peroxide and superoxide anion (phagocyte NADPH oxidase), and

TABLE 2.1. Proteins Involved in the Complement Cascade

Binding to Ag:Ab complexes	C1q
Activating Enzymes	C1r, C1s, C2b, Bd, D, MASP1,2
Membrane-binding opsonins	C4b, C3b, MBP
Mediators of inflammation	C5a, C3a, C4a
Membrane attack	C5b, C6, C7, C8, C9
Complement Receptors	CR1, CR2, CR3, CR4, C1qR
Complement-regulatory proteins	C1INH, C4bp, CR1, MCP, DAE, H, I, P, CD59

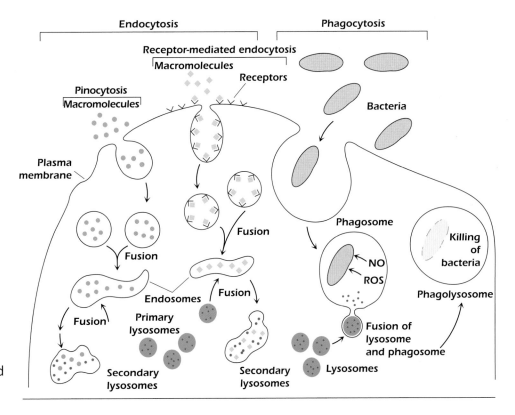

Figure 2.9. Endocytosis and phagocytosis by phagocytes.

hypochlorous acid (myeloperoxidase), each of which is toxic to bacteria. These microbicidal products can also damage host cells. Fortunately, a series of protective enzymes produced by phagocytes controls the action of these products so that their microbicidal activity is primarily limited to the phagolysosome (i.e., fused phagosomes and lysosomes; see Figure 2.9), thereby focusing their toxicity on ingested pathogens. These protective enzymes include catalase, which degrades hydrogen peroxide, and superoxide dismutase, which converts the superoxide anion into hydrogen peroxide and oxygen. The absence of, or an abnormality in, any one of the respiratory burst components from phagocytic cells results in a form of immunodeficiency that predisposes individuals to repeated infections (Chapter 18).

INFLAMMATION

An important function of phagocytic cells is their participation in inflammatory reactions. The word "inflammation" comes from the Latin *inflammare* (to set on fire). In some disorders, the inflammatory process, which under normal conditions is self-limiting, becomes continuous, and chronic inflammatory diseases develop subsequently.

Inflammation is a major component of the body's defense mechanisms. As a physiologic process, inflammation is typically initiated by tissue damage caused by endogenous factors (such as tissue necrosis or bone fracture) and by exogenous factors. The latter includes various types of damage, such as mechanical injury (e.g., cuts), physical injury (e.g., burns), chemical injury (e.g., exposure to corrosive chemicals), immunologic injury (e.g., hypersensitivity reactions; see Chapters 15–17) and biologic injury (e.g., infections caused by pathogenic microorganisms; see Chapter 21). Indeed, infection can be thought of as pathogen-induced injury when considering inflammatory responses, since the innate immune cells called into play and the inflammatory responses that manifest are essentially identical, regardless of the cause of injury. While perhaps paradoxical in light of the discomfort associated with certain types of inflammatory responses (e.g., hypersensitivity to poison ivy), inflammation is a normal immunologic process designed to restore immune homeostasis by bringing the injured tissue back to its normal state.

Hallmark Signs of Inflammation

The triad of clinical signs of inflammation are *pain*, *redness*, and *heat*. These can be explained by increased blood flow, elevated cellular metabolism, vasodilatation, release of soluble mediators, extravasation of fluids that move from the blood vessels to surrounding tissue, and cellular influx. Pain is caused by increased vascular diameter, which leads to increased blood flow, thereby causing heat and redness in the area. As discussed below, subsequent reduction in blood velocity and concomitant cytokine-induced and kinin-induced increased expression of adhesion molecules on the endothelial cells lining the blood vessel promote the binding of circulating leukocytes to the vessel. These events facilitate the attachment and entry of leukocytes into tissues and the recruitment of neutrophils and monocytes to the site of inflammation. Another major change in the local blood vessels is increased vascular permeability. This results from the separation of previously tightly joined endothelial cells lining the blood vessels leading to the exit of fluid and proteins from the blood and their accumulation in the tissue. These events account for the swelling (*edema*) associated with inflammation, which contributes significantly to the pain, and to the attendant redness and heat associated with the accumulation of cells to the site.

Most of the cells involved in inflammatory responses are phagocytic cells, consisting mainly of the polymorphonuclear leukocytes that accumulate within 30 to 60 minutes, phagocytize the intruder or damaged tissue, and release their lysosomal enzymes in an attempt to destroy the intruder. If the cause of the inflammatory response persists beyond this point, within 4 to 6 hours, the area harboring the invading microorganism or foreign substance will be infiltrated by macrophages and lymphocytes. The macrophages supplement the phagocytic activity of the polymorphonuclear cells, thus adding to the defense of the area. They also participate in the processing and presentation of antigens expressed by the invading pathogen or foreign substance to T cells, which then generate antigen-specific responses. Activated T cells synthesize and release a variety of cytokines that proactively stimulate antigen-specific B cells, thus facilitating antibody production. Within 5 to 7 days, antibodies produced by these B cells are detectable as serum antibodies and thus become part of the humoral immune defense arsenal.

Within minutes after injury, the inflammatory process begins with activation of innate immune cells responding to microbes expressing PAMPs. As discussed earlier, activation is stimulated by ligation of PRRs and results in the release of proinflammatory cytokines such as IL-1, IL-6, and tumor necrosis factor-α (TNF-α). These cytokines travel through the blood and stimulate hepatocytes in the liver to secrete *acute phase proteins* that function as soluble PRRs (Figure 2.10). Other consequences of the acute phase response include increased white blood cell production (neutrophils demarginate first; consequently their numbers increase quickly), increased synthesis of hydrocortisone and adrenocorticotropic hormone (ACTH). Systemic inflammatory responses also include the induction of *fever* (discussed below) due to the ability of the hypothalamus to respond to elevated levels of acute phase proteins.

Table 2.2 provides a list of the major acute phase proteins. Among these proteins, *C-reactive protein* (CRP) is capable of binding to the membranes of certain microorganisms and

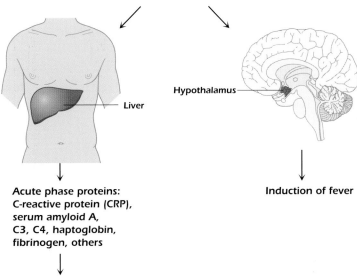

Acute phase response

Triggered by activated inflammatory cells that produce cytokines: IL-1, IL-6, TNF-α

Hypothalamus

Liver

Acute phase proteins:
C-reactive protein (CRP),
serum amyloid A,
C3, C4, haptoglobin,
fibrinogen, others

Induction of fever

Figure 2.10. The acute phase response stimulated by cytokines produced by innate immune cells.

Increased plasma viscosity and consequently, increased erythrocyte sedimentation rate (ESR)

activating the complement system (Chapter 14). This results in the lysis of the microorganism, enhanced phagocytosis by phagocytic cells, and several other important host defense functions, as we shall see later. It is noteworthy that acute phase responses are commonly assessed clinically by measuring blood levels of CRP as well as *erythrocyte sedimentation rate* (ESR). CRP is considered a nonspecific marker of inflammation and is therefore used as a marker to detect or monitor significant inflammation in an individual who is suspected of having an acute condition such as serious bacterial infections (e.g., sepsis), fungal infections, or pelvic inflammatory disease, just to name a few. Measuring CPR is also useful in monitoring people with chronic inflammatory conditions to detect flare-ups and/or to determine if treatment is effective. Examples include inflammatory bowel disease, some forms of arthritis, and autoimmune diseases (e.g., systemic lupus erythematosus [SLE]). Increased ESR associated with increased plasma viscosity can also be due to increased concentrations of acute phase proteins and is therefore an indicator of nonspecific inflammation. However, moderately elevated ESR may also occur with anemia and pregnancy (the latter due to increased levels of fibrinogen during pregnancy. A very high ESR may also be due to a marked increase in globulins as a result of severe infection but also myeloma and other lymphoid malignancies.

Localized Inflammatory Responses

Localized inflammatory responses are generated, in part, as a result of the activation of the *kinins* and the *coagulation*

system. Once activated, the *kinins* have several important localized effects on cells and organ systems. Together with the locally released cytokines, they (1) act directly on local smooth muscle and cause muscle contraction; (2) act on axons to block nervous impulses, leading to a distal muscle relaxation; and (3) act on vascular endothelial cells causing them to contract and leading to increase in vascular permeability.

Kinins are very potent nerve stimulators and are the molecules most responsible for pain (and itching) associated with inflammation. They are rapidly inactivated after their activation by proteases, which are generated during these localized responses.

Following kinin-induced damage to blood vessels, the *coagulation pathway* gets activated. Plasma enzymes are activated in a cascading manner contributing to the inflammatory response by forming a physical barrier with platelets (*clot* or *thrombus*) that prevents microorganisms from entering the bloodstream. The simultaneous activation of kinins and the coagulation system during inflammatory responses thus produce inhospitable conditions for invading pathogens as well as new physical barriers to limit their ability to use the circulatory system to gain entry to distal tissues and organs.

Transendothelial Migration of Leukocytes. All of this occurs within a local milieu that also contains chemotactic cytokines such as interleukin-8 (IL-8) and other cytokines (IL-1, TNF-α), which induce increased expression of *endothelial cell adhesion molecules* (ECAMs) and ligands on leukocytes to which ECAMs bind. Together, the

TABLE 2.2. Acute Phase Proteins

Protein	Immune System Function
C-reactive protein	• Binds to phosphocholine expressed on the surface of dead or dying cells and some types of bacteria • Opsonin
Serum amyloid P component	Opsonin
Serum amyloid A	• Recruitment of immune cells to inflammatory sites • Induction of enzymes that degrade extracellular matrix
Complement factors	• Opsonization, lysis, and clumping of target cells • Chemotaxis
Mannan-binding lectin	Mannan-binding lectin pathway of complement activation
Fibrinogen (α β globulin), prothrombin, factor VIII, von Willebrand factor	• Coagulation factors • Trapping invading microbes in blood clots. • Some cause chemotaxis
Plasminogen	Degradation of blood clots
Alpha 2-macroglobulin	• Inhibitor of coagulation by inhibiting thrombin. • Inhibitor of fibrinolysis by inhibiting plasmin
Ferritin	Binding iron, inhibiting microbe iron uptake
Hepcidin	Stimulates the internalization of ferroportin, preventing release of iron bound by ferritin within intestinal enterocytes and macrophages
Ceruloplasmin	Oxidizes iron, facilitating for ferritin, inhibiting microbe iron uptake
Haptoglobin	Binds hemoglobin, inhibiting microbe iron uptake
Orosomucoid (Alpha-1-acid glycoprotein, AGP)	Steroid carrier
Alpha 1-antitrypsin, Alpha alpha 1-antichymotrypsin	Serpin, downregulates inflammation

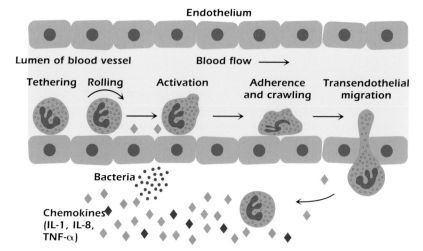

Figure 2.11. Leukocyte adhesion to endothelium leads to their adhesion, activation, and extravasation from the blood to tissue where they are needed to help destroy (e.g., phagocytize) pathogens such as bacteria that initiate this response.

increased vascular permeability, leukocyte endothelial adherence and rolling results in *transendothelial migration* (*extravasation*) of these cells from the blood to local tissue where the inciting inflammatory microbe (e.g., bacteria) is located (Figure 2.11). Leukocyte extravasation is now envisioned as a process that undergoes the following sequential steps: tethering, rolling, activation, adhesion, crawling, and transmigration, with each step relying on the function of a defined set of molecules. This is discussed further in Chapter 12.

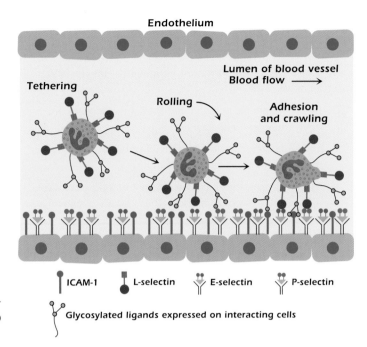

Figure 2.12. Adhesion molecules involved in leukocyte tethering, rolling, and adhesion to endothelium leading to transendothelial migration from blood to tissue.

Figure 2.12 illustrates the importance of adhesion molecules in this process. The expression of L-selectin by leukocytes and P- and E-selectin by activated endothelial cells are mostly responsible for the tethering and rolling of leukocytes on the luminal endothelial blood surface. Selectins interact with glycosylated ligands expressed by the interacting cells. Leukocyte activation and firm adhesion to the endothelium is then rapidly induced by the engagement of leukocyte chemotactic receptors by chemotactic factors immobilized on glycosaminoglycans or heparin sulphates present in the milieu. Chemotactic factors include PAMPs such as formylated peptides, complement proteins (e.g., C5a and C3a), lipids, and chemokines such as IL-8.

Chronic Inflammation

Many substances activated during the inflammatory process participate in repairing the injury. During this remarkable process, many cells, including leukocytes, are being destroyed. The macrophages present in the area phagocytize the debris, and the inflammation subsides, and a state of homeostasis at the site of injury is restored. Under these conditions, the tissue returns to its normal state or scar tissue may be formed.

Sometimes it is difficult or impossible to remove the causes of inflammation. This results in chronic inflammation, which occurs in situations of chronic infection (e.g., tuberculosis) or chronic activation of the immune response (e.g., rheumatoid arthritis and glomerulonephritis). In these cases, the inflammatory response continues and can be only temporarily modified by the administration of anti-inflammatory agents, such as aspirin, ibuprofen, and cortisone. These and other drugs and biological therapies act on several of the metabolic pathways involved in the elaboration and activation of the pharmacologic mediators of inflammation. However, they do not affect the root cause of the inflammation, so when they are withdrawn, the symptoms may return.

Fever

Although fever is one of the most common manifestations of infection and inflammation, there is still limited information about the significance of fever in the course of infection in mammals. In addition to the effects of acute phase proteins on the hypothalamus during inflammatory responses, fever is caused by many bacterial products, most notably the **endotoxins** (lipopolysaccharide [LPS]) of Gram-negative bacteria. Exposure of innate immune cells (monocytes and macrophages) to LPS causes their release of cytokines called **endogenous pyrogens**. Examples of cytokines with endogenous pyrogenic properties include IL-1 and certain interferons (see Chapter 12). Cells in other tissues can also produce these cytokines. For example, the keratinocytes present in skin contain IL-1. Interestingly, when the skin is overexposed to the ultraviolet rays of the sun (sunburn), keratinocytes are physically damaged, causing them to release their contents, including IL-1. Within a few hours, IL-1 induces the hypothalamus to raise body temperature (fever)—a phenomenon many have experienced after a summer day at the beach, with accompanying chills and malaise. Fortunately, the ultraviolet rays can be blocked by a variety of topical products to prevent skin damage. Many tissues also synthesize substances that are harmful to microorganisms. Examples include degradative enzymes, toxic free radicals, and, as noted above, acute-phase proteins

SUMMARY

1. There are two forms of immunity: innate and adaptive.

2. Innate immunity is broad and immune responses are rapid (minutes to hours).

3. Unlike adaptive immunity, innate immunity does not exhibit memory to antigenic exposure.

4. Many elements participate in innate immunity, including various physical barriers (e.g., skin), chemical barriers (e.g., low pH in stomach), cellular components (e.g., phagocytes, NKT cells), and germline-encoded pattern recognition receptors (e.g., TLRs, NLRs).

5. Macrophages constitute an essential part of the reticuloendothelial system and function to trap, process, and present antigen to T cells, thus assuming an important function in both innate and adaptive immunity.

REFERENCES AND BIBLIOGRAPHY

Aderem A, Underhill DM. (1999) Mechanisms of phagocytosis in macrophages. *Ann Rev Immunol* 17: 593.

Akira S, Takeda K, Kaiso T. (2001) Toll-like receptors: critical proteins linking innate and acquired immunity. *Nature Immunol* 2: 675.

Bernink J, Mjösberg J, Spits H. (2013) TH1- and TH2-like subsets of innate lymphoid cells. *Immunol Rev* 252: 133.

Beutler B, Jiang Z, Georgel P, Crozat P, Croker B, Rutschmann S, Du X, Hoebe K. (2007) Genetic analysis of host resistance: Toll-like receptor signaling and immunity at large. *Ann Rev Immunol* 24: 353.

Furster R, Sozzani S. (2013) Emerging aspects of leukocyte migration. *Europ J Immunol* 43(6): 1404.

Lanier, LL. (1998) NK cell receptors. *Ann Rev Immunol* 16: 359.

Mills KH, Dungan LS, Jones SA, Harris J. (2013) The role of inflammasome-derived IL-1 in driving IL-17 responses. *J Leukoc Biol* 93: 489.

Pancer Z, Cooper MD. (2007) The evolution of adaptive immunity. *Ann Rev Immunol* 24: 497.

Ricklin D, Lambris JD. (2013) Complement in immune and inflammatory disorders: pathophysiological mechanisms. *J Immunol* 190: 3831.

Song DH, Lee JO. (2012) Sensing of microbial molecular patterns by Toll-like receptors. *Immunol Rev* 205: 216.

Stekel DJ, Parker CE, Nowak MA. (1997) A model for lymphocyte recirculation. *Immunol Today* 18: 216.

REVIEW QUESTIONS

For each question, choose the ONE BEST answer or completion.

1. Which of the following generally does not apply to bone marrow (a primary lymphoid organ) but does apply to secondary lymphoid organs?
   A) cellular proliferation
   B) differentiation of lymphocytes
   C) cellular interaction
   D) antigen-dependent response

2. Which of the following is involved in recognition of intracellular pathogens in innate immune cells?
   A) Toll-like receptors (TLRs)
   B) antibody
   C) NOD-like receptors (NLRs)
   D) complement

3. Which of the following is a correct statement about NK cells?
   A) They proliferate in response to antigen.
   B) They kill target cells by phagocytosis and intracellular digestion.
   C) They are a subset of polymorphonuclear cells.
   D) They kill target cells in an extracellular fashion.
   E) They are particularly effective against certain bacteria.

4. Mature dendritic cells are capable of which of the following?
   A) activating naïve antigen-specific T cells
   B) removing red blood cells
   C) producing bradykinin
   D) extracellular killing of target cells

5. Killer-cell inhibitory receptors (KIRs) expressed by NK cells bind to which of the following to prevent killing of normal cells:
   A) complement receptors
   B) MHC class I
   C) immunoglobulin
   D) Toll-like receptors

ANSWERS TO REVIEW QUESTIONS

1. *D.* Cellular proliferation, differentiation of lymphocytes, and cellular interactions can take place in bone marrow. However, antigen-dependent responses occur in the secondary lymphoid organs, such as the spleen and lymph nodes.

2. *C.* The NLRs are a group of cytosolic innate receptors that recognize microbes that infect cells. Once ligated, they initiate a set of cellular activities that facilitate inflammatory responses and other host defense mechanisms.

3. *D.* NK cells are large granular lymphocytes. Their number does not increase in response to antigen. Their killing is extracellular, and their target cells are virus-infected cells or tumor cells. They are not particularly effective against bacterial cells.

4. *A.* When immature dendritic cells are activated following their engulfment of pathogens (phagocytosis), they mature and become more efficient at antigen presentation and, in fact, can activate antigen-specific naïve T cells.

5. *B.* NK cells express KIRs, which allow them to bind to MHC class I molecules expressed on all nucleated cells that would otherwise be targets for killing when infected with certain viruses that downregulate MHC class I expression.

3

ADAPTIVE IMMUNITY

Under circumstances in which infectious organisms are not eliminated by innate immune mechanisms, adaptive immune responses ensue, with the generation of *antigen-specific lymphocytes* (effector cells) and *memory cells* that can prevent reinfection with the same organism. These responses (sometimes called *adaptive immunity*) are attributes of virtually every living organism in one form or another; adaptive immunity is a more specialized form of immunity. It developed late in evolution and is found only in vertebrates. As discussed in Chapter 2, the various elements that participate in innate immunity exhibit broad specificity against the foreign agents they encounter through their recognition of antigens that display molecules not found in the host (e.g., N-formylated peptides). By contrast, adaptive immunity always exhibits antigenic specificity. As its name implies, adaptive immunity is a consequence of an encounter with a foreign substance. The first encounter with a particular foreign substance that has penetrated the body triggers a chain of events that induces an immune response with specificity against that foreign substance. Details of how this happens within the B- and T-cell lineages will be presented in the chapters that follow.

CELLS AND ORGANS INVOLVED IN ADAPTIVE IMMUNITY

In contrast with innate immunity, adaptive immune responses develop only after exposure to or immunization with a given substance or antigen. As we have already discussed, the effector cells responsible for adaptive immune responses are the B

and T cells. Unlike innate immune cells that use germline-encoded receptors to detect and respond to microbes and other foreign antigens, B and T cells express somatically generated antigen-specific receptors that are not germline encoded but rather are the translational products of multiple genes that are pieced together by gene rearrangements that occur during their development. B cells expressing antigen-specific B-cell receptors (BCRs) synthesize and secrete antibody into the bloodstream. This is often termed *humoral immunity*. T cells also exhibit antigen specificity by virtue of their expression of antigen-specific T-cell receptors (TCRs). In the case of T cells, their participation in adaptive immune responses is as varied as the T-cell subsets and cytokines they produce. Historically, T-cell mediated responses have been referred to as *cell-mediated responses* or *cellular immunity*.

Unlike B cells expressing BCRs that bind directly to antigens for which they are specific, T cells are incapable of binding to antigens directly. Instead, they recognize and bind to antigenic peptides when they come in contact with *antigen-presenting cells* (APCs) such as macrophages and dendritic cells that display processed, major histocompatibility complex (MHC)-bound peptides derived from the antigen (see Chapter 9). However, even this APC-dependent recognition of peptides is insufficient to activate the responding T cell. Indeed, two signals are required to activate T cells: (1) T-cell expression of peptide (epitope)-specific TCRs and, (2) ligation of T-cell expressed co-stimulatory molecules with complimentary membrane molecules expressed by APCs. The co-stimulatory signaling step initiates a cascade of intracellular and nuclear events that measurably change the behavior of responding T cells.

Immunology: A Short Course, Seventh Edition. Richard Coico and Geoffrey Sunshine.
© 2015 John Wiley & Sons, Ltd. Published 2015 by John Wiley & Sons, Ltd.
Companion Website: www.wileyimmunology.com/coico

Thus, T cells begin to express and release new gene products (e.g., cytokines), they undergo clonal expansion to increase the number of TCR-expressing cells within the T-cell repertoire, and they differentiate to create a pool of memory cells. These events occur in the secondary lymphoid organs (lymph nodes and spleen) as we will discuss in the next section of this chapter.

T-cell activation greatly facilitates the activation and differentiation of B cells responding to antigen. This is principally achieved by the action of T-cell–derived cytokines that bind to specific cytokine receptors expressed by B cells. Functional consequences of this T-cell help include B-cell proliferation, generation of memory B cells, and diversification of the kinds of immunoglobulins produced (immunoglobulin class switching). The recurring theme of cytokine involvement in normal immune responses is underscored by the fact that B cells are dependent on T cells for optimal antibody responses to most antigens. The term *T-cell–dependent antigens* is often used to characterize these antigens.

The Lymphatic Organs

The lymphatic system includes organs in which lymphocyte maturation, differentiation, and proliferation take place.

They are generally divided into two categories: (1) *primary* and (2) *secondary organs*. The primary or central lymphoid organs are those in which the maturation of B and T lymphocytes into antigen-recognizing lymphocytes occurs. In other words, these are the organs where gene rearrangements occur to generate functional antigen-specific BCR and TCR expressed by B and T cells, respectively. Mature B cells differentiate to fully mature cells within the *bone marrow*. Historically, the term "B cell" is derived from developmental studies in birds that demonstrated that antibody-forming lymphocytes differentiate within an organ unique to birds called the *bursa of Fabricius* (hence, "B" for bursa). In contrast, T cells differentiate only partially within the bone marrow. Precursor cells destined to become mature T cells undergo final maturation within the *thymus gland* (hence, "T" for thymus). Histological characteristics of the thymus are discussed in the next section.

Mature B and T cells migrate through the bloodstream and lymphatic system to the peripheral lymphoid tissues, including the lymph nodes and spleen. Collectively, these are referred to as the *secondary lymphoid organs* and this is where antigen-driven activation (proliferation and differentiation) of B and T cells takes place (Figure 3.1). Histological properties of the secondary lymphoid organs are also presented below.

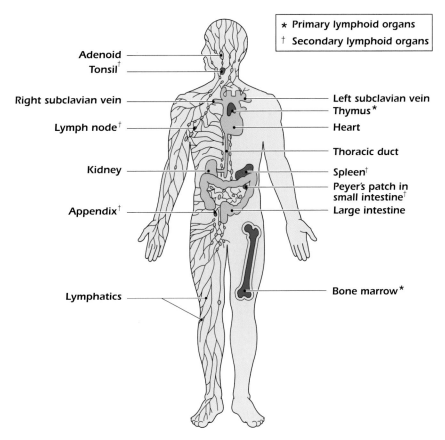

Figure 3.1. Distribution of lymphoid tissues in the body.

Thymus Gland. The thymus gland is a bilobed structure, derived from the endoderm of the third and fourth pharyngeal pouches. During fetal development, the size of the thymus increases. The growth continues until puberty. Thereafter, the thymus undergoes atrophy with aging.

The thymus is a ***lymphoepithelial*** organ and consists of epithelial cells organized into cortical (outer) and medullary (central) areas that are infiltrated with lymphoid cells (***thymocytes***) (Figure 3.2A). The cortex is densely populated with lymphocytes of various sizes, most of which are imma-

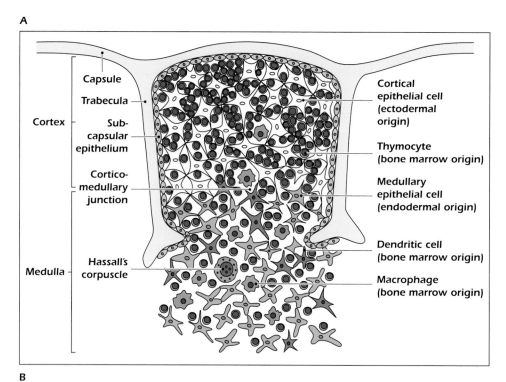

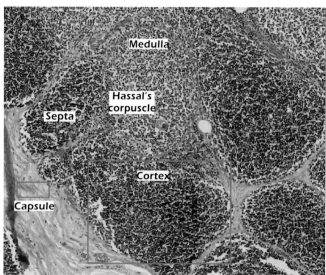

Figure 3.2. (A) Cellular organization of the thymus. (Rosen FS and Geha RS 2007. Reproduced with permission of Taylor & Francis.) (B) Section of an adolescent thymus showing capsule, septa, cortex, medulla, and Hassall's corpuscle. (Photograph by Dr. John Lewis, SUNY Downstate College of Medicine, New York.)

ture, and scattered macrophages involved in clearing apoptotic thymocytes. Figure 3.2B shows a section through normal human thymus tissue.

Secondary Lymphoid Organs. The secondary lymphoid organs have two major functions: (1) They are highly efficient in trapping and concentrating foreign substances, and (2) they are the main sites of production of antibodies and the induction of antigen-specific T lymphocytes. The major secondary lymphoid organs are the ***spleen*** and the ***lymph nodes***. In addition, tonsils, appendix, clusters of lymphocytes distributed in the lining of the small intestine (***Peyer's patches***), and lymphoid aggregates spread throughout mucosal tissue are considered secondary lymphoid organs. These secondary lymphoid organs are found in various areas of the body, such as the linings of the digestive tract, in the respiratory and genitourinary tracts, in the conjunctiva, and in the salivary glands, where mature lymphocytes interact with antigen and undergo activation. These mucosal secondary lymphoid organs have been given the name ***mucosa-associated lymphoid tissue*** (MALT). Those lymphoid tissues associated with the gut are ***gut-associated lymphoid tissue*** (GALT); those associated with the bronchial tree are termed ***bronchus-associated lymphoid tissue*** (BALT).

The Spleen. The spleen is the largest of the secondary lymphoid organs (Figure 3.3A). It is highly efficient in trapping and concentrating foreign substances carried in the blood. It is the major organ in the body in which antibodies are synthesized and from which they are released into the circulation. The spleen is composed of ***white pulp***, rich in lymphoid cells, and ***red pulp***, which contains many sinuses as well as large quantities of erythrocytes and macrophages, some lymphocytes, and a few other cell types. Figure 3.3B shows a section of human spleen showing red and white pulp areas.

The areas of white pulp are located mainly around small arterioles, the peripheral regions of which are rich in T cells; B cells are present mainly in ***germinal centers***. Approximately 50% of spleen cells are B lymphocytes; 30–40% are T lymphocytes. After antigenic stimulation, the germinal centers contain large numbers of B cells and plasma cells. These cells synthesize and release antibodies.

Lymph Nodes. Lymph nodes are small ovoid structures (normally less than 1 cm in diameter) found in various regions throughout the body (Figure 3.1). They are close to major junctions of the lymphatic channels, which are connected to the thoracic duct. The thoracic duct transports lymph and lymphocytes to the vena cava, the vessel that carries blood to the right side of the heart (Figure 3.4), from where it is redistributed throughout the body.

Lymph nodes are composed of a medulla with many sinuses and a cortex, which is surrounded by a capsule of connective tissue (Figure 3.5A). The cortical region contains primary lymphoid follicles. After antigenic stimulation, these structures enlarge to form secondary lymphoid follicles with germinal centers containing dense populations of lymphocytes

(mostly B cells) that are undergoing mitosis (Figure 3.5B). In response to antigen stimulation, antigen-specific B cells proliferating within these germinal centers also undergo a process known as ***affinity-maturation*** to generate clones of cells with higher affinity receptors (antibody) for the antigenic epitope that triggered the initial response (see Chapter 8). The remaining antigen-nonspecific B cells are pushed to the outside to form the mantle zone. The deep cortical area or paracortical region contains T cells and dendritic cells. Antigens are brought into these areas by dendritic cells, which present antigen fragments (peptides) to T cells, events that result in activation of the T cells. The medullary area of the lymph node contains antibody-secreting plasma cells that have traveled from the cortex to the medulla via lymphatic vessels.

Lymphocyte Migration and Recirculation

Lymph nodes are highly efficient in trapping antigen that enters through the ***afferent lymphatic vessels*** (Figure 3.5A). Within the lymph node, antigens interact with macrophages, T cells, and B cells, and that interaction brings about an immune response, manifested by the generation of antibodies and antigen-specific T cells. Lymph, antibodies, and cells leave the lymph node through the efferent lymphatic vessel, which is just below the medullary region. Blood lymphocytes enter the lymph nodes through ***postcapillary venules*** and leave the lymph nodes through ***efferent lymphatic vessels***, which eventually converge in the ***thoracic duct***. As noted above, the duct empties into the ***vena cava***, the vessel that returns the blood to the ***heart***, thus providing for the continual recirculation of lymphocytes.

The spleen functions in a similar manner. Arterial blood lymphocytes enter the spleen through the hilus and pass into the trabecular artery, which along its course becomes narrow and branched (Figure 3.3A). At the farthest branches of the trabecular artery, capillaries lead to lymphoid nodules. Ultimately, the lymphocytes return to the venous circulation through the trabecular vein. Like lymph nodes, the spleen contains efferent lymphatic vessels through which lymph empties into the lymphatics from which the cells continue their recirculation through the body and back to the afferent vessels.

The migration of lymphocytes between various lymphoid and nonlymphoid tissue and their homing to a particular site is highly regulated by means of various ***cell-surface adhesion molecules*** (CAMs) and receptors to these molecules. Thus, except in the spleen, where small arterioles end in the parenchyma, allowing access to blood lymphocytes, blood lymphocytes must generally cross the endothelial vascular lining of postcapillary vascular sites, termed ***high endothelial venules*** (HEVs) to enter tissues. This process is called ***extravasation***. Recirculating lymphocytes selectively bind to specific receptors on the HEVs of lymphoid tissue or inflammatory tissue spaces and appear to completely ignore other vascular endothelium. Moreover, it appears that a selective binding of finer specificity operates

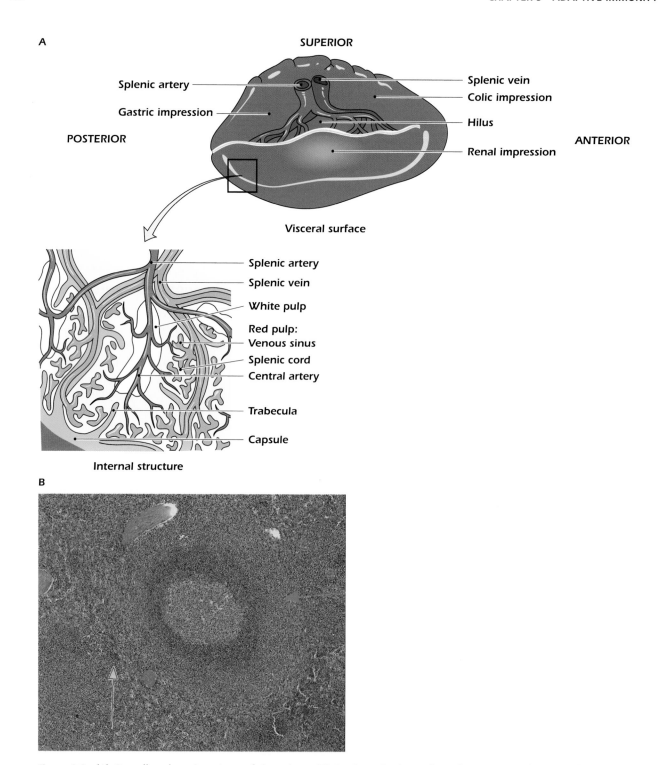

Figure 3.3. (A) Overall and section views of the spleen. (B) Section of spleen. The yellow arrow indicates red pulp. The green arrow points to white pulp showing a splenic nodule with a germinal center. (Photograph by Dr. Susan Gottesman, SUNY Downstate College of Medicine, New York.)

between the HEVs and various distinct subsets of lymphocytes, further regulating the migration of lymphocytes into the various lymphoid and nonlymphoid tissue. Recirculating monocytes and granulocytes also express adhesion molecule receptors and migrate to tissue sites using a similar mechanism.

The migration of lymphocytes between lymphoid and nonlymphoid tissue ensures that on exposure to an antigen,

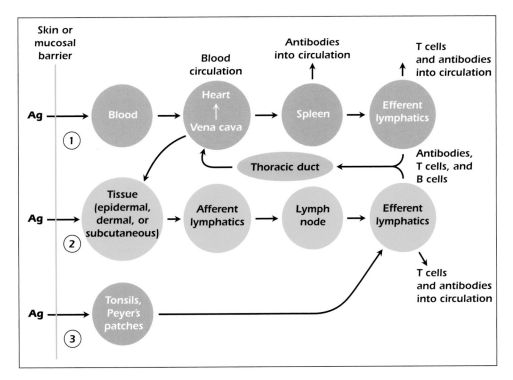

Figure 3.4. Circulation of lymph and fate of antigen following penetration through: (1) blood-stream, (2) skin, and (3) gastrointestinal or respiratory tract.

the antigen and the lymphocytes expressing antigen-specific receptors are sequestered in the lymphoid tissue, where the lymphocytes undergo proliferation and differentiation. This results in expansion of the antigen-specific B-cell population and the generation of circulating antibody-secreting plasma cells as well as long-lived, antigen-specific memory B cells. The latter are disseminated throughout the secondary lymphoid tissues to ensure long-lasting immunity to the antigen.

THE FATE OF ANTIGEN AFTER PENETRATION

The *reticuloendothelial system* is designed to trap foreign antigens that have penetrated the body and to subject them to ingestion and degradation by the phagocytic cells of the system. Also, there is constant movement of lymphocytes throughout the body, and this movement permits deposition of lymphocytes in strategic places along the lymphatic vessels. The system not only traps antigens but also provides loci (the secondary lymphoid organs) where antigen, macrophages, T cells, and B cells can interact within a very small area to initiate an immune response.

The fate of an antigen that has penetrated the physical barriers and the cellular and antibody components of the ensuing immune response are shown in Figure 3.4. Three major routes may be followed by an antigen after it has penetrated the interior of the body:

(1) Antigens may enter the body through the bloodstream. In this case, they are carried through circulatory system to the spleen where they interact with APCs, such as dendritic cells and macrophages. As we have discussed earlier, a major function of these APCs is to take up, process, and then present components of the antigen to the T cells that express the appropriate antigen-specific TCR. This interaction, together with the other co-stimulatory signals derived from cell–cell interaction, activates the T cells. Splenic B cells expressing antigen-specific BCRs are also activated following exposure to antigen, a process facilitated by the cytokines produced by antigen-activated T cells.

(2) Antigens may lodge in the epidermal, dermal, or subcutaneous tissues to stimulate inflammatory responses. From these tissues, the antigen, either free or trapped by APCs, is transported through the afferent lymphatic channels into the regional draining lymph node. In the lymph node, the antigen, macrophages, dendritic cells, T cells, and B cells interact to generate an immune response. Eventually, antigen-specific T cells and antibodies,

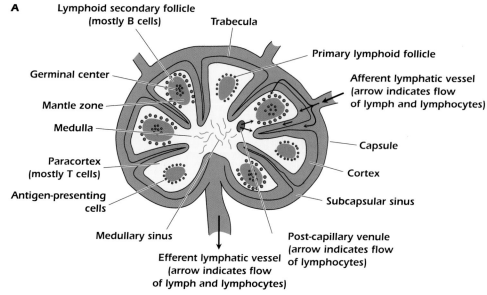

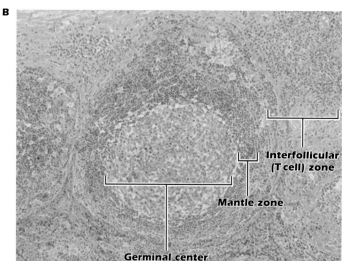

Figure 3.5. (A) Section of lymph node. Arrows show flow of lymph and lymphocytes. (B) Section through a lymph node showing T-cell zone, mantle zone, and germinal center.

which have been synthesized in the lymph node, enter the circulation and are transported to the various tissues. Antigen-specific T and B cells, and antibodies also enter the circulation via the thoracic duct.

(3) The antigen may enter the gastrointestinal or respiratory tract, where it lodges in the MALT and BALT, respectively. There it will interact with macrophages and lymphocytes. Antibodies synthesized in these organs are deposited in the local tissue. In addition, lymphocytes entering the efferent lymphatics are carried through the thoracic duct to the circulation and are thereby redistributed to various tissue.

Frequency of Antigen-Specific Naïve Lymphocytes

It has been estimated that in a naïve (nonimmunized) animal, only one in every 10^3–10^5 lymphocytes is capable of recognizing a typical antigen. Therefore, the probability that an antigen will encounter these cells is very low. The problem is compounded by the fact that for synthesis of antibody to ensue, two different kinds of lymphocytes—the T lymphocyte and B lymphocyte—each with specificity against this particular antigen, must interact.

Statistically, the chances for the interaction of specific T lymphocytes with their particular antigen, and then with B lymphocytes specific for the same antigen, are very low.

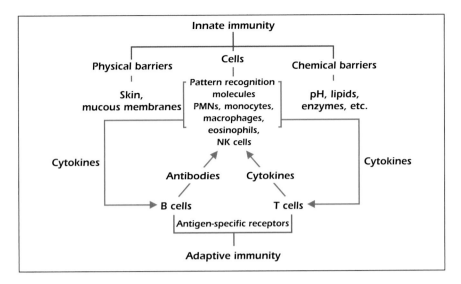

Figure 3.6. Interrelationship between innate and adaptive immunity.

However, nature has devised an ingenious mechanism for bringing these cells into contact with antigen: The antigen is carried via the draining lymphatics to the secondary lymphoid organs. In these organs, the antigen is exposed on the surface of fixed specialized cells. Because both T and B lymphocytes circulate at a rather rapid rate, making the rounds every several days, some circulating lymphocytes with specificity for the particular antigen should pass by the antigen within a relatively short time. When these lymphocytes encounter the antigen for which they are specific, the lymphocytes become activated, and the adaptive immune response, with specificity against this antigen, is triggered.

INTERRELATIONSHIP BETWEEN INNATE AND ADAPTIVE IMMUNITY

The innate and adaptive arms of the immune system have developed a beautiful interrelationship. The intricate and ingenious communication system through the various cytokines and cell adhesion molecules allows components of innate and adaptive immunity to interact, send each other signals, activate each other, and work in concert toward the final goal of destroying and eliminating the invading microorganism and its products. The interrelationship between innate and adaptive immunity is shown in Figure 3.6.

SUMMARY

1. Two major types of cells participate as effector cells in adaptive immunity: B cells and T cells.

2. B and T cells express antigen-specific receptors, namely BCRs and TCRs, respectively.

3. Precursor cells of the B and T lineages are found in the bone marrow—a primary lymphoid organ. B lymphocytes fully differentiate to become mature, albeit naïve, B cells.

4. T cells are derived from the same lymphoid progenitor cells as B cells and differentiate in the thymus to become functional cells before migrating to the peripheral lymphoid organs.

5. Mature B and T lymphocytes differentiate and proliferate in response to antigenic stimulation. These events generally take place in secondary lymphoid organs.

6. B lymphocytes synthesize and secrete antibodies. T lymphocytes participate in cell-mediated immunity; they help B cells make antibodies by providing them with soluble growth and differentiation factors (cytokines) needed for B-cell activation. They also participate in various other regulatory aspects of the immune response by releasing cytokines.

7. Lymphocytes continuously recirculate between the blood, lymph, lymphoid organs, and tissues. Receptors on lymphocytes interact with CAMs located on specialized HEVs, facilitating extravasation to tissue sites where immune-cell activation occurs.

REVIEW QUESTIONS

For each question, choose the ONE BEST answer or completion.

1. Which of the following applies uniquely with respect to B cells found in secondary lymphoid organs?
   A) present as precursor B cells
   B) express only IgM
   C) terminally differentiate into plasma cells
   D) undergo proliferation

2. The germinal centers found in the cortical region of lymph nodes and the peripheral region of splenic peri-arteriolar lymphatic tissue
   A) support the development of immature B and T cells
   B) function in the removal of damaged erythrocytes from the circulation
   C) act as the major source of stem cells and thus help maintain hematopoiesis
   D) provide an infrastructure that on antigenic stimulation contains large populations of B lymphocytes and plasma cells
   E) are the sites of natural killer T (NKT)-cell differentiation

3. Which of the following sequence correctly describes lymphocyte migration from lymph nodes to blood?
   A) postcapillary venules, efferent lymphatic vessels, thoracic duct, vena cava, heart
   B) postcapillary venules, afferent lymphatic vessels, thoracic duct, vena cava, heart
   C) postcapillary venules, efferent lymphatic vessels, vena cava, thoracic duct, heart
   D) postcapillary venules, afferent lymphatic vessels, vena cava, thoracic duct, heart

4. Clonal expansion of which of the following cells occurs following their direct interaction with the antigen for which they are specific?
   A) macrophages
   B) basophils
   C) Bcells
   D) T cells
   E) mast cells

ANSWERS TO REVIEW QUESTIONS

1. *C.* Terminal differentiation of B cells into plasma cells occurs only in secondary lymphoid organs, such as the spleen and lymph nodes. Circulation of lymphocytes and cellular proliferation (but not antigen-dependent responses of terminal differentiation) also take place in the primary lymphoid organs, such as the bursa of Fabricius, or its equivalent, and the thymus. The bone marrow is the site where pluripotential stem cells differentiate into precursor B and T cells.

2. *D.* On antigenic stimulation, the germinal centers contain large populations of B lymphocytes undergoing mitosis and plasma cells secreting antibodies. Virgin immunocompetent lymphocytes are developed in the primary lymphoid organs, not in the secondary lymphoid organs, such as the spleen and lymph nodes. Germinal centers do not participate in the removal of damaged erythrocytes,

nor are they a source of stem cells; the latter are found in the bone marrow.

3. *A.* Blood lymphocytes enter the lymph nodes through the afferent lymphatic vessel via postcapillary venules. They leave the lymph nodes through efferent lymphatic vessels, which eventually converge in the thoracic duct. This duct empties into the vena cava, the vessel that returns the blood to the heart, thus providing for the continual recirculation of lymphocytes.

4. *C.* B cells bind directly to antigens recognized by their B-cell receptors (BCRs). In contrast, T cells expressing T-cell receptors (TCRs) are incapable of binding to antigen unless they are presented by antigen-presenting cells in the context of MHC class I (cytotoxic T cells) or MHC class II (helper T cells).

4

IMMUNOGENS AND ANTIGENS

INTRODUCTION

Immune responses arise as a result of exposure to foreign stimuli. The compound that evokes the response is referred to either as **antigen** or as **immunogen**. The distinction between these terms is functional. An antigen is any agent capable of binding specifically to components of the immune system, such as the B cell receptor (BCR) on B lymphocytes and soluble antibodies. By contrast, an immunogen is any agent capable of inducing an immune response and is therefore **immunogenic**. The distinction between the terms is necessary because there are many compounds that are incapable of inducing an immune response, yet they are capable of binding with components of the immune system that have been induced specifically against them. Thus all immunogens are antigens, but not all antigens are immunogens. This difference becomes obvious in the case of low molecular weight compounds, a group of substances that includes many antibiotics and drugs. By themselves, these compounds are incapable of inducing an immune response but when they are coupled with much larger entities, such as proteins, the resultant conjugate induces an immune response that is directed against various parts of the conjugate, including the low molecular weight compound. When manipulated in this manner, the low molecular weight compound is referred to as a **hapten** (from the Greek *hapten*, which means "to grasp"); the high molecular weight compound to which the hapten is conjugated is referred to as a **carrier**. Thus a hapten is a compound that, by itself, is incapable of inducing an immune response but against which an immune response can be induced by immunization with the hapten conjugated to a carrier.

Immune responses have been demonstrated against all the known biochemical families of compounds, including carbohydrates, lipids, proteins, and nucleic acids. Similarly, immune responses to drugs, antibiotics, food additives, cosmetics, and small synthetic peptides can also be induced, but only when these are coupled to a carrier. In this chapter, we discuss the major attributes of compounds that render them antigenic and immunogenic.

REQUIREMENTS FOR IMMUNOGENICITY

A substance must possess the following characteristics to be immunogenic: (1) foreignness; (2) high molecular weight; (3) chemical complexity; and, in most cases, (4) degradability and interaction with host major histocompatibility complex (MHC) molecules.

Foreignness

Animals normally do not respond immunologically to self. Thus, for example, if a rabbit is injected with its own serum albumin, it will not mount an immune response; it recognizes the albumin as self. By contrast, if rabbit serum albumin is injected into a guinea pig, the guinea pig recognizes the rabbit serum albumin as foreign and mounts an immune response against it. To prove that the rabbit, which did not respond to its own albumin, is immunologically

Immunology: A Short Course, Seventh Edition. Richard Coico and Geoffrey Sunshine.
© 2015 John Wiley & Sons, Ltd. Published 2015 by John Wiley & Sons, Ltd.
Companion Website: www.wileyimmunology.com/coico

competent, it can be injected with guinea pig albumin. The competent rabbit will mount an immune response to guinea pig serum albumin because it recognizes the substance as foreign. Thus, the first requirement for a compound to be immunogenic is foreignness. The more foreign the substance, the more immunogenic it is. In general, compounds that are part of self are not immunogenic to that individual. However, there are exceptional cases in which an individual mounts an immune response against his or her own tissues. This condition is termed *autoimmunity* (see Chapter 3).

High Molecular Weight

The second feature that determines whether a compound is immunogenic is its molecular weight. In general, small compounds that have a molecular weight of less than 1,000 Da (e.g., penicillin, progesterone, aspirin) are not immunogenic; those of molecular weights between 1,000 and 6,000 Da (e.g., insulin, adrenocorticotropic hormone [ACTH]) may or may not be immunogenic; and those of molecular weights greater than 6,000 Da (e.g., albumin, tetanus toxin) are generally immunogenic. In short, relatively small substances have decreased immunogenicity whereas large substances have increased immunogenicity.

Chemical Complexity

The third characteristic necessary for a compound to be immunogenic is a certain degree of physicochemical complexity. Thus, for example, simple molecules such as homopolymers of amino acids (e.g., a polymer of lysine with a molecular weight of 30,000 Da) are seldom good immunogens. Similarly, a homopolymer of poly-γ-D-glutamic acid (the capsular material of *Bacillus anthracis*) with a molecular weight of 50,000 Da is not immunogenic. The absence of immunogenicity is because these compounds, although of high molecular weight, are not sufficiently chemically complex. However, if the complexity is increased by attaching various moieties (such as dinitrophenol or other low molecular weight compounds), which, by themselves, are not immunogenic, to the epsilon amino group of polylysine, the entire macromolecule becomes immunogenic. The resulting immune response is directed not only against the coupled low molecular weight compounds but also against the high molecular weight homopolymer. In general, an increase in the chemical complexity of a compound is accompanied by an increase in its immunogenicity. Thus copolymers of several amino acids, such as polyglutamic, alanine, and lysine (poly-GAT), tend to be highly immunogenic.

Because many immunogens are proteins, it is important to understand the structural features of these molecules. Each of the four levels of protein structure contributes to the molecule's immunogenicity. The acquired immune response recognizes many structural features and chemical properties of compounds. For example, antibodies can recognize various structural features of a protein, such as its primary structure (the amino acid sequence), secondary structures (the structure of the backbone of the polypeptide chain, such as an α-helix or β-pleated sheet), and tertiary structures (formed by the three-dimensional configuration of the protein, which is conferred by the folding of the polypeptide chain and held by disulfide bridges, hydrogen bonds, hydrophobic interactions, etc.) (Figure 4.1). They can also recognize quaternary structures (formed by the juxtaposition of separate parts, if the molecule is composed of more than one protein subunit) (Figure 4.2).

Degradability

In contrast to B cells, in order for antigens to activate T cells to stimulate immune responses, interactions with MHC molecules expressed on antigen-presenting cells (APCs) must occur (see Chapter 10). APCs must first degrade the antigen through a process known as antigen processing (enzymatic degradation of antigen) before they can express antigenic *epitopes* on their surface. Epitopes are also known as *antigenic determinants*. They are the part of an antigen that is recognized by the immune system and are the smallest unit of antigen that is capable of binding with antibodies and T-cell receptors. Once degraded and noncovalently bound to MHC, these epitopes stimulate the activation and clonal expansion of antigen-specific effector T cells. A protein antigen's susceptibility to enzymatic degradation largely depends on two properties: (1) it has to be sufficiently stable so that it can reach the site of interaction with B cells or T cells necessary for the immune response, and (2) the substance must be susceptible to partial enzymatic degradation that takes place during antigen processing by APCs. Peptides composed of D-amino acids, which are resistant to enzymatic degradation, are not immunogenic, whereas their L-isomers are susceptible to enzymes and are immunogenic. By contrast, carbohydrates are not processed or presented and are thus unable to activate T cells, although they can directly activate B cells.

In general, a substance must have all four of these characteristics to be immunogenic; it must be foreign to the individual, have a relatively high molecular weight, possess a certain degree of chemical complexity, and be degradable.

Haptens

As noted earlier, substances called *haptens* fail to induce immune responses in their native form because of their low molecular weight and their chemical simplicity. These compounds are not immunogenic unless they are conjugated to high molecular weight, physiochemically complex carriers. Thus an immune response can be evoked to thousands of chemical compounds—those of high molecular weight and

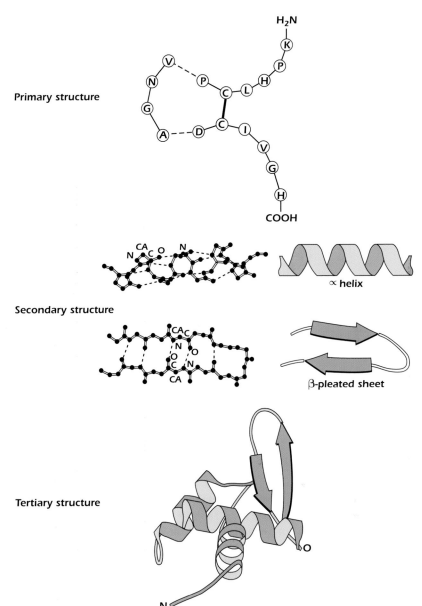

Figure 4.1. Levels of protein organizational structure. The primary structure is indicated by the linear arrangement of amino acids (using a single-letter code) and includes any intrachain disulfide bonds, as shown. The secondary structure derives from the folding of the polypeptide chain into α helices and β-pleated sheets. The tertiary structure, shown as a ribbon diagram, is formed by the folding of regions between secondary features. (Adapted with permission from P Sun and JC Boyington, *Current Protocols in Protein Science*, John Wiley and Sons, Inc., Hoboken, NJ.)

those of low molecular weight, provided the latter are conjugated to high molecular weight complex carriers.

Further Requirements for Immunogenicity

Several other factors play roles in determining whether a substance is immunogenic. The genetic makeup (genotype) of the immunized individual plays an important role in determining whether a given substance will stimulate an immune response. Genetic control of immune responsiveness is largely controlled by genes mapping within the MHC. Another factor that plays a crucial role in the immunogenicity of substances relates to the B- and T-cell repertoires of an individual. Acquired immune responses are triggered following the binding of antigenic epitopes to antigen-specific receptors on B and T lymphocytes. If an individual lacks a particular clone of lymphocytes consisting of cells that bear the identical antigen-specific receptor needed to respond to the stimulus, an immune response to that antigenic epitope will not take place. Finally, practical issues such as the dosage and route of administration of antigens play a role in determining whether the substance is immunogenic.

Insufficient doses of antigen may not stimulate an immune response either because the amount administered fails to activate enough lymphocytes or because such a dose renders the responding cells unresponsive. The latter phenomenon induces a state of tolerance to that antigen (see Chapter 13). Besides the need to administer a threshold amount of antigen to induce an immune response, the

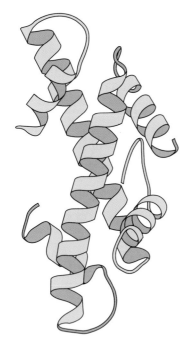

Figure 4.2. The quarternary structure of proteins results from the association of two or more polypeptide chains, which form a polymeric protein. (Adapted with permission from P Sun and JC Boyington, *Current Protocols in Protein Science*, John Wiley and Sons, Inc., Hoboken, NJ.)

number of doses administered also affects the outcome of the immune response generated. As discussed below, repeated administration of antigen is required to stimulate a strong immune response.

Finally, the route of administration can affect the outcome of the immunization strategy, because this determines which organs and cell populations will be involved in the response. Antigens administered via the most common route—namely, *subcutaneously*, generally elicit the strongest immune responses. This is due to their uptake, processing, and presentation to effector cells by Langerhans cells present in the skin, which are among the most potent APCs. Responses to subcutaneously administered antigens take place in the lymph nodes draining the injection site. *Intravenously* administered antigens are carried first to the spleen, where they can either induce immune unresponsiveness or tolerance, or, if presented by APCs, generate an immune response. Orally administered antigens (*gastrointestinal route*) elicit local antibody responses within the intestinal lamina propria but often produce a systemic state of tolerance (antigen unresponsiveness) (see Chapter 13 for a detailed discussion about tolerance). Finally, administration of antigens via the respiratory tract (*intranasal route*) often elicits allergic responses (see Chapter 15).

Since immune responses depend on multiple cellular interactions, the type and extent of the immune response is affected by the cells populating the organ to which the antigen is ultimately delivered. The stringent requirements given above constitute a portion of the delicate control mechanisms, expanded and elaborated in subsequent chapters, which, on one hand, trigger the adaptive immune response and, on the other hand, protect the individual from responding to substances in cases where such responses are detrimental.

PRIMARY AND SECONDARY RESPONSES

The first exposure of an individual to an immunogen is referred to as the *primary immunization*, which generates a primary response. As we shall see in subsequent chapters, many events take place during this primary immunization: cells process antigen, triggering antigen-specific lymphocytes to proliferate and differentiate; T-lymphocyte subsets interact with other subsets and induce the latter to differentiate into T lymphocytes with specialized function; T lymphocytes also interact with B lymphocytes, inducing them to synthesize and secrete antibodies.

A second exposure to the same immunogen results in a *secondary response*. This may occur after the response to the first immune event has leveled off or has totally subsided (within weeks or even years). The secondary response differs from the primary response in many respects. Most notably and biologically relevant is the much quicker onset and the much higher magnitude of the response. In a sense, this secondary (and subsequent) exposure behaves as if the body remembered that it had been previously exposed to that same immunogen. In fact, secondary and subsequent responses exploit the expanded number of antigen-specific lymphocytes generated in response to the primary immune response. Thus the increased arsenal of responding lymphocytes accounts, in part, for the magnitude of the response observed. The secondary response is also called the *memory* or *anamnestic response*, and the B and T lymphocytes that participate in the memory response are termed *memory cells*.

ANTIGENICITY AND ANTIGEN-BINDING SITE

An immune response induced by an antigen generates antibodies or lymphocytes that react specifically with the antigen. The antigen-binding site of an antibody or a receptor on a lymphocyte has a unique structure that allows a complementary fit to some structural aspect of the specific antigen. The portion of the immunoglobulin that specifically binds to the antigenic determinant or epitope is concentrated in several hypervariable regions of the molecule, which form the complementarity-determining region (CDR). Additional structural features of the immunoglobulin molecule are described in Chapter 5.

Various studies indicate that the size of an epitope that combines with the CDR on a given antibody is approximately equivalent to five to seven amino acids. These dimensions were calculated from experiments that involved the binding of antibodies to polysaccharides and to peptide epitopes. Such dimensions would also be expected to correspond roughly to the size of the complementary antibody-combining site (termed ***paratope***), and indeed this expectation has been confirmed by X-ray crystallography. The small size of an epitope (peptide) that binds to a specific T-cell receptor (TCR) (peptides with 8–12 amino acids) is made functionally larger, since it is noncovalently associated with MHC proteins of the antigen-presenting cell. This bimolecular epitope–MHC complex then binds to the TCR, forming a trimolecular complex (TCR–epitope–MHC).

EPITOPES RECOGNIZED BY B CELLS AND T CELLS

There is a large body of evidence pointing out that the properties of many epitopes recognized by B cells differ from those recognized by T cells (Table 4.1). In general, membrane-bound antibody present on B cells recognizes and binds free antigen in solution. Thus, these epitopes are typically on the outside of the molecule, accessible for interaction with the B-cell receptor. Terminal side chains of polysaccharides and hydrophilic portions on protein molecules generally constitute B-cell epitopes. An example of an antigen with five ***linear*** B-cell epitopes located on the exposed surface of myoglobulin is shown in Figure 4.3. B-cell epitopes may also form as a result of the folded conformation of molecules as shown in Figure 4.4. Such epitopes are called ***conformational*** or ***discontinuous epitopes***, where noncontiguous residues along a polypeptide chain are brought together by the folded conformation of the protein as shown in Figure 4.3. In contrast to B cells, T cells are unable to bind soluble antigen. The interaction of an epitope with the TCR requires APC processing of the antigen in which enzymatic degradation takes place to yield small peptides, which then associate with the MHC. Thus, T-cell epitopes can only be ***continuous*** or ***linear*** because they are composed of a single segment of a polypeptide chain. Figure 4.5 illustrates the structural organization of a class I MHC with an antigenic peptide bound to it. Generally such processed epitopes are internal denatured linear hydrophobic areas of proteins. Polysaccharides do not yield such areas and indeed are not known to bind or activate T cells. Thus, polysaccharides contain solely B-cell recognizable epitopes, whereas proteins contain both B- and T-cell recognizable epitopes (Table 4.1). Antigenic epitopes may have the characteristics shown schematically in Figure 4.6. Thus, they may consist of a single epitope (hapten) or have varying numbers of the same epitope on the same molecule (e.g., polysaccharides). The most common antigens (proteins) have varying numbers of different epitopes on the same molecule.

TABLE 4.1. Antigen Recognition by B and T Cells

Characteristic	B Cells	T Cells
Antigen interaction	B-cell receptor (BCR) binds antigen (Ag)	T-cell receptor (TCR) binds antigenic peptides bound to MHC
Nature of antigens	Protein, polysaccharide, lipid	Peptide
Binding soluble antigens	Yes	No
Epitopes recognized	Accessible, sequential, or nonsequential	Internal linear peptides produced by antigen processing (proteolytic degradation)

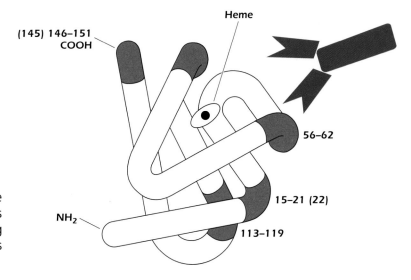

Figure 4.3. Example of antigen (sperm whale myoglobin) containing five linear B-cell epitopes (red), one of which is bound to antibody-binding site of antibody specific for amino acid residues 56–62.

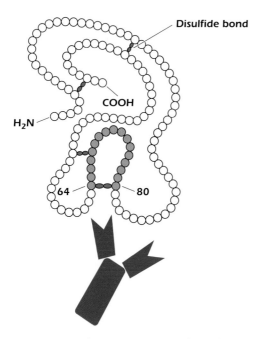

Figure 4.4. Antigen showing amino acid residues (circles), which form nonsequential epitope "loop" (blue) resulting from disulfide bond between residues 64 and 80. Note the binding of an epitope-specific antibody to the nonsequential amino acids that constitute the epitope.

MAJOR CLASSES OF ANTIGENS

The following major chemical families may be antigenic:

1. **Carbohydrates** (polysaccharides). Polysaccharides are only immunogenic when associated with protein carriers. For example, polysaccharides that form part of more complex molecules—glycoproteins—will elicit an immune response, part of which is directed specifically against the polysaccharide moiety of the molecule. An immune response, consisting primarily of antibodies, can be induced against many kinds of polysaccharide molecules, such as components of microorganisms and of eukaryotic cells. An excellent example of antigenicity of polysaccharides is the immune response associated with the ABO blood groups, which are polysaccharides on the surface of the red blood cells.

2. **Lipids.** Lipids are rarely immunogenic, but an immune response to lipids may be induced if the lipids are conjugated to protein carriers. Thus, in a sense, lipids may be regarded as haptens. Immune responses to glycolipids and to sphingolipids have also been demonstrated.

3. **Nucleic acids.** Nucleic acids are poor immunogens by themselves, but they become immunogenic when

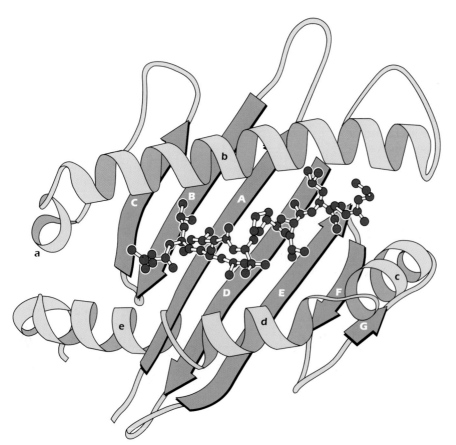

Figure 4.5. Structure of MHC class I molecule (ribbon diagram) with antigenic peptide (ball-and-stick model).

	Description	Example
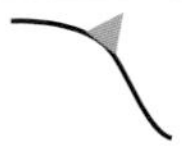	One epitope	Haptens
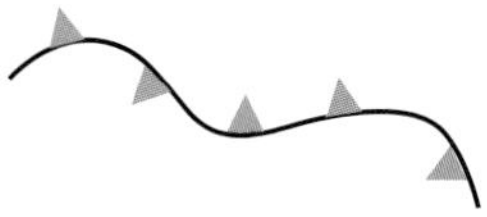	Many epitopes of the same specificity	Many polysaccharides, homopolymers
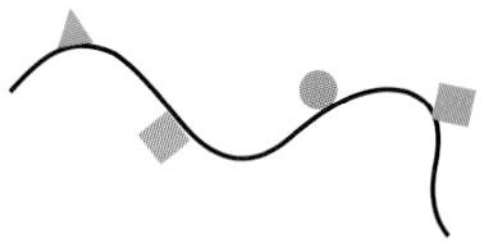	Many epitopes of different specificities	Proteins

Figure 4.6. Some possible antigenic structures containing single and multiple epitopes.

they are conjugated to protein carriers. DNA, in its native helical state, is usually nonimmunogenic in normal animals. However, immune responses to nucleic acids have been reported in many instances. One important example in clinical medicine is the appearance of anti-DNA antibodies in patients with systemic lupus erythematosus (discussed in detail in Chapter 13).

Read the related case: **Systemic Lupus Erythematosus**
In *Immunology: Clinical Case Studies and Disease Pathophysiology*

4. *Proteins.* Virtually all proteins are immunogenic. Thus, the most common immune responses are those to proteins. Furthermore, the greater the degree of complexity of the protein, the more vigorous will be the immune response to that protein. Because of their size and complexity, proteins contain multiple epitopes.

BINDING OF ANTIGEN WITH ANTIGEN-SPECIFIC ANTIBODIES OR T CELLS

The binding between antigen and antibodies is discussed in detail in Chapter 6. The interactions of antigen with both B and T cells and subsequent activation events are discussed in Chapter 11. At this point, it is important to emphasize only that the binding of antigen with antibodies or TCRs does not involve covalent bonds. The *noncovalent binding* may involve *electrostatic interactions*, *hydrophobic interactions*, *hydrogen bonds*, and *van der Waals forces*. Since these interactive forces are relatively weak, the fit between antigen and its complementary site on the antigen receptor must occur over an area large enough to allow the summation of all the possible available interactions. This requirement is the basis for the exquisite specificity observed in immunologic interactions.

CROSS-REACTIVITY

Since macromolecular antigens contain several distinct epitopes, some of these antigens can be altered without totally changing the immunogenic or antigenic structure of the entire molecule. This concept is important in relation to immunization against highly pathogenic microorganisms or highly toxic compounds. Obviously, immunization with the pathogenic toxin is unwise. However, it is possible to destroy the biologic activity of such toxins and a broad variety of other toxins (e.g., snake venoms) without appreciably affecting their immunogenicity. A toxin that has been modified to the extent that it is no longer toxic but still maintains some of its immunochemical characteristics is called a *toxoid*. Thus we can say that a humoral immune response to a toxoid *cross-reacts* immunologically with the toxin. Accordingly, it is possible to immunize individuals with the toxoid and thereby induce immune responses to some of the epitopes that the toxoid still shares with the native toxin because these epitopes have not been destroyed by the modification. Although the molecules of toxin and toxoid differ in many physicochemical and biologic respects, they nevertheless cross-react immunologically: They share enough epitopes to allow the immune response to the toxoid to mount an effective defense against the toxin itself. An immunologic reaction in which the immune components, either cells or antibodies, react with two molecules that share epitopes but are otherwise dissimilar, is called a *cross-reaction*. When two compounds cross-react immunologically, the compounds will have one or more epitopes in common, and the immune response to one of the compounds will recognize one or more of the same epitope(s) on the other compound and react with it. Another form of cross-reactivity is seen when antibodies or cells with specificity to one epitope bind, usually more weakly, to another epitope that is not quite identical but has a structural resemblance to the first epitope. To denote that the antigen used for immunization is different from the one with which the induced immune components are then allowed to react, the terms *homologous* and *heterologous* are used. **Homologous** denotes that the antigen and the immunogen are the same; **heterologous** denotes that the substance used to induce the immune response is different from the substance that is then used to react with the products of the induced response. In the latter case, the heterologous antigen may or may not react with the immune components. If reaction does take place, it may be concluded that the heterologous and homologous antigens exhibit immunologic cross-reactivity.

Although the hallmark of immunology is specificity, immunologic cross-reactivity has been observed on many levels. This does not mean that the immunologic specificity has been diminished but rather that the substances that cross-react share **antigenic determinants** (epitopes). In cases of cross-reactivity, the antigenic determinants of the cross-reacting substances may have identical chemical structures, or they may be composed of similar but not identical physicochemical configurations. In the example described above, a toxin and its corresponding toxoid represent two molecules: the toxin is the native molecule and the toxoid is a modified molecule, the response to which cross-reacts with the native molecule.

There are other examples of immunologic cross-reactivity, wherein the two cross-reacting substances are unrelated to each other except that they have one or more epitopes in common, specifically, one or more areas that have similar three-dimensional characteristics. These substances are referred to as **heterophile antigens**. For example, human blood group A antigen reacts with antiserum raised against pneumococcal capsular polysaccharide (type XIV). Similarly, human blood group B antigen reacts with antibodies to certain strains of *Escherichia coli*. In these examples of cross-reactivity, the antigens of the microorganisms are referred to as the *heterophile antigens* (with respect to the blood group antigen).

ADJUVANTS

To enhance the immune response to a given immunogen, various additives or vehicles are often used. An **adjuvant** (from the Latin, *adjuvare*, "to help") is a substance that, when mixed with an immunogen, enhances the immune response against the immunogen. It is important to distinguish between a carrier for a hapten and an adjuvant. A hapten will become immunogenic when conjugated covalently to a carrier; it will not become immunogenic if mixed with an adjuvant. Thus an adjuvant enhances the immune response to immunogens but does not confer immunogenicity on haptens.

Adjuvants have been used to augment immune responses to antigens for more than 80 years. Interest in the identification of adjuvants for use with vaccines is growing because many new vaccine candidates lack sufficient immunogenicity. This is particularly true of peptide-based vaccines.

Adjuvant mechanisms include (1) increasing the biological or immunological half-life of vaccine antigens; (2) increasing the production of local inflammatory cytokines; and (3) improving antigen delivery and antigen processing and presentation by APCs, especially the dendritic cells. Empirically, it has been found that adjuvants containing microbial components (e.g., mycobacterial extracts) are the best adjuvants. Pathogen components induce macrophages and dendritic cells to express co-stimulatory molecules and to secrete cytokines. More recently, it has been shown that such induction by microbial components involves pattern recognition molecules (e.g., Toll-like receptors [TLRs]) expressed by these cells. Thus binding of microbial components to TLRs signals the cells to express co-stimulatory molecules and to release cytokines.

Over the past decades, strategies for the development and delivery of vaccine antigens have expanded. Some of these antigens are weakly immunogenic and require the presence of adjuvants for the induction or enhancement of an adequate immune response. Vaccines with aluminum-based adjuvants have been extensively used in immunization programs worldwide and a significant body of safety information has accumulated for them. As knowledge of immunology and the mechanisms of adjuvant action have expanded, the number of vaccines containing novel adjuvants being evaluated in clinical trials has increased. Vaccines containing adjuvants other than aluminum-containing compounds have been authorized for use in several countries, and a number of vaccines with novel adjuvants are currently under development, including, but not limited to, vaccines against human papillomavirus (HPV), human immunodeficiency virus (HIV), malaria, and tuberculosis, as well as next- generation vaccines against influenza and other diseases. However, the development and evaluation of new adjuvants, as well as so-called adjuvanted vaccines (compound reagents administered as a single reagent as compared with vaccines used with adjuvants that are mixed with an adjuvant right before they are used for vaccination), present regulatory challenges. Vaccine manufacturers and regulators have questions about the type of information and extent of data that would be required to support proceeding to clinical trials with adjuvanted vaccines and to their eventual authorization. Obviously, this is beyond the scope of our discussion here, but it is important to understand that we face scientific and regulatory challenges in our efforts to develop new, efficacious, and safe adjuvants for future use.

While many adjuvants have been developed in animal models and tested experimentally in humans, only one type of adjuvant has been US Food and Drug Administration (USFDA) approved in the United States for routine vaccination. Currently, aluminum hydroxide and aluminum phosphate (alum) are the major adjuvants used for licensed human vaccines administered to normal individuals in the United States. As an inorganic salt, alum binds to proteins, causing them to precipitate and elicits an inflammatory response that nonspecifically increases the immunogenicity of the antigen. When injected, the precipitated antigen is released more slowly at the injection site than antigen alone. Moreover, the increased size of the antigen, which occurs as a consequence of precipitation, increases the probability that the macromolecule will be phagocytized.

Many adjuvants have been used in experimental animals. One commonly used adjuvant is **Freund's complete adjuvant** consisting of killed *Mycobacterium tuberculosis* or *M. butyricum* suspended in oil, which is then emulsified with an aqueous antigen solution. The oil-emulsified state of the adjuvant–antigen mixture allows the antigen to be released slowly and continuously, helping sustain the recipient's exposure to the immunogen. Other microorganisms used as adjuvants are bacille Calmette–Guerin (BCG) (an

attenuated *Mycobacterium*), *Corynebacterium parvum*, and *Bordetella pertussis*. In reality, many of these adjuvants exploit the activation properties of microbe-expressed molecules including lipopolysaccharide (LPS), bacterial DNA containing unmethylated CpG dinucleotide motifs, and bacterial heat-shock proteins. Many of these microbial cell adjuvants bind to pattern-recognizing signaling receptors such as the TLRs. Ligation of TLRs indirectly activates adaptive B- and T-cell responses. Dendritic cells are important APCs involved in the activity of microbial adjuvants. They respond by secreting cytokines and expressing co-stimulatory molecules that, in turn, stimulate the activation and differentiation of antigen-specific T cells. Table 4.2 lists the majority of currently used adjuvants, some of which are still being tested in clinical trials.

TABLE 4.2. Adjuvants: Currently Licensed for Use in the United States and Those Being Tested in Clinical Trials

Adjuvant Name (Year Licensed)	Adjuvant Class	Components	Vaccines (Disease)
Adjuvants licensed for use in human vaccines			
Alum*(1924)	Mineral salts	Aluminum phosphate/Aluminum hydroxide	Various
MF (Novartis; 1997)	Oil in water emulsion	Squalene, polysorbate 80 (Tween 80; ICI Americas), sorbitan trioleate (Span 85; Croda International)	Fluad (seasonal influenza), Aflunov (prepandemic influenza)
AS03 (GlaxoSmithKline; 2009	Oil in water emulsion	Squalene, Tween 80, α-tocopheral	Pandremix (pandemic influenza), Prepandrix (pre-pandemic influenza)
Virosomes (Berna Biotech; 2000	Liposomes	Lipids, hemagglutinin	Inflexal (seasonal influenza), Epaxal (hepatitis A)
AS04* (GlaxoSmithKline; 2005)	Alum-absorbed TLR4 agonist	Aluminum hydroxide, MPL	Fendrix (hepatitis B), Cervarix (human papilloma virus)
Adjuvants being tested in clinical trials but not licensed for use			
Cp 7909, CpG 1018	TLR agonist	CpG oligonucleotides alone or combined with alum/emulsions	—
Imidazoquinolines	TLR7 and TLR8 agonists	Small molecules	—
PolyI:C	TLR3 agonist	Double-stranded RNA analogs	—
Pam3Cys	TLR2 agonist	Lipopeptide	—
Flagellin	TLR5 agonist	Bacterial protein linked to antigen	—
Iscomatrix	Combination	Saponin, cholesterol, dipalmitoylphosphatidylcholine	—
AS01	Combination	Liposome, MPL, saponin (QS21)	—
AS02	Combination	Oil in water emulsion, MPL, saponin (QS21)	—
AF03	Oil in water emulsion	Squalene, Montane 80, Eumulgin B1 PH	—
CAF01	Combination	Liposome, DDA, TDB	—

*Adjuvants licensed in the United States. AF03 adjuvant formulation 03; CAF01, catonic adjuvant formulation 01; DDA, dimethyldioctadecylammonium; MPL, monophosphoryl lipid A; Pam3Cys, tripalmitoyl-S-gylceryl systeine; PolyI:C, polyinosinic-polycytidylic acid; TDB trehalose dibehenate; TLR, Toll-like receptor.

SUMMARY

1. Immunogenicity is the capacity of a compound to induce an immune response. Immunogenicity requires that a compound (a) be foreign to the immunized individual, (b) possesses a certain minimal molecular weight, (c) possesses a certain degree of chemical complexity, and (d) be degradable or susceptible to antigen processing and presentation through its interaction with MHC.

2. *Antigenicity* refers to the ability of a compound to bind with antibodies or with cells of the immune system. This binding is highly specific; the immune components are capable of recognizing various physicochemical aspects of the compound. The binding between antigen and immune components involves several weak forces operating over short distances (van der Waals forces, electrostatic interactions, hydrophobic interactions, and hydrogen bonds); it does not involve covalent bonds.

3. The smallest unit of antigen that is capable of binding with antibodies and T cells is called an **antigenic determinant** or **epitope**. Compounds may have one or more epitopes capable of reacting with immune components. The immune response against these compounds involves the production of antibodies or the generation of cells with specificities directed against most or all of the epitopes.

4. B-cell membrane immunoglobulin or secreted antibody tends to recognize amino acid sequences that are accessible, usually hydrophilic, and mobile. These can be contiguous or noncontiguous amino acids (conformational determinants), which are brought into proximity by the three-dimensional folding of the protein. B-cell membrane immunoglobulins and antibody are capable of recognizing polysaccharides and lipids.

5. T cells recognize internal amino acid sequences of proteins in the context of MHC class I or class II molecules. Peptide fragments of protein antigens generated by antigen processing may associate with MHC molecules and be presented to T cells.

6. Immunologic cross-reactivity denotes a situation in which two or more substances, which may have various degrees of dissimilarity, share epitopes and would, therefore, react with the immune components induced against any one of these substances. Thus a toxoid, which is a modified form of toxin, may have one or more epitopes in common with the toxin. Immunization with the toxoid leads to an immune response capable of reacting not only with the toxoid but also with the native toxin.

7. Adjuvants are substances that can accelerate, prolong, and enhance the quality of specific immune responses. When administered with antigens, adjuvants facilitate immune responses that are specific for the antigen (not for adjuvant itself) since the adjuvant nonspecifically amplifies the response. The principle mechanisms include increased antigen presentation by APCs (especially dendritic cells), induction of co-stimulatory molecules, and induction of local inflammatory cytokine responses.

REFERENCES AND BIBLIOGRAPHY

Ahmed SS, Plotkin SA, Black S, Coffman RL. (2011) Assessing the safety of adjuvanted vaccines. *Sci Transl Med* 3(93): 9.

Atassi MZ. (1977) *Immunochemistry of Proteins*, Vols 1 and 2. New York: Plenum.

Benjamin DC, Berzofsky JA, East IJ, Gurd FRN, Hannum C, Leach SJ, Margoliash E, Michael JG, Miller A, Prager EM, Reichlin M, Sercarz EE, Smith-Gill SJ, Todd PE, Wilson AC. (1984) The antigenic structure of proteins: a reappraisal. *Annu Rev Immunol* 2: 67.

Berzofsky JA, Cease KB, Cornette JL, Spouge JL, Margalit H, Berkower IJ, Good FM, Miller LH, DeLisi C. (1987) Protein antigenic structures recognized by T cells: potential applications to vaccine design. *Immunol Rev* 98: 9.

Christian RR, Mandl W, Black S, De Gregorio E. (2011) Vaccines for the twenty-first century society. *Nat Rev Immunol* 11: 865.

Davis DR and Cohen GH. (1996) Interactions of protein antigens with antibodies. *Proc Natl Acad Sci USA* 93: 7.

Davis MM, Boniface JJ, Reich Z, Lyons D, Hampl J, Arden B, Chien Y. (1998) Ligand recognition by αβ T cell receptors. *Annu Rev Immunol* 16: 523.

Freund J, Calals J, and Hosmer EP. (1937) Sensitization and antibody formation after injection of tubercle bacilli and paraffin oil. *Proc Soc Exp Biol Med* 37: 509.

Global Advisory Committee on Vaccine Safety, June 2012. (2012) *Wkly Epidemiol Rec* 87(30): 281.

Mastelic B, Ahmed S, Egan WM, Del Giudice G, Golding H, Gust I, Neels P, Reed SG, Sheets RL, Siegrist CA, Lambert PH. (2010) Mode of action of adjuvants: implications for vaccine safety and design. *Biologicals* 38(5): 594.

Novotny J, Handschumacher H, Bruccoleri RE. (1987) Protein antigenicity: a static surface property. *Immunol Today* 8: 26.

Rothbard JB, Gefter ML. (1991) Interactions between immunogenic peptides and MHC proteins. *Annu Rev Immunol* 9: 527.

Watts C. (1997) Capture and processing of exogenous antigens for presentation on MHC molecules. *Annu Rev Immunol* 15: 821.

REVIEW QUESTIONS

For each question, choose the ONE BEST answer or completion.

1. A large glycoprotein has been enzymatically digested in the laboratory to yield a mixture of glycopeptides ranging in size from 4 to 6 amino acids in length. Which of the following would be expected if the peptide mixture were administered to an experimental animal together with an adjuvant such as complete Freund's adjuvant?
   A) peptide-specific antibodies would be generated using the peptide mixture alone
   B) carbohydrate-specific antibodies would be generated only if an adjuvant were administered with the peptide mixture
   C) peptide-specific antibodies would be generated only if they were injected with a separate uncoupled protein carrier
   D) peptide-specific and carbohydrate-specific antibody and T-cell responses would be generated using the peptide mixture alone
   E) there would be neither a humoral nor cell-mediated immune response to the peptides in the mixture

2. The protection against smallpox virus infection afforded by prior infection with cowpox virus represents
   A) antigenic specificity
   B) antigenic cross-reactivity
   C) enhanced viral uptake by macrophages
   D) innate immunity
   E) passive protection

3. Converting a toxin to a toxoid
   A) makes the toxin more immunogenic
   B) reduces the pharmacological activity of the toxin
   C) enhances binding with antitoxin
   D) induces only innate immunity
   E) increases phagocytosis

4. Haptens
   A) require carrier molecules to be immunogenic
   B) react with specific antibodies when homologous carriers are not employed
   C) interact with specific antibody even if the hapten is monovalent
   D) cannot stimulate secondary antibody responses without carriers
   E) all of the above

5. An adjuvant is a substance that
   A) increases the size of the immunogen
   B) enhances the immunogenicity of haptens
   C) increases the chemical complexity of the immunogen
   D) enhances the immune response to the immunogen
   E) enhances immunologic cross-reactivity

6. A polyclonal antibody made against a large protein antigen reacts with it even when it is denatured by disrupting all disulfide bonds. Another monoclonal antibody against the antigen fails to react when it is similarly denatured. The most likely explanation can be stated as follows:
   A) The polyclonal antibody contains antibodies specific for several non-conformational epitopes expressed by the antigen.
   B) The monoclonal antibody recognizes both conformational and non-conformational epitopes.
   C) The monoclonal antibody is specific for disulfide bonds.
   D) The polyclonal antibody has a higher affinity for the antigen.

ANSWERS TO REVIEW QUESTIONS

1. *E.* Peptides ranging from 4 to 6 amino acids in length are low molecular weight molecules that are unable to generate antibody responses or T-cell responses due to their small size. If these peptides were coupled or bound to a protein carrier, they could be immunogenic. T cells do not generate T-cell responses to carbohydrates; therefore **D** is incorrect.

2. *B.* The protection against smallpox provided by prior infection with cowpox is an example of antigenic cross-reactivity. Immunization with cowpox leads to the production of antibodies capable of reacting with smallpox because the two viruses share several identical, or structurally similar, determinants.

3. *B.* Conversion of a toxin to a toxoid is performed in order to reduce the pharmacological activity of the toxin so that sufficient toxoid can be injected to induce an immune response.

4. *E.* Haptens are substances, usually of low molecular weight and univalent that by themselves cannot induce immune responses (primary or secondary), but can do so if conjugated to high molecular weight carriers. The haptens can and do interact with the induced antibodies without it being necessary that they be conjugated to the carrier.

5. *D.* An immunologic adjuvant is a substance that, when mixed with an immunogen, enhances the immune response against that immunogen by mechanisms that depend upon the specific adjuvant used (e.g., enhanced antigen presentation, delayed release of antigen, etc.). It does not increase its size or chemical complexity. In addition, it does not enhance the immune response against a hapten, which requires its conjugation to an immunogenic carrier to induce a response against the hapten. The adjuvant has no relevance to possible toxicity of an immunogen.

6. A. Polyclonal antibodies are a mixture of antibodies produced by multiple B-cell clones with B-cell receptors that react with specific antigenic epitopes expressed by the antigen. Antibodies can recognize single epitopes formed by primary sequence structures, or secondary, tertiary, and quaternary conformational structures. Denaturing a protein by disrupting disulfide bonds generally destroys conformational determinants. Therefore it is likely that the polyclonal antibody reacts with non-conformational epitopes present on both native and denatured antigen, while the monoclonal antibody reacts with a conformational determinant only on the native antigen.

5

ANTIBODY STRUCTURE AND FUNCTION

INTRODUCTION

One of the major functions of the immune system is the production of soluble proteins that circulate freely and exhibit properties that contribute specifically to immunity and protection against foreign material. These soluble proteins are the *antibodies*, which belong to the class of proteins called globulins because of their globular structure. Initially, owing to their migratory properties in an electrophoretic field, they were called γ-globulins (in relation to the more rapidly migrating albumin, α-globulin, and β-globulin); today they are known collectively as *immunoglobulins* (Igs).

Immunoglobulins can be membrane-bound or secreted. Membrane-bound antibody is present on the surface of B cells where it serves as the antigen-specific receptor. The membrane-bound form of antibody is associated with a heterodimer called Igα/Igβ to form the *B-cell receptor* (BCR). As will be discussed in Chapter 8, the Igα/Igβ heterodimer mediates the intracellular signaling mechanisms associated with B-cell activation. Secreted antibodies are produced by plasma cells—the terminally differentiated B cells that serve as antibody factories that reside largely within the bone marrow.

The structure of immunoglobulins incorporates several features essential for their participation in the immune response. The two most important of these features are specificity and biologic activity. *Specificity* is attributed to a defined region of the antibody molecule containing the hypervariable or *complementarity-determining region* (CDR). This restricts the antibody to combine only with those substances that contain a particular antigenic structure. The existence of a vast array of potential antigenic determinants, which, as we discussed in Chapter 4, are also known as *epitopes*, prompted the evolution of a system for producing an enormous repertoire of antibody molecules, each of which is capable of combining with a particular antigenic structure. Thus, antibodies collectively exhibit great diversity, in terms of the types of molecular structures with which they are capable of reacting, but individually they exhibit a high degree of specificity, since each is able to react with only one particular antigenic structure.

Despite the large numbers of antigen-specific antibodies, the biologic effects of antigen–antibody reactions are rather few in number. Depending on the nature of the antigen to which the antibody is specific, these include neutralization of toxins; immobilization of microorganisms; neutralization of viral activity; agglutination (clumping together) of microorganisms or of antigenic particles (see Chapter 6); or binding with soluble antigen, leading to the formation of precipitates. The latter is an example of how the adaptive immune system collaborates with the innate immune system since precipitated antigens are readily phagocytized and destroyed by phagocytic cells (see Chapter 2). Other examples of this collaboration, which occurs once antibodies react with antigens, include activation of complement to facilitate the lysis of microorganisms (see Chapters 2 and 14), and complement-mediated opsonization, which also results in phagocytosis and destruction of microbes. Still another important biologic function of antibodies is the

Immunology: A Short Course, Seventh Edition. Richard Coico and Geoffrey Sunshine.
© 2015 John Wiley & Sons, Ltd. Published 2015 by John Wiley & Sons, Ltd.
Companion Website: www.wileyimmunology.com/coico

ability of certain classes of immunoglobulins to cross the placenta from the mother to the fetus. This is discussed in more detail later in this chapter.

The differences in the various biologic activities of antibodies are attributed to structural properties conferred by the germline-encoded portions of the Ig molecule. Thus, not all antibody molecules are equal in the performance of all of these biologic tasks. In simplest terms, antibody molecules contain structural components that are shared with other antibodies within their *class*, and an antigen-binding component that is unique to a given antibody. This chapter deals with these structural and biologic properties of immunoglobulins.

ISOLATION AND CHARACTERIZATION OF IMMUNOGLOBULINS

Serum is the antibody-containing component of blood. It is the liquid portion left when blood has been withdrawn and allowed to clot. Unless measures are taken to prevent clotting of blood in the vacutainer in which blood is collected (e.g., the addition of heparin), clotting factors will be activated and cause a cellular clot to form. When the serum component is subjected to *electrophoresis* (separation in an electrical field) at slightly alkaline pH (8.2), five major components can normally be visualized (see Figure 5.1). The slowest, in terms of migration toward the anode, called γ-globulin, contains the immunoglobulins. This original demonstration entailed the simple comparison of the electrophoretic pattern of antiserum from a hyperimmune rabbit (one that had received multiple immunizations with the same test antigen) before and after the test antigen-specific antibody had been removed by precipitation with the antigen. Only the size of the γ-globulin fraction was diminished by this procedure. Analysis showed that when this fraction was collected separately, all measurable antibodies were contained within it. Later it was shown that antibody activity is present not only in the γ-globulin fraction but also in a slightly more anodic area. Consequently, all globular proteins with antibody activity are generically referred to as immunoglobulins, as exemplified by the γ peak (see Figure 5.1).

From the broad electrophoretic peaks, it is clear that a heterogeneous collection of immunoglobulin molecules with slightly different charges is present. This heterogeneity was one of the early obstacles in attempts to determine the structure of antibodies, since analytical chemistry requires homogeneous, crystallizable compounds as starting material. This problem was solved, in part, by the discovery of *myeloma proteins*, which are homogeneous immunoglobulins produced by the progeny of a single plasma cell that has become neoplastic in the malignant disease called *multiple myeloma*. This is demonstrated by the γ-globulin spike in the electrophoretic pattern of serum proteins of a patient

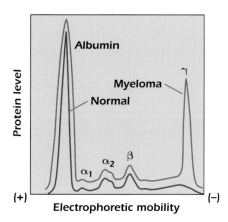

Figure 5.1. Electrophoretic mobility of serum proteins obtained from a normal individual (lower tracing in blue) and from a patient with IgG myeloma (upper tracing in red).

with multiple myeloma (see Figure 5.1). When it became clear that some myeloma proteins bound antigen, it also became apparent that they could be dealt with as typical immunoglobulin molecules.

Another aid to structural studies of antibodies was the discovery of *Bence Jones proteins* in the urine. These homogeneous proteins, produced in large quantities by some patients with multiple myeloma, are dimers of immunoglobulin κ or λ light chains. They were very useful in the determination of the structure of this portion of the immunoglobulin molecule. Today, the powerful technique of cell–cell hybridization (hybridomas), which allows for the *in vitro* immortalization of antibody-producing B-cells, permits the production of large quantities of homogeneous preparations of monoclonal antibody of virtually any specificity (see Chapter 6).

STRUCTURE OF LIGHT AND HEAVY CHAINS

Analysis of the structural characteristics of antibody molecules really began in 1959 with two discoveries that, for the first time, revealed that the molecule could be separated into analyzable parts suitable for further study. In England, Porter found that proteolytic treatment with the enzyme *papain* split the immunoglobulin molecule (molecular weight 150,000 Da) into three fragments of about equal size (see Figure 5.2). Two of these fragments were found to retain the antibody's ability to bind antigen specifically, although, unlike the intact molecule, they could no longer precipitate the antigen from solution. These two fragments are referred to as *Fab* (fragment antigen-binding) fragments and are considered to be univalent, possessing one binding site each and being in every way identical to each other. The third fragment could be crystallized out of solution, a property indicative of its apparent homogeneity. This fragment

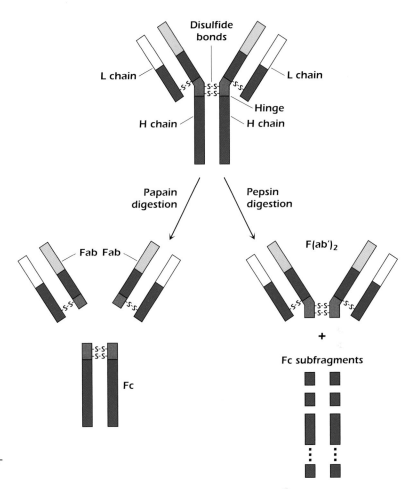

<u>Figure 5.2.</u> Proteolytic digestion of immunoglobulin using papain and pepsin.

is called the ***Fc fragment*** (fragment crystallizable). It cannot bind antigen, but as was subsequently shown, it is responsible for the biologic functions of the antibody molecule after antigen has been bound to the Fab part of the intact molecule.

At about the same time, Edelman in the United States discovered that when γ-globulin was extensively reduced by treatment with mercaptoethanol (a reagent that breaks disulfide bonds), the molecule fell apart into four chains: two identical light chains with a molecular weight of about 22,000 Da each and two others of about 53,000 Da each. The larger molecules were designated ***heavy chains*** (often abbreviated as ***H chains***) and the smaller ones, ***light chains*** (often abbreviated as ***L chains***). On the basis of these results, the basic unit structure of immunoglobulin molecules, as depicted in Figure 5.2, was proposed. This model was subsequently shown to be essentially correct, and Porter and Edelman shared the Nobel Prize for the elucidation of antibody structure. Thus, all immunoglobulin molecules consist of a basic unit of four polypeptide chains, two identical heavy chains and two identical light chains, held together by several disulfide bonds. It should be noted that papain digestion of the immunoglobulin molecule results in cleav-

age N-terminally to the disulfide bridge between the heavy chains at the hinge region, yielding two monovalent Fab fragments and an Fc fragment. On the other hand, ***pepsin*** digestion results in cleavage C-terminally to the disulfide bridge, resulting in a divalent fragment referred to as ***F(ab')₂***, consisting of two ***Fab fragments*** joined by the disulfide bond and several Fc subfragments. A more detailed diagram of a generic immunoglobulin molecule, consisting of two glycosylated heavy chains and two light chains, is shown in Figure 5.3. Note that in addition to the interchain disulfide bonds that hold the chains together, the heavy and light chains each contain intrachain disulfide bonds to create the ***immunoglobulin-fold domains*** to create the antiparallel β-pleated sheet structure characteristic of antibody molecules. As discussed later in this chapter, other molecules belonging to the so-called ***immunoglobulin superfamily*** share this structural feature.

As one might expect, immunoglobulins of one species are immunogenic in another species. In other words, the use of immunoglobulins of a given species as immunogens in another species allows for the production of antisera that can then be used to investigate the various features of different immunoglobulin chains. This serologic approach to

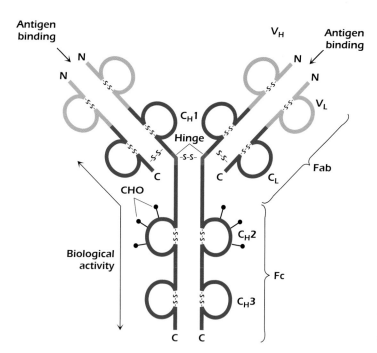

Figure 5.3. Schematic representation of an immunoglobulin molecule showing immunoglobulin-fold domains formed by intrachain disulfide bonds.

studying immunoglobulins, together with several biochemical strategies, revealed important insights into the structural properties of these molecules. For example, it demonstrated that almost all species studied have two major classes of light chains, called κ and λ. Any one individual of a species produces both types of light chain, but the ratio of κ chains to λ chains varies with the species (mouse: 95% κ; human: 60% κ). However, in any one immunoglobulin molecule, the light chains are always either both κ or both λ, never one of each.

Another important characteristic of immunoglobulins revealed in this early work was that the heavy chains of immunoglobulins of virtually all species studied can be divided into five different classes or *isotypes*. The five classes of immunoglobulins include IgM, IgD, IgG, IgA, and IgE. These are distinguished from one another based upon so-called *constant regions* of the heavy chains, which differ from one another with regard to their protein sequences, carbohydrate content, and size. As noted earlier, these portions of the various Ig classes also confer different biologic functions associated with each isotype. The Ig heavy chains, whose constant regions are derived from Ig heavy chain genes (discussed in detail in Chapter 7) are designated with Greek letters as shown in Table 5.1.

Therefore, the genes encoding these **constant** (C) **regions** responsible for the μ, δ, γ, α, and ε heavy chains are called Cμ, Cδ, Cγ, Cα, and Cε, respectively. Any individual of a species makes all five Ig isotypes, in proportions characteristic of the species, but, just as the case with light chains described above, in any one antibody molecule both heavy chains are always identical (e.g., 2γ or 2ε, etc.). Thus, an antibody molecule of the IgG class could have the structure

TABLE 5.1. Immunoglobulin Heavy Chain Isotopes

Immunoglobulin	Heavy chain gene
IgM	μ
IgD	δ
IgG	γ
IgA	α
IgE	ε

$\kappa2\gamma2$ with two identical kappa light chains and two identical gamma heavy chains. Alternatively, it could have the structure $\lambda2\gamma2$ with two identical lambda light chains and two identical γ heavy chains. In contrast, an antibody of the IgE class could have the structure $\kappa2\varepsilon2$ or $\lambda2\varepsilon2$. In each case, it is the nature of the heavy chains that confers on the molecule its unique biologic properties, such as its half-life in the circulation, its ability to bind to certain receptors, and its ability to activate complement (see Chapter 14) on combination with antigen.

Further characterization of these isotypes by specific antisera has led to the designation of several subclasses that have more subtle differences among themselves. Thus, the major class of human IgG can be subdivided into the **subclasses** IgG$_1$, IgG$_2$, IgG$_3$, and IgG$_4$. IgA has been divided similarly into two subclasses, IgA$_1$ and IgA$_2$. The subclasses differ from one another in numbers and arrangement of interchain disulfide bonds, as well as by alterations in other structural features. These alterations, in turn, produce some changes in functional properties that will be discussed later.

DOMAINS

Early in the study of the structure of immunoglobulins, it became apparent that in addition to interchain disulfide bonds that hold together light and heavy chains, as well as the two heavy chains, intrachain disulfide bonds exist that form loops within the chain. The ***globular structure*** of immunoglobulins, and the ability of enzymes to cleave these molecules at very restricted positions into large entities instead of degrading them to oligopeptides and amino acids, is indicative of a very compact structure. Furthermore, the presence of intrachain disulfide bonds at regular, approximately equal intervals of about 100–110 amino acids leads to the prediction that each loop in the peptide chains should form a compactly folded ***globular domain***. In fact, light chains have two domains each, and heavy chains have four or five domains, separated by a short unfolded stretch (see Figure 5.3). These configurations have been confirmed by direct observation and by genetic analysis (see Chapter 7).

Immunoglobulin molecules are assemblies of separate domains, each centered on a disulfide bond, and each having so much homology with the others as to suggest that they evolved from a single ancestral gene, which duplicated itself several times and then changed its amino acid sequence to enable the resultant different domains to fulfill different functions. Each domain is designated by a letter that indicates whether it is on a light chain or a heavy chain and a number that indicates its position. As we shall soon discuss in more detail, the first domain on light and heavy chains is highly variable, in terms of amino acid sequence, from one antibody to the next, and it is designated V_L or V_H accordingly (see Figure 5.3). The second and subsequent domains on both heavy chains are much more constant in amino acid sequence and are designated C_H1, C_H2, and C_H3 (Figure 5.3). In addition to their interchain disulfide bonding, the globular domains bind to each other in homologous pairs, largely by hydrophobic interactions, as follows: V_HV_L, C_H1C_L, C_H2C_H2, and C_H3C_H3.

HINGE REGION

The hinge region of immunoglobulins is composed of a short segment of amino acids (relatively long in the case of IgD and IgE) and is found between the C_H1 and C_H2 regions of the heavy chains (see Figure 5.3). This segment is made up predominantly of cysteine and proline residues. The cysteines are involved in formation of interchain disulfide bonds, and the proline residues prevent folding in a globular structure. This region of the heavy chain provides an important structural characteristic of immunoglobulins. It permits flexibility between the two Fab arms of the Y-shaped antibody molecule. It allows the two Fab arms to open and close to accommodate binding to two identical antigenic epitopes, separated by a fixed distance, as might be found on the surface of a bacterium. Additionally, since this stretch of amino acids is open and as accessible as any other nonfolded peptide, it can be cleaved by proteases, such as papain, to generate the Fab and Fc fragments described above (see Figure 5.2).

VARIABLE REGION

As we have discussed earlier, in contrast to the constant region of immunoglobulins, the ***variable region*** of immunoglobulins constitutes the part of the molecule that binds to the antigen for which the antibody is specific. A major problem for immunologists was to determine how so many individual specificities, which are required to meet the enormous variety of antigenic challenges, are generated from the variable region gene. As we shall see in Chapter 7, this issue has been largely resolved and is explained by the phenomenon of gene rearrangement associated with B cells (and T cells for the TCR as we shall in Chapter 10). We will briefly introduce the concept of hypervariability regions of immunoglobulins in this section, as it relates to the concept of antibody specificity, since it is important for topics covered later in this chapter.

When the amino acid sequences of immunoglobulin molecules derived from sera or urine of individuals suffering with multiple myeloma were examined, significant insights into the antigen-binding region of antibodies were obtained. Why were these sera and urine samples chosen for examination? As discussed earlier in this chapter, the sera in multiple myeloma patients often contains copious amounts of immunoglobulin molecules, all identical in structure and specificity by virtue of their production by the neoplastic plasma cells causing the disease. In addition, urine from such patients contains large amounts of light chain molecules associated with these myeloma proteins (i.e., Bence Jones proteins). Using these sera and urine samples, it was found that the greatest variability in sequence existed in the N-terminal 110 amino acids of both the light and heavy chains. Kabat and Wu compared the amino acid sequences of many different V_L and V_H regions. They plotted the variability in the amino acids at each position in the chain and showed that the greatest amount of variability (defined as the ratio of the number of different amino acids at a given position to the frequency of the most common amino acid at that position) occurred in three regions of the light and heavy chains. These regions are called ***hypervariable regions***. The less variable stretches, which occur between these hypervariable regions, are called ***framework regions***. It is now clear that the hypervariable regions participate in the binding with antigen and form the region complementary in structure to the antigen. Consequently, hypervariability regions are termed ***complementarity-determining regions*** (CDRs) of the light and heavy chains: CDR1, CDR2, and CDR3 (see Figure 5.4).

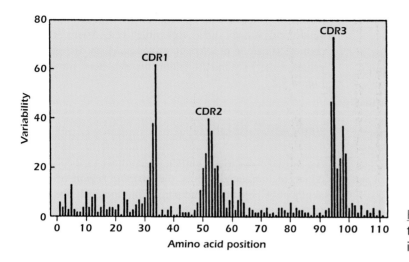

Figure 5.4. Variability of amino acids representing the N-terminal residues of V_H in a representative immunoglobulin molecule.

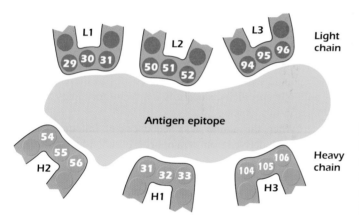

Figure 5.5. A schematic representation of the complementarity between an epitope and the antibody-combining site consisting of the hypervariable areas of the L and H chains. Numbered letters denote CDR of heavy and light chains; circled numbers denote the number of the amino acid residue in the CDRs.

The hypervariable regions, although separated in the linear, two-dimensional model of the peptide chains, are actually brought together in the folded form of the intact antibody molecule, and together they constitute the combining site, which is complementary to the epitope (Figure 5.5). The variability in these CDRs provides the diversity in the shape of the combining site that is required for the function of antibodies of different specificities. All the known forces involved in antigen–antibody interactions are weak, noncovalent interactions (e.g., ionic, hydrogen-bonding, van der Walls forces, and hydrophobic interactions). It is therefore necessary that there be a close fit between antigen and antibody over a sufficiently large region to allow a total binding force that is adequate for stable interaction. Contributions to this binding interaction by both heavy and light chains are involved in the overall association between epitope and antibody.

It should now be apparent that two antibody molecules with different antigenic specificities must have different amino acid sequences in their hypervariable regions and that those with similar sequences will generally have similar specificities. However, it is possible for two antibodies with different amino acid sequences to have specificity to the same epitope. In this case, the **binding affinities** of the antibodies with the epitope will probably be different because there will be differences in the number and types of binding forces available to bind identical antigens to the different binding sites of the two antibodies.

An additional source of variability involves the size of the combining site on the antibody, which is usually (but not always) considered to take the form of a depression or cleft. In some instances, especially when small, hydrophobic haptens are involved, the epitopes do not occupy the entire combining site, yet they achieve sufficient affinity of binding. It has been shown that antibodies specific for such a hapten may, in fact, react with other antigens that have no obvious similarity to the hapten (e.g., dinitrophenol and sheep red cells). These dissimilar antigens bind either to a larger area or to a different area of the combining site on the antibody (see Figure 5.6). Thus, a particular antibody-combining site may have the ability to combine with two (or more) apparently diverse epitopes, a property called **redundancy**. The ability of a single antibody molecule to cross-react with an unknown number of epitopes may reduce the number of different antibodies needed to defend an individual against the range of antigenic challenges.

TABLE 5.2. Most Important Features of Immunoglobulin Isotopes

Feature	Isotype				
	IgG	IgA	IgM	IgD	IgE
Molecular weight	150,000	160,000 for monomer	900,000	180,000	200,000
Additional protein subunits	—	J and S	J	—	—
Approximate concentration in serum (mg/mL)	12	1.8	1	0–0.04	0.00002
Percent of total Ig	80	13	6	0.2	0.002
Distribution	~Equal: intravascular and extravascular	Intravascular and secretions	Mostly intravascular	Present on lymphocyte surface	On basophils and mast cells present in saliva and nasal secretions
Half-life (days)	23	5.5	5	2.8	2.0
Placental passage	++	—	—		
Presence in secretion	—	++	—		
Presence in milk	+	+	0 to trace		
Activation of complement	+	—	+++		
Binding to Fc receptors on macrophages, PMN cells, and NK cells	++	—	—		
Relative agglutinating capacity	+	++	+++		
Antiviral activity	+++	+++	+		
Antibacterial activity (Gram-negative)	+++	++ (with lysozyme)	+++ (with complement)		
Antitoxin activity	+++	—	—		
Allergic activity	—	—	—	—	++

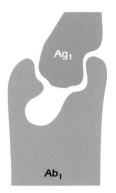 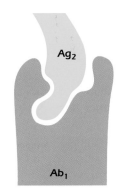

Figure 5.6. A representation of how an antibody of a given specificity (Ab) can exhibit binding with two different epitopes (Ag1 and Ag2).

IMMUNOGLOBULIN VARIANTS

Isotypes

We have already introduced the term *isotype* in this chapter. Why has the immune system evolved to provide this level of immunoglobulin diversity? To optimize humoral immune defenses against infectious pathogens and other foreign sub-

TABLE 5.3. Important Differences Among Human IgG Subclasses

Characteristic	IgG$_1$	IgG$_2$	IgG$_3$	IgG$_4$
Occurrence (% of total IgG)	70	20	7	3
Half-life	23	23	7	23
Complement binding	+	+	+++	—
Placental passage	++	±	++	++
Binding of monocytes	+++	+	+++	±

stances, a variety of mechanisms, each dependent on a somewhat different property or function of an immunoglobulin molecule, has developed. Thus, when a specific antibody molecule combines with a specific antigen such as a pathogen, several different effector mechanisms come into play. These different mechanisms derive from the different classes of immunoglobulin (isotypes), each of which may combine with the same epitope but each of which triggers a different biologic response. These differences result from structural variations in the constant regions of the heavy chains, which have generated domains that mediate a variety of functions. A summary of the properties of the immunoglobulin classes is given in Tables 5.2 and 5.3.

Allotypes

Another form of variation in the structure of immunoglobulins is *allotypy*. It is based on genetic differences between individuals. In other words, different *allelic forms* (allotypes) of the heavy or light chain constant region genes give rise to different forms of the same gene at a given locus. As a result of allotypy, a heavy or light chain constituent of any immunoglobulin can be present in some members of a species and absent in others. Bear in mind, however, that despite these allotypic differences among immunoglobulin classes within a species, the vast majority of the protein sequences of the constant regions (H or L) for a given class is highly conserved. Allotypic differences at known H- and L-chain gene loci usually result in changes in only one or two amino acids in the constant region of a chain. With a few exceptions, the presence of allotypic differences in two identical immunoglobulin molecules does not generally affect binding with antigen, but it serves as an important marker for analysis of Mendelian inheritance. Some known allotype markers constitute a group on the γ chain of human IgG (called *Gm* for IgG markers), a group on the κ chain (called *Km*), and a group on the α chain (called *Am*).

Allotypic markers have been found in the immunoglobulins of several species, usually by the use of antisera generated by immunization of one member of a species with antibody from another member of the same species. As with other allelic systems, allotypes are inherited as codominant Mendelian traits. The genes encoding these markers are expressed codominantly, so that an individual may be homozygous or heterozygous for a given marker.

Idiotypes

As we have seen, the combining site of a specific antibody molecule is made up of a unique combination of amino acids in the variable regions of the light and heavy chains. Since this combination is not present in other antibody molecules, it should be immunogenic and capable of stimulating an immunologic response against itself in an animal of the same species. This prediction was actually found to be accurate. If one immunizes mice to generate an antibody response to the immunogen and then isolates the antigen-specific antibodies from the immune sera, these antibodies are capable of stimulating anti-antibody responses in mice of the same strain. In fact, these anti-antibody responses are polyclonal in nature as they have been shown to be specific for several epitopes present on the antibodies used in the innoculation. Given the fact that the donors and recipients of the antiserum used in the immunization protocol were members of the same strain and therefore genetically identical, shouldn't the antibodies fail to stimulate a response due to the fact that they should be considered "self" antigens to which we are tolerant? The anti-antibody responses were, in fact, stimulated by the collective variable regions on the

H and L chains that constitute the antigen-specific regions of the antibody molecules contained in the inoculum. These portions of antibody molecules are called *idiotypes*. Thus, a more accurate designation of the antibodies produced in the antibody-immunized mice described above is *anti-idiotype antibodies*. Evidence has suggested that anti-idiotype responses occur normally within individuals. One proposed explanation for these findings is that anti-idiotypic antibodies play a physiologic role in regulating or turning off the antibody response to the antigen that stimulated the initial antibody response. Indeed, in some cases, anti-idiotypic sera prevent binding of the antibody with its antigen, in which event the idiotypic determinant is considered to be in or very near the combining site itself. Anti-idiotypic sera, which do not block binding of antibody with antigen, are probably directed against variable determinants of the framework area, outside the combining site (see Figure 5.7). Although this regulatory role for anti-idiotypic antibodies remains controversial, the concept is consistent with Jerne's network theory for immune regulation, discussed in subsequent chapters. In short, this theory postulates that antibodies respond primarily to each other and that foreign antigens merely perturb the normal equilibrium established between idiotypes. In 1984, Jerne was awarded the Nobel Prize in Medicine that he shared with Kohler and Milstein for their contributions to our understanding of development, specificity, and control of immune responses.

On theoretical grounds, it is possible to visualize that an anti-idiotypic antibody with a combining site complementary to that of the idiotype resembles the epitope, which is also complementary to the idiotypes' combining site. Thus, the anti-idiotype may represent a facsimile or an *internal image* of the epitope. Indeed, there are examples of immunization of experimental animals using anti-idiotypic internal images as immunogens. Such immunogens induce antibodies capable of reacting with the antigen that carries the epitope to which the original idiotype is

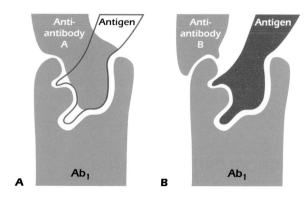

Figure 5.7. Two anti-idiotypic antibodies to Ab1. (A) The anti-idiotypic antibody on the left is directed to the combining site of Ab1, preventing binding of Ab1 with the antigen. (B) The anti-idiotypic antibody on the right binds with framework areas of Ab1 and does not prevent its binding with antigen.

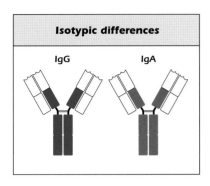
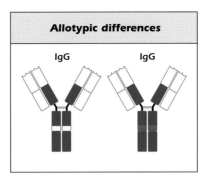
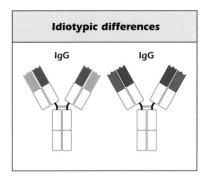

Figure 5.8. Different types of immunoglobulin variation.

directed. Thus, these antibodies are induced without the immunized animal ever having seen the original antigen.

In some instances, especially with inbred animals, anti-idiotypic antibodies react with several different antibodies that are directed against the same epitope and share idiotypes. These idiotypes are called *public* or *cross-reacting idiotypes*, and this term frequently defines families of antibody molecules. By contrast, sera that react with only one particular antibody molecule define a private idiotype.

Figure 5.8 summarizes the different types of variation between immuoglobulins. Differences between constant regions due to usage of different heavy and light chain constant region genes are called *isotypes*. Differences due to different alleles of the same constant region gene are called *allotypes*. Finally, within a given isotype (e.g., IgG), differences due to particular rearranged V_H and V_L genes are called *idiotypes*.

STRUCTURAL FEATURES OF IgG

IgG is the predominant immunoglobulin in blood, lymph fluid, cerebrospinal fluid, and peritoneal fluid. The IgG molecule consists of two γ heavy chains of molecular weight approximately 50,000 Da each and two light chains (either κ or λ) of molecular weight approximately 25,000 Da each, held together by disulfide bonds (Figure 5.9). Thus, the IgG molecule has a molecular weight of approximately 150,000 Da and a sedimentation coefficient of 7S. Electrophoretically, the IgG molecule is the least anodic of all serum proteins, and it migrates to the γ range of serum globulins, hence its earlier designation as γ-globulin or 7S immunoglobulin.

The IgG class of immunoglobulins in humans contains four subclasses designated *IgG$_1$*, *IgG$_2$*, *IgG$_3$*, and *IgG$_4$*, named in order of their abundance in serum (IgG$_1$ being the most abundant). Except for their variable regions, all the immunoglobulins within a class have about 90% homology in their amino acid sequences, but only 60% homology exists between classes (e.g., IgG and IgA). This degree of homology means that an antiserum made in mice against human IgG may include antibodies against all members of a given class (e.g., all members of the IgG class) while other antisera may be raised that are specific for determinants found in only one of the subclasses (e.g., in IgG$_2$). This variation was first detected antigenically by the use of antibodies against various γ chains. The IgG subclasses differ in their chemical properties and, more importantly, in their biologic properties, which are discussed below.

Biologic Properties of IgG

IgG present in the serum of human adults represents about 15% of the total protein (other proteins include albumins, globulins, and enzymes). IgG is distributed approximately equally between the intravascular and extravascular spaces.

Except for the IgG$_3$ subclass, which has a rapid turnover with a half-life of 7 days, the half-life of IgG is approximately 23 days, which is the longest half-life of all Ig isotypes. This persistence in the serum makes IgG the most suitable for passive immunization by transfer of antibodies. Interestingly, as the concentration of IgG in the serum increases (as in cases of multiple myeloma or after the transfer of very high concentrations of IgG), the rate of catabolism of IgG increases, and the half-life of IgG decreases to 15–20 days or even less. Recent studies have provided a clear explanation for the prolonged survival of IgG relative to other serum proteins and why its half-life decreases at high concentrations. A saturable IgG protection receptor (FcRp, also called the Brambell receptor) has been identified and shown to bind to the Fc region of this isotype. This receptor is found in cellular endosomes and selectively recycles endocytosed IgG (e.g., following endocytosis of antigen–antibody immune complexes) back to the circulation. Figure 5.10 illustrates how this mechanism operates to cleanse IgG antibody of antigen and harvest antigen for presentation without antibody destruction. Conditions associated with high IgG levels saturate the FcRp receptors rendering the catabolism of excess IgG indistinguishable from albumin or other Ig isotypes.

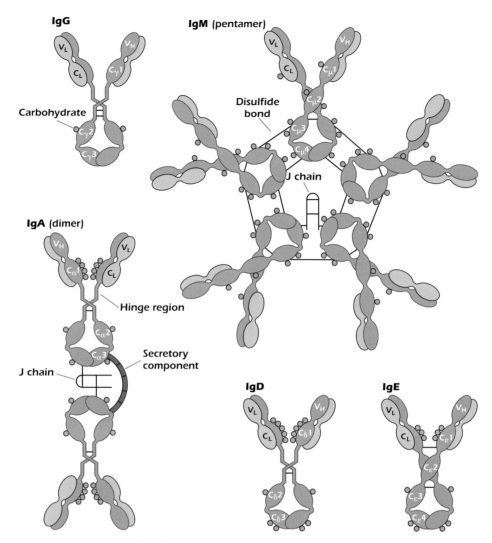

Figure 5.9. Structures of the five major classes of secreted antibody. Light chains are shown in green; heavy chains are shown in blue. Orange circles denote areas of glycosylation. The polymeric IgM and IgA molecules contain a polypeptide known as the J chain. The dimeric IgA molecule shown includes the secretory component (red).

Agglutination and Formation of Precipitate

IgG molecules can cause the *agglutination* or clumping of particulate (insoluble) antigens such as microorganisms. The reaction of IgG with soluble, multivalent antigens can generate *precipitates* (see Chapter 6). This property of IgG is undoubtedly of considerable survival value since insoluble antigen–antibody complexes are easily phagocytized and destroyed by phagocytic cells. IgG molecules may be made to aggregate by a variety of procedures. For example, precipitation with alcohol, a method employed in the purification of IgG, or heating at 56° C for 10 minutes, a method used to inactivate complement (see Chapter 14), causes aggregation. Aggregated IgG can still combine with antigen.

Many of the properties that are attributed to antigen–antibody complexes are exhibited by aggregated IgG (without antigen), for example, attachment to phagocytic

cells, as well as the activation of complement and other biologically active substances that may be harmful to the body. Such activation is due to the juxtaposition of Fc domains by the aggregation process in a way analogous to that produced by antigen-induced immune complex formation. It is therefore imperative that no aggregated IgG be present in passively administered IgG (e.g., gamma globulin preparations used to treat patients exposed to venomous snake bites, certain hepatitis viruses, etc.).

Passage through the Placenta and Absorption in Neonates

The IgG isotype (except for subclass IgG$_2$) is the only class of immunoglobulin that can pass through the placenta, enabling the mother to transfer her immunity to the fetus. Placental transfer is facilitated by expression of an IgG

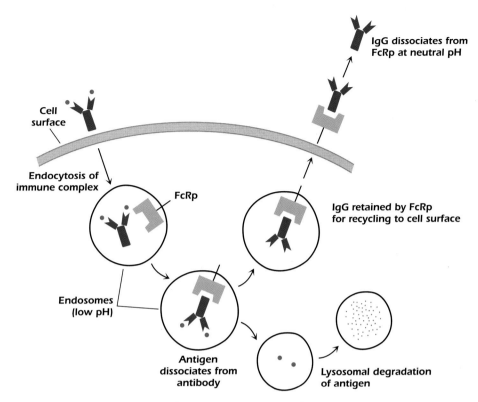

Figure 5.10. Recycling of IgG utilizing the protector receptor (FcRp). Circulating monomeric IgG plus antigen (immune complex) enters an antigen-presenting cell through the process of endocytosis. Within the endosome, the complex binds FcRp; IgG and Ag dissociate allowing the IgG to be directed to the cell surface for recycling. Antigen undergoes lysosomal degradation (antigen processing), and its proteolytic fragments are ultimately expressed on the cell surface in the context of MHC class II molecules.

protection receptor (FcRn) expressed on placental cells. FcRn was recently shown to be identical to the IgG protection receptor (FcRp) found in the cellular endosomes. Analysis of fetal immunoglobulins shows that at the third or fourth month of pregnancy there is a rapid increase in the concentration of IgG. This IgG must be of maternal origin, since the fetus is unable to synthesize immunoglobulins at this age. Then, during the fifth month of pregnancy, the fetus begins to synthesize IgM and trace amounts of IgA. It is not until 3 or 4 months after birth, when the level of inherited maternal IgG drops as a result of catabolism (the half-life of IgG is 23 days), that the infant begins to synthesize its own IgG antibodies. Thus, the resistance of the fetus and the neonate to infection is conferred almost entirely by the mother's IgG, which passes across the placenta. It has been established that passage across the placenta is mediated by the Fc portion of the IgG molecule; F(ab')$_2$ or Fab fragments of IgG do not pass through the placenta. It is of interest to note that the IgG protection receptor (FcRn) expressed on placental cells is transiently superexpressed in the intestinal tissue of neonates. Absorption of maternal IgG contained in the colostrum of nursing mothers is achieved by its binding to these high density receptors in intestinal tissue. FcRn are downregulated in intestinal tissue at 2 weeks of age.

While passage of IgG molecules across the placenta confers immunity to infection on the fetus, it may also be responsible for hemolytic disease of the newborn (erythroblastosis fetalis) (see Chapter 16). This is caused by maternal antibodies to fetal red blood cells. The maternal IgG antibodies, produced by a previously sensitized (immunized) Rh$^-$ mother, to Rh antigen, pass across the placenta and attack the fetal red blood cells that express Rh antigens (Rh$^+$).

Opsonization

IgG is an opsonizing antibody (from the Greek *opsonin*, which means "to prepare for eating") thereby facilitating phagocytosis. Thus, within a week to 10 days of generating an antibody response to a particular pathogen, IgG antibodies will be present that will bind to specific antigenic epitopes via their Fab portions. Once bound, it is the Fc portion of the IgG molecule that confers its opsonizing property. Many phagocytic cells, including macrophages and polymorphonuclear phagocytes, bear receptors for the Fc portion of the IgG molecule. These cells adhere to the antibody-coated bacteria by virtue of their Fc receptors. The net effect is a zipper-like closure of the surface

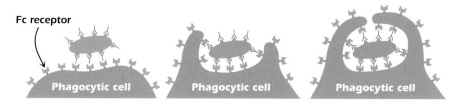

Fc receptor

Phagocytic cell   Phagocytic cell   Phagocytic cell

Figure 5.11. A diagrammatic representation of phagocytosis of a particle coated with antibodies.

membrane of the phagocytic cell around the organism, as receptors for Fc and the Fc regions on the antibodies continue to combine, leading to the final engulfing and destruction of the microorganism (see Figure 5.11).

Antibody-Dependent Cell-Mediated Cytotoxicity

IgG molecules play an important role in antibody-dependent, cell-mediated cytotoxicity (ADCC). In this form of cytotoxicity, the Fab portion of IgG binds with the target cell, whether it is a microorganism or a tumor cell, and the Fc portion binds with specific Fc receptors that are found on certain large granular lymphocytic cells called natural killer (NK) cells. By this mechanism, the IgG molecule focuses the killer cells on their target, and the killer cells destroy the target, not by phagocytosis but with the various toxic substances contained in cytoplasmic granules that they release.

Activation of Complement

We briefly introduced the basic components and functional outcomes associated with the three modes of complement activation in Chapter 2. Chapter 14 will discuss the major properties of complement. In brief, the complement system is a set of plasma proteins that can be activated either by binding to certain pathogens or by binding to antibody (e.g., pathogen-specific antibodies). Complement activation is often described as a series of cascading enzymatic events leading to the generation of specific complement components that cause *opsonization* and *phagocytosis* of infectious agents as well as direct *lysis* of the invading organism, among other important immunologic phenomena. Structural features of the early complement components involved in the activation cascade in which antibodies are involved dictate the antibody classes to which complement will bind.

As discussed in Chapter 2, IgG plays an important role in the classical activation of complement (also see Chapter 14). When the first protein in the complement series (C1q) is exposed to immune complexes composed of IgG–antigen, this initiates the classical activation pathway leading to a chain of downstream complement components as a result of proteolytic cleavage. This process ultimately results in the production of a membrane attack complex (MAC) that causes lysis of the microbe or cell. Some of the complement components activated along the way are also opsonins (e.g., C3b); they bind to the target antigen and thereby direct phagocytes, which carry receptors specific for these opsonins, to focus their phagocytic activity on the target antigen. Other components from the activation of complement are chemotactic; specifically, they attract phagocytic cells. All in all, the activation of complement by IgG has profound biologic effects on the host and on the target antigen, whether it is a live cell, a microorganism, or a tumor cell.

Neutralization of Toxins

The IgG molecule is an excellent antibody for the ***neutralization*** of toxins such as ***tetanus*** and ***botulinus***, or for the inactivation of, for example, snake and scorpion venoms. Because of its ability to neutralize such poisons (mostly by blocking their active sites) and because of its long half-life, compared to that of other isotypes, the IgG molecule is the isotype of choice for ***passive immunization*** (i.e., gamma globulin injections discussed above) against toxins and venoms.

Immobilization of Bacteria

IgG molecules are efficient in immobilizing various motile bacteria. The reaction of antibodies specific for the flagella and cilia of certain microorganisms causes them to clump, thereby arresting their movement and preventing their ability to spread or invade tissue.

Neutralization of Viruses

IgG antibody is an efficient virus-neutralizing antibody. One mechanism of neutralization is that in which the antibody binds with antigenic determinants present on various portions of the virus coat, among which is the region used by the virus for attachment to the target cell. Inhibition of viral attachment effectively arrests infection. Other antibodies are thought to inhibit viral penetration or shedding of the viral coat required for release of the viral DNA or RNA needed to induce infection.

The versatility in function of the IgG molecule makes it a very important molecule in the immune response. Its importance is underscored in those immune deficiency disorders in which an individual is unable to synthesize IgG molecules (see Chapter 18). Such individuals are prone to infections that may result in toxemias and death.

STRUCTURAL FEATURES OF IgM

As we shall see later in this chapter, IgM is the first immunoglobulin produced following immunization. Its name derives from its initial description as a macroglobulin (M) of high molecular weight (900,000 Da). It has a sedimentation coefficient of 19S, and it has an extra C_H domain. In comparison to the IgG molecule, which consists of one four-chain structure, IgM is a pentameric molecule composed of five such units, each of which consists of two light and two heavy chains, all joined together by additional disulfide bonds between their Fc portions and by a polypeptide chain termed the *J chain* (see Figure 5.9). The J chain, which, like light and heavy chains, is synthesized in the B cell or plasma cell, has a molecular weight of 15,000 Da. This pentameric ensemble of IgM, which is held together by disulfide bonds, comes apart after mild treatment with reducing agents such as mercaptoethanol.

Surprisingly, each pentameric IgM molecule appears to have a valence of 5 (i.e., five antigen-combining sites), instead of the expected valence of 10 predicted by the 10 Fab segments contained in the pentamer. This apparent reduction in valence is probably the result of conformational constraints imposed by the polymerization. It is known that pentameric IgM has a planar configuration, such that each of its 10 Fab portions cannot open fully with respect to the adjacent Fab, when it combines with antigen, as is possible in the case of IgG. Thus, any large antigen bound to one Fab may block a neighboring site from binding with antigen, making the molecule appear pentavalent (or of even lesser valence).

BIOLOGIC PROPERTIES OF IgM

IgM present in adult human serum is found predominantly in the intravascular spaces. The half-life of the IgM molecule is approximately 5 days. In contrast to IgG, the IgM antibodies are not very versatile; they are poor toxin-neutralizing antibodies, and they are not efficient in the neutralization of viruses. IgM in monomeric form is also found on the surface of mature B cells together with IgD (see below), where it serves as an antigen-specific BCR. Once the B cell is activated by antigen following ligation of the BCR, it may undergo class switching (see Chapter 7) and begin to secrete and express other membrane Ig isotypes (e.g., IgG).

Complement Fixation

Because of its pentameric form, IgM is an excellent complement-fixing or complement-activating antibody (see Chapters 2 and 14). Unlike other classes of immunoglobulins, a single molecule of IgM, upon binding to antigen with at least two of its Fab arms, can initiate activation of the classical pathway of complement, making it the most efficient immunoglobulin as an initiator of the complement-mediated lysis of microorganisms and other cells. This ability, taken together with the appearance of IgM as the first class of antibodies generated after immunization or infection, makes IgM antibodies very important as providers of an early line of immunologic defense against bacterial infections.

Neonatal Immunity and First Line of Humoral Defense

Unlike IgG, IgM antibodies do not pass through the placenta; however, since this is the only class of immunoglobulins that is synthesized by the fetus beginning at approximately 5 months of gestation, elevated levels of IgM in the fetus are indicative of congenital or perinatal infection.

IgM is the isotype synthesized by children and adults in appreciable amounts after immunization or exposure to T-independent antigens, and it is the first isotype that is synthesized after immunization (see Figure 5.12). Thus, elevated levels of IgM usually indicate either recent infection or recent exposure to antigen.

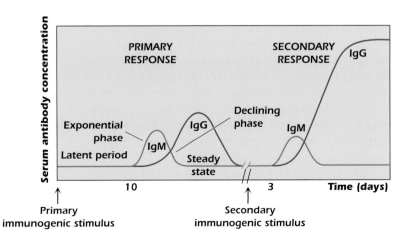

Figure 5.12. The kinetics of an antibody response.

Agglutination

IgM molecules are efficient agglutinating antibodies. Because of their pentameric form, IgM antibodies can form macromolecular bridges between epitopes on molecules that may be too distant from each other to be bridged by the smaller IgG antibodies. Furthermore, because of their pentameric form and multiple valence, the IgM antibodies are particularly well suited to combine with antigens that contain repeated patterns of the same antigenic determinant, as in the case of polysaccharide antigens or cellular antigens, which are multiply expressed on cell surfaces.

Isohemagglutinins

The IgM antibodies include the *isohemagglutinins*—the naturally occurring antibodies against the red blood cell antigens of the ABO blood groups. These antibodies are presumed to arise as a result of immunization by bacteria in the gastrointestinal and respiratory tracts, which bear determinants similar to the oligosaccharides of the ABO blood groups. Thus, without known prior immunization, people with the type O blood group have isohemagglutinins to the A and B antigens; those with the type A blood group have antibodies to the B antigens; and those with the B antigen have antibodies to the A antigen. An individual of the AB group has neither anti-A nor anti-B antibodies. Fortunately, the IgM isohemagglutinins do not pass through the placenta, so incompatibility of the ABO groups between mother and fetus poses no danger to the fetus. However, transfusion reactions, which arise as a result of ABO incompatibility, and in which the recipient's isohemagglutinins react with the donor's red blood cells, may have disastrous consequences.

STRUCTURAL AND BIOLOGIC PROPERTIES OF IgA

IgA is found in the serum as a monomeric molecule. It is also the major immunoglobulin in external secretions such as saliva, mucus, sweat, gastric fluid, and tears as a dimeric molecule. It is, moreover, the major immunoglobulin found in the colostrum of milk in nursing mothers, and it may provide the neonate with a major source of intestinal protection against pathogens during the first few weeks after birth. The IgA molecule consists of either two κ light chains or two λ light chains and two α heavy chains. The α chain is somewhat larger than the γ chain. The molecular weight of monomeric IgA is approximately 165,000 Da, and its sedimentation coefficient is 7S. Electrophoretically it migrates to the slow β or fast γ region of serum globulins. Dimeric IgA has a molecular weight of 400,000 Da.

The IgA class of immunoglobulins contains two subclasses: IgA_1 (93%) and IgA_2 (7%). It is interesting to note that if all production of IgA on mucosal surfaces (respiratory, gastrointestinal, and urinary tracts) is taken into account, IgA would be the major immunoglobulin in terms of quantity.

Biologic Properties of IgA

Serum IgA, which has no known biologic function, has a half-life of 5.5 days. The IgA present in serum is predominantly monomeric (one four-chain unit) and has presumably been released before dimerization so that it fails to bind to the secretory component. Secretory IgA is very important biologically, but little is known of any function for serum IgA.

Most IgA is present not in the serum, but in secretions such as tears, saliva, sweat, and mucus, where it serves an important biologic function as part of the mucosa-associated lymphoid tissue (MALT) as mentioned in Chapter 3. Within mucous secretions, IgA exists as a dimer consisting of two four-chain units linked by the same joining (J) chain found in IgM molecules (see Figure 5.9). IgA-secreting plasma cells synthesize the IgA molecules and the J chains, which form the dimers. Such plasma cells are located predominantly in the connective tissue called *lamina propria* that lies immediately below the basement membrane of many surface epithelia (e.g., in the parotid gland, along the gastrointestinal tract in the intestinal villi, in tear glands, in the lactating breast, or beneath bronchial mucosa). When these dimeric molecules are released from plasma cells, they bind to the poly-Ig receptor expressed on the basal membranes of adjacent epithelial cells. This receptor transports the molecules through the epithelial cells and releases them into extracellular fluids (e.g., in the gut or bronchi). Release is facilitated by enzymatic cleavage of the poly-Ig receptor, leaving a large 70,000 Da fragment (i.e., the secretory component) of the receptor still attached to the Fc piece of the dimeric IgA molecule (see Figure 5.13). The secretory component may help to protect the dimeric IgA from proteolytic cleavage. It should also be noted that the secretory component also binds and transports pentameric IgM to mucosal surfaces in small amounts.

Role in Mucosal Infections

Because of its presence in secretions, such as saliva, urine, and gastric fluid, secretory IgA is of importance in the primary immunologic defense against local respiratory or gastrointestinal infections. Its protective effect is thought to be due to its ability to prevent the invading organism from attaching to and penetrating the epithelial surface. For example, in the case of cholera, the pathogenic Vibrio organism attaches to, but never penetrates beyond, the cells that line the gastrointestinal tract, where it secretes an exotoxin responsible for all symptoms. IgA antibody, which can prevent attachment of the organism to the cells, provides protection from the pathogen. Thus, for protection against local infections, routes of immunization that result in local

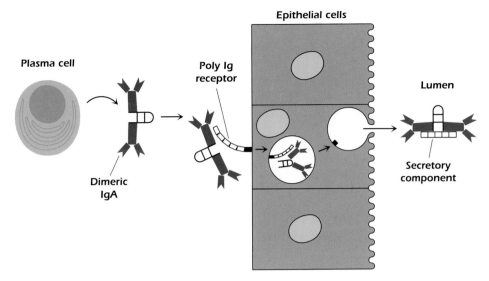

Figure 5.13. Transcytosis of dimeric IgA across epithelia. Plasma cells in close proximity to epithelial basement membranes in the gut, respiratory epithelia, salivary and tear glands, and lactating mammary glands, release dimeric IgA. The IgA binds to the poly-Ig receptor and the complex undergoes transcytosis within vesicles across the cell. The poly-Ig receptor is cleaved from the complex at the apical surface to release the IgA from the cell. After exiting the cell, a pentameric fragment of the poly-Ig receptor known as the secretory component remains attached to the dimeric IgA and is believed to protect the antibody within the lumen of several organs that are in contact with the external environment.

production of IgA are much more effective than routes that primarily produce antibodies in serum.

Bactericidal Activity

The IgA molecule does not contain receptors for complement, and thus IgA is not a complement-activating or complement-fixing immunoglobulin. Consequently, it does not induce complement-mediated bacterial lysis. However, IgA has been shown to possess bactericidal activity against Gram-negative organisms, but only in the presence of lysozyme, which is also present in the same secretions that contain secretory IgA.

Antiviral Activity

Secretory IgA is an efficient antiviral antibody, preventing the viruses from entering host cells. In addition, secretory IgA is an efficient agglutinating antibody.

STRUCTURAL AND BIOLOGIC PROPERTIES OF IgD

The IgD molecule consists of either two κ or two λ light chains and two δ heavy chains (see Figure 5.9). IgD is

present as a monomer with a molecular weight of 180,000 Da, it has a sedimentation coefficient of 7S, and it migrates to the fast γ region of serum globulins. No heavy chain allotypes (see below) or subclasses have been reported for the IgD molecule.

IgD is present in serum in very low and variable amounts because IgD-secreting plasma cells are rare and, among immunoglobulins, IgD is highly susceptible to proteolytic degradation due to its long hinge region. In addition, following B-cell activation, transcription of the δ heavy chain protein is rapidly downregulated, a phenomenon that also helps to explain the low serum IgD levels.

IgD is co-expressed with IgM on the surface of mature B cells and, like IgM, functions as an antigen-specific BCR. Its presence there serves as a marker of the differentiation of B cells to a more mature form. Thus, during ontogeny of B cells, expression of IgD lags behind that of IgM (see Chapter 8).

While the function of IgD has not been fully elucidated, expression of membrane IgD appears to correlate with the elimination of B cells with the capacity to generate self-reactive antibodies. Thus, during development, the major biologic significance of IgD may be in silencing autoreactive B cells. In mature B cells, IgD serves as an antigen-binding surface Ig together with co-expressed IgM.

STRUCTURAL AND BIOLOGIC PROPERTIES OF IgE

The IgE molecule consists of two light chains (κ or λ) and two heavy ε chains. Like IgM molecules, IgE has an extra C_H domain (see Figure 5.9). IgE has a molecular weight of approximately 200,000 Da, its sedimentation coefficient is 8S, and it migrates electrophoretically to the fast γ region of serum globulins.

Importance of IgE in Parasitic Infections and Hypersensitivity Reactions

IgE, also termed *reaginic antibody*, has a half-life in serum of 2 days, the shortest half-life of all classes of immunoglobulins. It is present in serum in the lowest concentration of all immunoglobulins. These low levels are due in part to a low rate of synthesis and to the unique ability of the Fc portion of IgE containing the extra C_H domain to bind with very high affinity to receptors (Fcε receptors) found on mast cells and basophils. Once bound to these high-affinity receptors, IgE may be retained by these cells for weeks or months. When antigen reappears, it combines with the Fab portion of the IgE attached to these cells, causing it to be cross-linked. The cells become activated and release the contents of their granules: histamine, heparin, leukotrienes, and other pharmacologically active compounds that trigger the immediate hypersensitivity reactions. These reactions may be mild, as in the case of a mosquito bite, or severe, as in the case of bronchial asthma; they may even result in systemic anaphylaxis, which can cause death within minutes (see Chapter 15).

IgE is not an agglutinating or complement-activating antibody; nevertheless, it has a role in protection against certain parasites, such as helminths (worms), a protection achieved by activation of the same acute inflammatory response seen in a more pathologic form of immediate hypersensitivity responses. Elevated levels of IgE in serum have been shown to occur during infections with ascaris (a roundworm). In fact, immunization with ascaris antigen induces the formation of IgE.

KINETICS OF THE ANTIBODY RESPONSE FOLLOWING IMMUNIZATION

Primary Response

As already mentioned, the first exposure of an individual to a particular immunogen is referred to as the priming immunization and the measurable response that ensues is called the primary response. As shown in Figure 5.12, the primary antibody response may be divided into several phases, as follows:

(1) *Latent or lag phase.* After initial exposure to an antigen, a period of 1 to 2 weeks follows before antibody is detectable in the serum. The actual length of time depends on the species immunized, the nature of the antigen used to stimulate the response, and other factors that will become apparent in subsequent chapters. The length of the latent period is also greatly dependent on the sensitivity of the assay used to measure the product of the response. As we shall see in more detail in subsequent chapters, the latent period includes the time taken for T and B cells to make contact with the antigen, to proliferate, and to differentiate. B cells must also secrete antibody in sufficient quantity so that it can be detected in the serum. The less sensitive the assay used for detection of antibody, the more antibody will be required for detection and the longer the apparent latent period will be.

(2) *Exponential phase.* During this phase, the concentration of antibody in the serum increases exponentially.

(3) *Steady state.* During this period, production and degradation of antibody are balanced.

(4) *Declining phase.* Finally, the immune response begins to shut down, and the concentration of antibody in serum declines rapidly.

The first class of antibody detected in primary responses is generally IgM, which, in some instances, may be the only class of immunoglobulin that is made. If production of IgG antibody ensues, its appearance is generally accompanied by a rapid cessation of production of IgM (see Figure 5.12).

Secondary Response

Although production of antibody after a priming contact with antigen may cease entirely within a few weeks (see Figure 5.12), the immunized individual is left with a pool of long-lived *memory cells* capable of mounting a secondary response as well as any other future responses to the antigen. Experimentally, this memory response (also called *anamnestic response*) becomes apparent when a response is triggered by a second injection of the same antigen used to stimulate a primary response. After the second injection, the lag phase is considerably shorter and antibody may appear in less than half the time required for the primary response. The magnitude of antibody produced in these responses is much greater than that seen in the primary response with significantly higher concentrations of antibody detectable in the serum. The production of antibody may also continue for a longer period, with persistent levels remaining in serum months, or even years, later.

There is a marked change in the type of antibody produced in the secondary response, as reflected in the appearance of different classes of immunoglobulins with the same antigen specificity. This shift is known as *class switching*, with IgG antibodies appearing at higher concentrations and with greater persistence, than IgM antibodies, which may be greatly reduced or disappear altogether. This may be also accompanied by the appearance of IgA and IgE. In addition, *affinity maturation* occurs, a phenomenon in which the average affinity (binding constant) of the antibodies for the antigen increases as the secondary response develops (see Chapter 8). The driving force for this increase in affinity may be a selection process during which B cells compete with free antibody to capture a decreasing amount of antigen. Thus, only those B cell clones with high-affinity Ig receptors on their surfaces will bind enough antigen to ensure that the B cells are triggered to differentiate into plasma cells. These plasma cells, which arise from preferentially selected B cells, synthesize this antibody with high affinity for antigen.

The capacity to make a secondary response may persist for a long time (years in humans), and it provides an obvious selective advantage for an individual who survives the first contact with an invading pathogen. Establishment of this memory for generating a specific response is, of course, the purpose of public health immunization programs.

THE IMMUNOGLOBULIN SUPERFAMILY

The shared structural features of immunoglobulin heavy and light chains that include the *immunoglobulin-fold domains* (see Figures 5.3 and 5.4) are also seen in a large number of proteins. Most of these have been found to be membrane-bound glycoproteins. Because of this structural similarity, these proteins are classified as members of the *immunoglobulin superfamily*. The redundant structural characteristic seen in these proteins suggests that the genes that encode them arose from a common primordial gene—one that generated the basic domain structure. Duplication and subsequent divergence of this primordial gene would explain the existence of the large number of membrane proteins that possess one or more regions homologous to the immunoglobulin-fold domain. Genetic and functional analyses of these immunoglobulin superfamily proteins have indicated that these genes have evolved independently, since they do not share genetic linkage or function. Figure 5.14 illustrates some examples of proteins that are members of the immunoglobulin superfamily. Numerous other examples are discussed in other chapters. As can be seen, each molecule contains the characteristic Ig-fold structure (loops) formed as a result of intrachain disulfide bonds and consisting of approximately 110 amino acids. These immunoglobulin-fold domains are believed to facilitate interactions between membrane proteins (e.g., CD4 molecules on helper T cells and class II major histocompatibility complex [MHC] molecules on antigen-presenting cells).

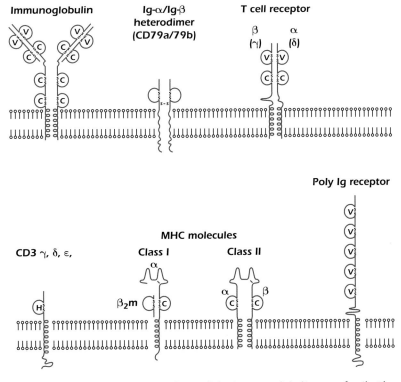

Figure 5.14. Representative members of the immunoglobulin superfamily. The immunoglobulin-fold domains (shown as circular loops in blue) form the common structural features of these molecules. In all cases, the carboxyl-terminal end of the molecules shown are anchored in the membrane.

SUMMARY

1. Immunoglobulins of all classes have a fundamental four-chain structure, consisting of two identical light (L) and two identical heavy (H) chains. Through disulfide bonds, each light chain is linked to a heavy chain, and the two heavy chains are linked to each other.

2. In the native state, L and H chains are coiled into domains stabilized by an intrachain disulfide bond. A group of other proteins (e.g., TCR, CD4, class I and class II MHC molecules) also contain these immunoglobulin-fold domains, making them all members of the immunoglobulin superfamily.

3. Immunoglobulins are expressed in two forms: a membrane-bound antibody present on the surface of B cells and a secreted antibody produced by plasma cells. Membrane-bound antibodies associate with a heterodimer called Igα/Igβ to form the B-cell receptor (BCR).

4. The N-terminal domains of both heavy and light chains are the variable (V) regions and contain the hypervariable regions, also called *complementarity-determining regions* (CDRs), which make up the combining site of the antibody and vary according to the specificity of the antibody.

5. The constant (C) region domains of L and H chains are similar within each of the L and H chain isotypes, respectively.

6. The Fc regions of the heavy chains are responsible for the different biologic functions carried out by each class of antibody.

7. Immunoglobulin heavy and light chain isotypes are distinguished by the structure of their constant regions. Differences in regions of the H chain constant regions are due to different genetic alleles causing even a one or two amino acid change. These are called *allotypes*, and they distinguish individuals within a species. By contrast, idiotypic markers are represented by the unique combinations of amino acids that make up the antigen-combining site of an antibody molecule; thus, they are unique for that particular antibody.

8. IgG is a versatile class of antibody, capable of carrying out numerous biologic functions that range from neutralization of toxins to activation of complement and opsonization. IgG is the only class of immunoglobulin that passes through the placenta and confers maternal immunity on the fetus. The half-life of IgG (23 days) is the longest of all immunoglobulin classes.

9. IgM is expressed on the surface of mature B cells (as a monomer) and is secreted as a pentameric antibody held together by a J chain; of all classes of immunoglobulin it functions as the best agglutinating and complement-activating antibody.

10. Monomeric IgA is found in serum, whereas dimeric IgA is found in secretions and is referred to as *secretory IgA*. Secretory IgA is an important antiviral immunoglobulin.

11. IgD is present on the surface of mature B cells and is co-expressed and shares antigen-specificity with IgM. The functional properties of IgD have not been fully elucidated.

12. IgE, also called *reaginic antibody*, is of paramount importance in allergic reactions. It also appears to be of importance in protection against parasitic infections. The Fc portion of IgE binds with high affinity to receptors on certain cells including mast cells. On contact with antigen, IgE triggers the degranulation of such cells, resulting in the release of pharmacologically active substances that mediate the hypersensitivity (allergic) reactions.

13. Following first exposure to an antigen, a primary antibody response occurs that consists mainly of the production of IgM antibodies. The second exposure to the same antigen results in a secondary or anamnestic (memory) response, which is more rapid than the primary response and in which the response shifts from IgM production to the synthesis of IgG and other isotypes. The secondary response lasts much longer than the primary response.

REFERENCES AND BIBLIOGRAPHY

Alzari PM, Lascombe MB, Poljak RJ. (1988) Three-dimensional structure of antibodies. *Annu Rev Immunol* 6: 555.

Capra D, Edmundson AB. (1977) The antibody combining site. *Sci Am* 236: 50.

Carayannopoulos L, Capra JD. (1998) Immunoglobulins: structure and function. In Paul WE. (ed) Fundamental Immunology, 4th ed. New York: Raven Press.

Davies DR, Metzger H. (1983) Structural basis of antibody function. *Annu Rev Immunol* 1: 87.

Eisen HN. (2001) Specificity and degeneracy in antigen recognition: Yin and yang in the immune response. *Ann Rev Immunol* 19: 1.

Jefferis R. (1993) What is an idiotype? *Immunol Today* 14: 19.

Junghans RP, Anderson CL. (1996) The protection receptor for IgG catabolism is the β2-microglobulin-containing neonatal intestinal transport receptor. *Proc Natl Acad Sci USA* 93: 5512.

Koshland ME. (1985) The coming of age of the immunoglobulin J chain. *Annu Rev Immunol* 3: 425.

Mestecky J, McGhee JR. (1987) Immunoglobulin A. (IgA) Molecular and cellular interactions involved in IgA biosynthesis and immune response. *Adv Immunol* 40: 153.

Stanfield RL, Fisher TM, Lerner R, Wilson IA. (1990) Crystal structure of an antibody to a peptide and its complex with peptide antigen at 2.8 D. *Science* 248: 712.

Tomasi TB. (1992) The discovery of secretory IgA and the mucosal immune system. *Immunol Today* 13: 416.

Williams AF, Barclay AN. (1988) The immunoglobulin superfamily. *Annu Rev Immunol* 6: 381.

REVIEW QUESTIONS

For each question, choose the ONE BEST answer or completion.

1. Functional properties of immunoglobulins such as binding to Fc receptors are associated with
   A) light chains
   B) J chains
   C) disulfide bonds
   D) heavy chains
   E) variable regions

2. The idiotype of an antibody molecule is determined by the amino acid sequence of the
   A) constant region of the light chain
   B) variable region of the light chain
   C) constant region of the heavy chain
   D) constant regions of the heavy and light chains
   E) variable regions of the heavy and light chains

3. Which of the following would generate a polyclonal rabbit antiserum specific for human γ heavy-chain, κ chain, λ chain, and Fc regions of Ig:
   A) Bench Jones proteins
   B) pooled IgG
   C) pepsin digested IgG
   D) purified Fab
   E) purified F(ab′)₂

4. A polyclonal antiserum raised against pooled human IgA will react with
   A) human IgM
   B) κ light chains
   C) human IgG
   D) J chain
   E) all of the above

5. An individual was found to be heterzygous for IgG₁ allotypes 3 and 12. The different possible IgG₁ antibodies produced by this individual will never have
   A) two heavy chains of allotype 12
   B) two light chains of either κ or λ
   C) two heavy chains of allotype 3
   D) two heavy chains, one of allotype 3 and one of allotype 12

6. Papain digestion of an IgG preparation of antibody specific for the antigen hen egg albumin (HEA) will
   A) lose its antigen specificity
   B) precipitate with HEA
   C) lose all interchain disulfide bonds
   D) produce two Fab molecules and one Fc fragment
   E) none of the above

7. If an individual who is highly allergic to cat dander is exposed to a pet cat in a friend's house, which class of immunoglobulin would most likely be found to be elevated soon after this exposure?
   A) IgA
   B) IgE
   C) IgG
   D) IgM
   E) IgD

8. Which of the following immunoglobulins can activate complement as a single molecule when bound to an antigen?
   A) IgA
   B) IgE
   C) IgG
   D) IgM
   E) IgD

9. The relative level of pathogen-specific IgM antibodies can be of diagnostic significance because
   A) IgM is easier to detect than the other isotypes
   B) viral infection often results in very high IgM responses
   C) IgM antibodies are more often protective against reinfections than are the other isotypes
   D) relatively high levels of IgM often correlate with a first and recent exposure to the inducing agent

10. Primary and secondary antibody responses differ in
    A) the predominant isotype generated
    B) the number of lymphocytes responding to antigen
    C) the time it takes for measurable amounts of antibodies to appear in the serum
    D) the biologic functions manifested by the Ig isotypes produced
    E) all of the above

11. In an individual predisposed to allergic responses, which of the following statement best describes the outcome of his/her exposure to an allergen:
    A) Within weeks of exposure, large amounts of allergen-specific IgM will be present in the serum.
    B) Clinical reactions such as wheezing and sneezing may soon manifest soon after exposure due to the presence of allergen-specific IgE that is retained by cells such as mast cells that express Fcε receptors.
    C) IgG responses will control the allergic responses by suppressing the ability of activated allergen-specific B cells to undergo IgE class switching.
    D) Circulating allergen-specific IgE will initiate an inflammatory response that may manifest as runny, itchy eyes.
    E) all of the above

ANSWERS TO REVIEW QUESTIONS

1. *D.* The C-terminal end of the constant region of the heavy contains the domains that are associated with biologic activity of immunoglobulins.

2. *E.* The idiotype is the antigenic determinant of an Ig molecule, which involves its antigen-combining site, which in turn consists of contributions from the variable regions of both L and H chains.

3. *B.* Only pooled IgG containing the a mixture of IgG molecules each expressing the γ heavy chain (thus the Fc region) and either the κ or λ light chains would generate an antiserum to each of these immunoglobulin components. None of the other answer choices would stimulate antibodies to all of these components. Bench Jones proteins are dimmers of light chains found in the urine of patients with multiple myeloma. Pepsin treatment of IgG results in the digestion of the Fc region. Purified Fab and F(ab′)₂ fragments lack the γ heavy chain (thus the Fc region).

4. *E.* All are correct statements. Antibody to IgA will have antibody specific for κ and λ light chains, which, of course, will react with IgG and IgM, both of which have κ and λ chains. Antibody will also be present against J chain if the IgA used for immunization was dimeric.

5. *D.* In any immunoglobulin produced by a single cell, the two heavy chains and the two light chains are identical. Therefore, any antibody molecule in this individual would have either allotype 3 heavy chains or allotype 12 heavy chains, not a mixture. Similarly, the antibody would have either two κ or two λ chains.

6. *D.* Papain digestion cleaves the IgG molecules above the hinge region, generating two Fab molecules and an Fc fragment. The Fab fragments can still bind to HEA, but since they are not held together by disulfide binds, they cannot precipitate the antigen. This contrasts with the effects of pepsin treatment of IgG, which cleaves below the hinge region, leaving intact one divalent F(ab′)₂ molecule capable of precipitating the antigen. Fragments of pepsin-treated HEA-specific antibody will have the same affinity for the antigen as the original Fab regions of the antibody, since the CDR regions of the molecules are preserved.

7. *B.* The major class of immunoglobulin produced in response to allergens is IgE.

8. *D.* Only IgM can activate or fix complement when a single molecule is bound to antigen. This is due to the pentameric form of this immunoglobulin class.

9. *D.* Only the last statement is correct. Relatively high levels of IgM often correlate with first recent exposure to an inducing agent, since IgM is the first isotype synthesized in response to an immunogen. All other statements are not true.

10. *E.* All are correct. The statements are self-explanatory.

11. *B.* Individuals predisposed to allergic responses produce large amounts of IgE antibodies with specificity for allergens. Once produced, the IgE becomes bound for long periods of time (weeks-to-months) to various cells that express high affinity Fcε receptors (e.g., tissue mast cells). When the allergens interact with the Fab portions of these IgE molecules, cross-linking the cell-bound antibodies, this results in destabilization of the cell membrane followed by degranulization of the cell. Finally, this results in the release of potent pharmacologically active agents that cause the clinical symptom associated with allergies.

6

ANTIGEN–ANTIBODY INTERACTIONS, IMMUNE ASSAYS, AND EXPERIMENTAL SYSTEMS

INTRODUCTION

In previous chapters, we have, by necessity, touched upon several techniques and assays that have been used to help us understand some fundamental aspects of innate and adaptive immunity. In this chapter we discuss, in greater detail, *in vitro* techniques, assays, and experimental systems that are used in research and diagnostic laboratories. Some of these are strictly antibody-based (e.g., ***serological methods***), whereas others employ molecular biological methods, genetic engineering, cell culture techniques, and *in vivo* animal models that have greatly contributed to our understanding of the physiology and pathophysiology of the immune system. Since the sequencing of the human genome in 2000, and with aggressive efforts to sequence microbial genomes, approaches that use bioinformatics and computational biology (so-called *in silico* analyses) have emerged as promising methods for the study of our immune system. Using information derived from genomic and proteomic databases, powerful software tools and algorithms, these technologies hold great promise for the field of immunology. This is particularly true with regard to important efforts to identify immunogenic epitopes expressed by pathogens that can be studied further as candidate vaccines. Although this topic is beyond the scope of this chapter, it is important to keep in mind that future progress in the field of immunology will come from a combination of *in vitro*, *in vivo*, and *in silico* approaches.

We begin this chapter with a discussion of physical dynamics of antigen–antibody interactions.

ANTIGEN–ANTIBODY INTERACTIONS

The reaction between antigen and antibodies serves as the basis for many immune assays. Because of the exquisite specificity of the immune response, the interaction between antigen and antibody *in vitro* is widely used for diagnostic purposes, for the detection and identification of either antigen or antibody. An example of the use of serological methods for the identification and classification of antigens is the ***serotyping*** of various microorganisms by the use of specific antisera.

The interaction of antigen with antibodies may result in a variety of outcomes, including ***precipitation*** (if the antigen is soluble), ***agglutination*** (if the antigen is particulate), and ***activation of complement***. All of these outcomes are caused by the interactions between multivalent antigens and antibodies that have at least two combining sites per molecule. The consequences of antigen–antibody interaction listed above do not represent the primary interaction between antibodies and a given antigen but rather depend on secondary phenomena, which result from the interactions between multivalent antigens and antibodies. Such phenomena as the formation of precipitate, agglutination, and complement activation would not occur if the antibody with two or more combining sites reacted with a hapten (i.e., a unideterminant, univalent antigen), nor would they occur as a result of the interaction between a univalent fragment of antibody, such as Fab, and an antigen, even if the antigen is multivalent. The reasons for these differences are depicted in Figure 6.1. ***Cross-linking*** of various antigen molecules by antibody is required for precipitation, agglutination, or complement activation, and it is possible only if the antigen is multivalent and the antibody is divalent [either intact, or F(ab')$_2$]. Figure 6.1 illustrates several different types of antigens and their interactions with antibody molecules or fragments thereof [Fab versus F(ab')$_2$]. Figure 6.1E illustrates a typical multivarient antigen, one that expresses multiple antigenic determinants or *epitopes* (in this case, epitopes A, B, and C) to which antibody responses have been generated (anti-A, anti-B, and anti-C, respectively). Pathogenic microorganisms are good examples of multivariant antigens since they express an array of epitopes to which B and T cells respond during an immune response to these pathogens. The assembly of immune complexes resulting from cross-linking facilitates several goals of the immune system that are collectively aimed at destroying, neutralizing, and eliminating the pathogenic organism. As we have discussed in earlier chapters, immune complexes activate the classical complement pathway leading to the assembly of a membrane attack complex and lysis of the organism. In addition, the immune complex brings together a high density of Fc regions of the antibodies interacting with antigen, which increases the chance that phagocytic cells expressing Fc receptors will bind to these Fc regions to initiate phagocytosis of the antigen. Finally, since complement activation also generates C3b components that also bind to immune complexes, red blood cells expressing CR1 receptors on their surface bind to the C3b-decorated immune complexes and transport them to phagocytes in liver and spleen for removal.

In contrast with multivalent antigens, Figure 6.1A shows molecules expressing a single low molecular weight *hapten* (A). If an antibody response is generated to this hapten (recall that this would require immunization using the molecule expressing the hapten together with a carrier protein in order to make the hapten immunogenic), the interactions between the anti-A antibodies and the antigen expressing the single hapten would result in complexes that are not cross-linked. Similarly, if one were to combine Fab fragments of an antibody specific for a unideterminant, multivalent antigen shown in Figure 6.1C, cross-linking of antibody–antigen complexes would not occur. Finally, in the case of unideterminant (epitope A), multivalent antigens shown in Figure 6.1B–D, cross-linking will occur when this antigen interacts with intact anti-A antibodies (Figure 6.1B) or divalent F(ab')$_2$ anti-A fragments (Figure 6.1C) but not with monovalent anti-A Fab fragments (Figure 6.1D).

PRIMARY INTERACTIONS BETWEEN ANTIBODY AND ANTIGEN

No covalent bonds are involved in the interaction between antibody and an antigen. Consequently, the binding forces are relatively weak. They consist mainly of *van der Waals forces*, *electrostatic forces*, and *hydrophobic forces*, all of

which require a very close proximity among the interacting moieties. Thus the interaction requires a very close fit between an epitope and the antibody, a fit that is often compared to that between a lock and a key. Because of the low levels of energy involved in the interaction between antigen and antibody, antigen–antibody complexes can be readily dissociated by low or high pH, by high salt concentrations, or by chaotropic ions, such as cyanates, which efficiently interfere with the hydrogen bonding of water molecules.

Association Constant

The reaction between an antibody and an epitope of an antigen is exemplified by the reaction between antibody and a univalent hapten. Because an antibody molecule is symmetric, with two identical Fab antigen-combining sites, one antibody molecule binds with two identical monovalent hapten molecules, each Fab binding in an independent fashion with one hapten molecule. The binding of a monovalent antigen (Ag) with each site can be represented by the equation:

$$Ag + Ab \underset{k_{-1}}{\overset{k_1}{\rightleftharpoons}} AbAg,$$

where k_1 represents the forward (association) rate constant and k_{-1} represents the reverse (dissociation) rate constant. The ratio of k_1/k_{-1} is the association constant K, a measure of affinity. It can be calculated by determining the ratio of bound AbAg complex to the concentration of unbound antigen and antibody. Thus,

$$K = \frac{k_1}{k_{-1}} = \frac{[AbAg]}{[Ab][Ag]}.$$

The association constant (K) is really a measure of the affinity of the antibody for the epitope (see below). When all the antibody molecules that bind a given hapten or epitope are identical (as in the case of monoclonal antibodies), then K represents the intrinsic association constant. However, because serum antibodies, even those binding to a single epitope, are heterogeneous, an average *association constant* of all the antibodies to the epitope is referred to as K_0. The interaction between antibodies and each epitope of a multivalent antigen follows the same kinetics and energetics as those involved in the interaction between antibodies and haptens because each epitope of the antigen reacts with its corresponding antibody in the same manner as that described above.

The association constant K can be determined using the method of *equilibrium dialysis*. In this procedure, a dialysis chamber is used in which two compartments are separated by a semipermeable membrane allowing the free passage of appropriately sized molecules from one side to the other. Antibody is placed on one side of the semipermeable

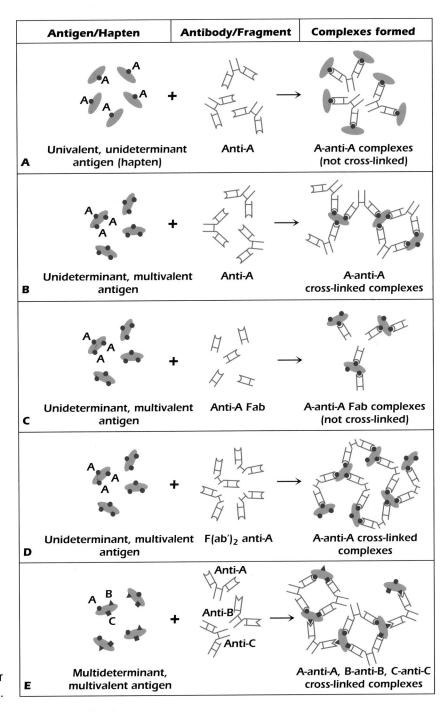

Antigen/Hapten	Antibody/Fragment	Complexes formed

A Univalent, unideterminant antigen (hapten) + Anti-A → A-anti-A complexes (not cross-linked)

B Unideterminant, multivalent antigen + Anti-A → A-anti-A cross-linked complexes

C Unideterminant, multivalent antigen + Anti-A Fab → A-anti-A Fab complexes (not cross-linked)

D Unideterminant, multivalent antigen + F(ab')₂ anti-A → A-anti-A cross-linked complexes

E Multideterminant, multivalent antigen + Anti-A, Anti-B, Anti-C → A-anti-A, B-anti-B, C-anti-C cross-linked complexes

Figure 6.1. Reactions between antibody or antibody fragments and antigens or hapten.

membrane and cannot pass through due to its size. On the antigen side of the membrane, a known amount of small, permeable, radiolabeled hapten molecules, oligosaccharides, or oligopeptides comprising the epitope of the complex carbohydrate or protein is added. At time zero, the hapten or antigenic epitope used (referred to as the *ligand* hereafter) will then diffuse across the membrane, and at equilibrium, the concentration of free ligand will be the same on both sides. However, the total amount of ligand will be greater on the side containing Ab because some of the ligand

will be bound to the antibody molecules. The difference in the ligand concentration in the two compartments represents the concentration of the ligand bound to antibody (i.e., the [AgAb] complex). The higher the affinity of the antibody, the more ligand is bound.

Since the concentration of antibody added to the equilibrium dialysis chamber can be predetermined and kept constant, varying concentrations of ligand can also be used in this analysis. This approach facilitates the so-called *Scatchard analysis* of the antibody. This is useful in determining whether a given antibody preparation is homogeneous (e.g., monoclonal antibody) or heterogeneous (e.g., polyclonal antiserum) and in measuring the average affinity constant (K_0).

Affinity and Avidity

As noted above, the intrinsic association constant that characterizes the binding of an antibody with an epitope or a hapten is termed *affinity*. When the antigen consists of many repeating identical epitopes or when antigens are multivalent, the association between the entire antigen molecule and antibodies depends not only on the affinity between each epitope and its corresponding antibody but also on the sum of the affinities of all the epitopes involved. For example, the affinity of binding of anti-A with multivalent A (shown in Figure 6.1) may be four or five orders of magnitude higher than between the same antibody (i.e., anti-A) and univalent A (Figure 6.1). This is because the pairing of anti-A with A (where A is multivalent) is influenced by the increased number of sites on A with which anti-A can react.

While the term *affinity* denotes the intrinsic association constant between antibody and a univalent ligand such as a hapten, the term *avidity* is used to denote the overall binding energy between antibodies and a multivalent antigen. Thus, in general, IgM antibodies are of higher avidity than IgG antibodies, although the binding of each Fab in the IgM antibody with ligand may be of the same affinity as that of the Fab from IgG.

SECONDARY INTERACTIONS BETWEEN ANTIBODY AND ANTIGEN

Agglutination Reactions

Referring again to the representations given in Figure 6.1, the reactions of antibody with a multivalent antigen that is *particulate* (i.e., an insoluble particle) results in the cross-linking of the various antigen particles by the antibodies. This cross-linking eventually results in the clumping or agglutination of the antigen particles by the antibodies.

Titer. The agglutination of an antigen as a result of cross-linking by antibodies is dependent on the correct proportion of antigen to antibody. A method sometimes used to measure the level of serum antibody specific for a particulate antigen is the agglutination assay. More sensitive, quantitative assays (e.g., enzyme-linked immunosorbent assay [ELISA], discussed later in this chapter) have largely replaced this approach for measuring antibody levels in serum. Indeed, the agglutinating titer of a certain serum is only a semiquantitative expression of the antibodies present in the serum; it is not a quantitative measure of the concentration of antibody (weight/volume). The assay is performed by mixing twofold serial dilutions of serum with a fixed concentration of antigen. High dilutions of serum usually do not cause antigen agglutination because at such dilutions there are not enough antibodies to cause appreciable, visible agglutination. The highest dilution of serum that still causes agglutination, but beyond which no agglutination occurs, is termed the *titer*. It is a common observation that agglutination may not occur at high concentrations of antibody, even though it does take place at higher dilutions of serum. The tubes with high concentrations of serum, where agglutination does not occur, represent a *prozone*. In the prozone, antibodies are present in excess. Agglutination may not occur at high ratio of antibody to antigen because every epitope on one particle may bind only to a single antibody molecule, preventing cross-linking between different particles.

Because of the prozone phenomenon, in testing for the presence of agglutinating antibodies to a certain antigen, it is imperative that the antiserum be tested at several dilutions. Testing serum at only one concentration may give misleading conclusions if no agglutination occurs, because the absence of agglutination might reflect either a prozone or a lack of antibody.

Zeta Potential. The surfaces of certain particulate antigens may possess an electrical charge, as, for example, the net negative charge on the surface of red blood cells caused by the presence of sialic acid. When such charged particles are suspended in saline solution, an electrical potential termed the *zeta potential* is created between particles, preventing them from getting very close to each other. This introduces a difficulty in agglutinating charged particles by antibodies, in particular red blood cells by IgG antibodies. The distance between the Fab arms of the IgG molecule, even in its most extended form, is too short to allow effective bridging between two red blood cells across the zeta potential. Thus, although IgG antibodies may be directed against antigens on the charged erythrocyte, agglutination may not occur because of the repulsion by the zeta potential. On the other hand, some of the Fab areas of IgM pentamers are far enough apart and can bridge red blood cells separated by the zeta potential. This property of IgM antibodies, together with their pentavalence, is a major reason for their effectiveness as agglutinating antibodies.

Through the years attempts were made to improve agglutination reactions by decreasing the zeta potential in various ways, none of which was universally applicable or effective. However, an ingenious method was devised in the 1950s by Coombs to overcome this problem. This method, described below, facilitates the agglutination of erythrocytes by IgG antibodies specific for erythrocyte antigens. It is also useful for the detection of nonagglutinating antibodies that are present on the surface of erythrocytes.

Coombs Test. The Coombs test employs antibodies to immunoglobulins (hence it is also called the *anti-immunoglobulin test*). It is based on two important facts: (1) that immunoglobulins of one species (e.g., human) are immunogenic when injected into another species (e.g.,

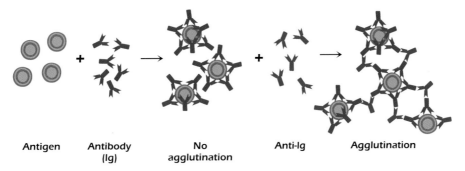

Figure 6.2. A representation of the anti-immunoglobulin (Coombs) test.

rabbit) and lead to the production of antibodies against the immunoglobulins, and (2) that many of the anti-immunoglobulins (e.g., rabbit anti-human Ig) bind with antigenic determinants present on the Fc portion of the antibody, and leave the Fab portions free to react with antigen. Thus, for example, if human IgG antibodies are attached to their respective epitopes on erythrocytes, then the addition of rabbit antibodies to human IgG will result in their binding with the Fc portions of the human antibodies bound to the erythrocytes by their Fab portion (see Figure 6.2). These rabbit antibodies not only bind with the human antibodies that are bound to the erythrocyte but also, by so doing, they cross-link (form bridges) between human IgG on relatively distant erythrocytes, across the separation caused by the zeta potential, and cause agglutination. The addition of anti-immunoglobulin brings about agglutination, even if the antibodies directed against the erythrocytes are present at sufficiently high concentrations to cause the prozone phenomenon.

There are two versions of the Coombs test: the ***direct Coombs test*** and the ***indirect Coombs test***. The two versions differ somewhat in the mechanics of the test but both are based on the same principle: using heterologous anti-immunoglobulins to detect a reaction between immunoglobulins and antigen. In the direct Coombs test, anti-immunoglobulins are added to the particles (e.g., red blood cells) that are suspected of having antibodies bound to antigens on their surfaces. For example, a newborn baby is suspected of having hemolytic disease of the newborn caused by maternal anti-Rh IgG antibodies that are bound to the baby's erythrocytes. If that suspicion proved to be correct, the direct Coombs test would have the following results: the addition of anti-immunoglobulin to a suspension of the baby's erythrocytes would result in the binding of the anti-immunoglobulin to the maternal IgG on the surface of the erythrocytes and would cause agglutination.

The indirect Coombs test is used to detect the presence, in the serum, of antibodies specific to antigens on a particle. The serum antibodies, when added to the particles, may fail to cause agglutination because of the zeta potential. The subsequent addition of anti-Ig will cause agglutination. A common application of the indirect Coombs test is in the

detection of anti-Rh IgG antibodies in the blood of an Rh⁻ woman (see Chapter 16). This consists, first, of the reaction of the woman's serum with Rh⁺ erythrocytes, and then the addition of the anti-immunoglobulin reagents (as in the direct Coombs test). Thus, the direct Coombs test, it measures Ab already bound to the red blood cells (RBCs) in the patient whereas the indirect test measures antibody in the serum of the patient.

Passive Agglutination. The agglutination reaction can be used with particulate antigens (e.g., erythrocytes or bacteria) and also with soluble antigens, provided that the soluble antigen can be firmly attached to insoluble particles. For example, the soluble antigen thyroglobulin can be attached to latex particles, so that the addition of antibodies to the thyroglobulin antigen will cause agglutination of the latex particles coated with thyroglobulin. Of course, the addition of soluble antigen to the antibodies before the introduction of the thyroglobulin-coated latex particles will inhibit the agglutination because the antibodies will first combine with the soluble antigen, and if the soluble antigen is present in excess, the antibodies will not be able to bind with the particulate antigen. This latter example is referred to as ***agglutination inhibition***. It should be distinguished from agglutination inhibition in which antibodies to certain viruses inhibit the agglutination of red blood cells by the virus. In these cases, the antibodies are directed to the area or areas on the virus that bind with the appropriate virus receptors on the red blood cells.

When the antigen is a natural constituent of a particle, the agglutination reaction is referred to as ***direct agglutination***. When the agglutination reaction takes place between antibodies and soluble antigen that had been attached to an insoluble particle, the reaction is referred to as ***passive agglutination***.

The agglutination reaction (direct or passive, either employing or not employing the Coombs test) is widely used clinically. In addition to the examples already given, major applications include erythrocyte typing in blood banks, diagnosis of various immunologically mediated hemolytic diseases such as drug-induced autoimmune hemolytic anemia, tests for rheumatoid factor (human IgM anti-human IgG), confirmatory test for syphilis, and the latex test for pregnancy, which involves the detection of human chorionic gonadotropin (HCG) in the urine of pregnant women.

Precipitation Reactions

Reaction in Solutions. In contrast to the agglutination reaction, which takes place between antibodies and particulate antigen, the ***precipitation reaction*** takes place when antibodies and soluble antigen are mixed. As in the case of agglutination, precipitation of antigen–antibody complexes occurs because the divalent antibody molecules cross-link multivalent antigen molecules to form a ***lattice***. When it reaches a certain size, this antigen–antibody complex loses its solubility and precipitates out of solution. The phenomenon of precipitation is termed the ***precipitin reaction***.

Figure 6.3 depicts a quantitative precipitin reaction. When increasing concentrations of antigen are added to a series of tubes that contain a constant concentration of antibodies, variable amounts of precipitate form. The weight of the precipitate in each tube may be determined by a variety of methods. If the amount of the precipitate is plotted against the amount of antigen added, a precipitin curve like the one shown in Figure 6.3 is obtained.

There are three important areas under the curve shown in Figure 6.3: (1) the zone of antibody excess, (2) the equivalence zone, and (3) the zone of antigen excess. In the equivalence zone, the proportion of antigen to antibody is optimal for maximal precipitation; in the zones of antibody excess or antigen excess, the proportions of the reactants do not lead to efficient cross-linking and formation of precipitate.

It should be emphasized that the zones of the precipitin curve are based on the amount of antigen–antibody complexes precipitated. However, the zones of antigen or antibody excess may contain soluble antigen–antibody complexes, particularly the zone of antigen excess where a minimal amount of precipitate is formed, but large amounts of antigen–antibody complexes are present in the supernatant. Thus, the amount of precipitate formed is dependent on the proportions of the reactant antigens and antibodies: the correct proportion of the reactions result in maximal formation of precipitate; excess of antigen (or antibody) results in soluble complexes.

In clinical laboratories, nephelometers are used to measure the amount of light scatter caused by antigen–antibody complexes in solution. They are also used to determine the levels of several blood plasma proteins, including complement. The technique is referred to as ***nephelometry*** and has largely replaced radial immunodiffusion (discussed later in this chapter). While both nephelometry and radial immunodiffusion measure immune complex formation, the former measures soluble immune complexes whereas the latter measures precipitated complexes. Therefore, these two approaches target different points on the precipitation curve.

Precipitation Reactions in Gels. Precipitation reactions between soluble antigens and antibodies can take place not only in solution but also in semisolid media such as agar gels. When soluble antigen and antibodies are placed in wells cut in the gel (Figure 6.4A), the reactants diffuse in the gel and form gradients of concentration, with the highest concentrations closest to the wells. Somewhere between the two wells, the reacting antigen and antibodies will be present at proportions that are optimal for formation of a precipitate.

If the antibody well contains antibodies 1, 2, and 3 specific for antigens 1, 2, and 3, respectively, and if antigens 1, 2, and 3, placed in the antigen well diffuse at different rates (with diffusion rates of $1 > 2 > 3$), then three distinct precipitin lines will form. These three precipitin lines form because anti-1, anti-2, and anti-3, which diffuse at the same rate, react independently with antigens 1, 2, and 3, respectively, to form three equivalence zones and thus three separate lines of precipitate (Figure 6.4B). Different rates of diffusion of both antibody, and antibody and antigen, result from differences in concentration, molecular size, or shape.

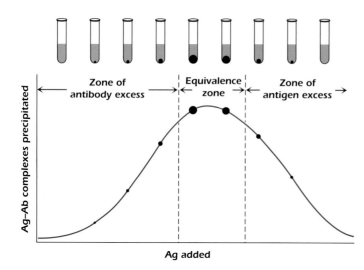

Figure 6.3. A representation of the precipitin reaction.

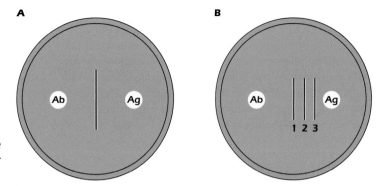

Figure 6.4. Gel diffusion by antibodies and a single antigen (A) and antibodies to antigens 1, 2, 3, and their respective antigens (B).

Radial Immunodiffusion. The radial immunodiffusion test, depicted in Figure 6.5, represents a variation of the double-diffusion test although it is not commonly used due to the availability of other more quantitative test options. The wells contain antigen at different concentrations, while the antibodies are distributed uniformly in the agar gel. Thus, the precipitin line is replaced by a precipitin ring around the well. The distance the precipitin ring migrates from the center of the antigen well is directly proportional to the concentration of antigen in the well. The relationship between concentration of antigen in a well and the diameter of the precipitin ring can be plotted as shown in Figure 6.5. If wells, such as F and G, contain unknown amounts of the same antigen, the concentration of that antigen in these wells can be determined by comparing the diameter of the precipitin ring with the diameter of the ring formed by a known concentration of the antigen.

Immunoelectrophoresis. Immunoelectrophoresis involves separating a mixture of proteins in an electrical field (electrophoresis) followed by their detection with antibodies diffusing into the gel. It is very useful for the analysis of a mixture of antigens by antiserum that contains antibodies to the antigens in the mixture. This is an extension of the protein electrophoresis described in Chapter 5 (Figure 5.1) in which proteins are separated and their presumed composition is determined by their position on the gel (e.g.,

albumin, gamma globulin regions). In immunoelectrophoresis or immunofixation electrophoresis, a specific protein is identified by the addition of a specific antibody following the separation. For example, in the clinical characterization of human serum proteins, a small drop of human serum is placed in a well cut in the center of a slide that is coated with agar gel. The serum is then subjected to electrophoresis, which separates the various components according to their mobilities in the electrical field. After electrophoresis, a trough is cut along the side of the slides, and antibodies to human serum proteins are placed in the trough. The antibodies diffuse in the agar, as do the separated serum proteins. At an optimal antigen-to-antibody ratio for each antigen and its corresponding antibodies, they form precipitin lines. The result is a pattern similar to that depicted in Figure 6.6. Comparison of the pattern and intensity of lines of normal human serum with the patterns and intensity of lines obtained with sera of patients may reveal an absence, overabundance, or other abnormality of one or more serum proteins. In fact, it was through the use of the immunoelectrophoresis assay that the first antibody-deficiency syndrome was identified in 1952 (Bruton's agammaglobulinemia) (see Chapter 18).

Western Blots (Immunoblots). In the Western blot (immunoblot) technique, antigen (or a mixture of antigens) is first separated in a gel. The separated material is then transferred onto protein-binding sheets (e.g., nitrocellulose) by using an electroblotting method. Antibody, which is then applied to the nitrocellulose sheet, binds with its specific antigen. The antibody may be labeled (e.g., with radioactivity), or a labeled anti-immunoglobulin may be used to localize the antibody and the antigen to which the first antibody

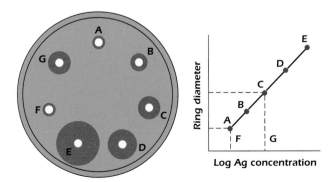

Figure 6.5. Radial diffusion, A, B, C, D, and E represent known concentrations of antigen; F and G represent unknown concentrations that can be determined from the graph.

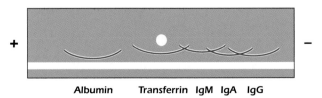

Figure 6.6. Patterns of immunoelectrophoresis of serum proteins.

is bound. These so-called Western blots are used widely in research and clinical laboratories for the detection and characterization of antigens. A particularly useful example is the confirmatory diagnosis of human immunodeficiency virus (HIV) infection by the application of a patient's serum to the nitrocellulose sheets on which HIV antigens are bound. The finding of specific antibody is strong evidence of infection by the virus (Figure 6.7).

IMMUNOASSAYS

Direct-Binding Immunoassays

While not routinely performed any longer due to the availability of alternative nonradioactive tests, radioimmunoassay (RIA) employs isotopically labeled molecules and permits measurements of extremely small amounts of antigen, antibody, or antigen–antibody complexes. The concentration of such labeled molecules is determined by measuring their radioactivity, rather than by chemical analysis. The sensitivity of detection is thus increased by several orders of magnitude. For the development of this highly sensitive analytical method that has tremendous application in hormone assays as well as assays of other substances found at low levels in biological fluids, Rosalyn Yalow received the Nobel Prize.

The principle of RIA is illustrated in Figure 6.8. A known amount of radioactively labeled antigen is reacted with a limited amount of antibody. The solution now contains antibody-bound labeled antigen, as well as some unbound labeled antigen. After separating the antigen bound to antibody from free antigen, the amount of radioactivity bound to antibody is determined.

The test continues with performance of a similar procedure in which the same amount of labeled antigen is premixed with unlabeled antigen (Figure 6.9). The mixture is reacted with the same amount of antibody as before, and the antibody-bound antigen is separated from the unbound antigen. The unlabeled antigen competes with the labeled

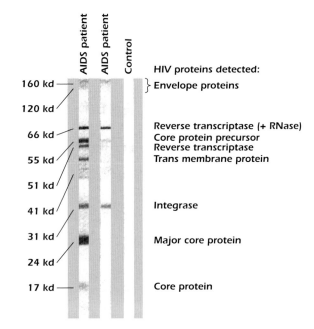

Figure 6.7. Western blots of serum samples from two HIV-infected individuals and one control subject. Note the presence of several bands in the acquired immune deficiency syndrome (AIDS) patient sample lanes indicating serum antibody reactions with HIV proteins.

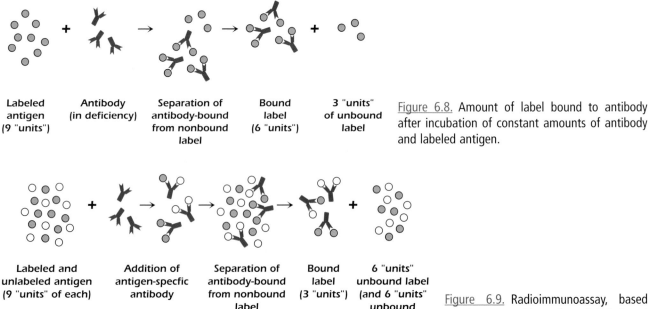

Figure 6.8. Amount of label bound to antibody after incubation of constant amounts of antibody and labeled antigen.

Figure 6.9. Radioimmunoassay, based on the competition of nonlabeled and labeled antigens for antibody.

antigen for the antibody, and as a result, less label is bound to antibody than in the absence of unlabeled antigen. The more unlabeled antigen present in the reaction mixture, the smaller the ratio of antibody-bound, radiolabeled antigen to free, radiolabeled antigen. This ratio can be plotted as a function of the concentration of the unlabeled antigen used for competition and is used to determine an unknown concentration of antigen in a solution. The ratio of bound to free radioactivity is compared with that obtained in the absence of unlabeled antigen (the latter value is set at 100%).

An important step in performing an RIA, as described above, is the separation of free antigen from that bound to antibody. Depending upon the antigen, this separation can be achieved in a variety of ways, principal among which is the anti-immunoglobulin procedure.

The anti-immunoglobulin procedure is based on the fact that antigen (labeled or unlabeled) bound to immunoglobulin will also be precipitated, following the addition of anti-immunoglobulin antibodies, so that only unbound antigen remains in the supernatant. Radioimmunoassays commonly employ rabbit antibodies to the desired antigens. These rabbit antibody–antigen complexes may be precipitated by the addition of goat antibodies raised against rabbit immunoglobulins.

Since the amounts of antigen and antibody required for RIA are extremely small, the antigen–antibody complexes reacted with anti-immunoglobulin would form only tiny precipitates. It is difficult, if not impossible, to recover these precipitates quantitatively by conventional means, in order to determine their radioactivity. To overcome this problem, it is customary to add immunoglobulins that are not specific for the antigen in the reaction mixture, thereby increasing the amount of total immunoglobulins to an amount that can easily be precipitated by anti-immunoglobulins and recovered quantitatively. Such precipitates consist mainly of nonspecific immunoglobulins to which radioactive antigen does not bind. However, they also contain the extremely small amount of antigen-specific immunoglobulin and any radioactive antigen bound to it.

An alternative method of separating complexes of antigen bound to antibody from free antigen is based on the fact that immunoglobulins become insoluble and precipitate in a solution containing 33% saturated ammonium sulfate. If the antigen alone does not precipitate in 33% ammonium sulfate, the addition of ammonium sulfate to 33% will cause the antibody complexed to antigen to precipitate, leaving the free antigen in solution. Here again, the amounts of antibodies reacting with antigen (or free antibodies) are small and unable to form precipitates. As described for the RIA where anti-immunoglobulins are used for the separation of antibody-bound antigen from free antigen, a sufficient amount of nonspecific immunoglobulins is added to the mixture; an appreciable precipitate will form at 33% saturation ammonium sulfate to enable the separation of free antigen from antigen bound to antibody.

Solid-Phase Immunoassays

Solid-phase immunoassay is one of the most widely used immunologic techniques. It is now automated and is widely used in clinical medicine for the detection of antigen or antibody. A good example is the use of solid-phase immunoassay for the detection of antibodies to HIV (see Chapter 18).

Solid-phase immunoassays employ the property of various plastics (e.g., polyvinyl or polystyrene) to adsorb monomolecular layers of proteins (antigen) onto their surface. Although the adsorbed molecules may lose some of their antigenic determinants, enough remain unaltered and can still react with their corresponding antibodies. The presence of these antibodies, bound to antigen adsorbed onto the plastic, may be detected by the use of antibodies conjugated to enzymes such as peroxidase. When chromogenic substrates are applied, the wells containing enzyme-conjugated antibodies bound to antigen will show a color change that can be detected quantitatively (Figure 6.10). More intense color signifies the presence of higher concentrations of antigen adsorbed to the well. Alternatively, unlabeled antibodies to the adsorbed antigens can be used followed by the addition of enzyme-conjugated anti-immunoglobulins. The test is called an *enzyme-linked immunosorbent assay* (ELISA). Fluorescent substrates can also be used in ELISAs and can provide increased sensitivity.

It should be emphasized that after coating the plastic surface with antigen, it is imperative to block any uncoated plastic surface to prevent it from absorbing the other reagents, most importantly the labeled reagent. Such blocking is achieved by coating the plastic surface with a high concentration of an unrelated protein, such as gelatin, after the application of the antigen.

Solid-phase immunoassay may be used to detect the presence of antibodies to the antigen that coats the plastic. Since the plastic wells are usually coated with relatively large amounts of antigen, the higher the concentration of antibodies bound with the antigen, the higher the amount of labeled anti-immunoglobulin that can bind to the antibodies. Thus, it is important always to use an excess of labeled anti-immunoglobulin to assure saturation.

Solid-phase immunoassay may be used for the qualitative or quantitative determinations of antigen. Such determinations are performed by mixing the antiserum with varying known amounts of antigen before adding the antiserum to the antigen-coated plastic wells. This preliminary procedure results in the binding of the antibodies with the soluble antigen, decreasing the availability of free antibodies for binding with the antigen that is coating the plastic. The higher the concentration of the soluble antigen that reacts with antibodies before the addition of the antibody to the wells, the lower the number of antibodies that can bind with the antigen on the plate, and the lower the number of labeled anti-immunoglobulin that can bind to these

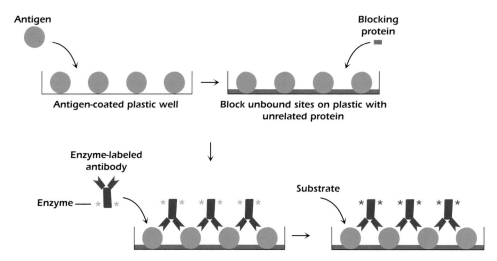

Figure 6.10. A representative ELISA using a well coated directly with antigen.

antibodies. The decrease in the amount of bound label as a function of the concentration of antigen used to cause this decrease can be plotted, and the amount of antigen in an unknown solution can then be determined from the graph by a comparison of the decrease in bound label caused by the unknown solution to the decrease caused by known concentrations of pure antigen.

IMMUNOFLUORESCENCE

A fluorescent compound has the property of emitting light of a certain wavelength when it is excited by exposure to light of a shorter wavelength. Immunofluorescence is a method for localizing an antigen by the use of fluorescently labeled antibodies. The procedure, originally described by Coombs, employs antibodies to which fluorescent groups have been covalently linked without any appreciable change in antibody activity.

One fluorescent compound that is widely used in immunology is fluorescein isothiocyanate (FITC), which fluoresces with a visible greenish color when excited by ultraviolet light. FITC is easily coupled to free amino groups. Another widely used fluorescent compound is phycoerythrin (PE), which fluoresces red and is also easily coupled to free amino groups. Fluorescence microscopes equipped with a UV light source permit visualization of fluorescent antibody on a microscopic specimen, and fluorescent antibodies are widely used to localize antigens on various tissues and microorganisms.

There are two important and related procedures that employ fluorescent antibodies: direct immunofluorescence and indirect immunofluorescence.

Direct Immunofluorescence

Direct immunofluorescence is primarily for detection of antigen and involves reacting the target tissue (or microorganism) with fluorescently labeled specific antibodies. It is widely used clinically for identifying lymphocytic subsets and for demonstrating the presence of specific protein deposition (e.g. auto-antibodies, complement) in certain tissues such as kidney and skin in cases of systemic lupus erythematosus (SLE) (see Chapter 13).

Indirect Immunofluorescence

Indirect immunofluorescence involves first reacting the target with unlabeled specific antibodies. This reaction is followed by subsequent reaction with fluorescently labeled anti-mmunoglobulin.

The indirect immunofluorescence method is more widely used than the direct method, because a single fluorescent anti-immunoglobulin antibody can be used to localize antibody of many different specificities. Moreover, since the anti-immunoglobulins contain antibodies to many epitopes on the specific immunoglobulin, the use of fluorescent anti-immunoglobulins significantly amplifies the fluorescent signal. An excellent example of the use of indirect immunofluorescence is the screening of patients' sera for anti-DNA antibodies in cases of SLE.

FLOW CYTOMETRY

A very powerful tool has been developed around the use of fluorescent antibody specific for cell-surface antigens. This is the technique of ***flow cytometric analysis*** and ***cell sorting***. Flow cytometry instruments are available as either analytical instruments that can measure the size, granularity, and expression of cell surface or intracellular proteins (analyzers) or as instruments that do all of these things and can also sort cells into distinct populations (cell sorters). A cell suspension labeled with specific fluorescent antibody is passed through an apparatus that forms a stream of small droplets,

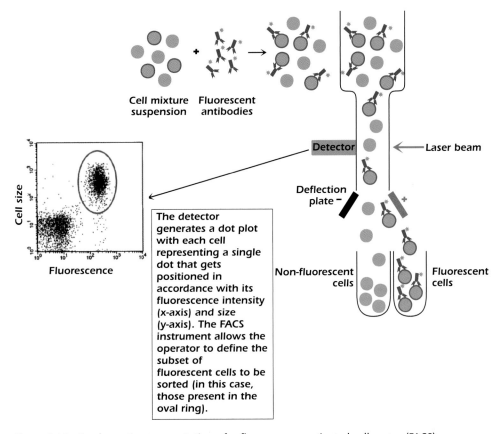

The detector generates a dot plot with each cell representing a single dot that gets positioned in accordance with its fluorescence intensity (x-axis) and size (y-axis). The FACS instrument allows the operator to define the subset of fluorescent cells to be sorted (in this case, those present in the oval ring).

Figure 6.11. A schematic representation of a fluorescence-activated cell sorter (FACS).

each containing one cell. These droplets are passed between a laser beam of ultraviolet light and a detector for picking up emitted fluorescence when a labeled cell is present in the droplet. This emitted signal is passed to an electrode that charges the droplet, leading to its deflection in an electro-magnetic field (Figure 6.11). Thus, as all droplets fall past the laser beam they are counted and can be sorted (e.g., unla-beled versus labeled) according to whether they emit a signal. The intensity of fluorescein-staining on each cell, which reflects the density of antigen expressed on the cell, may be determined by sophisticated electronics. With this type of apparatus it is now possible to rapidly develop a profile of a pool of lymphocytes based on their differential expression of cell-surface molecules, the relative amount of cell-surface molecule expressed on each cell, and the size distribution and percentage of each cell type. It is also possible to use the apparatus to sort a collection of cells stained with eight or more different fluorescent labels and obtain a very homoge-neous sample of a particular cell type. A variation of this technique uses fluorescent antibodies coupled to magnetic beads to separate cell populations. Cells that bind to the fluo-rescent antibody can be separated from unstained cells by a magnet. Both fluorescence-activated cell sorters (FACSs) and magnetic bead separation methods have resulted in the isolation of very rare cells such as hematopoietic stem cells.

The most common method for phenotyping and sorting cells involves the use of antibodies that react with cell-surface proteins identified as **clusters of differentia-tion (CD) antigens**. The CD nomenclature originates from studies using monoclonal antibodies (discussed later in this chapter) to phenotypically characterize cells. It was found that cell-surface markers (CD antigens) are associ-ated with distinct developmental stages. Moreover, these proteins have important biologic functions required for normal cell physiology. The developmental stages of B and T cells and functional subsets of these cells can now be phenotyped based on their expression of CD markers. It is also worth noting, however, that surface expression of a particular molecule may not be specific for just one cell or even for a cell lineage. Rather, it is the constellation of CD markers that determines a cell type. Nonetheless, cell-surface expression can be exploited for purification, as well as characterization, of cells. For practical purposes, the CD acronym is followed by an arbitrary number that identifies a specific cell-surface protein. CD numbers are assigned by the Nomenclature Committee of the Interna-tional Union of Immunologic Sciences. A list some of some of the more important CD antigens expressed by B cells, various T-cell subsets, and other cells can be found in the Appendix.

IMMUNOABSORPTION AND IMMUNOADSORPTION

Because of the specific binding between antigen and antibody, it is possible to trap, or selectively remove, an antigen against which an antibody is directed from a mixture of antigens in solution. Similarly, it is possible to trap, or selectively remove, the antigen-specific antibodies from a mixture of antibodies, using the specific antigen.

There are two general methods by which this removal can be achieved. The methods are related, but, in one method, the absorption is done with both reagents in solution (*immunoabsorption*); in the second method, it is performed with one reagent attached to an insoluble support (*immunoadsorption*). Immunoadsorption is of particular value because the adsorbed material can be recovered from the complex by careful treatments that dissociate antigen–antibody complexes, such as lowering the pH (HCl-glycine or acetic acid, pH 2–3) or adding chaotropic ions. This enables the effective purification of antigens or antibodies of interest.

CELLULAR ASSAYS

Other immune assays are used in the evaluation and study of the cellular components of the immune system. Among these are routine methods used to measure lymphocyte function. Assays designed to measure responses of B cells to antigenic or *mitogenic stimulation* are sometimes used clinically to assess humoral immunocompetence. In experimental settings, these assays help us to understand the regulatory and molecular mechanisms associated with B-cell activation. Similarly, assays for measuring T-cell function are used both clinically and experimentally to measure T-cell proliferative and effector responses and T-cell cytokine profiles. T-cell assays have contributed significantly to our understanding of T-cell functional diversity and to the identification of the many cytokines produced by cells belonging to a particular subset.

Assays of Lymphocyte Function

Assays used to assess lymphocyte function generally attempt to answer one of the following questions: (1) Do the B or T cells respond normally to mitogenic stimuli that activate cells to undergo a proliferative response? (2) Does mitogenic or antigen-driven stimulation result in antibody production (for B cells) or cytokine production (for T cells)? In addition, given the functional heterogeneity of T cells, T-cell assays can also be used to evaluate the functional integrity of a particular subset. This is particularly useful in the clinical evaluation of patients with suspected immunodeficiency diseases (see Chapter 18). In the case of T helper cell assays, the target cell receiving the T-cell help generally determines

the functional parameter to be measured. For example, the target population might be B cells in an assay designed to test the ability of T cells to help induce antibody responses. In this example, the assay would quantitate the level of antibody produced. Similarly, if one were interested in knowing whether T cells provide help needed to optimally activate macrophages, the parameters measured would focus on functional properties associated with these phagocytic cells. It is important to note that many of the assays used to assess helper T-cell function also rely upon the measurement of specific cytokines since the cells receiving help may be activated to produce cytokines themselves.

B-Cell and T-Cell Proliferation Assays

Mitogen-stimulated lymphocyte activation triggers biochemical signaling pathways that lead to gene expression, protein synthesis, cell proliferation, and differentiation. The proliferative responses generated in response to mitogens are polyclonal in nature. Mitogens, being by definition nonspecific stimuli, do not act through the antigen-specific receptor. Mitogens may selectively stimulate either B- or T-cell populations. Therefore, unlike immunogens that activate only the lymphocyte clones bearing the appropriate antigen receptor, polyclonal activators stimulate many B- or T-cell clones regardless of their antigenic specificity. Mitogens that selectively activate B cells, such as the *lipopolysaccharide* (LPS) component of Gram-negative bacterial cell walls, will cause polyclonal stimulation of B cells in mice and humans. Similarly, several sugar-binding proteins called *lectins*, including *concanavalin A* (Con A) and *phytohemagglutinin* (PHA), are very effective T-cell mitogens. *Pokeweed mitogen* (PWM) is another example of a lectin with potent mitogenic properties. However, unlike Con A and PHA, PWM stimulates polyclonal activation of both B and T cells. The magnitude of cell proliferation in response to mitogenic stimulation can be measured by adding nucleosides labeled with reagents that are detected based upon a color change (colorimetric assays) or fluorescence (flurometric assays). Older methods used radiolabeled nucleosides (e.g., tritiated thymidine) to monitor cell proliferation. In all cases, the labeled nucleosides are incorporated into the DNA of dividing cells.

Antibody Production by B Cells

Mitogenic stimulation of B and T cells results in the proliferation and differentiation of many clones of cells. Therefore, in the case of B cells, the polyclonal activators LPS or PWM can be used to assess the ability of a population of B cells to produce antibody. ELISAs are the most commonly used quantitative assays for measuring antibody levels. Alternatively, B cells can be stimulated with mitogens or specific antigens *in vitro*, then temporarily cultured in chambers directly on nitrocellulose membranes in a so-called enzyme-linked immunospot (ELISPOT) assay. The protein-binding property of nitrocellulose facilitates the capture of secreted antibody by individual B cells. This yields discrete foci of antibody bound to the nitrocellulose that can be detected using a secondary, enzyme-labeled antibody specific for the bound antibody, allowing for the enumeration of antibody-secreting cells.

Effector Cell Assays for T Cells and Natural Killer Cells

As noted above, the choice of effector cell assay used depends on the questions that need to be answered. T-cell assays are as varied as the functionally diverse T-cell subsets known to exist. Thus, various assays that measure T helper cell function, which focus on helper activity for B cells, macrophage activation, and even other T cells, can be used to measure the helper properties of CD4$^+$ T cells. Similarly, several assays which measure cytotoxic activity of CD8$^+$ T cells are available. One such assay (*cytotoxicity assay*) measures the ability of cytotoxic T cells to kill radiolabeled target cells expressing the antigen to which the cytotoxic T cells were sensitized. In a related assay, the natural killer (NK) cells are cultured with radiolabeled target cells bound to target cell-specific antibodies. The rationale for this approach is based on the fact that NK cells express membrane Fc receptors that bind to the Fc region of certain immunoglobulin isotypes. This method measures an important functional property of NK cells known as *antibody-dependent cell-mediated cytotoxicity* (ADCC).

CELL CULTURE

Several experimental systems have revolutionized our ability to investigate a myriad of questions about the development of the immune system, its functional and regulatory properties, and the pathologic mechanisms associated immunodeficiency and autoimmune diseases. Many of these experimental systems depend upon cell culture methods used to maintain cells *in vitro*. Cell culture systems have facilitated several major scientific breakthroughs including the development in the 1970s of B cell *hybridoma/monoclonal antibody technology* by Kohler and Milstein. Knowledge of the growth factors required to maintain lymphoid cells has made it possible to clone and grow functionally competent cells *in vitro*. Moreover, recombinant DNA techniques have permitted the transfer of genes to cloned cell lines thereby allowing researchers to answer many questions related to the gene under investigation. Similarly, recombinant DNA techniques have made it possible to develop genetically engineered immune molecules and receptors, which can be transferred into cells that are then used to elucidate the biologic consequences of receptor expression and receptor triggering (e.g., ligand binding).

These *in vitro* systems continue to be used to advance our knowledge of the immune system and, in some cases, to develop new biologic therapies and vaccines for clinical use.

Primary Cell Cultures and Cloned Lymphoid Cell Lines

As with many other fields of biologic science, cell culture systems have served as an essential investigational tool to facilitate our understanding of many developmental or maturational and physiologic properties of cells. The ability to culture primary lymphoid cells consisting of heterogeneous populations of T and/or B cells (albeit for limited periods of time) has allowed immunologists to study the biochemical and molecular mechanisms controlling many important biologic features of B and T cells, including gene rearrangement. Advances in cell culture systems have evolved rapidly over the past few decades leading to the development of cell cloning techniques. Transformation of B and T cells derived from a specific parent cell to generate cloned, immortal cell lines has been achieved using a variety of methods including exposure of cells to certain carcinogens or viruses (e.g., Epstein–Barr virus for the transformation of B cells; human T-cell leukemia virus type 1 for the transformation of T cells). It should be noted that many cell lines are derived from tumors arising either spontaneously or experimentally (as a result of exposure of cells to carcinogens or certain viruses). The major advantage of using cloned cell lines is that large numbers of cells can be generated for investigation. A disadvantage in the use of carcinogen- or virus-transformed cells is that they are, by definition, abnormal. Indeed, many transformed cells have abnormal numbers of chromosomes and often display phenotypic and functional properties not seen in normal cells. A major advance in the generation of cloned lymphoid cells came in the late 1970s with the discovery that nontransformed antigen-specific T-cell lines and antigen-specific T-cell clones could be grown indefinitely when a T-cell growth factor (interleukin-2) was included in the culture together with a source of antigen and antigen-presenting cells. This approach offered several advantages over the use of transformed cells since the cells derived from such cultures were, for all intents and purposes, normal. Thus, large numbers of nontransformed antigen-specific T cells could be generated for investigation. Indeed, many of these cloned T-cell lines have been used in the identification and biochemical characterization of cytokines, leading to the ultimate cloning of genes that encode these proteins.

The combined use of cell cloning systems, gene transfer methods, and animal models has helped us to understand how lymphoid cells develop self-tolerance as well as how they can escape tolerance-inducing mechanisms to become disease-causing autoreactive cells. In short, cell culture systems have served as a gateway for research endeavors to shed light on both the physiologic and pathophysiologic properties of lymphoid cells. As will be discussed below, cell culture systems have also been productively exploited with the development of many useful diagnostic and therapeutic reagents, such as monoclonal antibodies.

B-Cell Hybridomas and Monoclonal Antibodies

The specificity of the immune response has served as the basis for serologic reactions in which antibody is used for the qualitative and quantitative determination of antigen. The discriminating power of serum antibody is not without limitations, however, because the immunizing antigen, which usually has many epitopes, leads to production of antisera that contain a mixture of antibodies with varying specificity for all the epitopes. Indeed, even antibodies to a single epitope are usually mixtures of immunoglobulins with different fine specificities, and therefore different affinities for the determinant. Furthermore, immunization with an antigen expands various populations of antibody-forming lymphocytes. These cells can be maintained in culture for only a short time (on the order of days), so it is impractical, if not impossible, to grow normal cells and obtain clones that produce antibodies of a single specificity. A quantum leap in the resolution and discriminating power of antibodies took place in the 1970s with the development of methods for the generation of *monoclonal antibodies* by Kohler and Milstein, who shared the Nobel Prize for this achievement. Monoclonal antibodies are homogeneous populations of antibody molecules, derived from the progeny of a single antibody-producing cell, in which all antibodies are identical and of the same precise specificity for a given epitope. In this procedure, malignant non-immunoglobulin-producing plasma cells (immortal in cell culture) are used. The cells are engineered to be deficient in an enzyme (hypoxanthine guanine phosphoribosyl transferase [HGPRT]) and therefore will not survive in culture unless this enzyme is added to the media in which the cells are grown. These cells are fused (hybridized) with a source of freshly harvested B cells from a mouse recently immunized with antigen (e.g., spleen cells) (Figure 6.12). The fusion is often accomplished by the use of polyethylene glycol (PEG). Following fusion, the cells are cultured in media lacking HGPRT. Since the antibody-producing B cells produce HGPRT, only hybridoma cells consisting of malignant plasma cells fused with B cells will survive in the absence of supplemented HGPRT in the culture medium. Within days, non-fused HGPRT-negative malignant plasma cells soon die as do all non-fused B cells. Those hybrid cells synthesizing specific antibody are selected by a test for antigen reactivity (e.g., ELISA) and then cloned from single cells and propagated in tissue culture, each clone synthesizing antibodies of a single specificity. Those highly specific, monoclonal antibodies are used for numerous procedures, ranging from specific diagnostic tests to biologic agents used in immunotherapy of cancer (see Chapter 20). In immunotherapy, various drugs or toxins can be conjugated to monoclonal antibodies, which, in turn, deliver these substances to the tumor cells against which the antibodies are specifically directed.

T-Cell Hybridomas

It is important to note that hybridoma technology is not limited to the production of monoclonal immunoglobulins. In the late 1970s, methods for producing hybridomas were also developed for T cells, fusing lines of malignant T cells with nonmalignant, antigen-specific T lymphocytes whose populations had been expanded by immunization with antigen. T-cell hybridomas have been useful for studying the relationship between T cells of a single specificity with their corresponding epitope.

Genetically Engineered Molecules and Receptors

To date most of the monoclonal antibodies are made in mouse cells. These are suitable for diagnostic and many other purposes. However, their administration into humans carries the complication that the patient will form antibodies to the mouse immunoglobulins. Attempts to develop *in vitro* human monoclonal antibodies have, by and large, not been very successful.

Human monoclonal antibodies are currently being produced by genetic engineering utilizing several approaches. One method utilizes the technology of recombinant DNA to produce a chimeric mouse–human monoclonal antibody. These so-called *humanized antibodies* consist of the constant region of human immunoglobulin and a variable region of a mouse immunoglobulin. A similar method is used to construct humanized antibodies consisting of a human constant region and a variable region containing a mouse hypervariable region and a human framework region. Another method utilizes the polymerase chain reaction (PCR) to generate gene libraries of heavy and light chains from DNA obtained from hybridoma cells or plasma cells, joining at random numerous heavy and light chains and screening the resulting Fab clones for antibody activity against a desired antigen. With this technology it is now possible to produce millions of clones of different specificities, to rapidly screen them for the desired specificity, and generate the desired monoclonal Fab constructs without immunization and without the difficulties encountered with the production of monoclonal antibodies, especially human monoclonal antibodies.

Genetic engineering of immune proteins is not limited to the production of monoclonal antibodies. Many genes encoding membrane receptors expressed on lymphoid and nonlymphoid cells have been cloned and, in some cases, genetically engineered to allow for gene transfer to cells that do not normally express these receptors. The expression of certain co-stimulator molecules facilitates cell–cell

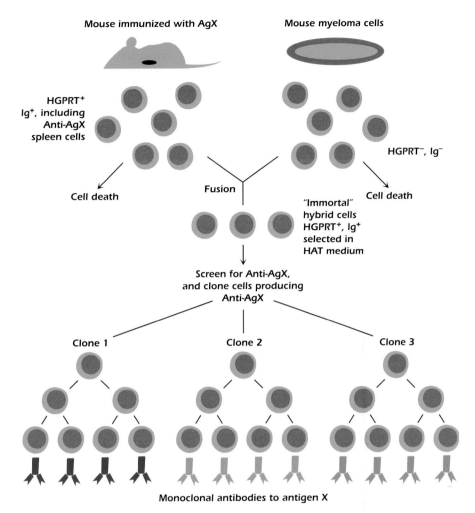

Figure 6.12. A schematic representation of the production of monoclonal antibodies.

interactions (e.g., the physical contact between cytotoxic T cells and target cells, which results in the killing of the latter). The expression, through gene transfer, of such co-stimulator molecules (e.g., B7) on tumor cells significantly enhances the ability of T cells to recognize and kill these cells. Experimental vaccination strategies (a form of immunotherapy) have demonstrated that immunization of tumor-bearing animals with their own tumor cells, which have been removed and transfected with the B7 gene, can potentiate T cells to recognize and destroy the parent tumor cells. It should be noted that a similar strategy using tumor cells transfected with certain cytokine genes has also been used with some success in animal models. Immunotherapeutic strategies used to treat a variety of diseases are discussed in several chapters of this book (see Chapters 18–20).

EXPERIMENTAL ANIMAL MODELS

Several important *in vivo* animal models have been developed with experimental value and clinical payoffs similar to

those emerging from the use of the *in vitro* systems noted above. These *in vivo* systems rely on the use of inbred mouse strains with a variety of genetic profiles, some of which are genetically engineered. Some inbred stains have an innate predisposition for developing a particular disease (e.g., mammary cancer, leukemia, autoimmune disease, severe combined immunodeficiency disease). Genetically altered animals, on the other hand, have been developed to either express a particular cloned foreign gene (transgenic mice) or by interfering with the expression of targeted genes (knockout mice). Such strains are useful in the study of the expression of a particular transgene or in determining the consequences of gene silencing in knockout mice. We begin with a discussion of inbred strains of animals.

Inbred Strains

Many of the classic experiments in the field of immunology have been performed using inbred strains of animals such as mice, rats, and guinea pigs. Selective inbreeding of littermates for more than 20 generations usually leads to the production of an inbred strain. All members of inbred strains of animals are genetically identical. Therefore, like identical twins, they are said to be *syngeneic*. Immune responses of inbred strains can be studied in the absence of variables associated with genetic differences between animals. As will be discussed in Chapter 19, organ transplants between members of inbred stains are always accepted since their major histocompatibility complex (MHC) antigens are identical. Indeed, knowledge of the laws of transplantation and the fact that the MHC is the major genetic barrier to transplantation was made possible through the use of inbred strains. Experiments using inbred strains led to the identification of class I and class II MHC genes whose main function is to deliver peptide fragments of antigen to the cell surface thus allowing them to be recognized by antigen-specific T cells. Subsequent chapters will elaborate on the important role of the MHC in (1) the generation of normal immune responses; (2) T-cell development; (3) disease susceptibility; and, (4) organ transplantation.

Adoptive Transfer

Protection against many diseases is conferred through *cell-mediated immunity* by antigen-specific T cells as opposed to antibody-mediated (humoral) immunity. The distinction between these two arms of the immune response can be readily demonstrated by adoptive transfer of T cells or by passive administration of antiserum or purified antibodies. Adoptive transfer of T cells is usually performed using genetically identical donor and recipients (e.g., inbred strains) and results in long-term adoptive immunization following antigen priming. By contrast, passive transfer of serum containing antibodies can be performed across MHC barriers and is effective as long as the transferred antibodies remain active in the recipient. This type of transfer is therefore called *passive immunization*.

SCID Mice

Severe combined immunodeficiency disease (SCID) is a disorder in which B and T cells fail to develop, causing the individual to be compromised with respect to lymphoid defense mechanisms. Chapter 18 discusses various causes of SCID in humans. In the 1980s, an inbred strain of mice spontaneously developed an autosomal recessive mutation, resulting in SCID in homozygous *scid/scid* mice. Because of the absence of functional T and B cells, SCID mice are able to accept cells and tissue grafts from other strains of mice or other species. SCID mice can be engrafted with human hematopoietic stem cells to create *SCID–human chimeras*. Such chimeric mice develop mature, functional T and B cells derived from the infused human stem-cell precursors. This animal model has become a valuable research tool, since it allows immunologists to manipulate the human immune system *in vivo* and to investigate the development of various lymphoid cells. Moreover, SCID–human mice can be used to test candidate vaccines, including those that might useful in protecting humans from HIV infection.

Thymectomized and Congenitally Athymic (Nude) Mice

The importance of the thymus in the development of mature T cells can be demonstrated by using mice that have been neonatally thymectomized, irradiated, and then reconstituted with syngeneic bone marrow. Such mice fail to develop mature T cells. Similarly, mice homozygous for the recessive *nude* gene mutation also fail to develop mature T cells because the mutation results in an athymic (and hairless, hence the term *nude mouse*) phenotype. In both situations, T-cell development can be restored by grafting these mice with thymic epithelial tissue. Like SCID mice, these animal models have been useful in the study of T-cell development. They have also been useful for the *in vivo* propagation of tumor cell lines and fresh tumor explants from other strains and other species due to the absence of T cells required to reject such foreign cells.

TRANSGENIC MICE AND GENE TARGETING

Transgenic Mice

Another significant animal system used extensively in immunologic research is the transgenic mouse. *Transgenic mice* are made by injecting a cloned gene (*transgene*) into fertilized mouse eggs. The eggs are then microinjected into pseudopregnant mice (Figure 6.13). The success rate of this technique is rather low, with approximately 10% to 30% of the offspring expressing the transgene. Since the transgene is integrated into both somatic and germline cells, it is transmitted to the offspring as a Mendelian trait. By constructing a transgene with a particular promoter, it is possible to control the gene's expression. For example, some promoters function only in certain tissues (e.g., the insulin promoter only functions in the pancreas), whereas others function in response to biochemical signals that can be supplied, in some cases, as a dietary supplement (e.g., the metallothionine promoter that functions in response to zinc, which can be added to the drinking water). Transgenic mice have been used to study genes that are not usually expressed *in vivo* (e.g., oncogenes), as well as the effects of transgenes encoding particular immunoglobulin molecules, T-cell receptors, MHC class I or class II molecules, and a variety of cytokines. Transgenic mice have also been developed in which the entire mouse immunoglobulin locus has been replaced by human immunoglobulin genes. These are useful in generating "human" antibodies in the mouse. It should be noted that a disadvantage of the transgenic method is that the transgene integrates randomly within the genome. This

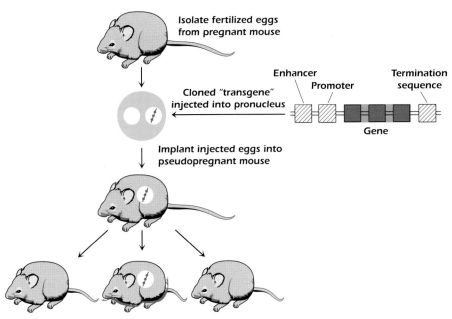

Figure 6.13. A general procedure for producing transgenic mice.

limitation, together with the fact that it is unphysiologic to express high quantities of transgenes in the wrong tissues, forces investigators to use great care in interpreting results obtained in transgenic mice.

Knockout and Knock-in Mice

Sometimes, it is of interest to determine how the removal of a particular gene product affects the immune system. Using a *gene targeting* method, it is possible to replace a normal gene with one that has been mutated or disrupted to generate so-called *knockout mice*. Thus, unlike the method used to generate transgenic mice, knockout mice express transgenes that integrate at specific endogenous genes through a process known as *homologous recombination*. Virtually any gene for which a mutated or altered transgene exists can be targeted this way. Knockout mice have been generated by using mutated or altered transgenes that target, and therefore silence, the expression of a variety of important genes, including those encoding particular cytokines and MHC molecules. They have also been used to identify the parts of genes essential for normal gene function. This is done by determining whether function can be restored by introducing different mutated copies of the gene back into the genome by transgenesis.

Gene knock-ins refers to a genetic engineering method that involves the insertion of a protein coding cDNA sequence at a particular locus in an organism's chromosome. Typically, this is done in mice because mouse embryonic stem cells are easily manipulated. The difference between knock-in technology and transgenic technology is that a knock-in involves a gene inserted into a specific locus and is therefore a targeted insertion. Knock-in technology is commonly used to create disease models that allow investigators to study, for example, the function of the regulatory machinery (e.g. promoters) that governs the expression of the natural gene being replaced. This is accomplished by observing the new phenotype of the organism in question.

ANALYSIS OF GENE EXPRESSION

Microarrays to Assess Gene Expression

Microarrays, or *gene chips*, are powerful tools for examining the level of expression of thousands of genes simultaneously. The microarray comprises thousands of DNA fragments, each with a unique sequence, attached in an ordered arrangement to a glass slide or other surface. These DNA fragments, in the form of complementary DNA (cDNA, generally 500 to 5,000 base pairs long) or oligonucleotides (20 to 80 base pairs long), can represent genes from all parts of the genome; alternatively, specialized microarrays can be prepared that use DNA from genes thought to be of particular interest. To perform a microarray assay, a sample of total messenger RNA (mRNA)—the product obtained from transcription of all active genes—from a cell or tissue is commonly tested with a reference sample to compare gene expression among various samples. For example, different cell types or tissues can be compared, cells can be compared at different stages of differentiation, or tumor cells can be compared with their

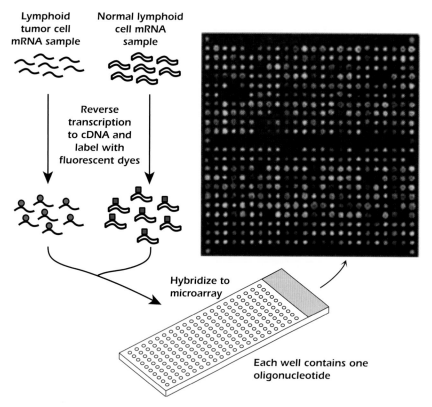

Figure 6.14. Microarray assay comparing samples of mRNA from lymphoid tumor cells and normal lymphoid cells.

normal counterparts with the goal of assessing differential gene expression within the tested samples. The samples that are added to the microarray are generally not mRNA; rather, the total mRNA is reverse transcribed into cDNA, which is then labeled with a fluorescent material (a fluorochrome). Different colored fluorochromes are used to distinctly label the different sources of cDNAs. Figure 6.14 illustrates how microarrays are used to compare gene expression in a lymphoid tumor cell population and a normal cell counterpart. A red fluorochrome is used to label experimental tumor cell cDNAs, and a green fluorochrome for cDNAs prepared from their control normal counterparts. The labeled cDNAs are washed over the microarray and allowed to hybridize by base pairing with matching fragments. The cDNA samples derived from both control samples and experimental samples are added together to the microarray so that they compete for binding to the microarray. Unhybridized material is washed away, leaving pockets of fluorescence where matching has occurred. At the end of the hybridization reaction, the microarray is laser scanned to reveal red, green, or yellow spots, indicating higher levels of the experimental tumor cell cDNA (which was labeled with a red fluorochrome in the example given), higher levels of the control cDNA (labeled green), or equal levels of DNA in the two samples (yellow), respectively. To interpret the results, a fluorescence scanner examines each spot on the slide for the precise level of fluorescence. The data are then analyzed by a computer program that typically combines the fluorescence information with a genetic database to determine which genes are overexpressed or underexpressed in the tested samples. Characterizing the pattern and amount of binding to the microarray has many potential uses in the field of immunology including clinical diagnosis of lymphoid tumors, drug development (e.g., testing candidate immunosuppressive drugs for their effects on cytokine gene expression), and new gene discovery.

SUMMARY

1. The reaction between an antibody and an antigen does not involve covalent forces; it involves weak forces of interaction such as electrostatic, hydrophobic, and van der Waals forces. Consequently, for a significant interaction, the antibody combining site and the antigen require a close steric fit like a lock and key.

2. Only the reaction between a multivalent antigen and at least a bivalent antibody can bring about antigen–antibody reactions that result in the cross-linking of antigen molecules by antibodies. These reactions do not take place with haptens or monovalent Fab.

3. The interaction between a soluble antibody and an insoluble particulate antigen results in agglutination. The extent of agglutination depends on the proportions of the interacting antibody and antigen. At high antibody levels, agglutination may not occur. This is referred to as a *prozone*. The term *titer* refers to the highest serum dilution at which agglutination still takes place and beyond which, at higher dilution, no agglutination occurs.

4. Precipitation reactions occur upon the mixing, at the right proportions, of soluble multivalent antigen and (at least) divalent antibodies. The precipitation reaction may take place in aqueous media or in gels.

5. The reaction in gels between soluble antigen and antibodies may be used for the qualitative and quantitative analysis of antigen or antibody. Examples of such reactions are seen in gel diffusion, radial diffusion, and immunoelectrophoresis.

6. Radioimmunoassay (RIA) is a very sensitive test used to quantitate antibody or antigen. It employs the use of radiolabeled antigen or antibody and is based on competitive inhibition of nonlabeled and labeled antigen. Antibody-bound antigen must be separated from nonbound labeled antigen. Separation is usually achieved by precipitation with anti-immunoglobulins.

7. Solid-phase immunoassay is a test that employs the property of many proteins to adhere to plastic and form a monomolecular layer. Antigen is applied to plastic wells, antibodies are added, the well is washed, and any antibodies bound to antigen are measured by the use of radiolabeled or enzyme-linked anti-immunoglobulins.

8. The enzyme-linked immunosorbent assay (ELISA) is essentially a solid-phase immunoassay in which an enzyme is linked to the anti-immunoglobulin. Quantitation is achieved by colorimetric evaluation after the addition of a substrate which changes color on the action of the enzyme.

9. Immunofluorescence is a method in which an antigen is detected by the use of fluorescence-labeled immunoglobulins. In direct immunofluorescence, the antibody to the antigen in question carries a fluorescent label. In indirect immunofluorescence, the antigen-specific antibody is not labeled; it is detected by the addition of fluorescently labeled anti-immunoglobulin. Fluorescence-activated cell sorters (FACSs) are instruments that can be used to quantitate and sort fluorescently labeled cells.

10. Assays used to assess lymphocyte function typically measure their proliferative responses or effector functions. For example, B cells can be functionally assessed by measuring their ability to proliferate and produce antibodies in response to B cell mitogens such as LPS. T cells are often assessed by measuring their ability to provide help for other cells (in the case of $CD4^+$ cells) or to kill antigen-bearing targets (in the case of $CD8^+$ cells). In addition, T cells can be assessed by measuring their ability to proliferate and produce certain cytokines in response to T cell mitogens such as PHA or Con A.

11. Monoclonal antibodies are highly specific reagents consisting of homogeneous populations of antibodies, all of precisely the same specificity toward an epitope.

REFERENCES AND BIBLIOGRAPHY

Camper SA. (1987) Research applications of transgenic mice. *Biotechniques* 5: 638.

Channing-Rodgers RP. (1994) Clinical laboratory methods for detection of antigens and antibodies. In Stites DP, Terr AI, Parslow TG (eds). *Basic and Clinical Immunology, 8th ed.* E Norwalk, CT: Appleton & Lange.

Gibson G. (2004). *A Primer Of Genome Science, 2nd Ed.* Sunderland, MA: Sinauer. p. 308.

Harlow E, Lane D. (1988) *Antibodies: A Laboratory Manual.* Cold Spring Harbor, NY: Cold Spring Harbor Laboratory Press.

Hudson L, Hay FC. (1989) *Practical Immunology, 3rd ed.* Oxford, UK: Blackwell.

Johnstone A, Thorpe R. (1987) *Immunochemistry in Practice.* Oxford, UK: Blackwell.

Köhler G, Milstein, C. (1975). Continuous cultures of fused cells secreting antibody of predefined specificity. *Nature* 256: 495.

Koller BH, Smithies O. (1992) Altering genes in animals by gene targeting. *Annu Rev Immunol* 10: 705.

Mayforth RD. (1993) *Designing Antibodies.* San Diego, CA: Academic Press.

Mishell BB, Shiigi SM. (1980) *Selected Methods in Cellular Immunology.* New York: Freeman.

Thompson KM. (1988) Human monoclonal antibodies. *Immunol Today* 9: 113.

Weir DM. (1986) *Handbook of Experimental Immunology, Vol. 12, 4th Ed.* Oxford, UK: Blackwell.

Winter G, Griffith AD, Hawkins RE, Hoogenboom HR. (1994) Making antibodies by phage display technology. *Annu Rev Immunol* 12: 433.

REVIEW QUESTIONS

For each question, choose the ONE BEST answer or completion.

1. Which of the following is required to ensure the integrity and stability of immunoglobulin molecules but is not associated with interactions between antigens and antibodies?
   A) covalent bonds
   B) van der Waals forces
   C) hydrophobic forces
   D) electrostatic forces
   E) a very close fit between an epitope and the antibody

2. If an IgG antibody preparation specific for hen egg lysosome (HEL) is treated with papain to generate Fab fragments, which of the following statements concerning the avidity of such fragments is true?
   A) They will have a lower avidity for HEL as compared with the intact IgG.
   B) They will have a higher avidity for HEL as compared with the intact IgG.
   C) They will have the same avidity for HEL as the intact IgG.
   D) They will have lost their avidity to bind to HEL.
   E) They will have the same avidity but will have a lower affinity for HEL.

3. Western blot assays used to test serum samples for the presence of antibodies to infectious agents, such as HIV, are particularly useful as diagnostic assays because
   A) They are more sensitive than ELISA.
   B) Antibodies specific for multiple antigenic epitopes can be detected.
   C) They provide quantitative data for sample analysis.
   D) They allow multiple samples to be tested simultaneously.
   E) They are less expensive and take less time to perform as compared with ELISA.

4. The major difference between transgenic mice and knockout mice is that
   A) Transgenic mice always employ the use of cloned genes derived from other species.
   B) Transgenic mice have foreign genes that integrate at targeted loci through homologous recombination.

C) Transgenic mice have a functional foreign gene added to their genome.
   D) Knockout mice always have a unique phenotype.

5. SCID mice have a genetic defect that prevents development of functional
   A) hematopoietic cells
   B) B cells and T cells
   C) T cells and NK cells
   D) pluripotential stem cells
   E) myeloid cells

6. Which of the following statements regarding B cell hybridomas is true?
   A) They are immortal cell lines that produce antibodies with more than one specificity.
   B) They are derived from B cells that are first cloned and grown in cell culture for short periods.
   C) They contain two nuclei.
   D) They are derived by fusing B cells with malignant plasma cells that are unable to secrete immunoglobulin.

7. An ELISA designed to test for the presence of serum antibody for a new strain of pathogenic bacteria is under development. Initially, a monoclonal antibody specific for a single epitope of the organism was used both to sensitize the wells of the ELISA plate and as the enzyme-labeled detecting antibody in a conventional sandwich ELISA. The ELISA failed to detect the antigen despite the use of a wide range of antibody concentrations. What is the most probable cause of this problem?
   A) The antigen used in the assay is too large.
   B) The antibody has a low affinity for the antigen.
   C) The monoclonal antibody used to sensitize the wells is blocking access of the epitope; thus when the same antibody is enzyme-labeled, it cannot bind to the antigen.
   D) The enzyme-labeled antibody used should have been a different isotype than the sensitizing antibody.
   E) The monoclonal antibody used is probably unstable.

ANSWERS TO REVIEW QUESTIONS

1. A. No covalent bonds are involved in the interaction between antibody and antigen. The binding forces are relatively weak and include van der Waals forces, hydrophobic forces, and electrostatic forces. A very close fit between an epitope and the antibody is required.

2. A. Avidity denotes the overall binding energy between antigens and multivalent antigens. Since the valency of the Fab fragments is 1 as compared with the HEL-specific IgG molecule, which has a valence of 2 (due to the presence of two Fab regions), the avidity of the fragments will be lower. Choice **E** is incorrect since the affinity of the Fab fragments will be the same as each of the Fab regions of the intact IgG molecule.

3. ***B.*** In Western blot assays, electrophoretic separation techniques are used to resolve the molecular mass of a given antigen or mixtures of antigens. Since antibody responses to infectious agents generate polyclonal responses by virtue of the complex antigenic determinants expressed by such agents, Western assays can confirm the presence of these antibodies, which react with the electrophoretically separated antigens of known molecular weights.

4. ***C.*** Cloned foreign genes from either the same or other species are introduced into mice to generate a transgenic strain. Integration is random and occurs in both somatic and germline cells. Choice **D** is incorrect because sometimes knockout mice do not have a phenotype unique caused by the replacement of a functional gene with one that is nonfunctional, probably due to the activity of redundant or compensatory mechanisms.

5. ***B.*** SCID mice possess an autosomal recessive mutation that causes a disorder in which B and T cells fail to develop. Like their human counterparts, SCID mice are compromised with respect to lymphoid defense mechanisms. Pluripotential stem cells present in SCID mice can give rise to other hematopoietic lineages, including cells in the myeloid lineage and NK cells.

6. ***D.*** The method used to generate B cell hybridomas employs the fusion of B cells (e.g., from the spleen and lymph nodes) harvested from immunized mice with a selected population of malignant plasma cells unable to secrete immunoglobulin. The process yields a monoclonal antibody secreted by cells that contain nuclei from the B cell and plasma cell that have fused.

7. ***C.*** In a sandwich ELISA, an antibody (often monoclonal) used to coat ELISA wells will bind to the epitope for which it is specific. In the example given, the same epitope-specific monoclonal antibody is used as enzyme-labeled detecting antibody. The sensitizing monoclonal is blocking access to the epitope by the enzyme-labeled monoclonal antibody; therefore it will not bind.

7

THE GENETIC BASIS OF ANTIBODY STRUCTURE

INTRODUCTION

In previous chapters we described the enormous diversity of the immune response, focusing on the diversity of antibodies: immunoglobulin (Ig) molecules that are the secreted forms of the antigen-specific receptors found on individual B lymphocytes. In later chapters we will also describe the similar scale of the diversity of antigen-specific T-cell receptors (TCR). Estimates of the number of B and T cells with different antigenic specificities that can be generated in a single individual are very high, in the range of 10^{11}; in other words, every person has the ability to generate 10^{11} or more different Ig or TCR molecules. However, from the sequencing of the human *genome* (inherited DNA) that has been conducted over the past few years, we now know that every person has only between 20,000 and 25,000 *genes*—stretches of DNA that code for a polypeptide (or RNA); the genomes of other mammalian species contain similar numbers of genes.

How do so few genes produce so many different antigen receptor molecules? Studies over the past 30 years have established that there are only a few hundred Ig and TCR genes, but they use a unique *rearrangement* or *recombination* strategy to produce millions or more possible protein sequences. In this way, genes, or in effect small gene segments, are combined to generate a single Ig or TCR molecule. A key feature of this rearrangement or recombination mechanism is that Ig and TCR genes change their positions along the DNA sequence, that is, move, during the development of B and T cells, respectively. This was first shown for

Ig genes by Susumu Tonegawa, who was awarded the Nobel Prize in 1987 for this work.

In this chapter we discuss how Ig genes are arranged in the genome and the key features of Ig synthesis, from the gene to the protein. We will also discuss the other mechanisms that contribute to the diversity of antigen-specific receptors, and how B cells generate the huge number of antigen-specific receptors that deal with the vast array of pathogens and harmless antigens that confront every individual.

A BRIEF REVIEW OF NONIMMUNOGLOBULIN GENE STRUCTURE AND GENE EXPRESSION

Before discussing how an Ig molecule is synthesized, we thought it helpful to review how a typical nonimmunoglobulin gene is organized and how a protein is synthesized from this gene. In Figure 7.1 and below we focus on a gene that codes for a prototypical protein expressed at the cell surface.

The gene has the characteristic structure shown in the top line of Figure 7.1: *exons*—sequences of base pairs that are later transcribed into mature messenger RNA (mRNA)—are separated from each other by *introns*—sequences of base pairs that are removed before a mature mRNA is produced. Typical of genes coding for proteins expressed at the cell surface (or those destined to be secreted or move into intracellular organelles), this gene also has a leader sequence (leader exon) at the 5′ end. This codes for a short sequence

Immunology: A Short Course, Seventh Edition. Richard Coico and Geoffrey Sunshine.
© 2015 John Wiley & Sons, Ltd. Published 2015 by John Wiley & Sons, Ltd.
Companion Website: www.wileyimmunology.com/coico

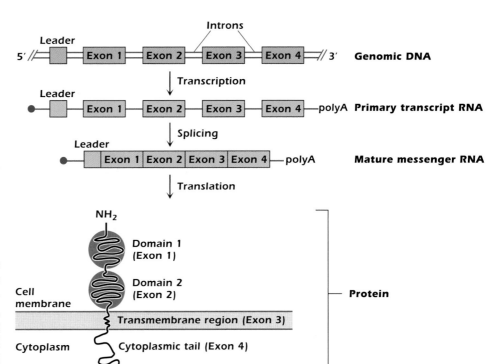

Figure 7.1. Prototypical gene that codes for a transmembrane protein: steps involved in expressing protein at the cell surface. The circle at the 5′ end of RNA is the methylguanosine "cap" and "polyA" is the polyadenylated "tail" at the 3′ end.

of about 10 mainly hydrophobic amino acids—the signal peptide—at the amino (N) terminus of the protein. Not shown in Figure 7.1 are regulatory sequences in front of (that is, 5′) the leader sequence that control gene transcription. These sequences of nucleotides bind proteins called *transcription factors* that initiate or modulate transcription. Transcription of the gene starts after RNA polymerase has bound to the transcription factor bound to the DNA.

When the gene shown in Figure 7.1 is transcribed into RNA, the entire stretch of DNA (exons plus introns) is transcribed into a primary RNA transcript. A "cap" (a single methylguanosine at the 5′ end) and "tail" (of about 250 adenines at the 3′ end) are added to the ends of the RNA transcript to protect it from degradation. Enzymes then modify the primary RNA transcript by *splicing* out the introns and bringing together all the exons. This yields a mature mRNA, which leaves the nucleus and is then translated into protein on ribosomes.

When the mRNA for a cell-membrane-associated protein is translated on ribosomes, the signal peptide directs the synthesis of the polypeptide chain to the endoplasmic reticulum. The nascent polypeptide chain is fed from the ribosomes into the interior of endoplasmic reticulum, where the signal peptide is cleaved off. The newly synthesized protein moves from the endoplasmic reticulum into the Golgi apparatus and then to the cell membrane.

Notice in Figure 7.1 the general feature that each exon codes for a discrete region or *domain* of an individual protein. In the example shown, the four exons code for the

two extracellular domains, a transmembrane region, and the cytoplasmic tail.

The surface molecule depicted in Figure 7.1 has some similarities to the structure of a membrane Ig molecule expressed at the surface of a B cell—shown for example in Figure 8.2—especially the extracellular N-terminal domains and transmembrane region. However, membrane Ig also differs in important ways from the structure of the depicted molecule. First, Ig is a four-chain glycoprotein. To make a complete Ig molecule, the newly synthesized individual heavy (H) and light (L) chains must be assembled and glycosylated inside the cell before the four-chain molecule reaches the cell surface. Second, each Ig chain has a very short cytoplasmic tail.

Other molecules involved in the immune response and expressed at the cell surface have different configurations; for example, the carboxy-terminal region can be extracellular and the N-terminus intracellular. Molecules such as CD81, expressed on B cells (see Chapter 8), loop multiple times through the membrane. Still others, such as leukocyte function-associated antigen 1 (LFA-1; CD58) and decay-accelerating factor (DAF; CD55), are completely extracellular; they are linked to the cell surface via a covalent bond to an oligosaccharide, which in turn is bound to a phospholipid (phosphatidylinositol) in the membrane. Thus these molecules are referred to as glycosylphosphatidylinositol (GPI)-linked membrane molecules. (The functions of LFA-1 and DAF are discussed in Chapters 11 and 14, respectively.)

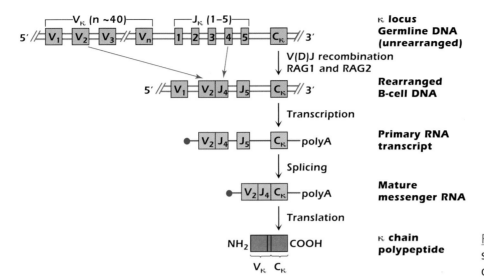

Figure 7.2. Gene rearrangement and subsequent steps in synthesis of a κ L chain.

Gene expression. Every diploid cell in the human body contains the same genes as every other cell. The only exceptions are lymphocytes, which, as we discuss shortly, differ from other cells and each other in the actual content of genes coding for their antigen-specific receptor.

Cells within an individual differ from one another because they transcribe and translate different genes. We say that these cells *express* different patterns of genes. The expression of a specific pattern of genes determines the cell's function. For example, every cell contains an insulin gene, but only pancreatic β cells express that gene, enabling them to make insulin. Similarly, all cells contain Ig genes; however, only B lymphocytes (and their differentiated form, plasma cells) express Ig genes and therefore synthesize Ig molecules. Like all other cells except B cells, T cells contain Ig genes but do not express them.

The control of gene expression exists at multiple levels, but many factors can either increase ("upregulate") or decrease ("downregulate") expression of a particular gene. Controls of gene expression include the activity of transcription factors, the rate of transcription, and the half-life of mRNA. Understanding the mechanisms that regulate gene expression in different cell types is an area of intense research interest. Genes occupy only a very small part (1–2%) of the total genome, and until recently, the rest of the DNA was not considered to have any function. Recent studies, however, have identified multiple gene switches throughout the genome, indicating that several sites in the genome outside of genes play a key role in the control of gene expression.

GENETIC EVENTS IN SYNTHESIS OF Ig CHAINS

The organization of genes coding for Ig H and L chains shows some similarities to, and some important differences from, the organization of genes for the prototypical cell surface membrane protein we described in the previous section. In addition, as we mentioned earlier in the chapter, genes coding for Ig (as well as genes coding for the TCR) have the unique property of moving—rearranging—during different stages of development of the cell. These properties are described in the sections that follow.

Organization and Rearrangement of Light-Chain Genes

General Features. We describe first the organization and rearrangement of Ig L-chain genes—κ and λ—because these are somewhat simpler than the organization and rearrangement of H-chain genes. We saw in Chapter 4 that each κ and λ L-chain polypeptide consists of two major domains, a variable region (V_L)—the approximately 108-residue amino-terminal portion of the L chain—and a constant region (C_L).

In the next sections we describe the following:

(a) Two different gene segments—*variable* (*V*) and *joining* (*J*) *segments*—code for the variable region of the L chain.

(b) A different gene, the C gene, codes for the constant region of the L chain.

(c) DNA coding for the L chain is cut and V and J gene segments are joined together in the genome by a complex of enzymes called ***V(D)J recombinase***. The joined VJ gene segments, together with the C gene, then synthesize a complete L chain.

The recombinase is called "V(D)J" because, as we describe later in the chapter, H chains use D gene segments as well as V and J segments, and the same recombinase is involved in cutting and joining H chain and L chain DNA. Thus, the mechanism of cutting and joining DNA coding for Ig genes is known as ***V(D)J recombination***.

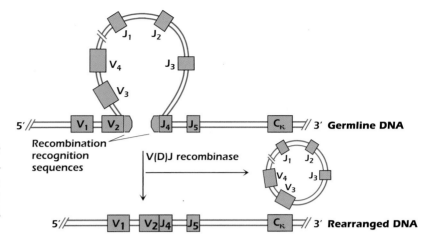

Figure 7.3. Involvement of V(D)J recombinase in rearrangement of DNA coding for a κ L chain. When the V(D)J recombinase joins the V_2 and J_4 gene segments at the recombination recognition sequences, the intervening DNA (V_3, V_4, etc.) is looped out and deleted.

κ-Chain Synthesis

The top line of Figure 7.2 shows the arrangement of the set of genes coding for human κ chains—referred to as the *κ locus* (located on chromosome 2)—in the *germline*, that is, in *any* cell in the body. There are approximately 40 different Vκ gene segments, arranged linearly and separated from each other by introns, 5 different Jκ segments downstream of the Vκ genes, and a single Cκ gene downstream of the Jκ genes. Each Vκ gene has its own leader sequence, which, for simplicity, has been omitted from the figure. The regions containing Vκ gene segments, Jκ gene segments, and the Cκ gene are separated from each other by long stretches of DNA.

Each Vκ gene segment has the ability to code for the N-terminal 95 amino acids of a κ variable region. Each of the smaller Jκ gene segments can code for the remaining 13 amino acid residues (96–108) of the κ variable region.

Figure 7.2 shows how a κ chain is synthesized by V(D)J recombination. Early in its development in the bone marrow (in the bursa in avian species), each B cell selects one of the Vκ genes from its DNA and physically joins it to one of the Jκ segments; in the B cell shown in the figure, V_2 rearranges to J_4. The mechanism of selection of V and J genes is unknown, but it is probably random. The stage in B cell development at which this occurs is explained in Chapter 8.

The rearrangement of Vκ to Jκ—and indeed the rearrangement of all Ig and TCR genes—is mediated by the V(D)J recombinase enzyme complex, which cuts and joins different gene segments in DNA. Some of the enzymes of the recombinase complex are involved in the repair of DNA strands in all cells of the body, but two of its components—*recombination-activating (RAG)-1 and RAG-2*—are expressed exclusively in developing lymphocytes. RAG-1 and RAG-2 are required for the initial

cutting of Ig (and TCR) DNA, and so RAG-1 and RAG-2 are critical for the development of B and T cells. Humans whose RAG-1 or RAG-2 gene product is defective lack mature B and T cells; this is one form of severe combined immunodeficiency (SCID) that is described in more detail in Chapter 18. Mice lacking either RAG-1 or RAG-2 genes ("RAG knockout") are also deficient in both B and T cells.

Figure 7.3 shows in more detail how the V(D)J recombinase-mediated cutting and joining of the κ locus DNA occurs. The V(D)J recombinase recognizes *recombination recognition sequences* that are located at the ends of the V and J gene segments. These recombination recognition sequences are conserved among all V, J (and D) gene segments used by Ig and TCR genes. The recombinase joins together the V_2 and J_4 gene segments, and the intervening DNA containing V_3, V_4 etc., is looped, cut out, and ultimately degraded. Note that the rearranged DNA in this early B cell still contains the gene segments V_1 and J_5 that were not affected by the recombination process.

After the DNA of a cell in the B-cell lineage has been rearranged (V_2 to J_4), a primary RNA transcript is made, which still contains introns (Figure 7.2). The primary transcript is then spliced to give a mature mRNA in which the Vκ, Jκ, and Cκ exons are brought together and the introns and additional J exons are removed. In the rough endoplasmic reticulum, this mRNA is translated into a complete κ polypeptide chain. The κ chain then moves into the lumen of the endoplasmic reticulum where the signal peptide (encoded by the leader sequence) is cleaved off, and the κ chain can now associate with a newly synthesized H chain to form an Ig molecule.

We explain in more detail below that every B cell has two sets of chromosomes—one set from each parent—and hence two κ loci. The rearrangement mechanism we have described occurs in a sequence. The cell first tries rearrangement at one of the two κ loci. If this results in a functional

Ig L chain (a "productive" rearrangement), rearrangement does not occur at either the other κ locus or the two λ loci; they remain in germline configuration. If the result of the rearrangement at the first κ locus is nonproductive, however, rearrangement at the other κ locus, and then the λ loci is tried sequentially.

λ-Chain Synthesis

The λ locus is found on chromosome 22 in the human, that is, on a chromosome distinct from the κ and the H-chain loci. Rearrangement of the λ locus occurs when rearrangement at both κ loci has been unsuccessful (nonproductive). The mechanism of λ locus rearrangement is similar to what we just described for κ chains. The synthesis of λ chains uses V and J gene segments and rearrangement of DNA mediated by V(D)J recombinase: one of about 30 Vλ gene segments is joined to one of the 4 Jλ gene segments. Each V_λ gene segment codes for the N-terminal region of a λ variable region, and each Jλ segment codes for the remaining 13 amino acids of the λ variable region. The organization of the λ locus is slightly different from that of the κ locus, which contains only one Cκ gene: each Jλ is associated with a different Cλ gene. Thus, each λ chain will have one of four possible Cλ regions. Note though that these different Cλ have similar functions, so they should not be considered the equivalent of different H-chain constant (C_H) regions, which we described in Chapter 5 as having different effector functions.

Once the V_λ and J_λ segments have rearranged in a particular B cell, the steps in the synthesis of a λ chain polypep-tide are very similar to those already described for the synthesis of a κ-chain polypeptide (see Figure 7.2).

Organization and Rearrangement of Heavy-Chain Genes

Figure 7.4 shows the organization of genes coding for immunoglobulin H chains—*the H-chain locus*. The human H chain locus is found on chromosome 14, distinct from either L-chain locus. The figure illustrates the similarities and differences of this locus with the L-chain loci. The first major difference is that the three different gene segments V_H, D_H, and J_H code for the variable region of the H chain. Thus, in addition to V_H and J_H segments, genes coding for the variable region of an H chain also use a *diversity* (**D**) *segment*. The D and J segments code for amino acid sequences in the third hypervariable region or *complementarity-determining region* (CDR3) of the H chain (see Chapter 5). The genes in the V region code for the first two hypervariable regions (CDR1 and 2). Figure 7.4 indicates that the human H-chain locus includes approximately 40 V_H genes, about 25 D_H gene segments, and 6 J_H gene segments.

The top line of Figure 7.4 also shows the second key feature of the H-chain locus: the presence in the germline of multiple genes coding for the C_H region of the immunoglobulin. Humans have nine C_H genes, one for each Ig class or subclass, clustered at the 3′ end of the H-chain locus; Cμ is closest to the V, D, and J segments. As described in Chapter 5, the C_H region determines the class—IgM, IgD, IgG, IgA or IgE—and hence biologic function of the particular antibody synthesized. H-chain synthesis uses the

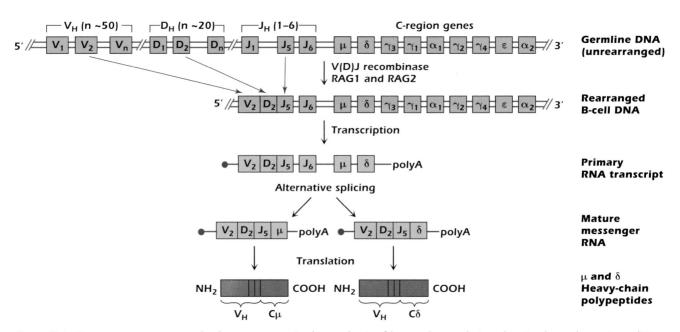

Figure 7.4. Gene rearrangements and subsequent steps in the synthesis of human heavy chains, showing how alternative splicing of B-cell RNA results in μ and δ chains of identical antigenic specificity.

same mechanisms of rearrangement described for L chains—namely, the use of the V(D)J recombinase and RAG-1 and RAG-2 gene products to mediate the cutting of DNA and joining of different gene segments. In the early stages of the life of a particular B cell, two rearrangements of germline DNA occur at one of the H-chain loci (line 2 of Figure 7.4). The first joins one D segment to one J segment, and the second brings one V segment next to the DJ unit ($V_2 D_2 J_5$ in Figure 7.4), fixing the antigen specificity of the H chain. If this rearrangement is successful, the other H-chain gene remains in germline configuration. As described in Chapter 8, in the stage of B cell differentiation known as the immature B cell, this VDJ unit is transcribed together with the closest C-region gene, Cμ, so the immature B cell expresses only IgM at the surface.

In the next stage of B-cell differentiation, the ***mature B cell*** shown in Figure 7.4 expresses both IgM and IgD at the surface. In this cell, the rearranged $V_2 D_2 J_5$ DNA is transcribed along with both the two closest C$_H$-region genes, Cμ and Cδ (line 3 of Figure 7.4). The primary transcript that contains both Cμ and Cδ RNA can be spliced in two different ways (***alternative splicing***) to yield either a VDJ-μ or a VDJ-δ mRNA; as a result, one mature B cell synthesizes both mRNAs. The two mRNAs are then translated in rough endoplasmic reticulum to yield either a μ or δ polypeptide. The individual H-chain polypeptides combine inside the cell with the L chain (either κ or λ) produced in the cell to form IgM and IgD, respectively, which traffic to the cell membrane. In this way, an individual mature B cell may express at its surface both IgM and IgD with identical antigenic specificity.

In addition to the form expressed at the surface of a B cell, IgM, IgG, IgA, and IgE (but not IgD) can also exist in a secreted form. This secreted Ig molecule is synthesized by a plasma cell, a cell that does not express Ig on its surface (see Chapter 8). The membrane and secreted forms of an Ig molecule are coded for by additional short exons at the 3′ end of each C$_H$ gene [not shown in Fig. 7.4].) For example, at the 3′ end of the Cμ gene, additional exons code for (a) the transmembrane region plus the cytoplasmic tail of the membrane form of Cμ, and (b) the C-terminal end of the secreted form of Cμ. All these exons are transcribed into one large primary transcript of the Cμ gene. Alternative splicing of this primary transcript results in two different mRNA species, one containing the RNA for the transmembrane region plus cytoplasmic tail that will be translated into the membrane form of the molecule, and one containing the RNA for the C-terminal end that will be translated into the secreted form of the same H chain.

Allelic Exclusion and the Regulation of Ig Gene Expression

Every B cell has many genes from which it can synthesize an Ig molecule: multiple V, D, and J genes to form the vari-

able regions and different genes for the κ and λ L chains. In addition, because a given B cell has two sets of chromosomes—one set from each parent—theoretically, Ig genes located on *both* chromosomes could code for Ig molecules. This could result in one B cell expressing multiple different antigen specificities. This does not occur. Each B cell expresses only one H-chain protein, which is synthesized by the rearranged H-chain locus located on either the maternal or paternal chromosome, and only one L-chain protein (either κ or λ), which is synthesized by the rearranged L-chain locus located on either the maternal or paternal chromosome. For example, the H chain may be coded for by genes on the paternal chromosome and the L chain (either κ or λ) by genes on the maternal chromosome.

This phenomenon of using genes from only one parental chromosome is known as ***allelic exclusion***; that is, only one of the two possible ***alleles***—alternative versions of a particular gene—in an individual's chromosomes is used to synthesize a polypeptide. In addition, the B cell synthesizes only one type of L chain so that the L-chain gene expression shows both isotype and allelic exclusion. The other alleles are "silenced." For nearly every other gene in the body, protein is synthesized from genes located on *both* parental chromosomes. As a result of allelic exclusion, one B cell synthesizes and expresses an Ig molecule of only a single antigenic specificity.

The steps in rearrangement, allelic exclusion, and synthesis of a complete Ig molecule are very tightly controlled. Rearrangement is tried first at one H-chain locus. If a successful or productive rearrangement of V, D, and J gene DNA occurs on one parental chromosome and an H-chain polypeptide is produced, the other parental H-chain locus stops rearranging as a result of a suppressive mechanism. If the attempt to rearrange the V, D, and J genes on the first parental chromosome is nonproductive (i.e., if it fails to produce a polypeptide chain), then the second parental chromosome begins H-chain locus rearrangement. The same process then occurs with the L-chain loci, first with the κ- and then with the λ-chain genes. Productive rearrangement resulting from the joining of a V segment to a J segment of any one of these genes causes the others to remain in germline form. In humans, the ratio of $\kappa:\lambda$ expressing B cells is approximately 2:1, suggesting that attempts at rearrangement are often successful at the κ locus. The developing B cell progresses through some or all of its chromosomal copies until it has successfully completed the productive rearrangement of genes for one H and one L chain. These chains then become the basis of the antibody specificity of that particular B cell. If a cell fails to productively rearrange any of its Ig genes, it dies.

In summary, only one H chain and one L chain are functionally expressed in a B cell, even though every B cell contains two chromosomes (paternally and maternally derived) that could code for the H chain and two chromosomes that could code for each L chain. This phenomenon of allelic exclusion ensures that an individual B cell expresses an Ig molecule (IgM, IgD, IgG, IgA, or IgE) on its cell surface of only one single antigen specificity. Similarly, the antibody molecule synthesized and secreted by that B cell will be specific for a single antigenic epitope.

CLASS OR ISOTYPE SWITCHING

As we have described above, one B cell makes antibody of a single specificity that is fixed by the nature of VJ (L-chain) and VDJ (H-chain) rearrangements. As we describe in detail in Chapter 8, these rearrangements occur in the absence of antigen in the early stages of B-cell differentiation.

Earlier in this chapter we described how a single mature B cell can synthesize IgM and IgD with the same antigenic specificity. If this IgM^+IgD^+ B cell is stimulated with antigen, it can undergo *class* or *isotype switching* via a mechanism known as *class switch recombination*, which is shown in Figure 7.5. The antigen-activated B cell literally switches its C_H genes by rearranging its DNA again, cutting out some of its C_H genes and transcribing a different, downstream C_H gene. Thus, this B cell switches to synthesizing an Ig molecule of a different class or isotype: IgG, IgE, or IgA. Class switching changes the effector function of the B cell but does not change the cell's antigenic specificity.

Figure 7.5 shows the key features of class switch recombination in an antigen-stimulated mature B cell. This

B cell expresses IgM and IgD of the same antigenic specificity, defined by the recombination events that brought together the $V_2 D_2 J_5$ unit. If this B cell is stimulated by antigen in the presence of signals from T cells (see below and further discussion in Chapters 8 and 11), it undergoes a further rearrangement of its DNA, juxtaposing the rearranged VDJ genes with a different H-chain C-region gene (γ_1 in Figure 7.5). The change in C region genes occurs at a *switch* (S) *region*, a stretch of repeating base sequences at the 5′ (upstream) end of every C_H gene, other than Cδ. In the figure, only the C_H genes γ_3, γ_1, and α_2 are shown, but other C_H genes further downstream may also be used. In so doing, the intervening C-region DNA, including the switch regions, is removed. Thus, at this stage, the cell loses its ability to make a class of antibody whose C-region gene has been deleted (IgM, IgD, or IgG_3 in this cell). After a primary RNA transcript is made from the rearranged DNA, the remaining introns are spliced out to give an mRNA coding for, in this example, the IgG_1 H chain. As a result of class switch recombination, this B cell now synthesizes an Ig molecule with a different H chain—IgG_1—but still specific for the original antigen that activated it.

Class switch recombination is unique to the Ig H-chain locus. It allows an antibody with a particular antigenic specificity to associate with a variety of different constant-region chains and thus have different effector functions. For example, an antibody with a VDJ unit specific for a bacterial antigen may be linked to Cγ to produce an IgG molecule;

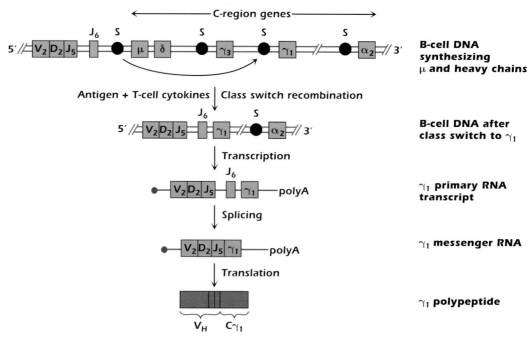

Figure 7.5. Class switch recombination. S = switch region, upstream of each H-chain constant region. In the presence of antigen and T-cell-derived cytokines, the VDJ unit that was closely linked to the closest H-chain constant regions—Cμ and Cδ—"switches," and is joined to the Cγ₁ H-chain constant region. This antigen-activated B cell now synthesizes a γ₁ polypeptide, and hence IgG₁, with identical antigenic specificity to the B cell that originally interacted with antigen.

this IgG antibody interacts via its Fc region with cells such as macrophages that express receptors for Fcγ. Alternatively, the same VDJ unit may be linked to Cε to produce an IgE molecule; IgE antibody interacts with cells such as mast cells that express receptors for Fcε. As we indicated above, isotype switching does not affect the antigen specificity of this B cell because Ig V region gene usage is not modified.

Class switch recombination generally occurs in the germinal center of a secondary lymphoid organ (discussed in more detail in Chapter 8). It requires antigen stimulation of the B cell through its receptor (BCR), paired interactions between the B- and T-cell surfaces, and T-cell-derived cytokines; in the absence of T-cell-derived signals there is little or no class switching by B cells. A further important feature of class switch recombination is that it requires the enzyme, *activation-induced cytidine deaminase* (AID), which is expressed by B cells activated in the germinal center of secondary lymphoid organs. As we also describe in more detail in Chapter 11, the cytokine present when antigen activates a B cells plays a key role in which C_H gene is selected; for example, in the presence of interferon-γ, the B cell rearranges its VDJ to the $C\gamma_3$ H chain, and the cell switches to IgG_3 synthesis. By contrast, in the presence of the cytokine IL-4, a B cell rearranges its VDJ to $C\gamma_4$ or Cε, and the cell switches to IgG_4 or IgE synthesis, respectively.

GENERATION OF ANTIBODY DIVERSITY

Thus far we have described the unique genetic mechanisms involved in generating an enormous variety of antibodies from a relatively small amount of DNA to cope with a multitude of antigens. Still more mechanisms exist for generating diversity, some of which are discussed briefly below.

Presence of Multiple V Genes in the Germline

The number of different genes for the V region in the germline constitutes the baseline from which antibody is derived and represents the minimum number of different antibodies that can be produced.

VJ and VDJ Combinatorial Association

As we have already described, any V gene segment can associate with any J gene segment to form an L-chain variable region. Similarly, any V gene segment can associate with any D or J gene segments in H-chain gene rearrangement. All of these distinct segments contribute to the structure of the variable region. As there are about 40Vκ and 5Jκ genes coding for the κ-chain variable region, assuming random association, then $40 \times 5 = 200$κ chains that can be formed; with 30Vλ and 4Jλ genes, 120λ chains can be

formed. Similarly, if there are about 40V genes, 25D genes, and 6J genes that can code for an H-chain variable region, and these may also associate in any combination, $40 \times 25 \times 6 = 6,000$ different H chains that can be formed.

Random Assortment of H and L Chains

In addition to VJ and VDJ combinatorial association, any H chain may associate with any L chain. Thus, a total of 1.2×10^6 different κ-containing Ig molecules $(200 \times 6,000)$ and 0.72×10^6 $(12 \times 6,000)$ λ-containing molecules can be generated from just 150 different genes (adding up all the H, κ, and λ segments)! This illustrates very effectively how a limited set of genes can generate a large number of different antibodies.

Junctional Diversity

DNA strands are cut and then rejoined as part of V(D)J recombination. However, the joining of V, D, and J segments is imprecise; that is, during the joining, small numbers of nucleotides can either be added or deleted at the end of the DNA strands. Consequently, the nucleotide sequence at the junctions can alter and in turn may change the amino acid sequence in the Ig polypeptide that is subsequently synthesized. Because imprecise recombination occurs in parts of the Ig hypervariable region where complementarity to antigen is determined, junctional diversity can result in changes in the amino acids in the antigen-binding site. All these changes are referred to as introducing *junctional diversity*. It has been calculated that about 80% of Ig molecules show some sort of junctional diversity, when compared to germline sequences.

One mechanism of adding nucleotides ("N-nucleotides") to the cut DNA is mediated by the enzyme *terminal deoxynucleotidyltransferase* (TdT). In addition, some nucleotides, called "P-nucleotides," can be introduced at the junctions of the cut DNA by mechanisms that do not involve TdT. During V(D)J recombination, nucleotides can also be deleted from the cut ends of DNA segments by enzymes known as exonucleases. The overall result of the addition and/or deletion of nucleotides is to make the junctions between V, D, and J segments highly variable, creating diversity in the antigen-binding site.

Somatic Hypermutation

Mutations that occur in V genes of H and/or L chains during the lifetime of a B cell also increase the variety and affinity of antibodies produced by the B-cell population. This results from *somatic hypermutation*, random point mutations in the recombined V(D)J unit of antibody H- or L-chain V region genes, changing individual amino acids. It is called "hypermutation" because it occurs at a rate at least 10,000 times higher than the normal rate of mutation.

Generally, antibodies of low affinity are produced in the primary response to antigen. As we describe in more detail in Chapter 8, however, the further development of the B-cell response to antigen in the germinal center of secondary lymphoid organs results in somatic hypermutation and an *increase* in the antibodies' affinity for antigen. This is referred to as **affinity maturation** of the immune response. Thus, somatic hypermutation increases both the variety and the affinity of antibodies produced by the B-cell population.

Somatic Gene Conversion

The paradigm that Ig diversity is generated by VDJ recombination and somatic hypermutation evolved from studies of mouse and human B cells. However, subsequent studies in other species, most notably in birds and rabbits, revealed that these animals use a different mechanism, known as **somatic gene conversion**, to generate a wide variety of diverse B-cell specificities. Somatic gene conversion involves the nonreciprocal exchange of sequences among genes: Part of the donor gene or genes is "copied" into an acceptor gene, but only the acceptor gene is altered. The precise mechanism by which this occurs is currently not clear. Figure 7.6 shows the chicken H-chain locus, which includes a single functional V_H gene that rearranges in all B cells, along with approximately 20 **pseudogenes**—gene segments that have mutations that prevent them from synthesizing a polypeptide. The bottom line of the figure shows that in this particular B cell a diversified variable gene unit is generated by incorporating two short sequences from pseudogene 3 and one from pseudogene 8 into the rearranged VDJ gene. Somatic gene conversion can also generate L-chain diversity.

Many species other than humans and mice rely on somatic gene conversion and somatic hypermutation to generate diversity within the *primary* Ig repertoire, that is, before antigen stimulation. For example, chickens use somatic gene conversion as a major mechanism to generate the primary repertoire, and sheep use somatic hypermutation. Other species, such as rabbit, cattle, and swine, use very limited VDJ recombination plus somatic gene conversion and somatic hypermutation to generate their primary Ig diversity.

All these mechanisms contribute to the formation of a huge library or **repertoire** of B lymphocytes that contains all the specificities required to deal with the multitude of diverse epitopes that antibodies could encounter. Estimates of the number of total Ig specificities that can be generated in an individual are on the order of 10^{11}, which is increased even more by somatic hypermutation.

ROLE OF ACTIVATION-INDUCED CYTIDINE DEAMINASE IN GENERATING ANTIBODY DIVERSITY

As we mentioned above, the enzyme **activation-induced cytidine deaminase** (AID) plays a key role in class switch recombination. As its name implies, AID removes amino groups from cytidine to convert it to uridine in the DNA in activated B cells. This generates U:G base pairs in DNA; the mismatched base pairs are then removed by one of several different enzymes. This, in turn, results in changes in the DNA, primarily in Ig V-region genes. Why AID interacts preferentially with Ig V-region genes is not currently well understood. A defect in this gene results in a deficiency known as hyper-IgM syndrome 2, characterized by high levels of IgM but little or no levels of other isotypes.

We also know that AID is also involved in somatic hypermutation and gene conversion. Thus, AID plays a role in the three major processes that generate diversity of antibodies. The precise function of AID in these three processes is currently under investigation. The role of AID in class switch recombination and somatic hypermutation in the germinal center is discussed further in Chapter 8.

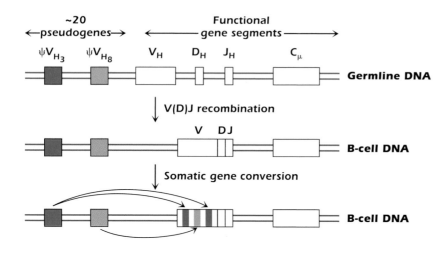

Figure 7.6. Somatic gene conversion generates diversity in the Ig genes of several species. The figure illustrates the phenomenon in the chicken Ig H-chain locus: short sequences of DNA from one or more pseudogenes (3 and 8 in the figure) are copied into the rearranged B-cell VDJ unit. Pseudogenes are gene segments with mutations that prevent them from synthesizing a polypeptide.

SUMMARY

1. B (and T) cells use a unique rearrangement (or recombination) mechanism in which a limited number of Ig (and TCR, in T cells) gene segments are combined—literally move and are joined together—in the genome of the developing lymphocyte. This mechanism is key in generating the enormous number of Ig (antibody) and TCR molecules found in every individual.

2. The joining of Ig and TCR gene segments is mediated by an enzyme complex, VDJ recombinase. Two components of the recombinase RAG 1 and RAG2 are specifically expressed in lymphocytes and are required for the cutting and joining of DNA in the developing lymphocyte.

3. Light chain synthesis: In a single B cell, the V region of an Ig L chain (κ or λ) is coded for by two gene segments, V_L and J_L; V_L codes for the first 95 amino acids of the V region and the J_L for the remaining 13 amino acids. A different gene codes for the constant region of the same L chain, C_L. The κ and λ loci—the genes coding for the κ and λ chains—are found on different chromosomes.

4. There are multiple V_L and J_L gene segments in every cell in the body. In a developing B cell, the VDJ recombinase complex physically joins, that is, rearranges, one V_L to one J_L, putting the VJ unit close to an L-chain constant-region gene. In a B cell committed to making a κ chain, the $V\kappa J\kappa$ unit is juxtaposed to the $C\kappa$ gene; in a B cell committed to making a λ chain, the $V\lambda J\lambda$ unit is juxtaposed to a $C\lambda$ gene.

5. Primary RNA transcripts are made from the rearranged DNA of the L-chain gene segments. Noncoding RNA is spliced out of the primary transcripts, resulting in mRNA. The mRNA is then translated into a κ or λ L chain.

6. Heavy chain synthesis: In a single B cell, the V region of an Ig H chain is coded for by three separate gene segments that are distinct from the gene segments used for L-chain synthesis chromosome. These gene segments are V_H (variable), D_H (diversity), and J_H (joining). A distinct gene segment codes for the constant region of the H chain, C_H; there are multiple C_H region genes: $C\mu$, $C\delta$, $C\gamma$, $C\alpha$, and $C\varepsilon$. The H-chain locus is found on a chromosome different from the κ and λ loci chromosomes.

7. There are multiple V_H, D_H, and J_H gene segments in every cell in the body. Similar to the rearrangements described for L-chain genes, the VDJ recombinase in a developing B cell physically joins one V_H gene segment to one D_H gene segment and one J_H gene segment. The joined VDJ unit codes for the entire variable region of the H chain. These gene rearrangements put the VDJ unit close to the H-chain constant-region genes.

8. In an immature B cell, the cell transcribes and translates the VDJ with the closest C_H, $C\mu$, and so synthesizes IgM. In a mature B cell, the cell transcribes VDJ-$C\mu C\delta$. At the primary transcript stage in mature B cells, alternative splicing of the H-chain RNA results in either a μ or δ chain; thus, one mature B cell synthesizes an IgM and an IgD molecule with identical antigenic specificity.

9. In a B cell, the H chain is coded for by the H-chain gene segments found on either the maternally derived chromosome or the paternally derived chromosome; the L chain is also coded for by the L-chain gene segments found on only one of these two chromosomes. This phenomenon, called allelic exclusion, ensures that a particular B cell produces an immunoglobulin of a single antigenic specificity.

10. After antigenic stimulation and in the presence of T-cell help and T-cell-derived cytokines in the germinal center, a mature B cell can undergo class switch recombination, and further rearrange its H-chain DNA. The VDJ unit of this cell, which was initially close to and transcribed with the $C\mu$ and $C\delta$ genes, can "switch" and be put close to another C-region gene, such as $C\gamma$, $C\alpha$, or $C\varepsilon$. As a result, the B cell that was synthesizing IgM and IgD can now synthesize antibody of a different isotype (IgG, IgA, or IgE) but with the same antigenic specificity.

11. Diversity in antibody specificity is achieved by the following:
    • Multiple inherited genes for the V regions of both L and H chains.
    • Rearrangement of V, D, and J segments in different combinations and random assortment of H and L chains.
    • Junctional diversity at the sites of V, D, and J gene segment joining caused by imprecise joining after nucleotide deletions or insertions (primarily mediated by terminal deoxynucleotidyltransferase (TdT).
    • Somatic hypermutation, which occurs after stimulation by antigen in germinal centers, changes

sequences in B cells' Ig V regions and hence alters the B cells' antigen-binding specificity. B cells with mutations in their V regions that endow the antibody with higher affinity for the antigen are selected.
- Somatic gene conversion in species other than the human or mouse: Short DNA sequences from non-rearranging genes are copied into a rearranged VDJ gene unit.

- These mechanisms allow a small number of genes to generate a vast number of antibody molecules with different antigenic specificities. One enzyme, activation-induced cytidine deaminase (AID), is involved in class switch recombination, somatic hypermutation, and gene conversion, the three major pathways that generate diversity of antibodies.

REFERENCES AND BIBLIOGRAPHY

Chaudhuri J, et al. (2007) Evolution of the immunoglobulin heavy chain class switch recombination mechanism. *Adv Immunol* 94: 157.

Di Noia JM, Neuberger MS. (2007) Molecular mechanisms of antibody somatic hypermutation. *Annu Rev Biochem* 76: 1.

Dudley DD, Chaudhuri J, Bassing CH, Alt FW. (2005) Mechanism and control of V(D)J recombination versus class switch recombination: Similarities and differences. *Adv Immunol* 86: 43.

Odegard VH, Schatz DG. (2006) Targeting of somatic hypermutation. *Nat Rev Immunol* 6: 573.

Petersen-Mahrt S. (2005) DNA deamination in immunity. *Immunol Rev* 203: 80.

Schatz DG, Spanopoulou E. (2005) Biochemistry of V(D)J recombination. *Curr Top Microbiol Immunol* 290: 49.

REVIEW QUESTIONS

For each question, choose the ONE BEST answer or completion.

1. The DNA for an H chain in a B-cell making IgG_2 antibody for diphtheria toxoid has the following structure: $5'\text{-}V_{17}D_5J_2 \; C\gamma_2\text{-}C\gamma_4\text{-}C\varepsilon\text{-}C\alpha_2\text{-}3'$. How many individual rearrangements were required to go from the embryonic DNA to this B-cell DNA?
   A) 1
   B) 2
   C) 3
   D) 4
   E) none

2. If you had 40 V, 25 D, and 6 J regions able to code for an H chain and 40 V and 5 J-region genes able to code for an L chain, you could have a maximum repertoire of:
   A) $76 + 45 = 121$ antibody specificities
   B) $76 \times 45 = 3{,}420$ specificities
   C) $(40 \times 5) + (40 \times 25 \times 6) = 6200$ specificities
   D) $(40 \times 5) \times (40 \times 25 \times 6) = 1{,}200{,}000$ specificities
   E) more than 1,200,000 specificities

3. The antigen specificity of a particular B cell:
   A) is induced by interaction with antigen
   B) is determined only by the L-chain sequence
   C) is determined by H+L-chain variable-region sequences

   D) changes after isotype switching
   E) is determined by the H-chain constant region

4. If you could analyze at the molecular level a plasma cell making IgA antibody, you would find all of the following *except*:
   A) a DNA sequence for V, D, and J genes translocated near the $C\alpha$ DNA exon
   B) mRNA specific for either κ or λ L chains
   C) mRNA specific for J chains
   D) mRNA specific for μ chains
   E) a DNA sequence coding for the T-cell receptor for antigen

5. The ability of a single B cell to express both IgM and IgD molecules on its surface at the same time is made possible by:
   A) allelic exclusion
   B) isotype switching
   C) simultaneous recognition of two distinct antigens
   D) alternative RNA splicing
   E) use of genes from both parental chromosomes

6. Which of the following statements concerning the organization of Ig genes is correct?
   A) V and J regions of embryonic DNA have already undergone a rearrangement.

B) Light-chain genes undergo further rearrangement after surface IgM is expressed.

C) V_H gene segments can rearrange with Jκ or Jλ gene segments.

D) The VDJ segments coding for an Ig V_H region may associate with different H-chain constant-region genes.

E) After VDJ joining has occurred, a further rearrangement is required to bring the VDJ unit next to the Cμ gene.

7. Which of the following does not contribute to the antigen-binding site diversity of B-cell antigen receptors?
A) multiple V genes in the germline
B) random assortment of L and H chains
C) imprecise recombination of V and J, or V, D, and J segments
D) inheritance of multiple C-region genes
E) somatic hypermutation

8. Which of the following statements regarding a B cell expressing both IgM and IgD on its membrane is incorrect?

A) The L chains of the IgM and IgD have identical amino acid sequences.

B) The constant parts of the H chains of the IgM and IgD have different amino acid sequences.

C) The IgM and IgD have different antigenic specificities.

D) If it is triggered by antigen and T-cell signals to proliferate and differentiate, it may differentiate into a plasma cell that may secrete IgG, IgE, or IgA antibodies.

E) The IgM on the surface will have either κ or λ L chains, but not both.

9. Which of the following plays a role in changing the antigen binding site of a B cell *after* antigenic stimulation?
A) junctional diversity
B) combinatorial diversity
C) germline diversity
D) somatic hypermutation
E) differential splicing of primary RNA transcripts

ANSWERS TO REVIEW QUESTIONS

1. C. Three DNA rearrangements are required. First, $D_5 \rightarrow J_2$ rearrangement occurs, followed by $V_{17} \rightarrow D_5 J_2$. This permits synthesis of IgM and IgD molecules using $V_{17} D_5 J_2$. The third rearrangement is the class switch of $V_{17} D_5 J_2 C\mu C\delta$ to $V_{17} D_5 J_2 C\gamma_2$, leading to the synthesis of IgG$_2$ molecules.

2. E. While 1,200,000 would be the product of all possible combinations of genes, many more antibody specificities are likely to be generated as a result of junctional diversity at the sites of V, D, and J gene segment joining (caused by imprecise joining, deletions, and nucleotide insertions) and somatic hypermutation.

3. C. The antigenic specificity is determined by the sequences and hence the structure formed by the combination of H- and L-chain variable regions.

4. D. As a consequence of the rearrangement of the VDJ to Cα in the IgA-producing cell, the Cμ gene will have been deleted. The other DNA sequences and mRNA species will be found in the cell.

5. D. The simultaneous synthesis of IgM and IgD is made possible by the alternative splicing of the primary RNA transcript 5′–VDJ–Cμ–Cδ–3′ to give either VDJCμ or VDJCδ mRNAs.

6. D. The association of VDJ segments coding for an Ig V_H region with different H-chain constant-region genes is the basis of isotype or class switching.

7. D. The presence of multiple C$_H$-region genes does provide the basis for functional diversity of Ig molecules but does *not* contribute to the diversity of antigen-specific receptors.

8. C. The IgM and IgD expressed on a single B cell use the same H- and L-chain V(D)J gene units and therefore have the same antigenic specificity.

9. D. Of the mechanisms described for generating diversity of Ig molecules, only somatic hypermutation affects the antigen binding site *after* antigen stimulation.

8

BIOLOGY OF THE B LYMPHOCYTE

INTRODUCTION

In previous chapters we described how B cells synthesize an enormous array of antibodies with different functions, with the function of the antibody—IgM, IgG, IgA or IgE—depending on the nature of the heavy chain. We also discussed the mechanisms B cells use to develop a vast *repertoire* that can respond to the universe of different antigenic specificities. These mechanisms explain two key features of the adaptive immune response (Chapter 1, Figure 1.1): *diversity*, the ability to respond to an enormous variety of different antigenic determinants (epitopes) even if the individual has not previously encountered them; and *specificity*, in which only the lymphocyte expressing the "correct" receptor among the universe of lymphocytes interacts with a particular epitope (clonal selection theory). With this enormous repertoire of potentially reactive B cells, it can almost be guaranteed that every person contains one or more clones of B cells able to interact with measles virus, one or more clones of B cells able to interact with a mycobacterium, and so on.

In this chapter we focus on the critical steps in B-cell development, from the earliest stages that take place in the absence of antigen through to the later stages that occur after the interaction with antigen and result in antibody synthesis. By these processes B cells acquire two other key features of the adaptive immune response: *discrimination between self and nonself*—the ability to respond to antigens that are "foreign" or nonself, and *not* to respond to antigens that are self; and *memory*—the ability to recall previous contact

with a particular antigen so that a subsequent interaction leads to a quicker, more effective secondary immune response.

DEVELOPMENT OF B LYMPHOCYTES

Overview

B lymphocytes acquired their name from early experiments in chickens. The synthesis of antibody was shown to require the presence of an organ called the *bursa of Fabricius* (an outpouching of the cloacal epithelium). Surgical removal of the bursa early in life prevented antibody synthesis. Thus the cells that developed into mature, antibody-forming cells were called *bursa-derived* or *B cells*. In contrast to chickens and other birds, mammals do not have a bursa; rather, the early stages of mammalian B-cell differentiation take place predominantly in the bone marrow throughout the life of the individual. Our understanding of B-cell differentiation has been facilitated by studies in animals in which the early embryonic stages can be easily manipulated. For this reason, B-cell differentiation is particularly well characterized in mice and chickens, but many of these differentiation steps are common to humans as well.

Figure 8.1 illustrates the key stages in the B-cell differentiation pathway, many of which are defined by specific immunoglobulin (Ig) gene rearrangements and by the expression of different surface markers (*CD markers*). As we describe below, many of the stages also represent

Immunology: A Short Course, Seventh Edition. Richard Coico and Geoffrey Sunshine.
© 2015 John Wiley & Sons, Ltd. Published 2015 by John Wiley & Sons, Ltd.
Companion Website: www.wileyimmunology.com/coico

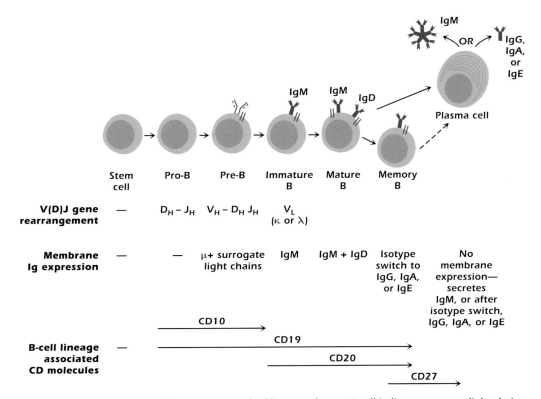

<u>Figure 8.1.</u> Stages in B-cell differentiation. Dashed lines on the pre-B cell indicate surrogate light chains. The two lines associated with the cell surface heavy chain represent the signaling molecules Igα and Igβ (CD79a and b). Not shown: CD10 also expressed by germinal center B cells.

developmental checkpoints—the signal received at these checkpoints determines whether the cell develops along one or another alternative pathway. The lack of a signal at this point may result in the death of the cell. Similar developmental checkpoints are also found in the differentiation of the T-cell lineage (see Chapter 10).

Sites of Early B-Cell Differentiation

B lymphocytes arise from *hematopoietic stem cells*. In mammals, the hematopoietic stem cells and the precursors of the B-cell lineage are found early in development of the fetus, at sites including the fetal liver. Later in fetal development, after birth and for the rest of life, the bone marrow is the main site of the early stages of B-cell differentiation. Thus in humans and other mammals, the bone marrow is the *primary lymphoid organ* for B-cell differentiation—the site at which the antigen-specific receptor is first expressed (see Chapter 3). B-cell differentiation occurs more or less throughout life, so the B-cell repertoire is continuously replenished.

During the early steps in the bone marrow, the *stroma*, the nonlymphoid cells that make up the framework or matrix of the marrow, provide critical adhesive interactions and produce cytokines such as interleukin (IL)-7 that promote the survival and enhance the proliferation of cells early in the B-cell lineage.

Pro-B and Pre-B Cells: First Ig Rearrangements

Pro-B cell: D to J Rearrangement. Figure 8.1 depicts the earliest distinguishable cell in the B lineage, the *pro-B cell*, which shows the first rearrangement of Ig genes: at the heavy-chain locus, a D_H gene segment rearranges to a J_H gene segment. This rearrangement is mediated by the V(D)J recombinase (also see Chapter 7). Pro-B cells express *CD19*, and CD19 is expressed on the surface of all subsequent stages of B-cell development except the plasma cell. CD19 is expressed almost exclusively on B cells, so expression of CD19 is a useful marker of all cells in the B-cell lineage up to the plasma cell. Pro-B cells also express *CD10*.

Pre-B Cell: V-DJ Rearrangement. In the next stage of B-cell differentiation, the *pre-B cell*, the Ig heavy-chain gene locus undergoes a second rearrangement. The V(D)J recombinase joins a heavy-chain V_H gene segment to the rearranged $D_H J_H$ segments, forming a VDJ unit. This rearranged VDJ is thus positioned close to Cμ, and the pre-B cell synthesizes a μ chain. No light-chain gene rearrangement has yet taken place. Like pro-B cells, pre-B cells express CD10 in addition to CD19.

The Ig heavy-chain gene rearrangements that occur during these early phases of B-cell differentiation follow an ordered sequence (Chapter 7): If the rearrangement at

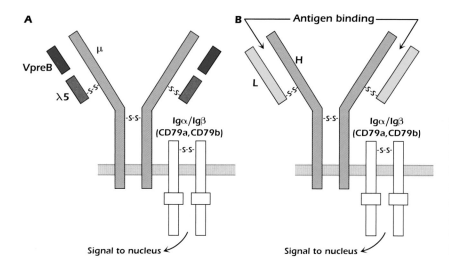

Figure 8.2. The pre-B-cell receptor (pre-BCR) (A), and B-cell receptor (BCR) (B). The heavy chain of the pre-BCR is a μ chain; the heavy chain of the BCR may be a μ, δ, γ, α, or ε chain. Igα/Igβ are signal transduction molecules associated with the pre-BCR and the BCR. The immunoreceptor tyrosine-based activation motif (ITAM) is depicted as a rectangle in the Igα and Igβ polypeptides.

the heavy-chain locus on the first of the two parental chromosomes is **productive**, that is, capable of being properly transcribed and translated into a μ chain, further rearrangement of heavy-chain gene segments is shut down. If the rearrangement is not productive on the first chromosome, rearrangement takes place on the second chromosome. If this rearrangement is productive, a μ chain is made.

The Pre-B Cell Receptor.   A key characteristic of the pre-B cell is that it expresses the **pre-B cell receptor** (pre-BCR) at the surface (Figure 8.2A). The expression of the pre-BCR is a key early developmental checkpoint in the B cell lineage; if the cell does not make a pre-BCR—because no heavy-chain rearrangement is productive—the cell dies by **apoptosis**, also known as **programmed cell death**.

The pre-BCR consists of the μ chain and two sets of tightly associated proteins: One set are the **surrogate light chains VpreB (CD179a)** and **λ5 (CD179b)** (Figure 8.2A) that bind to the μ chain on the outer side of the cell surface. VpreB is structurally similar to an IgV region and λ5 is structurally similar to the constant region of a λ light chain. λ5 and VpreB are the products of non-rearranging genes that are expressed only at this stage in B-cell development. λ5 and VpreB are associated but not covalently linked to each other; λ5, though, is covalently linked through disulfide bonds to the μ chain, similar to the binding of a light chain to a heavy chain.

The second set of proteins associated with the μ chain are **Igα (CD79a)** and **Igβ (CD79b)**, which are juxtaposed in the membrane with the Ig heavy-chain on all cells in the B-cell lineage, from the pre-B cell to the memory B cell (see Figure 8.1). Igα and Igβ form a disulfide bond-linked heterodimer (Igα/Igβ). Igα/Igβ do not bind antigen but act as **signal transduction molecules** for both the pre-BCR (Figure 8.2A) and the **B-cell receptor** (BCR) (Figure 8.2B), the complex of molecules that is expressed in cells of the B-cell lineage beyond the pre-B cell stage of development. Signal transduction molecules transmit signals into the cell that

activate intracellular pathways which ultimately reach the cell nucleus, leading to a change in the pattern of genes expressed. Similar signal transduction molecules are associated with the antigen-specific receptor on the T lymphocyte (Chapters 10 and 11). The signal transduction function of Igα/Igβ is mediated by their cytoplasmic regions, which contain sequences of amino acids known as **immunoreceptor tyrosine-based activation motifs** (ITAMs). The function of ITAMs is explained later in this chapter.

In B cells that express a BCR, Igα/Igβ transmit signals following antigen binding. It is currently unresolved, however, what molecules, if any, act as ligands for the pre-BCR to trigger signaling. Our current understanding is that in the pre-B cell, the signal from Igα/Igβ indicates that the cell has successfully rearranged its Ig heavy-chain genes and has made a functional μ chain. As a result of signaling through the pre-BCR, the pre-B cell further differentiates: It proliferates, shuts down surrogate light-chain synthesis, starts light-chain gene rearrangement mediated by the V(D)J recombinase, and stops further heavy-chain gene rearrangement.

Like heavy-chain gene rearrangements, light-chain gene rearrangement in the later phases of pre-B-cell development is sequential: the κ-chain genes rearrange first, but if neither of the chromosomes coding for κ chains rearranges successfully, λ gene rearrangement takes place. If no productive light-chain gene rearrangement occurs, the cell dies. The biological consequence of this use of genes from only one chromosome to make a heavy chain and genes from one chromosome to make a light chain—**allelic exclusion**—ensures that an individual B cell expresses on its cell surface an Ig molecule with only one single antigenic specificity (also see Chapter 7).

Bruton's tyrosine kinase (Btk) is an enzyme involved in a step in intracellular signaling from the pre-BCR (and BCR) that eventually leads to the nucleus. Btk plays a crucial role in the transition of pre-B cells to the next stage in B-cell differentiation: Boys with mutations in the *BTK* gene develop the immunodeficiency condition, *X-linked agammaglobulinemia*, in which B-cell differentiation is arrested at the pre-B-cell stage because of a lack of signaling (discussed in Chapter 18).

 Read the related case: **X-linked agammaglobulinemia**
In *Immunology: Clinical Case Studies and Disease Pathophysiology*

Immature B Cells

At the next stage of B-cell differentiation, the *immature B cell*, light chains pair with μ chains to form monomeric IgM, which is expressed at the cell surface in association with Igα/Igβ to form the BCR (Figure 8.1). Immature B cells express *CD20*, which is also expressed by cells in the next stages of B-cell differentiation; thus, CD20 is a marker for the later stages of B-cell development.

Negative Selection and the Development of Central Tolerance.

The immature B cell can respond to antigen; that is, the IgM expressed on the immature B cell can bind and respond to an individual antigenic epitope. Because the mechanisms used to generate this IgM—VDJ recombination and the pairing of heavy and light chains—are essentially random, some immature B cells that develop will express an IgM specific for a foreign (nonself) antigen and some will express an IgM specific for a self-antigen. If the immature B cell expresses a receptor for a nonself-antigen, it leaves the bone marrow and develops further to become a member of the huge repertoire of mature B cells specific for nonself-antigens.

However, allowing a B cell that has too high a reactivity to a self-molecule to leave the bone marrow runs the risk of developing autoimmune problems in the tissues. Thus, if an immature B cell expresses a receptor specific for a self-antigen and interacts with that self-antigen in the bone marrow, it is eliminated or *deleted*, by apoptosis (Figure 8.3). The self-antigens that are recognized by immature B cells are likely molecules expressed by stromal cells in the bone marrow.

This elimination or deletion of self-reactive B lymphocytes during development in the bone marrow is known as *negative selection*. It is a fundamental feature of the clonal selection theory and the development of *central tolerance*: the development of tolerance to self in the primary lymphoid organ, the organ or tissue in which lymphocytes acquire their antigen-specific receptor. As a consequence of negative selection, the lymphocytes that survive and leave the primary lymphoid organ to move into the periphery are tolerant to self but reactive to foreign antigens. Negative selection is also a critical feature of T-cell development in the thymus. Negative selection and central tolerance are discussed further in Chapters 10 and 13.

However, not all self-reactive immature B cells are deleted as soon as they react with self-antigen (Figure 8.3). Some self-reactive cells have the opportunity to change their receptor, via *receptor editing*. In this pathway, the

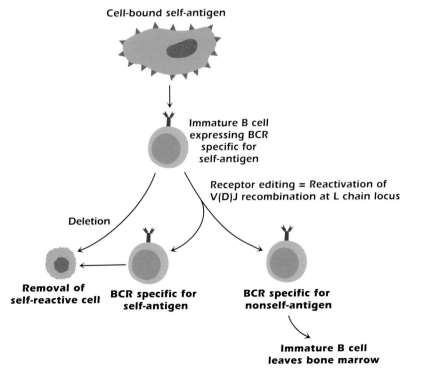

Figure 8.3. Alternative fates of an immature B cell interacting with self-antigen in the bone marrow. Cells that express a receptor (BCR) for a self-antigen (self-reactive) are deleted by apoptosis. In some self-reactive cells, interaction with self-antigen reactivates V(D)J recombinase, and receptor editing ensues. If, after receptor editing, the immature B cell expresses a BCR reactive to a self-antigen, the cell is deleted. If receptor editing generates a BCR that is not self-reactive, the cell survives and leaves the bone marrow.

interaction of self-antigen with the BCR expressed on the immature B cell reactivates the cell's V(D)J recombinase, and Ig light-chain genes undergo a secondary rearrangement that uses unrearranged V and J light-chain segments. For example, in the rearrangement of the B cell's κ locus shown in Figure 7.3 in Chapter 7, V_1 and J_5 are unrearranged gene segments that may be recombined during receptor editing. Receptor editing does not occur on the heavy chain because the initial rearrangement deletes D_H segments and the V_H and J_H segments that remain cannot be combined without a D_H.

If receptor editing generates an Ig specific for a nonself-antigen, the immature B cell survives and is able to leave the bone marrow; it becomes part of the repertoire of B cells responsive to nonself-antigens. If, however, receptor editing generates a specificity for the same or a different self-molecule, the immature B cell is deleted via apoptosis. In this way, B cells with the potential for high reactivity to self-molecules are prevented from exiting the bone marrow and entering the bloodstream and tissues. In some mouse models, self-reactive immature B cells that interact with self-antigen are not always deleted. They survive but are not able to respond to antigen; these B cells are said to be *anergic*; this is described further in Chapter 13.

Transitional B cells

Immature B cells that survive negative selection in the bone marrow have gone through a second critical developmental checkpoint. They remain in the bone marrow for approximately 24 hours, and then move out through blood to the spleen. These cells are known as *transitional B cells*. At this stage they start to express IgD together with IgM at the cell surface.

Transitional B cells are the first stage in the B-cell differentiation pathway to express a receptor for, and so respond to, the cytokine BAFF (B lymphocyte factor belonging to the tumor necrosis factor family, also known as B lymphocyte stimulator [BLyS]). BAFF, which is synthesized by multiple cell types including monocytes, dendritic cells and bone marrow stromal cells, is a survival signal for transitional B cells, as well many later stages in the B cell lineage. High BAFF levels have been reported in patients with the autoimmune conditions rheumatoid arthritis and systemic lupus erythematosus, and one current therapy for those diseases is targeted at reducing BAFF levels (see Chapter 13).

Mature B Cells

The next stage in the B-cell differentiation pathway is the *IgM⁺ IgD⁺ mature B cell*, which expresses higher levels of IgD than does the transitional B cell. These mature B cells that have not yet been exposed to antigen are referred to as *naïve*, and their interaction with antigen in the secondary lymphoid tissues generally results in activation, leading to the formation of memory cells or plasma cells and the production of antibody.

The IgM and IgD expressed on a single B cell have identical antigenic specificity as a result of having the same V region in the heavy chains and using the same light chain (see Figure 7.4). The function of IgD on the mature B cell is not well understood and is downregulated following antigen exposure. In addition to IgM and IgD, the mature B cell expresses several other molecules on its surface, which play key roles in interactions with other cells, particularly T cells, or that have other essential roles in transmitting signals into the B cell nucleus (see below).

Most naïve mature B cells circulate through the blood to secondary lymphoid organs, primarily to lymph nodes throughout the body and to mucosa-associated lymphoid tissue (MALT). These B cells are referred to as *follicular B cells* because they are found in primary and secondary follicles (see Chapter 3). The circulation time of about 12 hours quickly brings a B cell with the "correct" antigenic specificity in contact with antigen if it is present. Some mature B cells move to the marginal zone of the spleen, where they develop into *splenic marginal zone B cells*, which do not recirculate through the blood.

The recombination mechanisms operating during differentiation and throughout the life of the individual generate a vast repertoire of B-cell antigen specificities, more or less guaranteeing a response to any antigen that a person may encounter. The repertoire is so extensive that most mature B cells do not interact with antigen during their lifetime but remain as resting unstimulated IgM⁺ IgD⁺ B cells.

Plasma Cells

Plasma cells (Figure 8.1) synthesize and secrete Ig molecules and are the terminally differentiated stage of B-cell development. They do not express a membrane form of Ig. An individual plasma cell secretes antibody of a single antigenic specificity—the same antigenic specificity as the immunoglobulin on the surface of the B cell that developed into that plasma cells and that was initially triggered by antigen—and of a single isotype: IgM, IgG, IgA, or IgE. Plasma cells (and memory cells) express high levels of CD27, which is not expressed on other cells in the B cell lineage, but they do not express the markers CD10, CD19, or CD20 that characterize earlier stages of the B-cell lineage.

In responses to the major set of antigens known as *thymus-dependent* (TD)—because they require *helper T cells* (see below and Chapter 11)—plasma cells are generated at two major sites: in the *germinal center* of lymph nodes and spleen, and in MALT. Responses to TD antigens generally involve synthesis of antibodies of more than one isotype (that is, IgM plus IgG, IgA, or IgE) and antibodies specific for more than one epitope of a particular antigen. Thus, the population of plasma cells responding to an antigenic challenge is diverse and produces a mixture of immunoglobulins (a *polyclonal response*).

Both short-lived (days to weeks) and long-lived (up to years) plasma cell populations develop in the germinal centers of lymph nodes outside MALT synthesize and secrete IgG, IgA, or IgE. Long-lived plasma cells migrate primarily to the bone marrow, where they synthesize high levels of IgG and monomeric IgA that provide protection against a subsequent exposure to infectious agents such as viruses and bacteria. Long-lived IgE-synthesizing plasma cells are also found in the bone marrow. Plasma cells that develop in MALT synthesize and secrete the dimeric IgA at mucosal sites such as the gastrointestinal and respiratory tracts (see Figure 5.13), as well as salivary and tear glands and lactating mammary glands.

Some antigens do not require T-cell help for the B cell to make antibody. These are referred to as *thymus-independent* (TI) *antigens*. The polysaccharide components of bacterial capsules are one clinically important set of TI antigens. Responses to TI antigens are generally rapid (within a few days after exposure to antigen) and almost exclusively involve synthesis of IgM antibodies. The IgM synthesized in response to TI antigens is made by short-lived plasma cells in the marginal zone of the spleen. This IgM can agglutinate the antigen and activate the complement system, providing crucial early protection against many bacterial infections, even in people who lack T cells (discussed further in Chapter 18). Sites of IgM production are also discussed later in this chapter.

In Chapter 6 we described how plasma cells can be transformed and "immortalized" in cell culture. They can be used to generate *monoclonal antibodies*—antibodies specific for a single antigen epitope—that have a wide range of clinical and diagnostic functions.

Memory B Cells

Memory B cells develop in germinal centers of secondary organs after TD-antigen activation of the mature B cell. They express isotypes other than IgM (IgG, IgA, or IgE) on their surface and do not express IgD. Memory cells express CD27, as do plasma cells. Memory B cells are nonproliferating, generally long-lived cells, that can be activated for a subsequent (*secondary*) and more rapid response to antigen. When reactivated, memory cells can be converted into plasma cells. Memory B cells leave the lymphoid organ in which they were generated. Rather than circulating through lymphoid organs as naive B cells do, memory B cells move into tissues.

SITES OF ANTIBODY SYNTHESIS

The major function of B cells—specifically plasma cells—is to synthesize Ig molecules. In the sections that follow we describe in more detail the main sites in the body where Ig synthesis occurs, and the different types of responses to antigen that occur at those sites.

Interaction of Antigen, B Cells, and Helper T Cells in the Lymph Node

We described above that antibody responses to TD antigens require helper T cells. These helper T cells express the surface marker CD4 and so are referred to as CD4$^+$ T cells (see Chapters 10 and 11). The CD4$^+$ T and B cell that cooperate in the response to TD antigens are both specific for the same antigen; we say these are *cognate* T and B cells. How do these rare cells find each other? Antigen that penetrates the body and enters a tissue arrives at a draining lymph node by passive transport through lymphatic vessels or after being taken up, catabolized ("processed") and transported by antigen-presenting cells, particularly dendritic cells (see below). Naïve B cells circulate through the node increasing the chance of encountering "free" antigen. In the B cell area of the node, the follicle, a B cell with the appropriate receptor "captures" the antigen via its membrane Ig (Figure 8.4). Interaction with antigen activates the B cell, and it moves toward the boundary of the follicle with the T-cell region of the node.

The CD4$^+$ T cell specific for the same antigen also localizes to the boundary of the follicle and T-cell area. This T cell has been activated by the same antigen; however, to activate the T cell, the protein component of the antigen has been taken up and processed by dendritic cells in the tissue, and the antigen-bearing dendritic cell moves to the T-cell area of the node (Figure 8.4, and described further in Chapter 11). Naïve CD4$^+$ T cells also circulate through the node, and interaction with the antigen-bearing dendritic cell activates the CD4$^+$ T cell with the "right" T-cell receptor (TCR). The interaction of antigen-bearing dendritic cells with CD4$^+$ T cells is described in more detail in Chapter 11.

The CD4$^+$ T cell and cognate B cell interact at the boundary of the follicle and T-cell area of the node. In this interaction, the B cell acts as an antigen-presenting cell to the T cell. As we describe more fully in Chapter 11, once the B cell has captured the antigen, it takes it into the cell, processes it into peptides, and presents some of the peptides on its surface for recognition by the T cell. Contact between the CD4$^+$ T cell and the B cell takes place over several hours. Approximately 48 hours after the initiation of this interaction the B cell differentiates into a plasma cell that synthesizes IgM. Thus, IgM is the class of antibody synthesized earliest in the response.

Events in the Germinal Center

After being in contact for about 48 hours the antigen-activated CD4$^+$ T helper and B cells migrate back into the

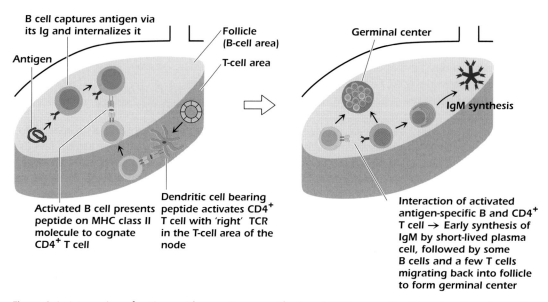

Figure 8.4. Interaction of antigen with an antigen-specific B and CD4+ helper T cell in a lymph node, leading to early synthesis of IgM and the development of a germinal center.

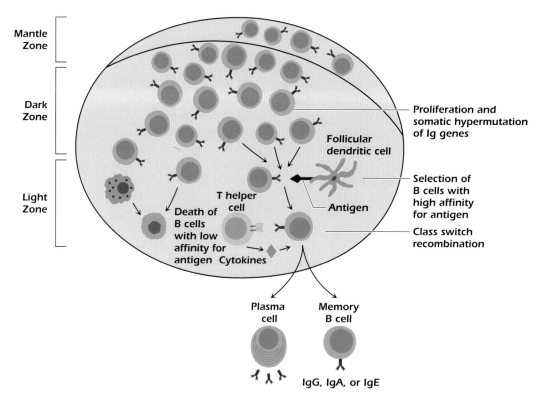

Figure 8.5. Key events in the germinal center: somatic hypermutation, class switch recombination, and development of plasma cells and memory B cells. Interactions of antigen, B cells, CD4+ helper T cells, and follicular dendritic cells are shown, as well as macrophages that ingest unselected B cells that die in the germinal center.

B-cell area, the follicle, and develop a ***germinal center***. Several key events occur in the germinal center in the synthesis of antibody in TD responses: somatic hypermutation, selection of high affinity B cell responders, and class switching (Figure 8.5).

Somatic Hypermutation. Most antigen-activated B cells rapidly and extensively proliferate in an area of the germinal center known as the *dark zone*. (B cells in the primary follicle that are not specific for the antigen move out of the area of proliferation and form a *mantle zone* around the proliferating cells.) During proliferation in the dark zone, B cells with mutations in their Ig variable-region genes are generated at a much higher rate than normal—about 100,000-fold greater than in other genes. This *somatic hypermutation* (described in Chapter 7) results in the development of B cells that synthesize and express Ig molecules with altered affinity for the activating antigen—either higher or lower affinity than the starting population.

The activation of B cells in the germinal center induces the enzyme activation-induced cytidine deaminase (AID), which changes nucleotides in the DNA of Ig variable-region genes. AID is involved in both somatic hypermutation and class switch recombination (see below).

Selection of B Cells with Higher Affinity for Antigen.

Following somatic hypermutation, B cells enter the *light zone* of the germinal center, where they interact with two different types of cells: CD4⁺ T cells specific for the antigen that initiated the response (discussed below) and antigen-bearing *follicular dendritic cells*. These latter cells are characterized by long processes that bind antigen in *antigen–antibody complexes* (antigen bound to antibody and complement components). They retain antigen on their surface for long periods, and present it to B cells in the germinal center. Follicular dendritic cells are not related to the dendritic cells that play a major role in presenting antigen to T cells (Chapters 9–11).

B cells in the light zone compete for the antigen presented by follicular dendritic cells: those B cells with Ig variable-region genes mutated to synthesize antibody with the *highest affinity* for the activating antigen are clonally selected and expanded. B cells with mutations that result in lower affinity antibodies are *not* selected and may die; some B cells without mutations in their variable regions do survive. Thus there is extensive cell death by apoptosis in the germinal center. Macrophages remove the dead cells by phagocytosis, and these *tingible body macrophages* are characteristic of a reactive follicle.

As a result of somatic hypermutation and competition for antigen in the germinal center, the B cells that emerge synthesize antibodies that overall have higher affinity for the activating antigen than the original population of B cells. This phenomenon is known as *affinity maturation* of the response to antigen.

Class Switch Recombination—Development of Plasma Cells and Memory Cells.

Antigen-activated B cells in the light zone interact with CD4⁺ T cells; these are referred to as *T follicular helper cells* (Tfh), and described in more detail in Chapter 11. The sustained interaction between pairs of molecules on the Tfh and B-cell surface as well as the action of T-cell derived cytokines results in *class switch recombination* (see Chapter 7 and Figure 7.5). As a result, this B cell switches to synthesizing Ig of a different isotype: IgG, IgA or IgE. The enzyme AID induced in ger-

minal center B cells is also essential for class switch recombination.

The transcription factor *Bcl-6* is essential for germinal center formation, and B cells require Bcl-6 for their development into germinal center B cells. It represses several genes and inhibits differentiation into plasma cells or memory cells. After the germinal center B cell has successfully completed somatic hypermutation and class switching, Bcl-6 expression is turned off, and the cell proceeds to the next step in its maturation, to become either a plasma cell or memory cell. The mechanisms that lead to the differentiation to plasma cells as opposed to memory cells are currently unclear.

Plasma cells produced in germinal centers may be very long-lived (up to years); they migrate to other lymphoid organs, particularly the bone marrow, where they continue to synthesize antibody. The antibodies secreted by the plasma cells in the bone marrow are thought to produce the bulk of the IgG and monomeric IgA found in serum; these antibodies provide protection against toxins (such as tetanus and diphtheria). These antibodies can also prevent reinfection by many types of pathogen, even in the absence of a secondary immune response. Long-lived IgE-synthesizing plasma cells are also found in the bone marrow.

Memory B cells are generally long-lived and nonproliferating; reexposure to antigen (usually requiring T cells) activates a secondary response to antigen that is more rapid than the primary response. Memory B cells proliferate and give rise to plasma cells and additional memory B cells expressing isotypes other than IgM.

Given the importance of the germinal center reaction in the response to thymus-dependent antigens, defects in its formation or function can have serious consequences; this may result from either deficiency in the activity of AID or from mutations in the expression of surface molecules by follicular B or Tfh. As a result of these deficiencies, somatic hypermutation and class switch recombination do not occur, memory B and class switched plasma cells do not develop, and the predominant antibody formed is IgM. Clinical consequences such as hyper-IgM syndromes can result (discussed further in Chapter 18).

 Read the related case: **Hyper-IgM syndrome**
In *Immunology: Clinical Case Studies and Disease Pathophysiology*

Antibody Synthesis in Mucosal Tissue

IgA plays a key role in the protection of the mucosal surfaces, such as those found in the respiratory and gastrointestinal tracts, salivary and tear glands, and lactating mammary glands. Plasma cells close to the epithelial basement membrane of mucosal tissue in these mucosal areas synthesize and secrete dimeric IgA (see Chapter 5 and

molecule CD5, which is not expressed on other sets of B cells.

In adults, B-1 cells synthesize predominantly low-affinity IgM *polyspecific* antibodies (those that are reactive with many different antigens) early in the TI primary response to many bacteria. In addition, B-l cells are considered responsible for synthesizing most "natural" antibody, generally IgM antibodies that are detected in the blood in the absence of specific antigen priming. These antibodies are broadly cross-reactive and most likely have been stimulated by prior bacterial exposure. Thus, B-l cells are thought to play a role as a first line of defense against systemic bacterial and viral infections. Some of the polyspecific IgM antibodies synthesized by B-1 cells react with self-antigens, and so B-1 cells may have a role in autoimmune diseases; high levels of B-1 cells have been reported in some conditions, such as systemic lupus erythematosus.

In mice, B-1 cells also produce a significant amount of the IgA that is found in serum and at mucosal surfaces. B-1 IgA synthesis is unusual because the switch to IgA synthesis occurs in the absence of T cells. B-1 cells show limited diversity in their receptor repertoire—reduced N region

diversity and somatic hypermutation—and so are more "germline" than conventional B cells.

B-CELL MEMBRANE PROTEINS

In the following paragraphs and in Figures 8.7–8.10 we briefly describe some of the key molecules that play a key role in B cell function.

Stage-Specific Markers

As noted earlier, different molecules are expressed at different stages in B-cell development and activation (Figure 8.1): CD10 is expressed by early cells in the lineage—pro-B and pre-B cells—as well as by germinal center B cells (not shown in Figure 8.1). CD19 is expressed on all cells in the B-cell lineage from the pro-B to memory B cell, but not the plasma cell. CD20 is expressed on all cells from the immature B cell to the memory B cell but not the plasma cell. CD27 is expressed exclusively on memory and plasma cells. CD5 characterizes the B-1 subset of B cells. In addition,

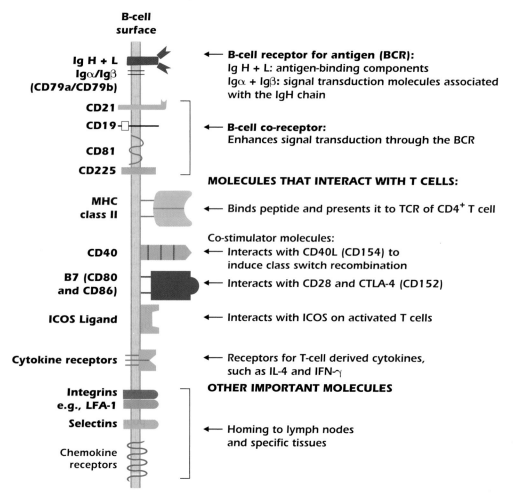

Figure 8.7. Important molecules expressed at the surface of B cells. See text for details.

several stages in B cell differentiation from the pre-B have surface receptors for and require interaction of the stromal cell-derived cytokines, particularly BAFF and IL-7, for survival.

Antigen-Binding Molecules: Membrane Immunoglobulin

The quintessential property of the B-lymphocyte lineage is the expression of Ig chains at the cell surface. (Note, however, that the pro-B cell—the most immature cell in the lineage—and the plasma cell—the end-stage cell of B-cell differentiation that secretes Ig—do not express immunoglobulin on their surfaces.) Because membrane-associated immunoglobulin binds antigen, the expression of surface immunoglobulin can be used both to identify B cells and to separate them from other lymphocytes and mononuclear cells.

Signal Transduction Molecules Associated with Membrane Immunoglobulin

Igα and Igβ. Ig H chains have very short intracellular domains and do not transmit a signal directly into the B cell after antigen binding. Rather, the activation signal is transmitted into the interior of the B-cell by the Igα/Igβ dimer (CD79a, CD79b) that is tightly associated in the membrane of B cells with Ig heavy chains to form the BCR (see Figure 8.2). The function of Igα/Igβ after antigen binding to Ig is explained later in this chapter.

B-Cell Co-Receptor. The ***B-cell co-receptor*** (Figures 8.7 and 8.8) consists of a set of four molecules—CD19, CD21, CD81 (also known as TAPA-1), and CD225 (or Leu13)—close to but not part of the BCR complex in the membrane. The B-cell co-receptor enhances the signal transmitted through the BCR after antigen stimulation. As a result of this enhanced signal, the co-receptor reduces the threshold of B-cell activation in response to an antigen; that is, less antigen is needed to stimulate an antibody response if the co-receptor is activated together with the BCR (estimated at 100–1000 times less) compared to activation through the BCR alone. Co-receptors with similar but not identical function, CD4 and CD8, are associated with the T-cell receptor (TCR) (see Chapter 10).

The role of the B-cell co-receptor in enhancing the signal through the BCR has been characterized best in the response to microbial pathogens that activate complement (see also Chapter 14). This is shown in Figure 8.8: a bacterium binds to the immunoglobulin of a B cell expressing the appropriate BCR; at the same time, the bacterium binds to ***C3dg***, a complement component that is generated in plasma early in the response to microbial pathogens (see Chapter 14). C3dg coats or "tags" the pathogen and binds to CD21, a component of the B-cell co-receptor. In this way the

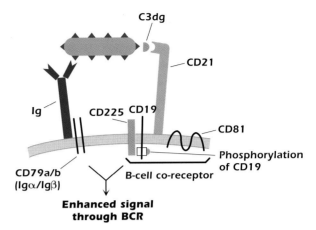

<u>Figure 8.8.</u> Enhancement of activation via the B-cell co-receptor CD19/CD21/CD81/CD225. Simultaneous binding of pathogen (a) to Ig on the B-cell surface and (b) to complement component C3dg bound to CD21 of the co-receptor enhances the activation signal delivered through the BCR alone and lowers the threshold for antigen needed to activate the B cell. The orange semicircle indicates phosphate groups added to activated CD19.

bacterium is attached to the B cell surface via both Ig and, through CD21, to the B-cell co-receptor. Thus, the simultaneous binding of pathogen to both the co-receptor and BCR enhances the signal to the B cell compared to the signal transmitted through the BCR alone.

Molecules Involved in T–B Cell Interactions

Earlier in the chapter we referred to production of antibody in response to TD antigens. In these responses, interactions between pairs of molecules on the B cell and T-helper cell surfaces are critical. As we describe more fully in Chapter 11, the B cell not only synthesizes immunoglobulin but also presents antigen and activates the helper (CD4⁺) T cell in these responses. Thus, B cells, and activated B cells in particular, share several important characteristics with other antigen-presenting cells that present antigen to CD4⁺ T cells. B cells express the following molecules on their surface.

Major Histocompatibility Complex Class II Molecules. Major histocompatibility complex (MHC) class II molecules selectively bind peptides derived from protein antigens following processing in the B cell and present them to CD4⁺ T cells. MHC class II molecules are expressed on all cells in the B-cell lineage except pro-B cells. The structure and function of MHC molecules are described in more detail in Chapter 9.

Co-Stimulator Molecules. Co-stimulator molecules are so called because they are required as a second signal to accompany the first signal (antigen interacting through the T-cell receptor) to activate naïve T cells (see Chapters 10 and 11). Co-stimulators are expressed at high levels on activated, rather than naïve, B cells. Several co-stimulators have been identified. One of the most studied is *B7*, now recognized as a family of several different molecules, which interacts with a family of molecules on the T cell that includes CD28. *CD40* is another important co-stimulator molecule expressed by B cells. CD40 interacts with CD40 ligand (CD40L or CD154) expressed on activated T cells. This interaction activates B cells and plays a critical role in class switch and somatic hypermutation. The importance of the CD40–CD154 interaction is underscored by a condition known as *human X-linked hyper-IgM syndrome*. Boys who have a mutation in their CD154 gene and whose activated T cells either do not express CD154 or have a nonfunctional version of the gene make only IgM antibodies; their B cells cannot undergo class switch.

Inducible Co-Stimulatory Ligand.

Inducible co-stimulatory (ICOS) ligand (ICOSL) is another important co-stimulatory molecule expressed by B cells. The interaction of ICOSL with ICOS expressed by activated T cells appears critical for the formation of the germinal center: People who lack functional ICOSL or ICOS make very low levels of IgG, IgA, and IgE. All these co-stimulator molecules are discussed in more detail in Chapters 10 and 11.

Receptors for Cytokines.

B cells express receptors for several T-cell-derived cytokines. A key aspect of TD-antigen responses is that the nature of the cytokine synthesized by T cells in the T–B interaction, for example IL-4 or interferon-γ, influences the class of antibody made by the B cell in the germinal center.

Homing

B cells at different stages of differentiation are found in different anatomical locations around the body. For example, naïve mature B cells are found in lymph nodes, but antigen-activated memory cells and plasma cells are found in different tissues (for example, long-lived plasma cells traffic predominantly to bone marrow, whereas memory cells enter specific tissues such as the lung or skin). The movement of B cells—as well as T cells and other leukocytes (see Chapters 11 and 12)—into lymph nodes and tissues around the body is tightly regulated.

Three sets of molecules expressed on the leukocyte surface are involved in *homing*: a *chemokine receptor* and two different types of *adhesion molecules*, which belong to families known as *integrins* and *selectins*. Chemokines are small cytokines produced by many types of cells that influence the movement of leukocytes including B and T lymphocytes (see Chapter 12). *Integrins*, such as LFA-1 (CD11 and CD18), are a family of two-chain adhesion molecules expressed on many cells including B and T cells. *Selectins*,

such as CD62L, are single-chain glycoproteins expressed on many cells including B and T cells; they bind to the carbohydrate portion of their glycoprotein ligands.

Our current model for homing is of an *address code*. To use the analogy of sending a letter to a particular address, the combination of chemokine receptor and adhesion molecules provides a degree of specificity to identify the recipient: The set of molecules expressed by a leukocyte interacts with molecules expressed on the surface of cells lining a particular tissue, specifically, molecules expressed by endothelial cells in a specialized region of the vascular endothelium (high endothelial venules [HEVs]) at the boundary of blood and a particular organ.

The pattern of B-cell (and T-cell) expression of adhesion molecules and chemokine receptors changes depending on the stage of development and whether or not the cell has interacted with antigen. As a result of these multiple paired interactions at the HEVs, the lymphocyte leaves the blood and enters that particular organ.

Intracellular Signaling in B Cells

In this final section we describe some of the key signaling pathways activated inside B cells by antigen stimulation. In Chapter 11 we show that T cells have similar activation pathways after they bind antigen.

Activation by Antigen.

The activation of B cells has been studied most extensively in the response to thymus-independent (TI) antigens, which directly activate the B cell (Figure 8.9). In brief, the recognition of antigen at the cell surface triggers multiple intracellular cascades that spread in an ordered manner from the surface of the cell through the cytoplasm and into the nucleus. Some events occur within seconds, others within minutes, and yet others within hours of the initial interaction. As a result of these events, the B cell changes its pattern of gene expression.

Activation is initiated by *receptor cross-linking*, bringing together more than one BCR complex in the cell membrane.

After antigen binds to the BCR, tyrosine residues in the ITAMs in the cytoplasmic domains of the closely associated Igα/Igβ are rapidly phosphorylated; that is, phosphate groups are added by the tyrosine kinases Fyn and Lyn, members of a family of tyrosine kinases known as Src. Phosphorylation of the Igα/Igβ ITAMs recruits another kinase, Syk, to the aggregated cluster of molecules, and Syk is phosphorylated and activated. (Syk is a member of another family of tyrosine kinases, which also contains the T-cell specific tyrosine kinase, ZAP-70, described further in Chapter 11.) Activated Syk in turn recruits and activates another tyrosine kinase, Btk, and B-cell linker protein (BLNK). BLNK is an *adaptor*—a protein that does not have enzymatic activity but contains multiple binding domains for other proteins. The recruitment, activation, and aggregation

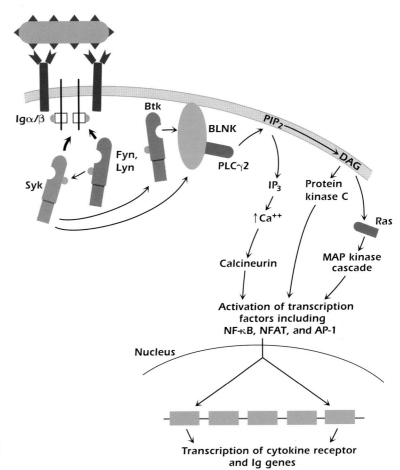

<u>Figure 8.9.</u> Intracellular events in B-cell activation. Orange semicircles indicate phosphate groups added to activated molecules. Thick arrows indicate movement of components after activation. See text for details.

of all these molecules result in the formation of a large signaling complex on the cytoplasmic side of the membrane associated with the BCR.

One of the key molecules that binds to BLNK is the enzyme ***phospholipase Cγ2*** (PLCγ2). The binding of PLCγ2 to BLNK activates three major signaling pathways inside the cell. The first pathway involves increasing intracellular calcium levels. This occurs as a result of the PLCγ2-catalyzed breakdown of the membrane phospholipid phosphatidylinositol 4,5 bisphosphate (PIP$_2$). PIP$_2$ is broken down into two products, one of which is inositol triphosphate (IP$_3$). IP$_3$ triggers the release of intracellular pools of calcium. The increased calcium level in turn activates the cytoplasmic molecule ***calcineurin***.

The second pathway leads to the activation of protein kinase C. This results from the formation in the membrane of ***diacylglycerol*** (DAG), the second product of the PLCγ2-catalyzed breakdown of PIP$_2$. DAG activates the enzyme ***protein kinase C*** (PKC), which in turn activates a cascade of molecules in the cytoplasm, ultimately activating the transcription factor, ***NF-κB***.

The third pathway results from DAG interacting with the GTPase, Ras. This activates the cytoplasmic cascade of mitogen-activated protein (MAP) kinases. Ras also interacts directly with molecules bound to the adaptor BLNK (not shown in the figure), also resulting in activation of the MAP kinase pathway.

All three intracellular pathways ultimately lead to the activation of transcription factors, including NF-AT, AP-1, and NF-κB, that enter the nucleus and alter gene expression. They promote the transcription of several genes involved in proliferation and the synthesis of Ig and cytokine receptors. Approximately 24–48 hours after contact between antigen and the BCR, the B cell starts to proliferate and differentiates into a plasma cell that synthesizes and secretes Ig.

Enhancement of B-Cell Signaling. The enhancement of activation signals that we described above and in Figure 8.8 to result from activation through the B-cell co-receptor occurs as a result of the rapid phosphorylation of the ITAM in the cytoplasmic domain of CD19 by a tyrosine kinase associated with the BCR. This phosphorylation in turn recruits a kinase, phosphatidylinositol-3 (PI$_3$) kinase, to CD19. This triggers intracellular pathways that augment the activation of transcription factors and their translocation into the nucleus.

Negative Regulation of B-Cell Signaling. Some molecules expressed on the B-cell surface have a *negative* effect on B-cell signaling. These include ***CD22***, which

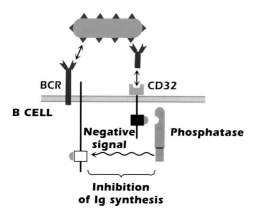

Figure 8.10. Antibody feedback inhibits B-cell activation. Simultaneous binding of the antigen and antibody components of an antigen–antibody complex to receptors on a single B cell (antigen to the Ig, and the Fc portion of the antibody component to the FcR, CD32) results in the binding of phosphatases to the ITIM (black rectangle) in the cytoplasmic region of CD32. Binding to the ITIM activates the phosphatases, which then remove phosphate groups from tyrosine residues in molecules activated in the signal transduction pathways associated with the BCR. As a result, the activating signal through the BCR is inhibited.

negatively regulates the CD19, CD81, and CD21 co-receptors, as well as **CD32**. CD32 is the low-affinity receptor for the Fc region of IgG (FcγRIIb), expressed on almost all mature B cells. CD32 can bind IgG that is part of an antigen–antibody complex. In this way, CD32 plays an important role in **antibody feedback**, which occurs after an antibody has been synthesized in response to an antigen: The antibody produced inhibits a further B-cell response to that antigen.

Figure 8.10 shows how the binding of CD32 to Ig in an antigen–antibody complex (IgG bound to a bacterium) leads to negative signaling inside the B cell. First, the Fc end of the antigen–antibody complex binds to CD32 and the antigen simultaneously binds to Ig expressed on the same B cell. The binding of the Fc end of the antibody to CD32 recruits one or more phosphatases to the intracellular domain of CD32; specifically, the phosphatases bind to a tyrosine-containing sequence of amino acids in CD32 that by analogy to the previously described ITAMs is known as an **immunoreceptor tyrosine-based inhibitory motif** (ITIM). Binding to the ITIM activates the phosphatases, which then remove phosphate groups from tyrosine residues in molecules activated in the signal transduction pathways associated with the BCR. As a result, the activating signal through the BCR is inhibited.

SUMMARY

1. In mammals, the early stages of B-cell differentiation take place in the bone marrow and throughout the life of an individual.

2. Different CD molecules are expressed at different stages of B-cell development.

3. The earliest recognizable cell in the B-cell lineage is the pro-B cell, in which the first stage of Ig H-chain gene rearrangement takes place: A D_H gene segment rearranges to a J_H gene segment.

4. The next stage is the pre-B cell, in which a V_H gene segment rearranges to the joined DJ segments to form a VDJ unit, positioning the rearranged VDJ close to the Cμ gene. The pre-B cell synthesizes a μ chain that is expressed on the surface in association with non-rearranging surrogate light chains plus the signal transduction molecules Igα (CD79a) and Igβ (CD79b). The complex of μ and surrogate light chains in conjunction with Igα/β is referred to as the pre-B-cell receptor.

5. In the next stage of differentiation, light-chain genes start to rearrange; surrogate light-chain synthesis is shut down, and a κ or λ chain is formed that associates with the cell's μ chain. This cell, the immature

B cell, expresses an IgM molecule in association with Igα/β on the surface of the cell. The complex of IgM and Igα/β is referred to as the *B-cell receptor*.

6. Because the V(D)J recombination mechanism is essentially random, some immature B cells express an IgM specific for a foreign (nonself) antigen and some an IgM specific for a self-antigen. Immature B cells with receptors specific for nonself-antigens leave the bone marrow and move to the spleen. Immature B cells with receptors specific for self-antigens are deleted by apoptosis. The deletion in bone marrow of immature B cells with potential reactivity to self is an important feature of central tolerance in the B-cell lineage.

   Not all self-reactive immature B cells are deleted immediately. Some undergo receptor editing: V(D)J rearrangement is reactivated and the light-chain genes undergo further rearrangement. If the cell generates a receptor that is specific for a nonself molecule, the cell is "rescued" and differentiates further. If the cell generates a receptor that is still reactive to a self-molecule, the cell is deleted.

7. In the next phase of B-cell differentiation, the mature B cell expresses IgM and IgD—with identical antigenic specificity—on the cell surface.

8. Further development of the mature B cell occurs outside the bone marrow as a result of exposure to antigen. Activation of the B cell leads to proliferation and differentiation into plasma cells, the cells that synthesize and secrete antibody. Some activated B cells differentiate into memory cells, which make more rapid responses and synthesize non-IgM isotypes in subsequent responses to antigen.

9. Thymus-dependent antigens require T-cell help to induce B-cell antibody synthesis. In the early phase of the response, IgM is synthesized, but in the later phases of the response other isotypes—IgG, IgA, or IgE—are synthesized.

10. The interaction of T-helper cells and B cells takes place predominantly in the germinal centers of secondary lymphoid organs. Events in the germinal center reaction include (a) somatic hypermutation of genes coding for antibody V regions, resulting in affinity maturation, and (b) class switch recombination, in which a B cell that was synthesizing IgM and IgD switches to synthesizing antibody of a different isotype (IgG, IgA, or IgE) with the same antigenic specificity. Cytokines synthesized by T cells influence the isotype of antibody synthesized by the B cell.

11. Germinal center B cells develop into memory B cells or plasma cells. Memory cells "home" to different tissues; plasma cells home predominantly to bone marrow where they continue to synthesize antibody for a long time.

12. In mucosa-associated lymphoid tissue, IgA-committed B cells develop at an inductive site, migrate out of the lymphoid tissue and home back via the blood to a different mucosal effector site, where they complete their differentiation to IgA-secreting plasma cells.

13. B-cell responses to thymus-independent antigens involve other sets of B cells—marginal-zone B cells and B-1 cells—and generate almost exclusively IgM.

14. Expression of membrane Ig is unique to B cells. CD10, CD19, CD20, and CD27 expression defines stages of B-cell differentiation. B cells also express a co-receptor, CD19/CD21/CD81/CD225, that enhances signals through the B-cell receptor and lowers the threshold for the level of antigen required to activate the B cell after binding to Ig.

15. Mature and activated B cells also express an array of surface molecules that play a vital role in interactions with other cells, particularly T cells. These include MHC class II molecules, the co-stimulatory molecules B7, CD40, and ICOSL, and receptors for cytokines. B cells, like other leukocytes, express homing molecules that allow the trafficking of cells to specific tissues.

REFERENCES AND BIBLIOGRAPHY

Amanna IJ, Carlson NE, Slifka MK. (2007) Duration of humoral immunity to common viral and vaccine antigens. *New Engl J Med* 357: 1903.

Corthésy B. (2007) Roundtrip ticket for secretory IgA: Role in mucosal homeostasis? *J Immunol* 178: 27.

Germain RN, Robey EA, Cahalan MD. (2012) A decade of imaging cellular motility and interaction dynamics in the immune system. *Science* 336: 1676.

Kamada N, Seo SU, Chen GY, Núñez G. (2013) Role of the gut microbiota in immunity and inflammatory disease. *Nat Rev Immunol* 13: 321.

Kunkel EJ, Butcher EC. (2002) Chemokines and the tissue-specific migration of lymphocytes. *Immunity* 16: 1.

Luger EO, Fokuhl V, Wegmann M, Abram M, Tillack K, Achatz G, Manz RA, Worm M, Radbruch A, Renz H. (2009) Induction of long-lived allergen-specific plasma cells by mucosal allergen challenge. *J Allergy Clin Immunol* 124: 819.

McHeyzer-Williams LJ, McHeyzer-Williams MG. (2005) Antigen-specific memory B cell development. *Annu Rev Immunol* 23: 487.

Martin F, Kearney JF. (2000) B cell subsets and the mature preimmune repertoire: Marginal zone and B1 B cells as part of a "natural immune memory." *Immunol Rev* 175: 70.

Pieper K, Grimbacher B, Eibel H. (2013) B-cell biology and development. *J Allergy Clin Immunol* 131: 959.

Salmi M, Jalkanen S. (2005) Lymphocyte homing to the gut: Attraction, adhesion, and commitment. *Immunol Rev* 206: 100.

Vinuesa CG, Linterman MA, Goodnow CC, Randall KL. (2010) T cells and follicular dendritic cells in germinal center B-cell formation and selection. *Immunol Rev* 237: 72.

REVIEW QUESTIONS

For each question, choose the ONE BEST answer or completion.

1. The earliest stages of B-cell differentiation:
   A) occur in the embryonic thymus
   B) require the presence of antigen
   C) involve rearrangement of κ-chain gene segments
   D) involve rearrangement of surrogate light-chain gene segments
   E) involve rearrangement of heavy-chain gene segments

2. Which of the following is expressed on the surface of the mature B lymphocyte?
   A) CD40
   B) MHC class II molecules
   C) CD32
   D) IgM and IgD
   E) all of the above

3. Which of the following statements is incorrect?
   A) Antibodies in a secondary immune response generally have a higher affinity for antigen than antibodies formed in a primary response.
   B) Somatic hypermutation of variable-region genes may contribute to changes in antibody affinity observed during secondary responses.
   C) Synthesis of antibody in a primary response to a thymus-dependent antigen occurs predominantly in the blood.
   D) Isotype switching occurs in the presence of antigen.
   E) Predominantly IgM antibody is produced in the primary response.

4. Immature B lymphocytes:
   A) have rearranged only D and J gene segments
   B) are progenitors of T as well as B lymphocytes
   C) express both IgM and IgD on their surfaces
   D) are at a stage of development where contact with antigen may lead to receptor editing and deletion
   E) must go through the thymus to mature

5. Antigen binding to the B-cell receptor:
   A) transduces a signal through the antigen-binding chains
   B) invariably leads to B-cell activation
   C) transduces a signal through the Igα and Igβ molecules
   D) results in macrophage activation
   E) leads to cytokine synthesis, which activates T cells

6. Which of the following would not be found on a memory B cell?
   A) Igα and Igβ
   B) γ heavy chains
   C) ε heavy chains
   D) surrogate light chains
   E) κ light chains

7. Germinal centers found in lymph nodes and spleen:
   A) support the development of immature B and T cells
   B) function in the removal of damaged erythrocytes from the circulation
   C) act as the major source of stem cells and thus help to maintain hematopoiesis
   D) are sites where antigen-activated mature B cells proliferate and differentiate
   E) exclude T cells

ANSWERS TO REVIEW QUESTIONS

1. *E.* The earliest events in B-cell differentiation take place in fetal liver and bone marrow in the adult and involve rearrangement of heavy-chain V, D, and J gene segments.

2. *E.* All the molecules are expressed on the surface of the mature B cell.

3. *C.* Antibody synthesis in the primary response to TD antigens occurs predominantly in secondary lymphoid organs—the spleen lymph nodes, and mucosa-associated lymphoid tissue.

4. *D.* In immature B cells, which express only IgM, contact with cell-bound self-antigen initiates receptor editing—secondary rearrangement of light-chain genes. If receptor editing results in a receptor specific for self, the B cell is deleted.

5. *C.* The molecules Igα and Igβ, which are associated with the surface Ig molecule, transduce a signal following antigen binding to surface Ig.

6. *D.* Surrogate light chains are expressed only at the pre-B-cell stage of B-cell differentiation.

7. *D.* Germinal centers are the areas of lymph node and spleen in which antigen-activated B cells interact with T cells, proliferate, undergo somatic hypermutation and class switch recombination, and ultimately differentiate into memory or plasma cells.

9

HOW T CELLS RECOGNIZE ANTIGEN: THE ROLE OF THE MAJOR HISTOCOMPATIBILITY COMPLEX

INTRODUCTION

Previous chapters have focused on the development and function of B cells, their antigen-specific receptors (immunoglobulin [Ig]), and the mechanisms by which B cells generate a huge array of clonally distributed receptors. Antibodies, the antigen-specific products of B cells, play a critical role in the interaction with antigens *outside* cells, such as viruses or bacteria encountered in blood or at mucosal surfaces. However, many pathogens—particularly viruses, parasites, and some bacteria—invade host cells and live at least part of their life cycle inside them. Antibodies do not enter cells, so once a pathogen gains entry to a host cell, antibodies are ineffective at defending the host. The immune response to pathogens inside host cells is the domain of T cells and their products. T cells also mount responses to "harmless" antigens—foreign agents that are not pathogenic but to which we need to respond and eliminate.

Antibodies bind to all types of antigens, regardless of whether the antigens are protein, carbohydrate, nucleic acid, or lipid. By contrast, T cells respond almost exclusively to proteins, or more precisely, small peptides derived from the catabolism of proteins. (Later in the chapter we describe additional types of antigens that some subsets of T cells respond to.) Proteins are major constituents of pathogens and are also the products of viral infection. In addition, most other antigens are protein in nature. Thus, T cells play a critical role in the response to nearly all potentially harmful agents and the myriad of other antigens to which an individual is exposed.

Because T cells deal with pathogens and antigens that infect or are taken into host cells, they use an antigen recognition system distinct from the one used by B cells: T cells interact with antigens expressed on the surface of host cells. However, like B cells, T cells express an antigen-specific receptor, the **T-cell receptor** (TCR).

Before we discuss the properties of the TCR (Chapter 10), in this chapter we describe how T cells recognize antigen, and the role played by **major histocompatibility complex** (MHC) **molecules** in this recognition. We will focus on antigen recognition by the major set of T cells, known as $\alpha\beta$ **T cells**, which express the two-chain molecule $\alpha\beta$ as their TCR. Unless otherwise indicated we will refer to these cells as simply "T cells." Later in the chapter we discuss antigen recognition by other subpopulations of T cells. We will also discuss the characteristics of the genes that code for MHC molecules, the enormous and unique diversity of these molecules within the population, and possible reasons for this diversity.

HOW THE MHC GOT ITS NAME

The term *major histocompatibility complex* derives from research in transplantation that started in the mid-twentieth century. These experiments provided insight into the rules governing the acceptance or rejection of tissues—literally, *histocompatibility*—when tissues were transplanted between different members of the same species (generally mice; see Chapter 19 for more discussion). Researchers interpreted

Immunology: A Short Course, Seventh Edition. Richard Coico and Geoffrey Sunshine.
© 2015 John Wiley & Sons, Ltd. Published 2015 by John Wiley & Sons, Ltd.
Companion Website: www.wileyimmunology.com/coico

their early findings to indicate that rapid rejection of such transplants was determined by a single gene, which they called the *major histocompatibility gene*. Because later studies indicated that this "gene" was in fact a **complex**—a set of closely linked genes inherited as a unit—it became known as the **major histocompatibility complex**. We know now that every vertebrate species has an MHC containing multiple genes. The human MHC is known as **HLA (human leukocyte antigen)**.

Other early studies of transplantation in mice indicated that T cells played an important role in the rejection response (see Chapter 19 for more details). Taken together, these transplantation studies demonstrated an important but not well-understood connection between the MHC and T-cell responses. Because individuals do not normally undergo transplants, the function of the MHC in "everyday" T-cell responses became the focus of intense investigation.

The everyday function of the MHC is described in the sections that follow.

MHC ROLE IN ANTIGEN PRESENTATION

The events that occur inside a host cell after a protein antigen has entered it are summarized in Figure 9.1. In summary:

- The protein is broken down (catabolized or "processed") to peptides—linear fragments—of varying length.

- Some of these peptides bind to an MHC molecule inside the cell. This binding is selective; that is, not all the peptides formed bind to MHC molecules.
- The MHC molecule with bound peptide moves to the cell surface.
- The combination of peptide bound to an MHC molecule is recognized at the cell surface by a T cell that expresses the "appropriate" or "correct" TCR—one of the billions of different TCRs the host can generate. Figure 9.2 shows the three critical components of T-cell recognition of antigen: peptide, an MHC molecule expressed on the surface of a host cell, and the TCR expressed on a T cell.

Thus, MHC molecules have two key functions: (1) to **selectively bind** to peptides produced when proteins are processed inside cells of the host, and (2) to **present** peptides on the surface of a host cell to a T cell with the appropriate TCR.

The critical role played by MHC molecules in binding processed antigen and presenting it in T-cell responses is referred to as the **MHC restriction of T-cell responses**.

Multiple copies of each MHC molecule are expressed on the surface of a host cell, and each MHC molecule can bind many peptides (one peptide at a time, as we explain later in the chapter). By binding to peptides inside the cell, MHC molecules "sample" the internal environment of host cells and present information on the cell surface that allows T cells to identify whether a particular host cell has been infected, or contains some foreign component. The combination of MHC molecule plus foreign peptide expressed on the surface of a host cell is a key signal to host T cells that they need to respond. An important corollary is that our T cells do *not* respond to host cells in the absence of foreign

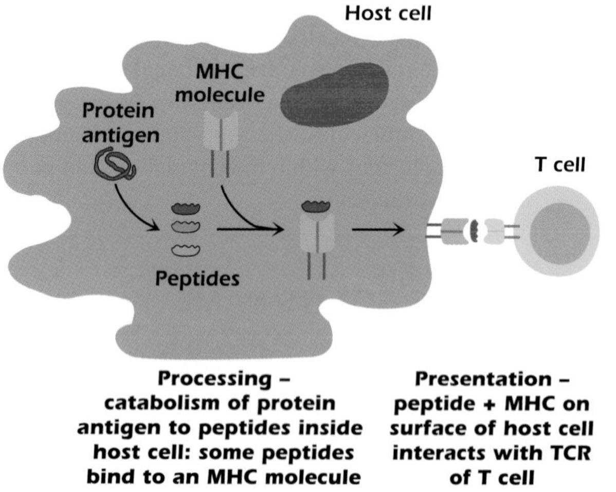

Figure 9.1. The role of MHC in antigen presentation to T cells. Protein antigens are catabolized—processed—to peptides inside host cells. Some peptides bind to MHC molecules and the peptide–MHC combination moves to the surface of the cell, where it is presented to a T cell with the "correct" T-cell receptor (TCR).

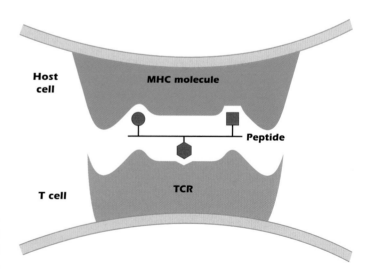

Figure 9.2. Interaction of an MHC molecule expressed on the surface of a host cell with bound peptide and a TCR.

peptide: our T cells focus on responding to infected cells (or cells that contain antigen) but do not respond to host cells that are uninfected.

MHC molecules also play a key role during the differentiation of T cells in the thymus (see Chapter 10). Thus, MHC molecules play important interrelated roles in both the differentiation of *immature* T cells and in the responses of *mature* T cells.

DIFFERENT MHC MOLECULES ARE EXPRESSED BY DISTINCT HOST CELLS AND INTERACT WITH DIFFERENT SETS OF T CELLS

Two major sets of MHC molecules—***MHC class I*** and ***MHC class II molecules***—direct distinct T cell responses (Figure 9.3).

MHC Class I

MHC class I molecules interact with CD8, whose expression defines the subset of T cells called **CD8$^+$ T cells**. Thus, to expand on the definition of MHC restriction of T-cell responses we introduced earlier, we say that *the responses of CD8$^+$ T cells are restricted by MHC class I molecules*.

MHC class I molecules are expressed on all nucleated cells (thus, not on red blood cells), any of which may be infected by a pathogen such as a virus, bacterium, or parasite. The main function of CD8$^+$ T cells is to kill pathogen-infected host cells, as well as tumors and transplanted tissue. Thus, MHC class I molecules and CD8$^+$ T cells play critical roles in the responses to pathogens that infect host cells.

In addition to their interaction with CD8 expressed on CD8$^+$ T cells, MHC class I molecules also interact with molecules expressed on natural killer (NK) cells. This interaction prevents NK cells from killing normal host cells.

MHC Class II

MHC class II molecules interact with CD4, whose expression defines the subset of T cells called **CD4$^+$ T cells**. In parallel with our definition in the previous section, we say that *the responses of CD4$^+$ T cells are restricted by MHC class II molecules*.

MHC class II molecules have a more limited distribution than MHC class I molecules: They are expressed **constitutively** (that is, under baseline conditions) only on **antigen-presenting cells** (APCs) but can be induced on other cell types. APCs are cells that take up antigen and present it to T cells. In humans, the principal APCs that express MHC class II are dendritic cells, macrophages, and B lymphocytes; thymic epithelial cells (discussed in the next chapter) also express MHC class II molecules. In the absence of inducing factors, most cells (for example, liver and kidney tissue cells) express MHC class I but not MHC class II molecules; by contrast, APCs constitutively express *both* MHC class I and class II molecules.

In response to activation, CD4$^+$ T cells synthesize a vast array of cytokines, and hence cooperate with multiple types of cells, including helping B cells synthesize antibody. Thus, MHC class II molecules and CD4$^+$ T cells play critical roles in the responses to agents—pathogens and antigens—that are taken into APCs.

The expression of both MHC class I and II molecules can be affected by many factors. Cytokines released during the response to infectious agents enhance the expression of MHC molecules: Interferon (IFN) α, β, and γ upregulate MHC class I expression, and IFN-γ upregulates MHC class II expression. As a consequence of this upregulation, MHC class II expression is *induced* on cells such as fibroblasts and endothelial cells that do not normally express it, and *increased* on APCs. Induction and increased expression of MHC class I and II molecules thus enhance T-cell responses to infectious agents. On the other hand, some virus infections and tumor development result in *decreased* expression of MHC molecules. We will discuss the regulation of expression of MHC class molecules in greater detail later in this chapter.

VARIABILITY OF MHC CLASS I AND MHC CLASS II MOLECULES

Before discussing the structures of MHC molecules, we note an important point: MHC class I and class II molecules differ from individual to individual within the population, and these differences are genetically determined; that is, MHC-distinct individuals express MHC molecules with somewhat different sequences.

These differences in MHC molecules from individual to individual arise from two sources: ***polygenicity*** and ***polymorphism***. *Polygenicity* means that MHC class I and II

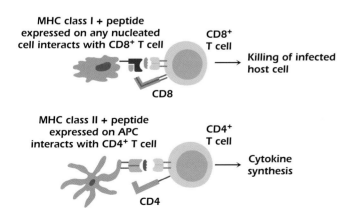

Figure 9.3. Cells expressing MHC class I interact with CD8$^+$ T cells, which kill infected host cells; cells expressing MHC class II interact with CD4$^+$ T cells, which synthesize cytokines.

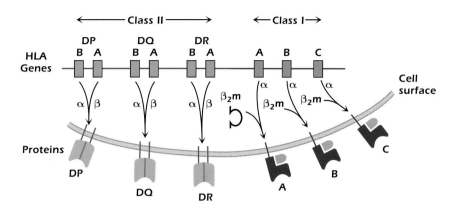

<u>Figure 9.4.</u> Simplified depiction of the human MHC, HLA, showing genes coding for polymorphic HLA class I (A, B, and C) and class II (DP, DQ, and DR) molecules. β2-microglobulin (β_2m) encoded outside MHC.

molecules are coded for by multiple independent genes. The human HLA complex (found on chromosome 6) contains three independent genes—**HLA-A**, **HLA-B**, and **HLA-C**—that code for MHC class I molecules (Figure 9.4).

As we explain below, each HLA class I molecule is expressed at the surface in association with a small molecule, **β_2-microglobulin** (β_2m), coded for outside the HLA complex. Because every cell has two sets of chromosomes (one paternally derived and one maternally derived), every nucleated cell may express up to six different HLA class I molecules, each capable of binding peptides. Similarly, the HLA complex codes for three different two-chain MHC class II molecules: **HLA-DP**, **HLA-DQ**, and **HLA-DR** (Figure 9.4). Thus, human APCs may express up to six different HLA class II molecules, each capable of binding to peptides.

Polymorphism means that multiple stable forms of each MHC gene exist in the population. The MHC is the most highly polymorphic gene system in the body and hence in the population: In humans over a thousand slightly different versions—*alleles*—of the gene that codes for the MHC class I molecule HLA-B and MHC class II molecule HLA-DRB have been identified. Other important examples of genetic polymorphism in humans are the different forms of the red blood cell antigens (A, B, and O) and of hemoglobin molecules. Recent studies comparing gene sequences from different individuals—by identifying single nucleotide polymorphisms—have found that many genes show allelic variation, for example, genes coding for cytokine receptors and liver detoxification enzymes. However, none of these genes is as variable within the population as HLA.

The extensive polymorphism of human MHC genes makes it very unlikely that two random individuals will express identical sets of HLA class I and class II molecules. As we describe in Chapter 19, the enormous diversity of MHC molecules and the genes that code for them is a major barrier to successful transplantation of organs and tissues. Later in this chapter we discuss why we believe the MHC evolved to be so diverse.

Note that the mechanisms used to generate the diversity of MHC structures differ from the mechanisms used to generate the diversity of the antigen-specific receptors of B and T cells (Ig and TCR, respectively) that arises from rearrangement of DNA and which produces one type of receptor per cell (Chapters 7 and 10). In contrast, although MHC molecules are diverse within the population, each cell in a particular individual (liver, kidney, lymphocytes, etc.) expresses the same set of HLA class I and class II molecules.

STRUCTURE OF MHC CLASS I AND CLASS II MOLECULES

In the sections below we refer to "typical" MHC class I and II molecules to illustrate the general features of their structure. These "typical" features mean they are common to humans and other vertebrate species (for example, mice, cats, and cattle).

MHC Class I

Parts A–D of Figure 9.5 show different ways to represent the key features of the structure of a typical MHC class I molecule and how it interacts with peptide and a TCR. An MHC class I molecule is a transmembrane glycoprotein (molecular weight approximately 43 kDa), expressed on the cell surface in noncovalent association with a small *invariant* (identical on all cells) polypeptide called *β_2-microglobulin* (β_2m; molecular weight 12 kDa). As we noted above, β_2m is encoded by a gene on a separate chromosome from the MHC. The MHC class I molecule is referred to as the α or heavy chain and comprises three extracellular Ig-like domains—α_1, α_2, and α_3. β_2m has a structure homologous to a single Ig domain; indeed, β_2m and MHC class I are members of the Ig superfamily described in Chapter 5. At the cell surface, MHC class I plus β_2m has the appearance of a four-domain molecule—α_1 paired with α_2 on the exterior of the MHC class I molecule and α_3 and β_2m paired closer to the membrane.

Figure 9.5B shows the most striking feature of all MHC class I molecules that have been examined by X-ray

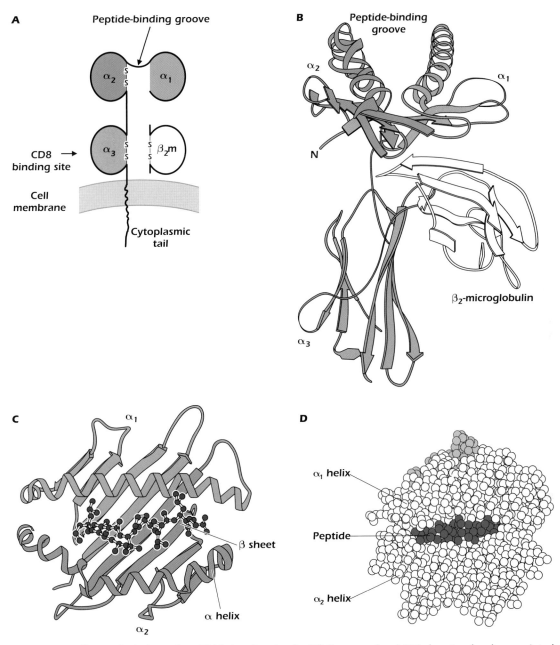

Figure 9.5. Different depictions of an MHC class I molecule. (A) Cartoon of an MHC class I molecule associated at the cell surface with β_2m. (B) Side view of MHC class I molecule with β_2m, showing peptide-binding groove. (Bjorkman PJ et al. 1987. Reproduced with permission of Nature Publishing Group.) (C) Top view of peptide-binding groove, showing bound peptide. (Bjorkman PJ et al. 1987. Reproduced with permission of Nature Publishing Group.) (D) Top view, space-filling model of peptide bound in the groove of an MHC class I molecule. (Delves P, et al. 2011. Reproduced with permission of John Wiley & Sons Ltd.)

crystallography: a deep groove or cleft—the ***peptide-binding groove***—in the part of the molecule farthest from the membrane that is composed of parts of the α_1 and α_2 domains. This groove can hold one peptide 8–9 amino acids in length in a linear array (see also Figure 4.5 of Chapter 4). Every MHC class I molecule can bind several different peptides, but only one at a time. Figure 9.5C shows that the groove

resembles a basket with an irregular floor (made up of amino acids in a β-pleated sheet structure) surrounded by walls (formed by α helices). The bound peptide fits inside the groove, as illustrated in both Figures 9.5C and 9.5D.

Selectivity of Peptide Binding to MHC Class I Molecules. We referred above to the tremendous

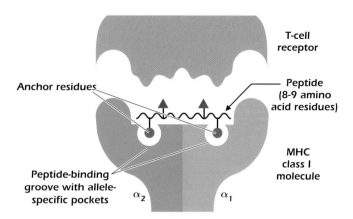

<u>Figure 9.6.</u> Peptide bound in the MHC class I molecule peptide-binding groove interacts with the MHC molecule and the T-cell receptor. Anchor residues in the peptide bind to the allele-specific pockets of the MHC molecule. (Rammensee HG, Falk K, Rötzschke O 1993. Reproduced with permission of Elsevier.)

variability of MHC class I molecules within the population. Looking at differences in sequence among MHC class I molecules, we find that most of the differences in amino acids are confined to a limited region in the extracellular α_1 and α_2 domains, and particularly in the floor and walls of the peptide-binding groove (see Figure 9.5C). These differences in amino acid sequence and hence structure of the binding groove play a critical role in determining which peptides bind to a particular MHC molecule. The pockets forming the floor of the groove also help to align peptides so they can be recognized by specific TCRs (Figure 9.6).

Thus, binding of peptide to an MHC class I molecule is selective: One MHC molecule will bind with high affinity to only certain peptides. A single MHC class I molecule preferentially binds peptides with specific *anchor residues*: invariant or closely related amino acids at certain positions in the 8- or 9-amino-acid sequence. As shown in Figure 9.6, a peptide that binds to an MHC class I molecule typically has two anchor residues, which interact with the allele-specific pockets in the MHC molecule. The other positions in the peptide may vary. As a result, one MHC molecule can bind a large number of peptides with different sequences. This helps explain how only a maximum of six MHC class I molecules in an individual can display many different peptide antigens. It also helps explain why with very few exceptions T-cell responses are made to at least one epitope from almost all proteins and why failure to respond to a protein antigen is so rare.

Figure 9.6 also shows that the peptide bound in this cleft and parts of the MHC class I molecule interact with the TCR. One to four amino acids in the peptide make contact with the TCR, indicating that only a small number of contacts with the peptide are critical for recognition by the TCR.

CD8 Binding to Invariant Region of MHC Class I Molecules. Outside the peptide-binding cleft the sequences of different MHC class I molecules are very similar. Thus an individual MHC class I molecule can be divided into a ***polymorphic*** or ***variable region*** (sequence unique to that molecule) in the area in and around the peptide-binding groove, and a ***nonpolymorphic*** or ***invariant region*** that is similar in all MHC class I molecules. CD8, the molecule that characterizes the CD8$^+$ T-cell subset, binds to the invariant region of all MHC class I molecules, specifically in the α_3 domain (see Figure 9.5A).

Structure of MHC Class II Molecules

Figure 9.7 shows different ways to represent the key features of a typical MHC class II molecule. Figure 9.7A shows that an MHC class II molecule is a transmembrane glycoprotein comprising two chains: α and β (molecular weight of approximately 35,000 and 28,000 Da, respectively). Like MHC class I molecules, every MHC class II molecule is expressed at the cell surface as a four-domain structure: the α_1 domain is paired with β_1, and α_2 with β_2. The chains α and β have cytoplasmic tails and extracellular Ig-like domains; they are also members of the Ig superfamily.

Like the MHC class I molecule, the MHC class II molecule contains a peptide-binding groove at the top of the molecule (shown in more detail in Figures 9.7B and 9.7C), which holds one peptide. However, in the MHC class II molecule, the groove is formed by interactions between the α_1 and β_1 domains. Figure 9.7C indicates that the floor and walls of the MHC class II cleft have the same β-pleated sheet and α-helical structures found in the MHC class I molecule.

In contrast to the 8- to 9-amino-acid peptides that bind to the cleft in the MHC class I molecule, the MHC class II groove binds peptides varying in length from 12 to approximately 17 linearly arranged amino acids. Figures 9.7C and 9.7D show that the ends of the peptide are outside the peptide-binding groove.

As with MHC class I molecules, each MHC class II molecule binds to peptides with specific anchor residues. Figure 9.8 shows that a peptide that binds to a typical MHC class II molecule has three (sometimes four) anchor residues in the central region of the peptide that bind to the allele-specific pockets of the MHC class II molecule. Because the other amino acids in the peptide outside the anchor residues may vary, MHC class II molecules are also capable of binding a wide selection of peptides. Between four and six of the peptide's amino acids contact the TCRs; only two are shown in Figure 9.8.

Like MHC class I molecules, MHC class II molecules are composed of variable or polymorphic regions, and invariant or nonpolymorphic regions. CD4, the molecule that characterizes the CD4$^+$ T-cell subset, binds to the invariant region of all MHC class II molecules, specifically in the β_2 domain (see Figure 9.7A).

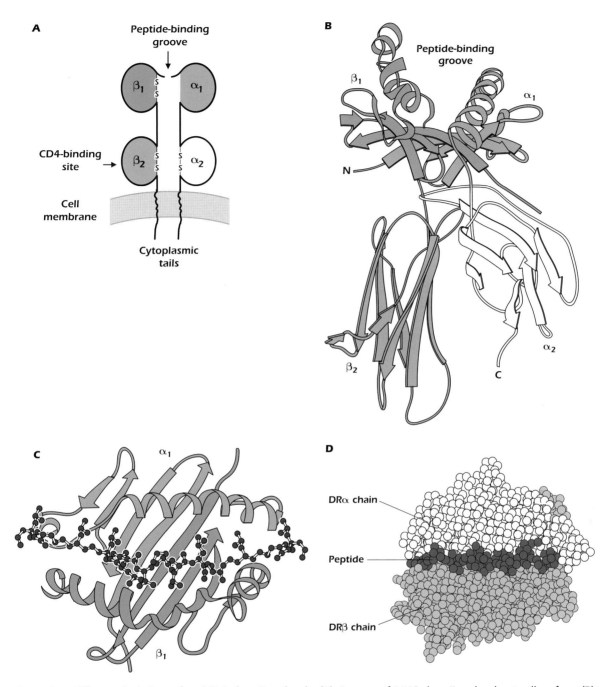

Figure 9.7. Different depictions of an MHC class II molecule. (A) Cartoon of MHC class II molecule at cell surface. (B) Side view of MHC class II molecule showing peptide-binding groove. (Stern LJ, Wiley, DC 1994. Reproduced with permission of Elsevier.) (C) Top view of peptide-binding groove showing bound peptide. (Stern LJ, Wiley, DC 1994. Reproduced with permission of Elsevier.) (D) Top view, space-filling model of peptide bound in the groove of an MHC class II molecule. (Delves P, et al. 2011. Reproduced with permission of John Wiley & Sons Ltd.)

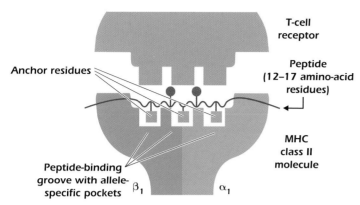

Figure 9.8. Peptide bound in MHC class II molecule peptide-binding groove interacts with the MHC molecule and the T-cell receptor. Anchor residues in the peptide bind to the allele-specific pockets of the MHC molecule. (Rammensee HG, Falk K, Rötzschke O 1993. Reproduced with permission of Elsevier.)

ANTIGEN PROCESSING AND PRESENTATION: HOW MHC MOLECULES BIND PEPTIDES AND CREATE LIGANDS THAT INTERACT WITH T CELLS

Exogenous Antigens and Generation of MHC Class II–Peptide Complexes

As the term implies, *exogenous antigens* are antigens that come from *outside* a host cell and are taken inside, normally by endocytosis or phagocytosis. Exogenous antigens can be derived from pathogens (such as bacteria or viruses) or from foreign proteins (such as vaccines) that do not injure the host but activate an immune response. As we noted earlier in this chapter, the specialized cells that take up exogenous antigens (and present it to T cells) are known as APCs. The main APCs are dendritic cells, macrophages, and B cells, all of which express MHC class II molecules constitutively.

Figure 9.8 shows the processing and presentation of a typical exogenous antigen, a protein injected as a component of an inactivated or "dead" virus vaccine. The protein is internalized, contained in an intracellular vesicle that fuses with endosomal or lysosomal vesicles that are highly acidic (pH approximately 4.0). These vesicles contain an array of degradative enzymes, including proteases and peptidases. Proteases, known as cathepsins, which function at low pH, cut proteins into peptides in these vesicles. Catabolism of a typical protein antigen yields several peptides (only three are shown in Figure 9.9).

The acid vesicles containing peptides intersect inside the cell with vesicles containing MHC class II molecules that have been synthesized on ribosomes of the rough endoplasmic reticulum. The MHC class II α and β chains are synthesized individually in the endoplasmic reticulum and are assembled there with **invariant chain (Ii, CD74)**. The invariant chain binds to the groove of the newly formed MHC class II molecule, preventing the binding of peptides that may be present in the endoplasmic reticulum, such as peptides derived from the processing of endogenous antigens (see below).

The invariant chain also acts as a **chaperone** for the newly synthesized MHC class II chains; that is, interaction with the invariant chain allows the MHC class II α and β chains to leave the endoplasmic reticulum and enter the Golgi complex, and from there they proceed into the acid vesicle endocytic pathway. Removal of invariant chain from the complex occurs in stages. Initially, the invariant chain is degraded proteolytically, leaving a fragment known as CLIP (class II-associated invariant polypeptide) bound to the MHC class II groove. Vesicles containing MHC class II with bound CLIP then fuse with the acid vesicles (endosomes or lysosomes) containing peptides derived from the catabolism of exogenous antigens. In this compartment, a molecule known as HLA-DM catalyzes the peptide exchange between the MHC class II–CLIP complex and peptides derived from the exogenous antigen. In this way, a peptide–MHC class II complex is generated, which moves to the cell surface where it is displayed and available to interact with—that is, be presented to—a CD4+ T cell expressing the appropriate antigen receptor.

Although catabolism of a typical protein yields several peptides, not all the peptides formed bind to MHC molecules because, as we described earlier in the chapter, MHC binding to peptides is *selective*. Figure 9.10 shows the situation with three of the many peptides that are derived from the catabolism of a larger protein. Peptides 35–48 and 110–122 (these numbers reflect to the position of amino acids in the protein sequence) bind to two different HLA class II molecules, HLA-DR4 and HLA-DP2, expressed in this individual. Only these peptides have the potential to induce a T-cell response in this particular person to this protein antigen. Because peptide 1–13 does not bind to this individual's MHC class II molecules, it does not trigger a CD4+ T-cell response. We say that peptides 35–48 and 110–122 are the **immunodominant** CD4+ T-cell epitopes of this protein in this person. Peptide 1–13 quite probably is an immunodominant epitope of this protein in a different individual expressing a completely different set of MHC molecules. Thus, we can say, almost without fail, that every person will make a T-cell response to this viral protein; however, because of the selectivity of peptide–MHC binding,

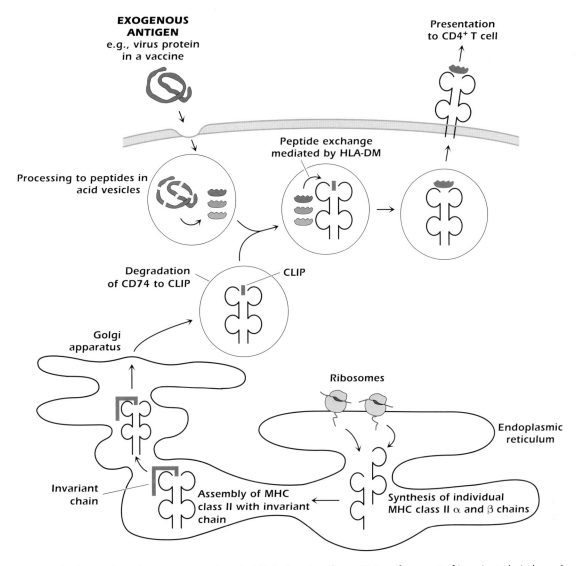

<u>Figure 9.9.</u> Processing of exogenous antigen in MHC class II pathway CLIP = fragment of invariant chain bound to MHC class II groove).

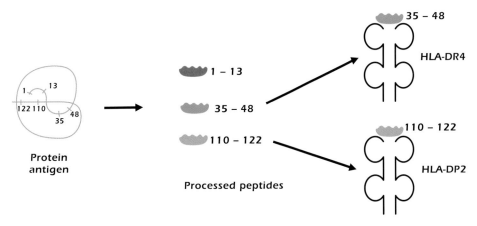

<u>Figure 9.10.</u> Selective binding of processed peptides by different MHC molecules. The numbers refer to the positions of amino acids in the sequence of the protein antigen.

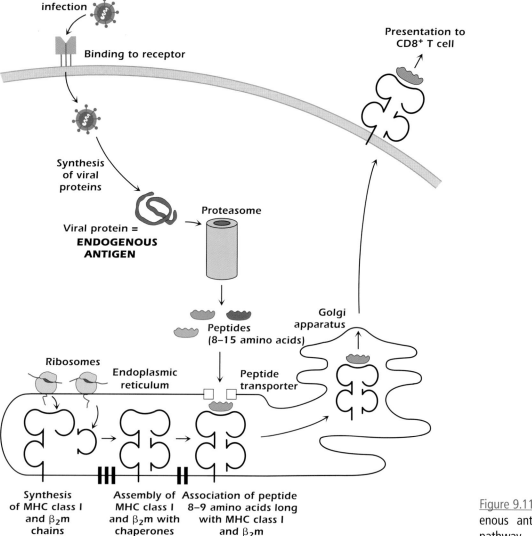

Figure 9.11. Processing of endogenous antigen in MHC class I pathway.

individuals who express different MHC molecules respond to different parts of the same protein.

Endogenous Antigens: Generation of MHC Class I–Peptide Complexes

Endogenous antigens are proteins synthesized *inside* a cell and are generally derived from pathogens (such as viruses, bacteria, and parasites) that have infected a host cell. Figure 9.11 illustrates the processing and presentation of a typical endogenous antigen, a viral protein synthesized after a cell has been infected by a virus. Processing occurs in the cytoplasm, and the major mechanism for generating peptide fragments is via a giant cytoplasmic protein complex known as the **proteasome**. The proteasome is also involved in normal turnover (the routine degradation) of cellular proteins and breaks them down into peptides about 15 amino

acids in length. Cytosolic enzymes (aminopeptidases) remove even more amino acids from the peptides. Some peptides are destroyed, but some, 8–15 amino acids in length (such as the three shown in Figure 9.11), are selectively transported into the endoplasmic reticulum by a two-chain peptide transporter (TAP).

Peptides transported from the cytoplasm into the endoplasmic reticulum bind to newly synthesized MHC class I molecules. MHC class I and β_2m chains are synthesized separately in the rough endoplasmic reticulum and associate in this cellular compartment. As with the synthesis of MHC class II molecules, chaperones stabilize the structure of the assembled MHC class I with their β_2m chains in the endoplasmic reticulum and direct transport of the complex through the cell.

As indicated earlier, MHC class I molecules preferentially bind peptides 8 to 9 amino acids in length. The normal fate of peptides that reach the endoplasmic reticulum is degradation by an aminopeptidase, which removes amino acids one at a time until the peptides are completely degraded; some peptides with the appropriate binding characteristics—that is, 8–9 amino acids in length and with sufficient affinity to bind to the MHC class I binding groove—are "rescued" from this fate by binding to a newly synthesized MHC class I molecule.

A peptide that binds to an MHC class I molecule in the endoplasmic reticulum moves via the Golgi apparatus to the cell surface, where it is displayed and presented to a CD8$^+$ T cell expressing the appropriate antigen receptor. As described above for the interaction of peptides with MHC class II molecules, only those peptides that bind to MHC class I molecules trigger CD8$^+$ T-cell responses. These are the immunodominant epitopes for the CD8$^+$ T-cell response specific for that antigen; one such immunodominant epitope is the peptide derived from the catabolism of the virus protein shown in green in Figure 9.11.

Because MHC class I molecules are expressed on all nucleated cells, the processing and presentation of endogenous antigens can occur in *every* nucleated cell in the body. Because pathogens can infect almost any cell in the body, CD8$^+$ T cells "scan" MHC class I and peptide combinations expressed on any nucleated host cell to identify whether it has been infected.

Decreased MHC Class I Expression in Virus-Infected and Tumor Cells: Role of NK Cells.

Factors such as cytokines synthesized in response to infectious agents induce or increase expression of MHC class I and class II molecules. This leads to enhanced immune responses to the pathogen that induced the response. In contrast, some viruses (such as the herpes simplex virus, adenovirus, and cytomegalovirus) synthesize proteins that interfere with steps in the pathway shown in Figure 9.11: They inhibit the synthesis of MHC class I molecules or interrupt the transport of peptide–MHC class I complexes to the cell surface. In this way the virus product *decreases* expression of MHC class I molecules and so subverts the potential host CD8$^+$ T-cell response to the virus. In addition, tumor cells frequently show decreased expression of MHC class I molecules compared to normal cells, so reducing a potential antitumor response by CD8$^+$ T cells.

Although the decrease in MHC class I expression may result in a reduced CD8$^+$ T-cell response, other immune responses come into play. In particular, the decrease in MHC class I expression triggers the response of NK cells to a virus-infected or tumor cell. As we described in Chapter 3, MHC class I molecules are *negative* regulators of NK cell function; that is, an MHC class I expressed on a normal host cell interacts with a killer-cell inhibitory receptor (KIR) expressed on an NK cell and so *prevents* the NK cell from killing the host cell. If a host cell does not express MHC class I (as in the case of tumors or virus-infected cells) and the KIR–MHC class I interaction does *not* occur, NK cells are activated and kill the MHC-deficient cells.

Cross-Presentation: Exogenous Antigens Presented in the MHC Class I Pathway

In addition to their ability to process exogenous antigens in the MHC class II pathway, APCs—and particularly dendritic cells—have a unique pathway, called **cross-presentation**, for generating peptides derived from exogenous protein antigens and presenting them to CD8$^+$ T cells (Figure 9.12). The dendritic cell takes up exogenous antigens (such as those derived from a virus-infected or dying cell) by either phagocytosis or pinocytosis. How peptides intersect with MHC class I molecules inside the cell is not completely understood; one pathway is thought to involve transferring antigen from acid compartments into the cytosol for processing by proteasomes. Peptides are then transported into the endoplasmic reticulum where they bind to newly synthesized MHC class I molecules. A second pathway involves the loading of peptides directly onto MHC class I molecules in acid vesicles, with peptide–MHC complexes then trafficking to the cell surface.

Cross-presentation is believed to play an important role in activating CD8$^+$ T cells to respond to tissue cells infected by some viruses that are not taken up by APCs (see Chapter 11). It is also thought to play a role in the response to dying cells.

In addition to this cross-presentation pathway in which exogenous antigens associate with MHC class I molecules, in some circumstances endogenous antigens may associate with MHC class II molecules. This may occur during **autophagy**, an intracellular pathway in which proteins in the cytoplasm are transported into lysosomes for degradation. Self-peptides can bind to MHC class II in these acid vesicles. Currently, however, there is very limited evidence that

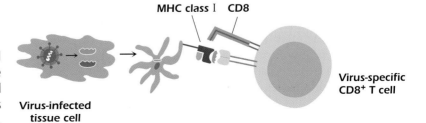

MHC class I   CD8

Virus-infected tissue cell

Virus-specific CD8$^+$ T cell

<u>Figure 9.12.</u> Cross-presentation. A dendritic cell takes up an exogenous antigen, for example derived from a virus-infected cell, but processed peptides associate with MHC class I molecules inside the cell and are presented to CD8$^+$ T cells.

TABLE 9.1. Comparison of Properties and Function of MHC Class I and II Molecules

Characteristic	MHC Class I	MHC Class II
Name	HLA-A, HLA-B, and HLA-C	HLA-DP, HLA-DQ, and HLA-DR
Structure	α chain $+ \beta_2$m	$\alpha + \beta$ chains
Cellular expression	All nucleated cells. Upregulated on many cell types by interferons. Downregulated by viruses and in some tumors	Constitutively on APC (dendritic cells, macrophages, B cells, thymic epithelial cells); induced on many cell types by interferon-γ
Peptide binding	Selectively to peptides 8–9 amino acids long. Groove formed by α_1 and α_2 domains	Selectively to peptides 12–17 amino acids long. Groove formed by α_1 and β_1 domains
MHC–peptide complex interacts with	TCR of a CD8$^+$ T cell	TCR of a CD4$^+$ T cell
Binds peptides derived from	(1) Endogenous antigens catabolized in the cytoplasm or (2) cross-presentation	Exogenous antigens catabolized in acid compartments
MHC molecule interacts with	CD8 (α3 domain), expressed on CD8$^+$ T cells; KIR expressed on NK cells	CD4 (β_2 domain), expressed on CD4$^+$ T cells

TABLE 9.2. Features Common to Both MHC Class I and Class II

- Both are polygenic (multiple independent genes) and highly polymorphic (enormous allelic variation within the population).
- Both bind selectively to peptides
- Both are coordinately and codominantly expressed.

autophagy results in the processing of foreign antigens to generate T cell responses.

Table 9.1 compares the characteristics of MHC class I and II molecules that we have described so far. Table 9.2 indicates features common to both MHC class I and II molecules.

Which Antigens Trigger Which T-Cell Responses?

We have described how exogenous protein antigens are taken up by APCs, processed in acid compartments that intersect with the MHC class II pathway, and presented to CD4$^+$ T cells. Thus, proteins from bacteria, most viruses, allergens, and completely harmless antigens all trigger CD4$^+$ T-cell responses. In contrast, only infectious pathogens, particularly viruses, create epitopes via the endogenous or cross-presentation pathways and are presented by MHC class I molecules; thus, they are the only types of antigen that activate CD8$^+$ T cells. Generally, but not always, infectious agents activate both CD4$^+$ T cells and CD8$^+$ T cells because these agents are taken up by APCs; however, as we describe in Chapter 11, some viruses do not evoke responses by CD4$^+$ T cells and activate CD8$^+$ T cells almost exclusively.

Transplantation responses—in which host T cells respond to nonself MHC molecules expressed on cells of the graft—generally activate both CD4$^+$ and CD8$^+$ T-cell responses (see Chapter 19). Immune responses to tumors are generally mediated by CD8$^+$ cells.

MHC Molecules Bind Peptides Derived from Self-Molecules

The phenomena of antigen processing and presentation described above—the catabolism of proteins and movement of products from compartment to compartment inside a cell—are all aspects of normal cell physiologic pathways. Thus, the proteins normally found inside cells, self-proteins, "turn over" and are catabolized using the same pathways described for the processing of protein antigens. For example, ribosomal and mitochondrial proteins are broken down inside cells and peptides derived from these molecules can associate with MHC molecules. Indeed, MHC molecules extracted from cells nearly always contain peptides derived from such self-proteins. From our description of protein processing, proteins from inside host cells would be expected to associate with MHC class I molecules, and indeed this is observed.

However, self-peptides bound to MHC molecules do not normally activate T cells. One reason is that T cells reactive to many self-molecules are removed or inactivated during differentiation in the thymus (see Chapter 10). However, we know that mature T cells with the potential to react with self-molecules are detectable outside the thymus. Why are these T cells not activated? Equally important, an individual's cells are bathed in a sea of self-proteins that they are continually processing and binding to their MHC molecules—how can a person respond to a tiny amount of foreign protein? These are critical issues; a T cell must be able to distinguish between a normal host cell, to which no response is required, and a cell that has been infected by a pathogen.

The answer appears to be that pathogens induce effects that activate the immune response over and above their ability to generate peptides for binding to MHC molecules. The major effect induced by pathogens is *co-stimulator function*—also referred to as *second signals*—in the specialized APCs that present antigen to T cells (this concept is discussed further in Chapters 10 and 11). These co-stimulator signals are required to activate naïve T cells. In contrast to APCs, normal tissue cells (such as those of the liver or pancreas) displaying peptides derived from self-molecules do not express co-stimulator function; thus, T cells are not activated when they encounter self-molecules in tissues.. Even if peptides derived from a self-molecule are presented by an APC in the tissue, T cells are not activated because in the absence of foreign antigen or an inflammatory response APCs in tissue do not express co-stimulator signals (see Chapter 11). This signaling requirement ensures that T cells do not normally respond to peptides derived from self-components but do respond to peptides derived from nonself, potentially harmful, antigens.

This also helps to explain why the induction of T-cell responses to even some foreign antigens, such as harmless antigens or some vaccines, can be difficult. To develop strong T-cell (and antibody) responses, such antigens are frequently administered with an *adjuvant* (literally, adding to the response). Adjuvants are generally products that activate APCs such as dendritic cells, macrophages, and B cells; they and are discussed further in Chapter 4.

Inability to Respond to an Antigen

As described in the preceding sections, limited numbers of different MHC class I and II molecules are expressed on the cells of any one person. For an antigen to generate a T-cell response, at least one peptide derived during processing must bind to one of these MHC molecules. A peptide that does not bind to an MHC molecule does not activate a T-cell response; thus, if an entire antigen fails to generate a single peptide able to bind to an MHC molecule, the individual will not mount a T-cell response to that particular antigen.

Naturally occurring pathogens are generally large and complex and contain multiple epitopes that stimulate responses by both T and B cells; thus, some sort of response to a pathogen is more or less certain. However, unresponsiveness to a large antigen can occur in the case of synthetic polymers of amino acids that contain a very limited number of epitopes. Another important situation is in the response to a small peptide, such as a vaccine comprising a single, small peptide. Since the population expresses many different types of MHC molecules, the MHC molecules expressed in some people may not bind this particular peptide. In vaccination, this problem has been circumvented by coupling

the peptide to a large protein, a *carrier*, which enhances the response to the peptide (described further in Chapter 11).

OTHER TYPES OF ANTIGEN THAT ACTIVATE T-CELL RESPONSES

Superantigens

Figure 9.13A shows the key characteristics of the set of protein antigens known as *superantigens*; in humans, these are predominantly exotoxins produced by pathogenic bacteria. Two examples are the enterotoxin released by staphylococcal organisms (the cause of food poisoning) and the toxin responsible for toxic shock syndrome. Superantigens are not processed, but the intact molecule binds to MHC class II molecules outside the peptide-binding groove and cross-links the MHC class II molecule with the variable region of the TCR β chain expressed by a CD4$^+$ T cell. Each superantigen binds to T cells expressing a particular Vβ TCR gene product. Since there are only about 50 different Vβ TCR genes in humans, and a superantigen may bind to more than one Vβ, superantigens are able to activate more than 10% of the total T-cell population. This is an enormous response compared to the triggering of a few T-cell clones by a peptide–MHC class II complex derived from a conventional antigen. Thus, the key biologic and clinical feature of superantigens is that they activate huge numbers of CD4$^+$ T cells, which proliferate and secrete high levels of cytokines, and can pass into the circulation. The systemic effects of the toxin activating so many T cells can have clinical consequences, including fever and cardiovascular shock, and can be fatal.

Lipids and Glycolipids

Some T cells can recognize lipids and glycolipids found in the cell walls of pathogens such as *Mycobacterium tuberculosis* that live inside macrophages; these T cells also respond to many host glycolipids. Lipids and glycolipids are presented by a family of molecules known as **CD1** (CD1a through CD1d), which is expressed by APCs such as macrophages and dendritic cells (Figure 9.13B). CD1 molecules are cell surface glycoproteins coded for outside the MHC region; like MHC class I molecules, they are expressed on the surface of APCs in association with β$_2$m. The structure of a CD1 molecule is similar to that of an MHC class I molecule, but CD1 contains a larger binding groove with a deep cavity. The cavity binds the hydrophobic backbone of a lipid antigen, exposing the polar region of the lipid or glycolipid for binding to the T-cell receptor. Binding of lipid antigens to CD1 is believed to take place in acidic cellular compartments, similar to the loading of exogenous peptides onto MHC class II molecules. Like the interaction of some viruses with MHC class I, recent evidence indicates that

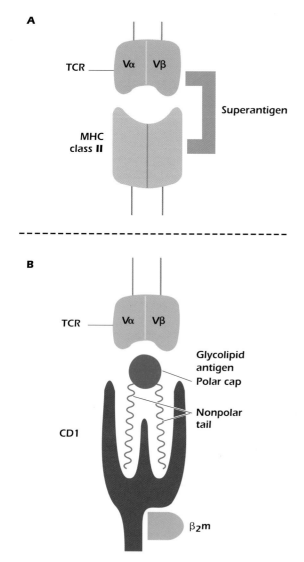

Figure 9.13. Interaction of TCRs with nonpeptide antigens: (A) superantigens bind outside MHC class II peptide-binding groove and interact with TCR Vβ; (B) CD1 presents glycolipid antigens.

herpes simplex virus 1 downregulates expression of CD1d, inhibiting glycolipid antigen presentation.

CD1a, b, and c present lipids and glycolipids to T cells that use an αβ TCR, but CD1d presents lipids and glycolipids to a subset of T cells, NKT cells, which express both NK- and T-cell characteristics (NKT cells are discussed further in Chapters 10 and 11).

Multiple Antigens Activate γδ T Cells

A subset of T cells uses a two-chain molecule known as γδ, rather than αβ as its TCR. γδ T cells (discussed further in Chapter 10) respond to many different types of antigens derived from both pathogens and damaged host cells. The antigens that γδ T cells respond to include phospholipids and other small nonprotein molecules, known as *phosphoantigens*, as well as *heat-shock proteins*: proteins that are synthesized when cells are heated or stressed in different ways. How these different antigens are presented to γδ T cells is not completely understood, but it does not appear to involve polymorphic MHC molecules. Lipid molecules are likely presented by CD1 molecules and heat-shock proteins by MHC class I-like molecules, such as MHC class I polypeptide-related sequence (MIC) A and MICB, discussed later in this chapter.

GENES OF THE HLA REGION

Scientists have recognized for a long time that MHC genes found in all vertebrate species are a complex group of tightly linked genes passed down as a unit. The MHC of the human and the mouse have both been mapped and shown to contain many more genes than the polymorphic MHC class I and class II molecules shown in Figure 9.4.

The class I region, in addition to the three genes that code for the polymorphic MHC class I molecules—HLA-A, HLA-B, and HLA-C—also contains the much less polymorphic MHC class Ib genes *HLA-E*, *HLA-F*, and *HLA-G*. The function of the protein products of the MHC class Ib genes are not well understood; they have a structure similar to the polymorphic class I gene products, but they do not present peptides to T cells. HLA-E and HLA-F are thought to be involved in the presentation of antigens to NK cells. The expression of HLA-G by placental trophoblast cells has been suggested as a potential mechanism preventing rejection of the fetus by the maternal host. *MICA* and *MICB* genes are also contained in this class I region; they code for stress-induced products that interact with NK and γδ T cells. MICA and MICB proteins have class I-like structures, but are not expressed on the cell surface in association with β2m and do not bind peptides.

The class II region includes pairs of genes that code for the polymorphic MHC class II molecules HLA-DP, HLA-DQ, and HLA-DR. Each of these MHC class II subregions contains an A gene and a B gene; these code for the α and β chain, respectively, of the two-chain MHC class II molecule (Figure 9.4). Thus, for example, the HLA-DPA1 gene codes for DPα of the HLA-DP molecule and the HLA-DPB1 gene codes for the other chain, DPβ, of the HLA-DP molecule. Some people have more than one DRB gene (DRB1, DRB2, etc.) that may be used to code for the DRβ chain, so they can express more than one pair of DRα and β chains. Thus, these individuals may express more than 6 HLA class II molecules on their surface.

We also note that some people may express fewer than six HLA class I or class II molecules on their surface. This can arise when both chromosomes express the identical allele, for example, for HLA-DR4. These individuals are *homozygous* for HLA-DR4. Most individuals, however, are *heterozygous* for their HLA genes; that is, they express different alleles on the two chromosomes.

The class II region also includes the gene **HLA-DM**, which codes for the molecule that is involved in peptide exchange in the exogenous antigen processing-MHC class II pathway. This region also contains genes coding for molecules involved in the MHC class I pathway: the peptide transporter molecules TAP-1 and TAP-2, and the major subunits of the proteasome.

Between the class I and class II regions is the **class III region**. This contains genes that code for serum complement components C2, C4, and factor B (described in Chapter 14). The human MHC class III region also contains genes coding for the cytokines tumor necrosis factor and lymphotoxin (TNF-α and TNF-β, respectively), heat-shock proteins hsp 70-1 and 70-2, and 21-hydroxylase (an enzyme involved in steroid metabolism).

Why all these genes are linked in a complex that is passed down as a unit with genes coding for molecules responsible for crucial cell interactions is currently unknown.

NOMENCLATURE OF POLYMORPHIC MHC MOLECULES

Originally, HLA molecules were characterized by serology, that is, using antibodies specific for different HLA class I or II molecules. This approach gave rise to a terminology that established differences among HLA antigens, for example, HLA-A2 differs from HLA-A25, and HLA-DR14 from HLA-DR16. The advent of polymerase chain reaction (PCR) technology has provided a much more detailed description of differences among HLA molecules. For example, current terminology refers to *HLA-DRB1*1301*, in which the letters to the left of the asterisk specify the HLA gene, in this case *DRB1*, and the four (or, in some cases, six or eight) numbers to the right of the asterisk define the particular allele. This more extensive and precise characterization of HLA alleles has been invaluable in trying to match transplant donors and recipients and for identifying individuals who may be at risk for different autoimmune conditions (see Chapters 19 and 13, respectively). Important examples of specific alleles associated with human autoimmune conditions are given in Table 13.2 in Chapter 13.

REGULATION OF EXPRESSION OF MHC GENES

Codominant Expression

MHC class I and II molecules are *codominantly expressed*, that is, every cell expresses MHC molecules transcribed from both the maternal and paternal chromosomes. Thus, every nucleated cell of a particular person expresses up to six different HLA class I and six different HLA class II molecules. As we noted above, some individuals may express more than six different HLA class II molecules (because they express more than one pair of DRα and β chains), and some individuals may express fewer than six different class I or class II molecules (because they are homozygous for a particular allele).

Coordinate Regulation

Expression of MHC molecules is *coordinately regulated*, meaning that all class I molecules and all class II molecules are expressed at the same time on a single cell. Thus, factors such as IFN-γ enhance expression of all class I molecules and induce all class II molecules on a particular cell. As the foregoing discussion has emphasized, MHC class I and II genes are regulated separately, because MHC class I molecules can be expressed in the absence of MHC class II molecules.

Rare people with *bare lymphocyte syndrome* lack the ability to express either HLA class I or class II molecules or both (see Chapter 18). Individuals who do not express HLA class II molecules have the most profound immunodeficiency, characterized by defective presentation of antigens to CD4+ T cells and decreased numbers of CD4+ T cells. These individuals have a mutation in one of the factors that controls the transcription of MHC class II genes.

Read the related case: **Bare Lymphocyte Syndrome**
In *Immunology: Clinical Case Studies and Disease Pathophysiology*

Inheritance of MHC Genes

The set of HLA class I plus class II genes expressed on an individual chromosome—referred to as a *haplotype*—is passed on to offspring as a unit (Figure 9.14). In this example, the cells of the father express HLA class I and II molecules coded for by his paternal and maternal chromosomes (haplotypes 1 and 2) and the cells of the mother express HLA class I and II molecules coded for by both her chromosomes (haplotypes 3 and 4). Because of the diversity of HLA genes and molecules in the population, it can almost be guaranteed that the HLA haplotypes 1 and 2 contributed by the father will differ from the haplotypes 3 and 4 contributed by the mother (represented by the different colors of the chromosomes in the figure).

The HLA haplotypes of a son or daughter differs from the haplotypes of his or her parents: Each parent expresses one HLA haplotype different from each child, and each child one HLA haplotype different from each parent. Every

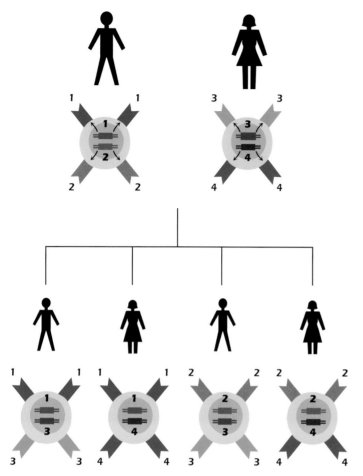

Figure 9.14. HLA genes are passed on as a unit from parent to child. Because HLA is highly polymorphic, it is likely that any two adults will have four distinct HLA haplotypes (father: 1 and 2, mother: 3 and 4). The children of these parents express four different haplotypes (1/3, 1/4, etc.). The different-colored structures expressed on the cell surface represent the combined set of HLA class I plus II molecules expressed by all the cells in that individual.

child in the family expresses a different set of HLA haplotypes, but there is a 1 in 4 chance that any two siblings will have identical HLA haplotypes. However, individuals within a family do not usually express identical MHC molecules, and the likelihood of finding individuals in the general population who are matched at all HLA alleles is extremely small.

MHC IN OTHER SPECIES

Every vertebrate species has an MHC. Generally, the names of the MHCs of other species are similar to the human MHC, HLA; for example, BoLA for the bovine system and SLA for swine. The mouse MHC, known as *H-2*, has been studied in great detail. The name H-2 differs because it was derived from the early studies of histocompatibility genes involved in transplantation responses. Intensive interest in H-2 developed because mice can be selectively bred to create *inbred strains* in which all members of the strain are genetically identical (a topic discussed in more detail in Chapter 6). Studies taking advantage of the genetic identity of inbred strains of mice and the identity of their MHC molecules have helped answer many fundamental immuno-

logic questions that could not be addressed easily in humans. The genes and protein products of the human and mouse MHCs show a high degree of homology, indicating a common ancestral origin.

H-2 is located on mouse chromosome 17. Unlike the single MHC class I region of human HLA, mouse MHC class I genes are found at both ends of H-2 (Figure 9.15). Three independent genes—*K, D,* and *L*—code for the murine MHC class I molecules, which are expressed at the cell surface in association with β_2m. H-2 contains a class II region that contains two pairs of genes (rather than the three found in humans) that code for the polymorphic MHC class II molecules, *I-A and I-E*; each of these is composed of an α chain and a β chain.

DIVERSITY OF MHC MOLECULES: MHC ASSOCIATION WITH RESISTANCE AND SUSCEPTIBILITY TO DISEASE

The extensive polymorphism of MHC genes and molecules is a great impediment to the acceptance of tissue transplanted between individuals, because it is highly unlikely that two random individuals are genetically identical (see

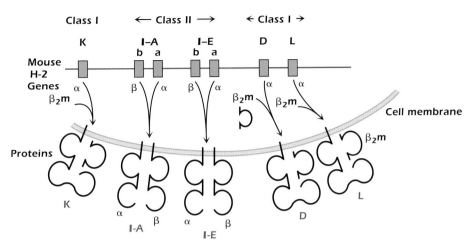

Figure 9.15. Simplified depiction of the mouse MHC, H-2, showing regions and genes coding for polymorphic MHC class I and II molecules expressed at the cell surface; β_2m encoded outside MHC. In mice, H-2 haplotypes are given superscript letters. For example, in the mouse strain H-2^b all the MHC class I and II genes and products are of type b (K^b, I-A^b, etc.), and in the MHC-distinct strain H-2^d all the MHC I and II genes are of type d (K^d, I-A^d, etc.).

Chapter 19). Because nearly every vertebrate species has developed a similarly diverse array of MHC genes and molecules, the maintenance of MHC diversity must have some major benefit to the species. However, to date no explanation for this phenomenon has been universally accepted.

One of the most likely explanations is that the diversity of MHC molecules provides protection to the species from the surrounding array of pathogenic organisms. Presumably, the variety of MHC molecules in the population enhances the probability that some pathogen-derived set of peptides will bind to MHC and activate a T-cell response in at least some individuals. To illustrate this point, imagine the extreme case if there were only one MHC molecule in the population. If a pathogen such as a virus synthesized peptides that did not bind to this MHC, no T-cell response would be mounted, and the entire species could be wiped out. Maintaining a large number of MHC genes and molecules in the species would greatly reduce the risk of such an event.

It is also apparent that the expression of a specific MHC allele is one of the important factors associated with susceptibility or resistance to different infectious agents. In humans, expression of specific HLA alleles has been associated with either susceptibility or resistance to a number of different infectious diseases, such as in the response to human T lymphotropic virus 1 (HTLV-1), hepatitis B, leprosy, malaria, tuberculosis, and rapid progression to acquired immune deficiency syndrome (AIDS). One important recent example is the association described between HLA-C and progression to AIDS in human immunodeficiency virus (HIV) infection: higher expression of HLA-C is associated with reduced viral load and reduced rate of progression to low CD4$^+$ T cell counts.

Similar MHC associations have been shown in infectious diseases afflicting other species. These include Marek's disease (a viral disease in chickens) and bovine leukemia virus infection in cows. In addition, individuals with certain HLA alleles have a higher risk of developing certain autoimmune or inflammatory diseases, although other genes and their products contribute to the development of these diseases.

Definitive mechanisms linking possession of a particular MHC gene or molecule with the onset or progress of disease have not been established for almost any of these diseases or conditions. Nonetheless, the onset and progression of many of these diseases are likely to be related in some way to the presentation of certain peptides by particular MHC molecules and result in the activation of either protective or, alternatively, "inappropriate" pathological T-cell responses. For example, the association described above between high HLA-C expression and improved control of HIV infection may result from a more effective CD8$^+$ T-cell response to the virus in these individuals than in others who do not express high levels of HLA-C.

SUMMARY

1. MHC molecules play a crucial role in the response of T cells to antigens that are taken into or live inside cells of the body: MHC molecules selectively bind peptides derived from protein antigens and present them to T cells with the appropriate receptor. Thus, T-cell responses are said to be MHC restricted.

2. The MHC is a complex set of genes inherited as a unit. The MHC codes for two major categories of cell surface transmembrane molecules, MHC class I and MHC class II:
   • *MHC class I* is expressed on all nucleated cells in association with a small invariant peptide, β_2-microglobulin; antigenic peptide bound to MHC class I interacts with the TCR of a $CD8^+$ T cell, so responses of $CD8^+$ T cells are MHC class I restricted.
   • *MHC class II* is expressed constitutively only on cells that present antigen to T cells: APCs such as dendritic cells, macrophages, and B cells. Peptide bound to MHC class II interacts at the cell surface with the TCR of a $CD4^+$ T cell. Thus, the response of $CD4^+$ T cells is MHC class II restricted.

3. The expression of MHC molecules is inducible on many cell types, particularly in response to cytokines generated in the response to infectious agents. This induction of expression enhances T-cell responses directed against the pathogen. Viruses inhibit MHC class I expression and so subvert the T-cell response directed against them.

4. Within one individual, the same MHC class I and II molecules are expressed on all cells of the body. Different individuals express different MHC class I and II molecules. This diversity arises because individuals within a species have a huge range of inheritable forms of MHC class I and II genes (genetic polymorphism)—the MHC is the most genetically diverse system in the population. Because of the extensive polymorphism of MHC genes, every individual has an almost unique array of inherited MHC genes.

5. The outer region of every MHC class I and II molecule contains a deep cleft called the peptide-binding groove that binds a peptide derived from the catabolism (processing) of protein antigens. The binding of peptides to MHC molecules is selective; that is, each MHC molecule binds a range of peptides but favors the binding of peptides with particular motifs.

6. MHC class I and II molecules bind peptides derived from proteins processed in different compartments inside the cell.
   • *MHC class I* molecules bind peptides 8–9 amino acids long derived from proteins catabolized in the cytoplasm ("endogenous antigens"); peptides are transported into the endoplasmic reticulum where they interact with newly synthesized MHC class I and β_2m chains.
   • *MHC class II* molecules bind peptides 12–17 amino acids long derived from proteins taken into cells ("exogenous" antigens) and catabolized in acid vesicles in APCs.
   Dendritic cells have a unique pathway—cross-presentation—in which antigen taken into the cell associates with MHC class I molecules and peptides are presented to $CD8^+$ T cells.

7. Because proteins are generally structurally complex, they usually generate at least one peptide able to bind to an MHC molecule, ensuring that a T-cell response is made to at least some part of a foreign antigen.

8. MHC class I molecules also interact with receptors on NK cells. This interaction prevents NK cells from killing normal cells of the host. Decreased expression of MHC class I after infection by certain viruses and in some tumors triggers NK cell killing of the altered host cell.

9. MHC molecules bind peptides derived from self-components as well as from foreign antigens, but self-components do not normally activate a T-cell response. This is because under normal conditions self-molecules do not generate the co-stimulator (second) signals needed to activate naïve T cells. The T-cell response is focused on the response to foreign molecules, particularly components of pathogens, which induce these co-stimulator signals.

10. Susceptibility and resistance to many autoimmune and inflammatory conditions are associated with the expression of a particular MHC molecule.

REFERENCES AND BIBLIOGRAPHY

Blum JS, Wearsch PA, Cresswell P. (2013) Pathways of antigen processing. *Annu Rev Immunol* 31: 443.

Bjorkman PJ, Saper MA, Samraoui B, Bennett WS, Strominger JL, Wiley DC. (1987) Structure of the human class I histocompatibility antigen, HLA-A2. *Nature* 329: 506.

Boyton RJ, Altmann DM. (2007) Natural killer cells, killer immunoglobulin-like receptors and human leucocyte antigen class I in disease. *Clin Exp Immunol* 149: 1.

Delves PJ, Martin SJ, Burton DR, Roitt IM. (2011) *Roitt's Essential Immunology*, 12th ed., John Wiley & Sons.

Joffre OP, Segura E, Savina A, Amigorena S. (2012) Cross-presentation by dendritic cells. *Nat Rev Immunol.* 12: 557.

Rammensee HG, Falk K, Rötzschke O. (1993) MHC molecules as peptide receptorss. *Curr Opin Immunol* 5: 35–44.

Stern LJ, Brown JH, Jardetzky TS, Gorga JC, Urban RG, Strominger JL, Wiley DC. (1994) Crystal structure of the human class II MHC protein HLA-DR1 complexed with an influenza virus peptide. *Nature* 368: 215.

Stern LJ, Wiley DC. (1994) Antigenic peptide binding by class I and class II histocompatibility proteins. *Structure* 2: 245.

Trowsdale J. (2005) HLA genomics in the third millennium. *Curr Opin Immunol* 17: 498.

REVIEW QUESTIONS

For each question, choose the ONE BEST answer or completion.

1. All the following are characteristics of both MHC class I and II molecules except:
   A) They are expressed codominantly.
   B) They are expressed constitutively on all nucleated cells.
   C) They are polypeptides with domain structure.
   D) They are involved in presentation of antigen fragments to T cells.
   E) They are expressed on the surface membrane of B cells.

2. MHC class I molecules are important for which of the following?
   A) binding to CD8 molecules on T cells
   B) presenting exogenous antigen (e.g., bacterial protein) to B cells
   C) presenting intact viral proteins to T cells
   D) binding to CD4 molecules on T cells
   E) binding to Ig on B cells

3. Which of the following is *incorrect* concerning MHC class II molecules?
   A) B cells may express different allelic forms of MHC class molecules on their surface.
   B) MHC class II molecules are synthesized in the endoplasmic reticulum of APCs.
   C) Genetically different individuals express different MHC class II alleles.
   D) MHC class II molecules are associated with β_2-microglobulin on the cell surface.
   E) A peptide that does not bind to an MHC class II molecule will not trigger a CD4$^+$ T-cell response.

4. The peptide transporter TAP
   A) binds β_2-microglobulin
   B) prevents peptide binding to MHC molecules
   C) is part of the proteasome
   D) transports peptides into the endoplasmic reticulum for binding to MHC class I
   E) transports peptides into the endoplasmic reticulum for binding to MHC class II

5. Which of the following statements about HLA genes is *incorrect*?
   A) They code for complement components.
   B) They code for both chains of every HLA class I molecule expressed.
   C) They code for both chains of every HLA class II molecule expressed.
   D) They are associated with susceptibility and resistance to different diseases.
   E) The total set of HLA alleles on the chromosome is known as the HLA haplotype.

6. Which of the following is found on the surface of every B cell, T cell, and pancreatic cell?
   A) MHC class II molecules
   B) a rearranged antigen-specific receptor
   C) immunoglobulin
   D) MHC class I molecules
   E) CD19

7. After a virus infects a boy's liver cells, which of the following about the processing and presentation of virus-derived proteins is correct?
   A) All the peptides derived from the processing associate with his HLA class I molecules.
   B) Processing occurs exclusively in acid vesicles.
   C) The virus-derived peptides that bind to his HLA class I molecules also bind to his sister's HLA class I molecules.
   D) Some virus-derived peptides are presented to CD8$^+$ T cells.
   E) His HLA class I molecules preferentially bind virus-derived peptides 12–17 amino acids long.

ANSWERS TO REVIEW QUESTIONS

1. *B.* MHC class I molecules are expressed on all nucleated cells, but the constitutive expression of MHC class II molecules is limited to APC such as B cells and dendritic cells. MHC class II expression can be induced on other cell types such as endothelial cells and fibroblasts by cytokines.

2. *A.* The interaction of CD8 expressed on the T cell and an invariant region of an MHC class I molecule expressed on a host cell plays a critical role in the triggering of CD8$^+$ T cells (see also Chapters 10 and 11).

3. *D.* The MHC class I molecule, not the MHC class II molecule, associates with β2-microglobulin.

4. *D.* The peptide transporter TAP selectively transports peptides generated in the cytoplasm into the endoplasmic reticulum where peptides 8–9 amino acids long, with the appropriate sequence, may bind to a newly synthesized MHC class I molecule.

5. *B.* HLA class I molecules are expressed at the cell surface with β_2-microglobulin; the gene coding for β_2-microglobulin is located outside the MHC, on a different chromosome.

6. *D.* MHC class I molecules are expressed on these cells, and all nucleated cells. MHC class II molecules are expressed constitutively on APCs such as B cells, but not on T cells or pancreatic cells. T cells and B cells express an antigen-specific receptor (see also Chapters 8 and 10) but pancreatic cells do not. Ig and CD19 are expressed by B cells (Chapter 8).

7. *D.* Because of the selectivity of binding of peptides to MHC molecules, some but not all of the peptides derived from processing the virus proteins are likely to associate with the boy's HLA class I molecules and activate a virus-specific CD8$^+$ T-cell response. The peptides that bind to HLA class I molecules are 8–9 amino acids long. Because the boy's sister is expected to have a different HLA haplotype, a distinct set of virus-derived peptides will bind to her HLA class I molecules.

10

BIOLOGY OF THE T LYMPHOCYTE

INTRODUCTION

Previous chapters focused on the characteristics of B lymphocytes and their receptor for antigen, immunoglobulin (Ig). In Chapter 9 we introduced the role of immune responses involving T lymphocytes (T cells) and discussed the key roles of MHC molecules in the recognition of antigen by T cells. Why do we need two sets of antigen-specific lymphocytes if we have B cells? B cells and their products—antibodies—are extremely effective at dealing with pathogens such as viruses, bacteria, and parasites in the body fluids but are *not* effective once the pathogens infect or are taken into cells. We believe that T cells evolved to deal with the crucial phase of the response to pathogens that takes place *inside* host cells. Because proteins are either major components of pathogens or are synthesized by pathogens, T cells play a critical role in the response to nearly all the harmful agents—and "harmless" antigens—to which an individual is exposed.

In this chapter we focus on the major characteristics of T cells. First we describe the T cell's receptor for antigen—*the TCR*—and compare its characteristics with those of the B-cell receptor (BCR), Ig, and then we will describe other important molecules on the T-cell surface. Next we explain the key steps in T-cell development in the thymus, the organ in which the developing T cell acquires its TCR, and describe the critical role played by MHC molecules in this process.

THE ANTIGEN-SPECIFIC T-CELL RECEPTOR

Molecules That Interact with Antigen

Like B cells, T cells express an antigen-specific receptor that is *clonally distributed*, i.e., every clone of T cells expresses a TCR with a unique sequence. The huge repertoire of TCR molecules, calculated to be 10^9 or more different possible structures, is generated by the same V(D)J gene rearrangement strategies described for Ig molecules in Chapter 7. The unique aspects of TCR gene rearrangement are discussed in more detail later in the chapter.

The αβ TCR. Figure 10.1 shows the form of the TCR expressed on the majority of mature T cells in humans and many other species. It comprises two disulfide-linked polypeptide chains, α and β, that span the cell membrane. A minor population of human T cells expresses an alternative TCR made of γ and *δ* chains, which we discuss later in the chapter.

The TCR α and β chains are both glycoproteins with short cytoplasmic tails; because of differences in the carbohydrate composition, the molecular weights of the chains vary between 40 and 60 kDa. The TCR α and β chains consist of variable (V) and constant (C) regions, analogous to the V and C regions of Ig molecules (see Figures 5.3 and 5.14 in Chapter 5). Each TCR V and C region folds into an Ig-like domain.

Immunology: A Short Course, Seventh Edition. Richard Coico and Geoffrey Sunshine.
© 2015 John Wiley & Sons, Ltd. Published 2015 by John Wiley & Sons, Ltd.
Companion Website: www.wileyimmunology.com/coico

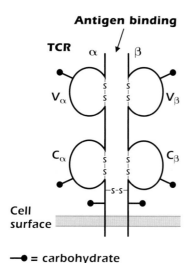

Antigen binding

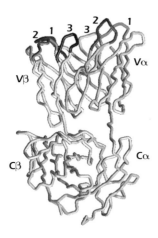

Figure 10.1. The αβ TCR, showing V and C regions and the antigen-binding site.

Figure 10.2. Structure of the αβ TCR (ribbon diagram) showing Vα and Cα, and Vβ and Cβ, and the three complementarity determining regions (1, 2, and 3) at the top of Vα (right side) and Vβ (left side).The number 4 indicates the fourth hypervariable (HV4) region in the β chain, which is not involved in binding to peptide-MHC complexes. The antigen is colored orange. (Garcia K et al. 1998. Reproduced with permission of American Association for the Advancement of Science.)

As shown in Figure 10.2, the TCR Vα and Vβ regions, like the Ig V_H and V_L regions, contain three complementarity-determining regions (CDR1, CDR2, and CDR3) that come together in the three-dimensional structure to form the antigen-binding site. (The β chain has an additional hypervariable region [HV4] that does not bind MHC + peptide, but does bind to superantigens, discussed in Chapter 11.)

The similarities between the structures of the TCR and Ig and the organization of the genes that code for these molecules suggest that the TCR and Ig evolved from a common ancestral gene. As we described in Chapter 5 and

illustrated in Figure 5.14, these genes belong to the **Ig gene superfamily**, and the molecules are referred to as members of the **Ig superfamily**.

Comparison of the αβ TCR and Ig.   Although the structures of the TCR and Ig are similar, they differ in several important ways (see Table 10.1).

Antigen Recognition.   Ig binds to many different types of antigen (carbohydrates, DNA, lipids, and proteins), which it encounters in fluids such as serum (see Chapters 5 and 6). Ig can also respond to linear *and* conformational epitopes in an antigen; thus, both the three-dimensional shape and the sequence of an antigen are important in eliciting antibody responses. By contrast, the αβ TCR interacts predominantly with small linear fragments of proteins (peptides) bound to an MHC molecule expressed on the surface of a host cell. Consequently, in contrast to the variety of structures and shapes recognized by Ig molecules, the antigen recognized by the αβ TCR is generally a combination of major histocompatibility complex (MHC) molecule (either MHC class I or II) and a small peptide (8–9 amino acids long for peptides bound to MHC class I or 12–17 amino acids long for peptides bound to MHC class II).

The TCR makes critical interactions with both the MHC molecule and the peptide bound in the MHC groove—the complex of MHC and peptide interacts with the CDRs of the TCR Vα and Vβ chains (Figure 10.3). Some sequences in the TCR contact the MHC molecule, while other sequences contact the peptide. In the TCR-peptide–MHC interaction shown in Figure 10.3, the TCR CDR3 contacts amino acids in the center of the peptide, with CDRs 1 and 2 interacting with the MHC molecule (not shown). This pattern is found in many TCRs but some show the reverse pattern, in which CDRs 1 and 2 interact with the peptide.

Valence and Conformation.   The four-chain Ig molecule has a hinge and two antigen-binding sites. When expressed at the surface of the B cell or in solution, these properties give the Ig molecule a flexibility that allows it to bind bivalently to antigens of different shapes and sizes. The TCR is a two-chain structure that forms a single binding site for antigen; in other words, the TCR is monovalent and resembles the monovalent Fab fragment of an antibody. The TCR also has a rigid conformation, which is appropriate for binding to the surface of other host cells.

Secretion of Receptor.   Unlike Ig, the TCR does not exist in a specifically secreted form and is not secreted as a consequence of T-cell activation. Thus, unlike Ig, the TCR does not have an "effector" function. Rather, T-cell activation results in cytokine secretion and/or the killing of infected host cells. By contrast, after antigen binds to membrane Ig and activates the B cell, the B cell differentiates into a plasma cell that secretes Ig with the same antigenic

TABLE 10.1. Comparison of the Properties of the TCR and the B Cell Receptor for Antigen, Immunoglobulin

T-Cell Receptor	B-Cell Receptor
Two chains	Four chains
One antigen binding site (monovalent)	Two antigen binding sites (bivalent)
Predominantly *protein* antigens (more specifically, *peptides*) recognized	Can recognize carbohydrate, DNA, lipid, or protein
Peptide recognized must be *bound to an MHC molecule*	Can recognize *free* antigen
Restricted to interacting with other cells	Can deal with any antigen *in body fluids*
Not secreted on activation	Secreted on activation
No change in TCR during response to antigen	Can undergo somatic hypermutation and class switch recombination

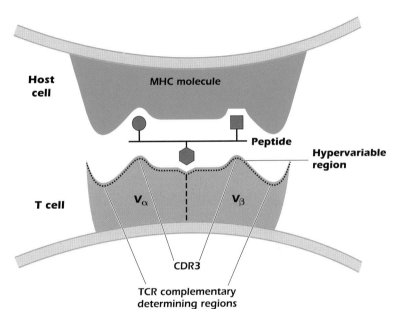

Figure 10.3. Interaction of the complementarity-determining regions (CDRs) of the TCR Vα and Vβ with an MHC molecule (class I or II) and bound peptide expressed on the surface of a host cell. CDR 3 binds to amino acids in the center of the bound peptide.

specificity expressed by the B cell that initially bound the antigen (see Chapters 7 and 8). Thus the effector molecule of the B cell is antigen specific, but the effector molecules secreted by T cells are not.

No Change in TCR During Response to Antigen.

Over the course of a response to antigen, Ig molecules undergo **somatic hypermutation** (with associated affinity maturation) and **class switching**, the linking of one set of genes coding for a particular V region to different C region genes. These mechanisms are unique to B cells: Once a T cell has acquired its TCR in the thymus, it does not undergo any further genetic alteration. Thus, the TCR does not change during the response to antigen.

The T-Cell Receptor Complex

The TCR is expressed on the surface of T cells in tight, noncovalent association with the molecule **CD3** and with

two identical ζ (**zeta**) chains (**CD247**, molecular weight 16 kDa; Figure 10.4).

The combination of TCR and CD3 and ζ is referred to as the **TCR complex**. CD3 consists of three polypeptides γ, δ, and ε (molecular weights 25, 20, and 20 kDa, respectively), which are expressed in the membrane as two sets of molecules: γε and δε. Note that the CD3 γ and δ molecules differ from the γ and δ chains of the TCR expressed by γδ T cells.

CD3 and ζ do not bind antigen. They are **signal transduction molecules** activated after antigen binding to the TCR; thus, they are analogous to the Igα/Igβ molecules associated with Ig in the B-cell antigen-specific receptor complex (Chapter 8).

Each chain of the CD3 complex contains one tyrosine-containing sequence referred to as an **immunoreceptor tyrosine-based activation motif** (ITAM) (also found in Igα and Igβ), and the ζ chain contains three. After antigen binds to the antigen-binding chains of the TCR, the ITAMs of the

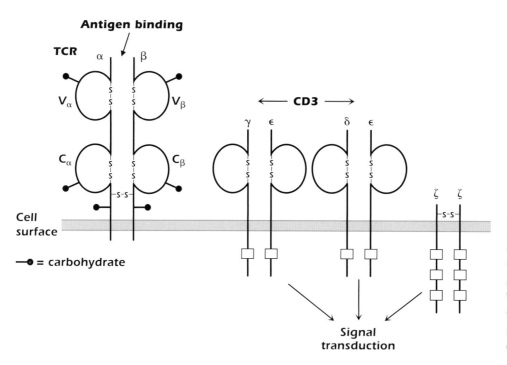

Figure 10.4. The TCR complex; α and β antigen binding chains with associated signal transduction molecules CD3 (γ, δ, and ε chains) plus the ζ homodimer. White boxes = immunoreceptor tyrosine-based activation motifs (ITAMs) in cytoplasmic domains.

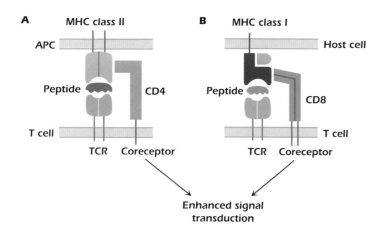

Figure 10.5. TCR co-receptors and their interaction with MHC molecules expressed on host cells: (A) CD4 with MHC class II expressed on APCs; (B) CD8 with MHC class I expressed on all nucleated cells.

CD3 and ζ chains play important roles in the early phases of T-cell activation (see Chapter 11).

CD3 has a second important function: It acts as a "chaperone" to transport a newly synthesized TCR molecule through the cell to the cell surface. Thus, it is always found in association with the TCR at the T-cell surface. Although the CD3ε chain is detectable in the cytoplasm of natural killer (NK) cells, the entire CD3 molecule is expressed exclusively only on the surface of T cells. Thus, surface expression of all CD3 polypeptides can be used as a marker to distinguish T cells from all other cells.

Co-Receptors

The TCR is expressed on the T-cell surface in close association with either **CD4** or **CD8**, which are known as

co-receptors (Figure 10.5). CD4 is a single-chain glycoprotein, and CD8 is a two-chain glycoprotein. CD4 and CD8 do not bind antigen but, as shown in Figures 10.5A and 10.5B, they bind to MHC class II and MHC class I molecules, respectively. Expression of either CD4 or CD8 splits the αβ TCR-expressing T-cell population into two major subsets, known as **CD4⁺ T cells** and **CD8⁺ T cells**; only immature T cells differentiating in the thymus express *both* CD4 and CD8. In addition to their expression on these major subsets of T cells, CD4 and CD8 are also expressed on other cells: CD4, by monocytes, macrophages and dendritic cells, and CD8 by dendritic cells and NK cells.

The function of CD4⁺ T cells is predominantly in producing cytokines and thus interacting with many other cell types. The function of CD8⁺ T cells is predominantly to kill infected cells. In healthy people, the ratio of CD4⁺ T cells to CD8$^+$ T cells in the circulation is approximately 2:1, but this ratio is decreased during viral infections (due to an increased number of CD8$^+$ T cells) and in conditions such as acquired immune deficiency syndrome (AIDS), in which the level of CD4$^+$ T cells is depleted (see Chapter 18).

CD4 and CD8 have several important functions, as follows:

- They act as specific **adhesion molecules** in T-cell interactions with host cells, and thus tighten the binding of T cells to host cells that express peptide in combination with an MHC molecule.

  CD4 binds selectively to all cells expressing MHC class II molecules (Figure 10.5A); CD4 binds outside the peptide-binding groove of the MHC class II molecules, to the invariant portion of the molecule. MHC class II molecules are expressed constitutively on antigen-presenting cells (APCs): dendritic cells, macrophages, B cells, and thymic epithelial cells. Thus, CD4$^+$ T cells interact with APCs expressing antigen bound to MHC class II.

  CD8 binds selectively to cells expressing MHC class I molecules (Figure 10.5B), which are expressed on the surface of all nucleated cells in the body. Thus, CD8$^+$ T cells interact with all host cells expressing antigen associated with MHC class I.

- They are **signal transduction** molecules that enhance the signal through the TCR after antigen binding. In this way, the co-receptor enhances the ability of antigen to activate T cells; that is, expression of the co-receptor *lowers the threshold* for antigen responses; therefore, less antigen is needed to stimulate the T cell than in the absence of the co-receptor. Thus, the T-cell co-receptor is analogous to the B-cell co-receptor, the complex of CD19, CD21, CD81, and CD225 (Chapter 8). The signaling function of CD4 and CD8 is carried out by the intracellular portion of each molecule, which is linked to protein tyrosine kinases that are important early components of the T-cell activation pathways. This concept will be discussed more fully in Chapter 11.

- A unique characteristic of the human CD4 molecule is that **HIV-1 binds to it**. This binding allows the virus to infect cells expressing CD4, eventually leading to AIDS (see Chapter 18). Because CD4 is expressed by monocytes, macrophages and dendritic cells as well as T cells, all these cell types may be infected by HIV-1.

Other Important Molecules Expressed on the T-Cell Surface

In the following paragraphs and in Figure 10.6 we describe molecules in addition to those associated with the TCR complex and T-cell co-receptors that play important roles in T-cell function.

Co-Stimulator Ligands. In order to be activated, *naïve T cells* (T cells that have not previously encountered antigen) need two signals. The *first signal* is the interaction between peptide and MHC expressed on the APCs and the TCR expressed by the T cell. *Second signals*, also known as *co-stimulator interactions*, are needed for full T-cell activation. These co-stimulator interactions enhance the signal delivered by the TCR complex.

Multiple pairs of such co-stimulator molecules have been defined on the T cell and APC surfaces. The best understood interaction is between *CD28* expressed on the T cell and the *B7 family* of molecules expressed on APCs. This interaction is critical for antigen-activated T cells to synthesize the cytokine IL-2, a T-cell growth factor, which is required for the proliferation of T cells (also see Chapter 11). We now know that there are several molecules in the CD28 family on T cells. These interact with either B7 or other molecules on the surface of an APC and have functions other than simply activation. One important member of the CD28 family is *CTLA-4 (CD152)* (Chapters 11 and 13). It is expressed on activated T cells and interacts with B7 molecules to impart a *negative* signal to the activated T cell, which helps to terminate the response.

T cells also express *CD40 ligand* (*CD40L* or *CD154*), which interacts with CD40 expressed on macrophages, dendritic cells, and B cells. This interaction enhances the B7-CD28 co-stimulator interaction. The CD40–CD40L interaction also plays a critical role in T-cell-dependent class switching and somatic hypermutation in B cells.

Molecules Involved in Adhesion and Homing
Adhesion. T cells make several adhesive interactions with molecules expressed on the surface of APCs. None of these molecules is specific to the T cell or APC. These interactions are important when the T cell enters a lymph node; the adhesive interactions slow down the movement of the T cell near the APCs, particularly dendritic cells, allowing the T cell time to "scan" the dendritic cells for the "correct" peptide + MHC combination. Key adhesion molecules expressed on the T cell include the following:

- *CD2*, which binds to *LFA-3* (*CD58*) expressed on APCs and many other cells; CD2 is expressed almost exclusively on T cells and is expressed by all mature and immature T cells, as well as NK cells.
- *LFA-1* (*CD11aCD18*), a member of the two-chain integrin family, which binds to several ligands, including *ICAM-1* (*CD54*), expressed on endothelial cells and APCs such as macrophages and dendritic cells.
- *ICAM-3* (*CD50*), which binds to LFA-1 expressed on APC.

Homing. Like B cells, T cells express surface molecules associated with **homing**, the preferential entry of

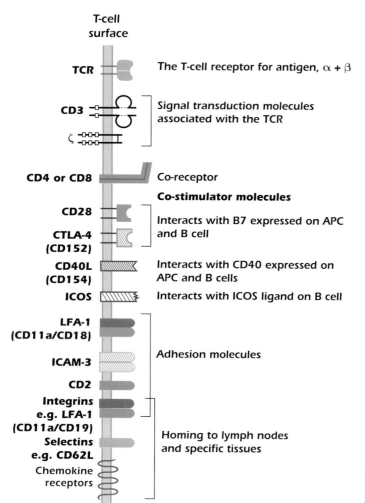

Figure 10.6. Important molecules expressed at the T-cell surface. Hatched bars indicate expression induced on activated T cells.

cells into specific tissues. Homing is tightly regulated by the expression pattern of adhesion molecules and chemokine receptors; their pattern of expression changes with the activation state of the cell. Naïve T cells, like naïve B cells, circulate through peripheral and mucosal lymph nodes. This enhances their ability to interact with antigen because naïve lymphocytes are not normally resident in tissues, where an individual is likely to be exposed to pathogens.

Entry of naïve T lymphocytes to lymph nodes is mediated by the expression of the same set of adhesion molecules and chemokine receptors expressed by naïve B cells. The critical adhesion molecules are **L-selectin** (**CD62L**) for entry to peripheral lymph nodes (those outside the mucosal associated lymphoid tissue) and the integrin **α4β7** for lymphoid tissue in the mucosa. These adhesion molecules bind to glycoproteins known as **addressins**, which are expressed on cells of the high endothelial venules, the specialized region of the vascular endothelium at the boundary of the nodes. Naïve T cells also express the chemokine receptor **CCR7**, which binds chemokines expressed by high endothelial venules of peripheral and mucosal nodes. Binding of the appropriate combination of adhesion

molecule and chemokine receptor to their ligands expressed by high endothelial venules allows naïve T cells to leave the circulation and enter a particular lymph node. The mechanisms by which lymphocytes enter tissues from the bloodstream are similar to those described for other leukocytes in Chapter 12.

Once T cells are activated in the nodes, the resulting **effector cells** and **memory T cells** change their pattern of expressing adhesion molecules and chemokine receptors, migrate out of the nodes, and home to specific tissues. The expression pattern of adhesion molecules and chemokine receptors provides an "address code" that identifies the tissue to which the T cell migrates. Generally, this homing takes the effector or memory T cell back to the region in which the T cell was originally activated; for example, cells that were initially activated in nodes draining the gut will home back to the gut.

γδ T Cells

Most human T cells use αβ chains as their TCR but a minor population expresses a distinct two-chain TCR known as γδ;

the cells expressing this receptor are referred to as $\gamma\delta$ **T cells**. The $\gamma\delta$ TCR is expressed in association with CD3 and ζ. Generally, $\gamma\delta$ T cells lack the CD4 and CD8 co-receptor molecules found on $\alpha\beta$-expressing T cells, but $\gamma\delta$ T cells found in the intestine express CD8.

$\gamma\delta$ T cells are found predominantly at mucosal epithelial sites such as the skin, gut, and lung, and are also found at proportionately much lower numbers than $\alpha\beta$ T cells in the circulation and secondary lymphoid organs of normal adult humans. About 10% of intraepithelial lymphocytes (IEL, see Figure 8.6 in Chapter 8) scattered throughout the mucosal epithelium are $\gamma\delta$ T cells, and in some parts of the lower intestine the proportion of $\gamma\delta$ T cells is even higher. $\gamma\delta$ T cells are present in all mammals at some level; the peripheral blood of ruminant species, which include the cow and deer, can have higher circulating levels of $\gamma\delta$ T cells than $\alpha\beta$ T cells.

Like TCR α and β chains, the γ and δ chains consist of V and C regions—$V\gamma + C\gamma$ and $V\delta + C\delta$, respectively—and the antigen-binding site is formed by the combined $V\gamma + V\delta$ regions. As described below, the $V\gamma$ and $V\delta$ regions are generated by recombination. However, unlike the enormous number of different receptors found in the $\alpha\beta$ TCR T cell population, the total number of different $\gamma\delta$ receptors is much smaller. In part this results from the smaller numbers of $V\gamma$ and $V\delta$ gene segments than $V\alpha$ and $V\beta$ gene segments in the germline (discussed below). In addition, the pairing of γ and δ chains is much more limited than the random pairing of α and β chains; that is, the $\gamma\delta$ T cells found in different mucosal tissues express a limited number of preferred combinations of $V\gamma$ and $V\delta$ chains.

$\gamma\delta$ T cells have some features associated with the adaptive immune response (use of antigen-specific receptors) but have several properties associated with the innate immune response. They respond rapidly (within hours as opposed to days for $\alpha\beta$ T cells) to pathogens such as mycobacteria, cytomegalovirus, and *Plasmodium falciparum*, the disease agent of malaria. The $\gamma\delta$ T-cell response includes synthesis of cytokines— particularly IFN-γ and tumor necrosis factor (TNF)—and cytotoxic function.

$\gamma\delta$ T cells do not generally respond to peptides associated with MHC molecules but do respond to phospholipids and other small nonprotein molecules, known as *phosphoantigens*. They also can respond to heat-shock proteins produced when host cells are shocked or stressed. Unlike $\alpha\beta$ T cells, $\gamma\delta$ T cells do not show memory responses. The antigen-binding site in the $\gamma\delta$ TCR is closer in shape to the antigen-binding site of an antibody molecule than to the corresponding structure in an $\alpha\beta$ TCR; presumably this difference between the two types of TCRs governs the molecules they can bind.

As we describe later in this chapter, the $\alpha\beta$ and $\gamma\delta$ lineages diverge early in intrathymic development, and $\gamma\delta$ T cells arise earlier in ontogeny than $\alpha\beta$ T cells. Thus, it has been suggested that $\gamma\delta$ T cells play a critical role in protecting the neonate from pathogens.

GENES CODING FOR T-CELL RECEPTORS

The organization of the human gene loci coding for the α, β, γ, and δ TCR chains (***TCRA, TCRB, TCRG,*** and ***TCRD,*** respectively) is shown in Figure 10.7.

Note the following features:

- The α and γ chains are constructed from V and J gene segments, like Ig light chains, but β and δ chains are constructed from V, D, and J gene segments, like Ig heavy chains.
- The β and γ TCR loci are found on different chromosomes, but the α and δ TCR loci are located on the same chromosome. In fact, genes coding for the δ chain of the TCR are flanked by genes coding for the α chain. Gene rearrangement mechanisms at the α and δ loci ensure that α and δ are not expressed on the same T cell.
- There are many more $V\alpha$ and $V\beta$ genes (approximately 40–50) than $V\gamma$ and $V\delta$ genes (5–10) in the germline.
- There are two different $C\beta$ genes ($C\beta_1$ and $C\beta_2$), but these genes and their products are virtually identical

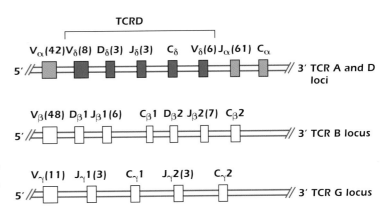

Figure 10.7. Organization of human α, β, γ, and δ genes coding for TCR chains: the TCRA, TCRB, TCRG, and TCRD loci. The number in brackets indicates the number of different gene segments in the germline. TCRB and TCRG loci are expressed on different chromosomes; TCRA and TCRD loci are expressed on a different chromosome; genes coding for the TCR δ chain are flanked by genes coding for the TCR α chain. Gene rearrangement mechanisms ensure that TCR α and δ are not expressed on the same T cell.

and have no known functional differences. Thus, they should not be confused with antibody isotypes, in which the Ig heavy-chain constant genes and products differ considerably and have different effector functions: the TCR C regions do not have effector function.

GENERATION OF T-CELL RECEPTOR DIVERSITY

The mechanisms for generating diversity in TCRs are very similar to the mechanisms of generating diversity in BCRs. The same fundamental principles of gene rearrangement described in Chapter 7 for Ig apply in the synthesis of the V and C regions of each chain of TCRs α, β, γ and δ. *Recombinases* and *recombination recognition sequences* are used to link up a VJ or a VDJ unit, generating the variable-region specificity of a particular TCR polypeptide chain. The same enzymes are involved in the recombination events in both B and T cells. As described in Chapters 7 and 8, the *recombination activation genes* (RAGs), *RAG-1* and *RAG-2*, play a crucial role in both early B cells and early T cells. In addition, like B cells (Chapter 7), T cells early in development express the enzyme terminal deoxynucleotidyltransferase (TdT), which inserts nucleotides at DNA strand breaks and so contributes to junctional and insertional diversity in TCR V regions.

In summary, TCR diversity is generated by (1) multiple V (D) and J genes in the germline, (2) random combination of chains, and (3) junctional and insertional variability. Junctional and insertional variability, which are important contributors to TCR diversity, result in an enormous number of different sequences for the CDR3 region of the TCR antigen binding site. However, as we pointed out earlier in the chapter, one important difference between the generation of diversity in TCRs and Ig molecules is that following antigenic stimulation, Ig genes undergo somatic hypermutation; TCR genes do not.

T-CELL DIFFERENTIATION IN THE THYMUS

The Thymus as Primary Organ for T-Cell Differentiation

T cells, like B cells, are derived from hematopoietic stem cells, which during early fetal development in mammals are found in the liver. Later in fetal development and after birth, precursors of the T-cell lineage are found in the bone marrow. Some of these precursor stem cells—***common lymphoid progenitor*** (CLP) cells—move through the blood to the thymus.

The thymus, located above the heart, is the primary lymphoid organ for the development of T cells (see also Chapter 3). In this organ, developing T cells acquire their TCR and other characteristics of T cells, and generate the

huge diversity of TCR structures that form the T-cell repertoire. Indeed, the thymus is a site of intense proliferation of developing T cells; however, as we describe later in the chapter, the vast majority of these cells—calculated to be around 95% of the cells produced daily—dies in the thymus.

The importance of the thymus is shown in ***DiGeorge syndrome***, in which children are born with a defect in the development of the thymic structure (as well as with cardiac anomalies and absence of the parathyroid (see also Chapter 18). In addition, the ***nude mouse*** is a strain that arose as a mutant that lacks hair but also has a defect in the development of thymic cells (specifically, thymic epithelial cells, whose function is described below). Mature T cells do not develop and T-cell responses are defective in both individuals with DiGeorge syndrome and in the nude mouse.

 Read the related case: **DiGeorge Syndrome**
In *Immunology: Clinical Case Studies and Disease Pathophysiology*

One major difference between T-cell and B-cell differentiation is that T-cell differentiation significantly diminishes after puberty. At this stage and subsequently, the size of the thymus decreases (***thymic involution***), presumably because of the increased synthesis of steroid hormones. Although some differentiation in the thymus occurs in adults, the majority of the T-cell repertoire is composed of a long-lived pool of T cells that was established before thymic involution. In some species, particularly the mouse, the mature T-cell population is drastically depleted if the thymus is removed within a few days after birth. Indeed, these were the pioneering observations that established the crucial role of the thymus in T-cell responses. Removing the thymus later in the development of the animal has much less impact on the mature T-cell population, because the repertoire of long-lived cells has already been established.

Thymic Nonlymphoid Cells in T-Cell Development. Figure 10.8 shows the detailed structure of the thymus and the cells within it.

Developing T lymphocytes in the thymus (***thymocytes***) are in contact with, and interact with, a mesh formed by the thymic nonlymphoid cells, the most important of which are (1) epithelial cells in the ***cortex*** and ***medulla*** (the outer and inner regions of the thymus, respectively) and (2) dendritic cells, found predominantly at the junction of the cortex and medulla. Thymic dendritic cells are derived from bone marrow stem cells and are members of the same family of cells that present antigens to T cells in other tissues and organs (see Chapters 9 and 11). Thymic epithelial cells and thymic dendritic cells express MHC class I *and* II molecules, a characteristic of APCs.

The nonlymphoid cells produce the cytokine ***IL-7***, which induces proliferation and survival of cells in the early

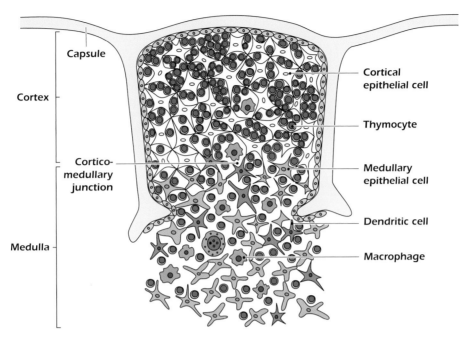

Figure 10.8. Cellular organization of the thymus. Reproduced with permission from Rosen FS, Geha RS (1996) *Case Studies in Immunology*, New York: Garland Publishing.

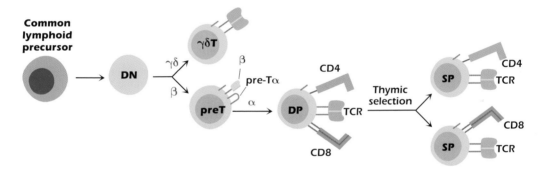

Figure 10.9. Key stages in development of $\alpha\beta$ and $\gamma\delta$ T cells in the thymus. The stage at which individual TCR genes start to rearrange is shown in red. The single line at the surface represents CD3 + ζ. DN = double-negative cell; DP = double-positive cell (CD4⁺CD8⁺); SP = single-positive cell (either CD4⁺ or CD8⁺).

stages of T-lymphocyte development (similar to the role IL-7 plays in B-cell development in the bone marrow, described in Chapter 8). The nonlymphoid cells also provide critical cell surface interactions required for thymic selection, which we describe below.

Key Steps in Thymic Differentiation

T-cell differentiation in the thymus is a complex multistep process. As with the early phases of B-cell differentiation, most of the information about the early phases of T-cell differentiation derives from work in nonhuman species such as the mouse. The key features of T-cell differentiation in the thymus are summarized in Figure 10.9 and described further in the sections that follow. We focus on critical

checkpoints in T-cell development, highlighting the sequence of TCR gene rearrangements, the expression of the co-receptor molecules CD4 and CD8, and thymic selection.

Early T-Cell Receptor Gene Rearrangements: Double-Negative Cells and Splitting Off of $\gamma\delta$ T Cells

Bone marrow-derived common lymphoid precursor cells enter the thymus at the junction of the cortex and medulla with their TCR genes in an unrearranged (germline) configuration. These cells move into the cortex, where they start to proliferate and differentiate. These precursors are not fully committed to the T-cell lineage; other cell types may also develop from these very early thymic precursor cells. At this stage the cells do not express either the CD4 or CD8 co-receptor and so are referred to as *double-negative* (*DN*) *cells* (See Figure 10.9.).

RAG1 and RAG2, the lymphocyte-specific components of the recombinase complex, are then transiently expressed, and rearrangement of TCR genes begins: TCR γ, δ, and β-chain genes start to rearrange more or less simultaneously. Terminal deoxynucleotidyltransferase (TdT), the enzyme that adds nucleotides to the ends of V, D, and J gene segments and so contributes to junctional diversity (see Chapter 7), is also expressed. The decision whether to become an αβ or a γδ T cell occurs at the DN stage, but the signals that determine the pathway chosen are not well understood.

DN cells that productively rearrange both a γ and a δ gene shut down β-gene rearrangement and express TCR γ and δ chains on the cell surface in association with the signal transduction molecules CD3 and ζ. These γδ TCR-expressing cells exit the thymus and form the pool of peripheral γδ T cells, which are found predominantly at epithelial sites round the body. Most γδ T cells arise early in development of the individual but are later swamped by the development of αβ T cells.

Pre-T Cells

Double-negative cells that productively rearrange a β gene from one of their chromosomes express the TCR β chain on the surface of the cell in tight association with CD3 and ζ and *pre-Tα* (see Figure 10.9). These cells are referred to as *pre-T cells*. Pre-Tα is invariant and not formed by rearrangement, so is analogous to the surrogate light chains expressed by pre-B cells at a similar stage of B cell development (see Chapter 8). The complex of β chain, pre-Tα, CD3, and ζ constitutes the *pre-T cell receptor* (pre-TCR), analogous to the pre-B-cell receptor expressed by pre-B cells. Cells that do not productively rearrange a β gene and so do not express the pre-TCR die via apoptosis.

Expression of the pre-TCR, like the expression of the pre-BCR in the B-cell lineage, is a critical checkpoint in the development of cells expressing α and β as their TCR. Signaling through the pre-TCR stops further rearrangement of TCRβ genes, ensuring that the cell expresses only one type of β chain (allelic exclusion), and stops further rearrangement of TCRγ genes.

Double-Positive Cells

After the pre-TCR is expressed, expression of pre-Tα is downregulated, *RAG1* and *RAG2* genes are reactivated, and α genes start to rearrange. As we noted previously, the δ TCR locus is flanked on both sides by gene segments of the α locus, so rearrangement of the α locus on a particular chromosome deletes the δ locus. Thus, a T cell that expresses αβ as its TCR cannot express γδ as its TCR. The TCR α

locus does not show allelic exclusion, so rearrangement of α genes may occur on both chromosomes. Rearrangement at the α locus occurs until after positive selection (see below).

Signaling through the pre-TCR also initiates cell proliferation and upregulation of both co-receptor molecules, CD4 and CD8. Thus, the next cell in the T-cell differentiation sequence expresses an αβ TCR (together with CD3 and ζ) and both CD4 and CD8 co-receptor molecules on its surface. This *αβ⁺CD3⁺CD4⁺CD8⁺* thymocyte (see Figure 10.9), referred to as a CD4⁺CD8⁺ or *double-positive* (*DP*) *cell*, comprises the largest population of thymocytes (over 80%) in the young mammalian thymus, and predominates in the thymic cortex.

Thymic Selection

Developing thymocytes undergo the critical two-step process known as *thymic selection*. As its name implies, thymic selection ensures that thymocytes with only specific characteristics are *selected* to develop further. The cells that survive thymic selection—a very small percentage of the initial double-positive population—ultimately leave the thymus to form the populations of mature CD4⁺ and CD8⁺ T cells.

During thymic selection the TCR complex plus CD4 and CD8 expressed by the thymocyte make critical interactions with MHC molecules plus peptides expressed by thymic nonlymphoid cells. These interactions are crucial checkpoints that determine the fate of the developing cell.

The two major stages of thymic selection are known as *positive selection* and *negative selection*. Most studies suggest that positive and negative selection take place on different thymic nonlymphoid cells and in different parts of the thymus, with positive selection preceding negative selection. We describe these selection processes in the paragraphs that follow and in Figures 10.10 and 10.11.

Positive Selection.   In the first stage, *positive selection*, double-positive cells interact with epithelial cells in the thymic cortex that express MHC class I and II molecules. These MHC molecules contain peptides derived from self-molecules present in the thymus, which are bound in their peptide-binding groove (Figure 10.10).

This interaction results in the survival of the double-positive cell. In addition, as a consequence of this interaction, the double-positive cell commits to developing into either a CD4⁺ or a CD8⁺ T cell. Details of this **lineage choice** are not fully worked out.

Thus, to survive and be positively selected, the double-positive T cell must have some affinity for *self-MHC*, the MHC molecules expressed by the individual's thymic epithelial cells. (For this person, all other types of MHC molecules are *nonself*.) The developing αβ T cell that passes through this developmental checkpoint becomes *educated* to the self-MHC molecules—either MHC class I or class

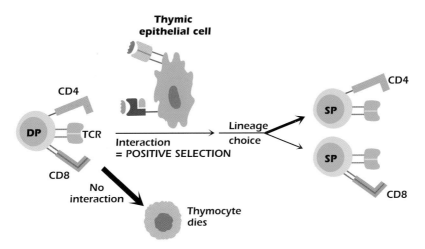

Figure 10.10. Positive selection and lineage choice. The double-positive (DP) thymocyte that interacts with MHC molecules (+ self-peptides) expressed by thymic epithelial cells is positively selected. If the DP cell does not interact with the MHC molecules expressed by the thymic epithelial cell, it dies (the fate of most DP cells). Positively selected cells then undergo lineage choice, committing to developing into either the CD4$^+$ or CD8$^+$ lineages. The single-positive (SP) CD4$^+$ T and CD8$^+$ cells that result are "educated" to the self-MHC molecules— MHC class II and class I, respectively—expressed by the thymic cortical epithelial cells.

II—expressed by the thymic cortical epithelial cells. This means that for the rest of the life of a particular αβ T cell, even as a mature cell when it leaves the thymus, it will respond to antigen *only* when the antigen is bound to the MHC molecule the developing T cell encountered in the thymus. Thus, a mature CD4$^+$ T cell will respond to peptide plus self-MHC class II, and a mature CD8$^+$ T cell to peptide plus self-MHC class I. This is the origin of the phenomenon of MHC restriction of T-cell responses we referred to in Chapter 9; more specifically, this key concept is *self-MHC restriction of T-cell responses*.

Positive selection also results in the downregulation of *RAG-1* and *RAG-2* gene expression, so no further gene rearrangement occurs. This stops further attempts at rearrangement by the TCR α genes. Consequently, even if a cell expresses two different α chains in combination with a β chain (as appears to be the case in some human and mouse T cells), positive selection of a developing T cell on one MHC–peptide complex ensures that only one of the expressed TCR αβ-chain combinations is functional.

Note that because of the essentially random nature of the gene recombination processes that generate TCRs, more than 90% of double-positive cells generated in the thymus express a TCR with no or very low affinity for self-MHC. Thus, most of the combinations of α and β chains expressed on double-positive cells do not have a high enough affinity to interact with the MHC and peptide combinations expressed by thymic cortical epithelial cells. Because the majority of DP cells generated in the thymus

do not make this interaction with cortical epithelial cells, they are not positively selected, and they die by apoptosis (Figure 10.10).

Negative Selection. Although a developing thymocyte needs to have some affinity for self-MHC to be positively selected, allowing a thymocyte with too high a reactivity to self-MHC to leave the thymus could result in undesirable autoimmune responses in tissues. This is prevented by *negative selection* (Figure 10.11): thymocytes with too high a reactivity to self-MHC are removed.

Negative selection is thought to occur when the thymocytes that have survived positive selection interact either with dendritic cells at the interface of the cortex and medulla or with epithelial cells in the medulla. These nonlymphoid cells express both MHC class I and II molecules (and associated peptides). A thymocyte that reacts with too high an affinity to the combination of MHC and peptide is deleted by apoptosis. Thus, negative selection removes T cells expressing TCRs with too high a reactivity to self-components; in other words, negative selection prevents T-cell reactivity to self-components. This is a critical feature of the development of ***central tolerance*** in T cells, analogous to the development of central tolerance in B cells (see Chapters 8 and 13).

To summarize the selection process, we can say that thymocytes with affinity that is either *too low* or *too high* for self-MHC do not survive thymic selection. Only thymocytes with some *intermediate* affinity for self-MHC survive thymic selection.

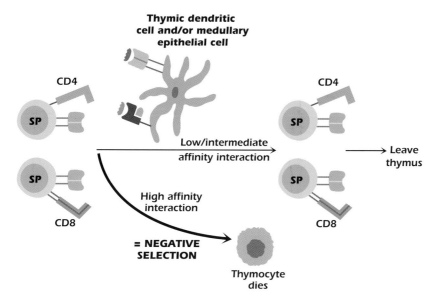

Figure 10.11. Negative selection. Thymocytes that have survived positive selection interact with self-MHC molecules (+ self-peptides) expressed by dendritic cells and/or thymic medullary epithelial cells. If the thymocyte interacts with too high an affinity for self-MHC, it is negatively selected and deleted. Cells that interact with low to intermediate affinity for self-MHC survive, leave the thymus and ultimately comprise the pool of SP CD4$^+$ or CD8$^+$ T cells outside the thymus (peripheral T cells).

Several questions remain about the mechanisms involved in thymic selection. The central issue is to understand how the signals delivered by the same pairs of molecules (MHC plus peptides and TCR plus co-receptors) differ in positive versus negative selection. The nature of the intracellular signals involved and the identification of thymic nonlymphoid cells involved in different stages of selection are areas of intense research activity. Another key question is whether the peptides expressed by thymic nonlymphoid cells differ in positive versus negative selection. Some evidence supports this possibility, but further studies will be needed to resolve the issue.

Role of AIRE Gene Product in Negative Selection. We described above that negative selection involves the presentation of peptides derived from self-molecules in the thymus. As a consequence, developing T cells potentially responsive to molecules found in the thymus are deleted. How, though, do we develop self-tolerance to molecules normally found outside the thymus? We now know that at least some tissue-specific self-molecules normally synthesized outside the thymus—including insulin, thyroglobulin, and myelin basic protein—are expressed in the thymus, and particularly by epithelial cells in the thymic medulla. Thus, T cells that develop with receptors specific for these self-antigens can be deleted in the thymus.

We also know that expression of these self-antigens by thymic medullary epithelial cells is controlled at least in part by the transcription factor *autoimmune regulator* (AIRE)—the rare individuals who lack an AIRE gene product are defective in negative selection. They develop a condition called autoimmune polyendocrinopathy-candidiasis-ectodermal dystrophy syndrome (APECED), in which multiple endocrine organs, particularly the adrenals, parathyroids and thyroid, are damaged.

Leaving the Thymus

Single-positive CD4$^+$ and CD8$^+$ T cells that have passed through positive and negative selection are the end points of the complex pathway of αβ TCR differentiation in the thymus; from studies in mice it has been determined that this process takes approximately 3 weeks. Single-positive T cells remain in the thymus for 2–3 days and then leave via the bloodstream. These naïve T cells express a pattern of adhesion molecules and chemokine receptors that allows them to circulate through all secondary lymphoid organs, where a cell with the appropriate receptor may encounter and respond to antigen. Naïve T cells may live for a long time (up to years) in a resting state without encountering antigen; recent studies suggest that mature T cells in the periphery that have not encountered antigen need signals (including the cytokine IL-7) to keep them alive.

Generation of the T-Cell Repertoire

Thymic differentiation of T cells expressing αβ as their TCR generates a huge repertoire of mature CD4$^+$ T cells and CD8$^+$ T cells in the periphery. The individual uses these to respond to the universe of nonself antigens. T-cell clones with the appropriate receptor for self-MHC plus peptide exist in the repertoire prior to exposure to antigen. As with B cells, the appropriate T-cell clone may never be triggered because the person may never be exposed to that particular virus or bacterium. Nonetheless, it can almost be guaranteed that the T cell (or B cell) with the "right" receptor is present and this receptor will be triggered by foreign antigen.

Characteristics of αβ T Cells Emerging from the Thymus

The thymus is a site of intense proliferation but also of the death of the overwhelming majority of developing thymocytes. The single-positive CD4$^+$ and CD8$^+$ T cells that emerge from the thymus are the survivors of many critical steps in the differentiation pathways. The surviving single-positive T cells have the following two important characteristics:

1. *T cells are self-MHC restricted.* Positive selection *educates* T cells to respond to antigen *only* when associated with the MHC molecule(s) that the developing T cell interacted with in the thymus. The MHC molecules that the developing T cell encounters define "self-MHC" for the rest of the life of the surviving T cell. Thus, a mature CD4$^+$ T cell responds to peptide plus self-MHC class II, and a mature CD8$^+$ T cell to peptide plus self-MHC class I. In the previous chapter, we referred to the MHC restriction of T-cell responses. More specifically, we say that T-cell responses are *self*-MHC restricted.

2. *T cells are self-tolerant.* Negative selection prevents the emergence from the thymus of T cells with too high a reactivity to self-molecules. Thus, mature CD4$^+$ and CD8$^+$ T cells do not respond to self-components.

Note that a developing T cell that survives thymic selection has been selected as a result of an interaction with self-MHC + *self*-peptide, that is, a peptide derived from a self-molecule expressed in the thymus. Nonetheless, the same T cell responds as a mature T cell to self-MHC + *nonself*-peptide, that is, derived from a "foreign" antigen. How does the same TCR respond to both self-peptides and nonself-peptides? The most likely explanation is that a single MHC molecule may bind different peptides; studies suggest that an MHC molecule's peptide-binding properties are flexible enough to allow peptides derived from self- or non-self-proteins to bind.

Further Differentiation of CD4$^+$ and CD8$^+$ T Cells Outside the Thymus

As will be described more fully in Chapter 11 and later chapters of the text, once a CD4$^+$ T cell or a CD8$^+$ T cell has been triggered by antigen, it differentiates into an **effector** T cell, that is, a cell able to perform a function without further activation. CD4$^+$ effector cells predominantly synthesize cytokines that affect the activity of a vast array of cell types. CD8$^+$ effector cells predominantly kill host cells infected with viruses. A small fraction of antigen-activated T cells become **memory** cells, long-lived cells that play a key role in the second or subsequent responses to antigen and help provide protection in second and subsequent exposures to many pathogens. It is not currently clear whether memory cells differentiate from effector cells or whether memory and effector cells diverge early after activation. Effector and memory T cells use the same types of "address codes" of adhesion molecules and chemokine receptors that are used by activated B cells (see Chapter 8) to home to tissues to combat infection, particularly to sites such as the skin and mucosa.

Differentiation of Other Cell Types in the Thymus

This chapter has focused on the development of the two major subsets of T cells, CD4$^+$ and CD8$^+$ T cells, which use α and β chains as their TCR. We also described the properties and differentiation in the thymus of T cells that use $\gamma\delta$ as their TCR. Described below are other sets of cells that develop in the thymus and are found outside the thymus.

Natural Killer T (NKT) Cells. NKT cells are a small subset of T cells (about 1% of peripheral blood mononuclear cells in humans) that express both a TCR and the surface molecule, NK1.1 (CD161c in humans) characteristic of NK cells. NKT cells respond to glycolipid antigens presented by CD1d, rather than MHC molecules. NKT cells regulate the function of other sets of T cells and are thought to have key roles in regulating conditions including autoimmunity, cancer, and infection. NKT cells arise in the thymus when the recombination events in the developing T cell generate a T cell with a TCR that interacts, by chance, with CD1d expressed by thymic nonlymphoid cells. Because most NKT cells use only one type of TCR Vα gene and a limited number of Vβ genes, their TCR usage is referred to as *semi-invariant*. Consequently, they are thought not to respond to a wide variety of antigens. Because of these characteristics, NKT cells are considered to have features of both the innate and adaptive immune defenses.

Treg Cells. Treg cells are a subset of CD4$^+$ T cells (approximately 10% of peripheral CD4$^+$ T cells) that inhibit the actions of other sets of T cells. They characteristically express the molecule CD25 and the transcription factor Foxp3 (discussed further in Chapters 11 and 13). Treg cells that develop in the thymus (natural Treg, or nTreg) are autoreactive; that is, they are T cells that recognize combinations of self-peptide and self-MHC but have survived negative selection in the thymus. Some Treg cells also develop outside the thymus (induced Treg, or iTreg). Treg cells play a role in inhibiting responses to both self *and* foreign antigens; in this way, they help to maintain and regulate self-tolerance and limit potentially damaging host responses to foreign antigens in tissues (see Chapter 13).

NK Cells. Recent studies indicate that most natural killer (NK) cells develop in the bone marrow, but some develop in the thymus from the lymphoid precursors that give rise to the T-cell lineage. In the thymus, the NK cell development pathway splits off from the T-cell lineage at an early stage of DN cells before TCR genes start to rearrange. Thus, NK cells do not express a TCR.

NK cells, which are involved in the early phase of the immune response and are considered part of the innate immune defenses, kill virus-infected and tumor cells (see Chapter 2). NK cells express the molecules CD16 and CD56, which are used to distinguish them from other cell types.

SUMMARY

1. T cells express a unique, clonally distributed receptor for antigen, known as the T-cell receptor (TCR). The same V(D)J recombination strategies and recombinase machinery used by B cells to generate Ig diversity are also used to generate a huge repertoire of T cells with different TCRs.

2. On the majority of human and mouse T cells, the TCR is a two-chain transmembrane molecule, $\alpha\beta$. The TCR comprises V and C regions, analogous to those of Ig molecules. The extracellular portion of the TCR resembles the Fab fragment of an antibody.

3. An $\alpha\beta$ TCR interacts with peptide bound to an MHC molecule on the surface of a host cell. The antigen-binding $\alpha\beta$ chains are expressed on the surface of the T cell in a multimolecular complex (the TCR complex) in association with CD3 and ζ polypeptides, which act as a signal transduction unit after antigen binding to $\alpha\beta$.

4. Co-receptor molecules are associated with the $\alpha\beta$ TCR. On mature T cells the co-receptor is either CD4 or CD8, dividing T cells into two major subsets, either $\alpha\beta^+CD4^+$ or $\alpha\beta^+CD8^+$. The functions of these co-receptor molecules are (a) to bind to the invariant portion of an MHC molecule on a host cell (CD4 with MHC class II and CD8 with MHC class I); (b) to tighten the adherence between the T cell and presenting cell; and (c) enhance signal transduction after activation through the TCR. The human CD4 molecule also binds to HIV.

5. The T cell also expresses on its surface molecules involved in (a) co-stimulation and signal transduction —CD28, CTLA-4 (CD152), and CD40 ligand; (b) adhesion to APCs—CD2, LFA-1 and ICAM-3; and (c) homing to specific tissues—a combination of integrins and selectins (adhesion molecules) and chemokine receptor.

6. $\gamma\delta$ is the TCR expressed on a minor population of human T cells, found predominantly at mucosal epithelial sites such as the intestine and skin. The γ and δTCR chains are also generated by V(D)J recombination and are expressed on the surface of the cell in association with CD3 and ζ. $\gamma\delta^+$ T cells play a role in the first line of defense against pathogens; thus, these cells have characteristics of both the innate and the adaptive immune response.

7. The thymus is the organ in which developing T cells acquire a TCR, either $\alpha\beta$ or $\gamma\delta$. The thymus is a site of intense proliferation and differentiation of developing T cells, but most die there. The few T cells that survive give rise to the population of mature T cells found in the circulation and tissues outside the thymus.

8. TCR gene rearrangement starts in early double-negative thymocytes in the thymus. The differentiation pathways of $\alpha\beta$ and $\gamma\delta$ T cells diverge during this double-negative stage. If $\gamma\delta$ TCR genes rearrange successfully, $\gamma\delta$T cells develop and exit the thymus.

9. Thymocytes that successfully rearrange TCR β genes express the β chain on their surface in association with a non-rearranged molecule, pre-Tα, in the pre-T cell. In the next stage of thymic development, TCR α genes rearrange, pre-Tα is downregulated, CD4 and CD8 co-receptor expression is upregulated, and a "double-positive" cell is formed. It expresses an $\alpha\beta$TCR (in association with CD3 and ζ) and both CD4 and CD8.

10. Double-positive cells undergo thymic selection, mediated by interactions of the TCR and co-receptor molecules on the double-positive cell with MHC molecules and peptides expressed by thymic nonlymphoid cells.

    Positive selection: The developing T cell interacts with MHC molecules (and peptides) expressed by thymic cortical epithelial cells. Lineage commitment to becoming either a CD4$^+$ T or CD8$^+$ T cell follows. In this way, the developing T cell is "educated," so that as a mature cell it responds to antigen *only* when presented by a cell that expresses the same MHC molecule that the T cell interacted with during differentiation in the thymus (self-MHC restriction of the T-cell response). Thus, a mature CD4$^+$ T cell responds to peptide plus self-MHC class II, and a mature CD8$^+$ T cell responds to peptide plus self-MHC class I.

    Negative selection: The developing T cell interacts with MHC molecules (and peptides) expressed by thymic dendritic cells and medullary epithelial cells. This removes T cells with too high an affinity for self, preventing potential reactivity to self-molecules, and ensuring self-tolerance. Thus, $\alpha\beta$TCR$^+$ T cells that emerge from the thymus are self-MHC-restricted and self-tolerant.

11. Single positive $\alpha\beta$TCR$^+$ CD4$^+$ or $\alpha\beta$TCR$^+$ CD8$^+$ T cells that survive positive and negative selection leave the thymus and form the repertoire of peripheral $\alpha\beta$T cells that respond to nonself antigen in blood, secondary lymphoid organs, and the tissues. After antigen activation, the $\alpha\beta$T cell differentiates into an effector cell; some activated T cells become memory CD4$^+$ or CD8$^+$ cells.

12. In addition to $\alpha\beta$ and $\gamma\delta$ T cells, NKT cells, Treg, and some NK cells also develop in the thymus.

REFERENCES AND BIBLIOGRAPHY

Anderson G, Lane PJ, Jenkinson EJ. (2007) Generating intrathymic microenvironments to establish T-cell tolerance. *Nature Rev Immunol* 7: 954.

Garcia KC, Degano M, Pease LR, Huang M, Peterson PA, Teyton L, Wilson IA. (1998) Structural basis of plasticity in T cell receptor recognition of a self peptide-MHC antigen. *Science* 279: 1166–1172.

Gallegos AM, Bevan MJ. (2006) Central tolerance: Good but imperfect. *Immunol Rev* 209: 290.

Kronenberg M, Engel I. (2007) On the road: Progress in finding the unique pathway of invariant NKT cell differentiation. *Curr Opin Immunol* 19: 186.

Laky K, Fowlkes BJ. (2005) Receptor signals and nuclear events in CD4 and CD8 T cell lineage commitment. *Curr Opin Immunol* 17: 116.

Lauritsen JP, Haks MC, Lefebvre JM, Kappes DJ, Wiest DL. (2006) Recent insights into the signals that control $\alpha\beta/\gamma\delta$-lineage fate. *Immunol Rev* 209: 176.

Mathis D, Benoist C. (2007) A decade of AIRE. *Nature Rev Immunol* 7: 645.

Rodrigo Mora J, von Andrian UH. (2006) Specificity and plasticity of memory lymphocyte migration. *Curr Top Microbiol Immunol* 308: 83.

Rudolph MG, Stanfield RL, Wilson IA. (2006) How TCRs bind MHCs, peptides, and coreceptors. *Annu Rev Immunol* 24: 419.

Van Laethem F, Tikhonova AN, Singer A. (2012) MHC restriction is imposed on a diverse T cell receptor repertoire by CD4 and CD8 co-receptors during thymic selection. *Trends Immunol* 33: 437.

Yin L, Scott-Browne J, Kappler JW, Gapin L, Marrack P. (2012) T cells and their eons-old obsession with MHC. *Immunol Rev* 250: 49.

REVIEW QUESTIONS

For each question, choose the ONE BEST answer or completion.

1. Which of the following statements concerning T-cell development is correct?
   A) Progenitor T cells that enter the thymus from the bone marrow have already rearranged their TCR genes.
   B) Interaction with thymic nonlymphoid cells is critical.
   C) Maturation in the thymus requires the presence of foreign antigen.
   D) MHC class II molecules are not involved in positive selection.
   E) Mature, fully differentiated T cells are found in the cortex of the thymus.

2. The development of self-tolerance in the T-cell compartment is important for the prevention of autoimmunity. Which of the following results in T-cell self-tolerance?
   A) allelic exclusion
   B) somatic hypermutation
   C) thymocyte proliferation
   D) positive selection
   E) negative selection

3. Which of the following statements is correct?
   A) The TCR chains transduce a signal into a T cell.
   B) A cell depleted of its CD4 molecule would be unable to recognize antigen.
   C) T cells with fully rearranged TCR chains are not found in the thymus.
   D) T cells expressing the TCR are found only in the thymus.
   E) CD4$^+$ CD8$^+$ T cells form the majority of T cells in the thymus.

4. Which of the following is *incorrect* regarding mature T cells that use $\alpha\beta$ as their antigen-specific receptor?
   A) They all express CD8 on the cell surface.
   B) They may be either CD4$^+$ or CD8$^+$.
   C) They interact with peptides derived from nonself antigens.
   D) They can further rearrange their TCR genes to express $\gamma\delta$ as their receptor.
   E) They circulate through blood and lymph and migrate to secondary lymphoid organs.

5. Which of the following statements is *incorrect* concerning TCR and Ig genes?
   A) In both B- and T-cell precursors, multiple V-, D-, J-, and C-region genes exist in an unrearranged configuration.
   B) Rearrangement of both TCR and Ig genes involves recombinase enzymes that bind to specific regions of the genome.
   C) Both Ig and TCR are able to switch C-region usage.
   D) Both Ig and the TCR use combinatorial association of V, D, and J genes and junctional imprecision to generate diversity.

6. Which of the following statements is *incorrect* concerning antigen-specific receptors on both B and T cells?

A) They are clonally distributed transmembrane molecules.

B) They have extensive cytoplasmic domains that interact with intracellular molecules.

C) They consist of polypeptides with variable and constant regions.

D) They are associated with signal transduction molecules at the cell surface.

E) They can interact with peptides derived from nonself antigens.

7. Which of the following is correct concerning the characteristics of T cells that exit the thymus?

A) They do not express CD4 or CD8 but express a TCR that has high affinity for MHC plus self-antigen.

B) They express CD4 and CD8 but no TCR and have low affinity for MHC plus self-antigen.

C) They express either CD4 or CD8 with a TCR that has high affinity for MHC plus self-antigen.

D) They express either CD4 or CD8 with a TCR that has low to moderate affinity for MHC plus self-antigen.

E) They express CD4, CD8, and a TCR that has high affinity for MHC plus self-antigen.

ANSWERS TO REVIEW QUESTIONS

1. *B.* Interaction of thymocytes with thymic nonlymphoid cells—cortical epithelial cells, dendritic cells and medullary epithelial cells—is critical in T-cell development.

2. *E.* Negative selection removes developing T cells with potential reactivity to self-molecules.

3. *E.* CD4$^+$ CD8$^+$ T cells form the majority of cells in the thymus.

4. *D.* The genes of T cells that use $\alpha\beta$ as their receptor cannot further rearrange to use $\gamma\delta$ as their receptor; TCR δ gene segments are interspersed with the α locus and are deleted when the α locus rearranges.

5. *C.* The ability to change the heavy-chain constant region while retaining the same antigen specificity is a property unique to Ig. The other features are common to both the TCR and Ig.

6. *B.* Both the TCR and Ig have short cytoplasmic tails. The signal transduction molecules associated with the antigen-binding chains interact with intracellular molecules.

7. *D.* T cells that use $\alpha\beta$ as their TCR and emerge as the end stage of differentiation in the thymus express either CD4 or CD8 (as well as a TCR) and, as a result of thymic selection, have a low to intermediate affinity for self-antigen associated with self-MHC (the MHC molecules expressed by the individual's thymic nonlymphoid cells).

11

ACTIVATION AND FUNCTION OF T CELLS

INTRODUCTION

In previous chapters we touched on the signals that are needed to activate the two major subsets of T cells CD4$^+$ and CD8$^+$ T cells. In this chapter we describe in more detail the cells and signals involved in T-cell activation, and how once T cells are activated they exert their *effector* functions. For CD4$^+$ T cells, we will focus on the cytokines produced by different subsets and their role as helper T cells in antibody synthesis by B cells. For CD8$^+$ T cells we will describe their role as **cytotoxic** or **killer T cells**. We will also describe how *memory cells* are formed and the termination of the T cell response. We end with descriptions of the roles of other subsets of T cells in the immune response.

A TWO-SIGNAL MODEL FOR THE ACTIVATION OF T CELLS

Figure 11.1 shows that two sets of signals are needed to activate naïve CD4$^+$ and CD8$^+$ T cells, that is, T cells that have not previously encountered antigen. The *first signal* is antigen-specific: peptide bound to major histocompatibility complex (MHC) on the surface of a host cell interacting with the T-cell receptor (TCR). The interaction of the T-cell co-receptor (CD4 or CD8) with the MHC molecule is considered part of this first signal. The *second signal* is not antigen-specific and is provided by **co-stimulator pair**s, molecules expressed on the surface of specialized antigen-presenting cells (APCs) interacting with molecules expressed

on the T-cell surface. Both the first and second signals send messages into the T-cell nucleus (i.e., trigger signal transduction) that change the pattern of the genes expressed by that T cell. Both signals are needed to activate naïve T cells; ultimately, they lead to survival, proliferation, and differentiation of the T cell. Note that the first signal by itself is necessary but not sufficient. Indeed, in the absence of a second signal, the first signal alone turns the T cell *off* rather than *on* (see Chapter 13).

However, we also now recognize that the activation and signaling processes within T cells are complex, and that the family of co-stimulator molecules is extensive. We now understand that some members of the co-stimulator family play important negative and regulatory roles in T cell activation. We discuss these molecules later in the chapter.

In the sections below we focus first on how CD4$^+$ T cells are activated and their function; later in the chapter we discuss the activation and function of CD8$^+$ T cells.

DENDRITIC CELLS ARE THE KEY APC FOR NAÏVE T CELLS

Only a few specialized, or "professional," APCs express MHC class II molecules, process protein antigens, and present selected catabolized linear fragments of the protein (peptides) to CD4$^+$ T cells (also see Chapter 9). Dendritic cells are one of these MHC class II expressing cells, and they are the principal APCs for initiating the primary

Immunology: A Short Course, Seventh Edition. Richard Coico and Geoffrey Sunshine.
© 2015 John Wiley & Sons, Ltd. Published 2015 by John Wiley & Sons, Ltd.
Companion Website: www.wileyimmunology.com/coico

responses of both CD4$^+$ and CD8$^+$ T cells. Dendritic cells, initially named for their dendritic star-shaped appearance under the microscope, are derived from the same hematopoietic precursor as monocytes and macrophages in bone marrow.

Two major subsets of dendritic cells have been distinguished based on their function (and expression of surface molecules). *Plasmacytoid dendritic cells* synthesize the interferons (IFNs) α and β in the early phases of an immune response and are major contributors to the innate phase of the response to pathogens such as viruses. *Myeloid den-*

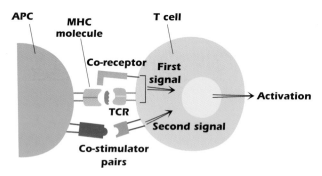

Figure 11.1. Activation of the naïve T cell requires two signals. First signal = TCR with peptide + MHC; T cell co-receptor (CD4 or CD8) with MHC is a component of the first signal. Second signal = co-stimulator pairs at the APC–T-cell surface.

dritic cells have a major role in the induction of T-cell responses and subsequently we use the term *dendritic cells* to refer to this set of cells. Dendritic cells are found in the circulation and in many tissues. Antigens can enter the body by several different routes—especially the airways, gastrointestinal tract, and skin—and dendritic cells are found in tissues close to these entry sites. Dendritic cells are also found in lymphoid organs. (In Chapter 10 we discussed the role of the dendritic cells resident in the thymus in negative selection of developing T cells, a key feature of the establishment of central tolerance in the T-cell population.) In addition, dendritic cells are also found in secondary lymphoid organs.

One of the key features of dendritic cells is that they can migrate from tissues to lymph node after encountering antigen. For example, the dendritic cell in the skin—known as the Langerhans cell—interacts with antigen and moves through lymph to the nearest draining node. Thus, dendritic cells can also be divided into "migratory" and "lymphoid organ resident." Migratory and lymphoid organ resident dendritic cells show some differences in surface molecule expression, but it is not currently clear that these are subsets with distinct functions. In this chapter we focus on the properties of the migratory dendritic cells.

The dendritic cell in tissues that has not interacted with antigen is referred to as an *immature dendritic cell* (Figure 11.2). It expresses low levels of MHC class II molecules. It

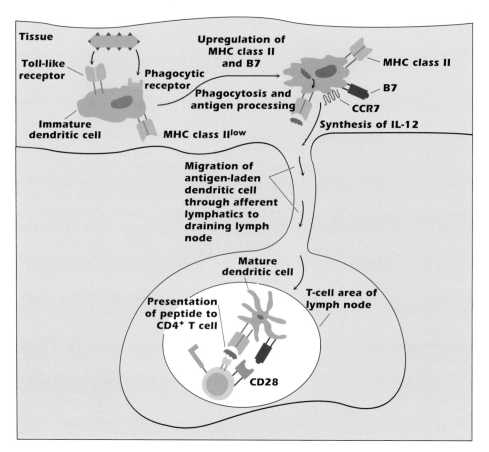

Figure 11.2. Dendritic cell maturation in response to pathogen: The immature cell interacts with a bacterium in a tissue; processes bacterial proteins; upregulates the expression of MHC class II and co-stimulator molecules, changes expression of chemokine receptors; migrates to the T-cell area of the lymph node draining the tissue; and presents peptides to the CD4$^+$ T cell with the appropriate TCR.

also expresses many different pattern recognition receptors (described in Chapter 2) that interact with components of several types of infectious microorganisms, particularly bacteria and viruses. Among these pattern recognition receptors are the Toll-like receptors (TLRs), a family of predominantly cell surface molecules that interact with bacterial DNA, lipoprotein, and lipopolysaccharide, as well as viral RNA and DNA. The immature dendritic cell also expresses phagocytic receptors, which enhance uptake of pathogen into the cell. Once the cell has taken up the pathogen it is also very efficient at catabolizing its protein components into peptides in the MHC class II pathway (Chapter 9).

The uptake and processing of a pathogen trigger development into a *mature dendritic cell*. This cell upregulates and expresses high levels of both MHC class II and co-stimulator molecules, particularly of the B7 family. Upregulation of MHC class II and co-stimulator molecules enhances the ability of the cell to present antigen to T cells. Interaction with bacterial pathogens also results in the synthesis and secretion of many cytokines, one of the most important being IL-12 (see below).

Interaction with pathogen also upregulates dendritic cell expression of the chemokine receptor CCR7, which binds to a ligand expressed by high endothelial venules at the entrance to lymph nodes. As a result, the dendritic cell with peptide bound to MHC class II molecules leaves the tissue in which it encountered pathogen and migrates through lymph vessels to the closest or "draining" lymph node. This mature dendritic cell then presents peptide to a T cell with the "correct" TCR in the T-cell region of the node (Figure 11.2).

The migration of an antigen-bearing dendritic cell to the draining node, combined with the ability of naïve T cells to recirculate through lymph nodes, increases the likelihood that the rare T cell expressing the appropriate TCR will be activated by the antigen-bearing dendritic cell. The interaction between the antigen-bearing dendritic cell and the T cell generally occurs within 8–10 hours of exposure to antigen.

Note that in the absence of signals induced by pathogens, immature dendritic cells express low levels of co-stimulator and MHC class II molecules. Thus, antigens that do *not* induce high levels of co-stimulator function do not activate naïve T cells. This is why we believe that the encounter of a dendritic cell with self-molecules in normal tissue does not lead to activation of either the dendritic cell or of T cells: co-stimulator function is not induced (see Chapter 9). Similarly, T-cell and antibody responses to many "harmless" foreign antigens (e.g., after injection with peptides or even small proteins in a vaccine) may evoke little or no response. For this reason proteins in many vaccinations are given with an *adjuvant* to ensure that a response is activated; components of the adjuvant enhance the activation of APCs, in particular by inducing the expression of co-stimulator molecules.

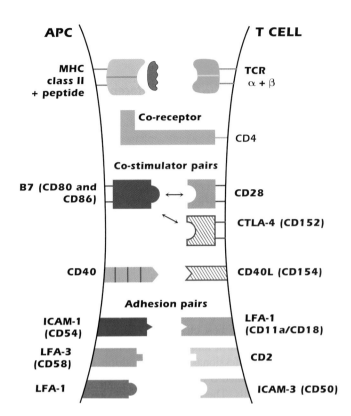

Figure 11.3. Paired interactions at the surface of an APC and a CD4⁺ T cell that lead to T-cell activation, cytokine synthesis, and proliferation. Hatching indicates expression upregulated by activation.

ACTIVATION OF CD4⁺ T CELLS

The lower part of Figure 11.2 shows the mature antigen-bearing dendritic cell interacting with a naïve CD4⁺ T cell in the T-cell area of the node. Figure 11.3 and the paragraphs below summarize the key pairs of interactions at the surface of the cells that result in the activation of the CD4⁺ T cell.

Paired Interactions at the Surface of the APC and CD4⁺ T Cell

Peptide/MHC and TCR. The interaction between peptide + MHC class II molecule expressed on the APC and the variable regions, $V\alpha + V\beta$, of the T-cell's TCR is the critical antigen-specific *first signal* for the activation of the CD4⁺ T cell. The TCR can detect a very small number of foreign peptides—as low as four peptide molecules out of the thousands of peptides expressed on a particular APC—so the T cell is very sensitive to foreign antigen. However, this interaction is of low affinity and has a rapid off-rate—the interacting components rapidly dissociate. The paired interactions described below both enhance the affinity of the interaction between the TCR and the peptide–MHC and stabilize the interaction between the two cells. Altogether

When Fyn and Lck are activated, they bind to regions of the CD3 and ζ chains that contain the previously described immunoreceptor tyrosine-based activation motifs (ITAMs) and phosphorylate them (Chapter 10). Because Lck is associated with CD4, this binding also pulls CD4 into close association with the TCR complex. The phosphorylated ITAMs in CD3 and ζ then act as docking sites for another tyrosine kinase, **ZAP-70** (belonging to a second tyrosine kinase family known as Syk), that is recruited to the complex. This step appears critical for T-cell activation, because T cells from the rare individuals who lack ZAP-70 do not respond to antigen; these individuals are profoundly immunodeficient (see Chapter 18). Because CD3 and ζ contain multiple ITAMs, more than one molecule of ZAP-70 is recruited into this complex of signaling proteins.

Lck activates ZAP-70 when it has joined the multiprotein signaling protein complex. Activated ZAP-70 phosphorylates **linker for activation of T cells** (LAT), which binds to the signaling complex already formed. LAT is an *adaptor*: a protein that does not have enzymatic activity but contains multiple binding domains for other proteins. LAT in turn recruits several more molecules, forming an even larger signaling complex. One of these is another adaptor molecule, SLP76, which activates the reorganization of actin molecules within the cell. SLP76 binds the enzyme *phospholipase Cγ1* (PLCγ1). In summary, a multiprotein complex of signal transduction molecules is assembled in sequence and activated on the cytoplasmic side of the T-cell membrane.

Activation of Intracellular Signaling Pathways.

Three major intracellular signaling pathways are activated in the cytoplasm after PLCγ1 is recruited to the signaling complex. Ultimately these pathways lead to the activation of transcription factors that enter the nucleus and alter gene expression.

The first pathway involves increasing intracellular calcium levels. This occurs as a result of the PLCγ1-catalyzed breakdown of the membrane phospholipid, phosphatidylinositol 4,5 bisphosphate (PIP$_2$), which is broken down into two products, one of which is inositol triphosphate (IP$_3$). IP$_3$ triggers the release of intracellular pools of calcium. The increased calcium level in turn activates the cytoplasmic molecule *calcineurin*, ultimately activating the transcription factor, **NFAT**. This pathway is clinically significant because the immunosuppressive agents cyclosporin A and tacrolimus (originally known as FK506) bind to and inhibit the function of calcineurin, particularly in T cells, thereby inhibiting the subsequent steps in T-cell activation. That is why these agents are extremely effective in preventing graft rejection when tissues are transplanted between genetically different individuals (see Chapter 19).

A second pathway leads to the activation in the cytoplasm of the transcription factor, **NF-κB**. This results from the formation of *diacylglycerol* (DAG), the second product of the PLCγ 1-catalyzed breakdown of PIP$_2$. DAG activates the enzyme *protein kinase C* (PKC), which in turn activates a cascade of kinases, ultimately activating NF-κB.

The third pathway is the *mitogen-activated protein* (MAP) kinase signaling pathway, ultimately leading to the activation of the transcription factor *AP-1*. This pathway is activated when DAG binds to a protein that in turn binds to and activates Ras, an enzyme that hydrolyzes guanosine triphosphate (i.e., it is a GTPase).

The activated transcription factors NF-κB, NFAT, and AP-1 enter the nucleus of the activated T cell and bind selectively to regulatory sequences of several different genes. Two important genes that are transcribed and translated in the activated T cell (within 24 hours of the onset of activation) are the genes for the cytokine IL-2 and for one of the chains of the IL-2 receptor: IL-2Rα (CD25). IL-2 is also known as **T-cell growth factor** and stimulates T-cell proliferation.

B7–CD28 Interaction.

After B7 and CD28 interact, one of the key early events inside the T cell is the recruitment of *phosphatidylinositol-3 (PI$_3$)* kinase to the cytoplasmic domain of CD28 (Figure 11.4). In addition, the B7–CD28 interaction mobilizes lipid rafts in the T-cell membrane, which brings tyrosine kinases and other molecules to the area of contact between the TCR and the APC. Ultimately these events lead to the activation and translocation into the nucleus of the transcription factors NF-AT and NF-κB. As described in the section above, these activated transcription factors upregulate expression of IL-2 and IL-2Rα.

The B7–CD28 co-stimulator interaction plays a critical role in IL-2 synthesis by increasing the rate of transcription of the IL-2 gene (via increased production of transcription factors) and increasing the half-life of IL-2 mRNA. The enhancement of IL-2 protein synthesis is calculated to be as much as 100-fold over and above the IL-2 synthesis induced by signaling through the TCR alone. This co-stimulator signal results in both survival—by suppressing apoptosis—and proliferation of the T cell.

Proliferation.

Figure 11.5 shows the events in the activated CD4$^+$ T cell after it starts to transcribe and translate the IL-2Rα and IL-2 genes. Synthesis of the IL-2Rα chain converts the low affinity two-chain IL-2 receptor (β + γ) on the resting T-cell surface into a three-chain (α, β, and γ) high-affinity IL-2 receptor on the activated T cell (see also Chapter 12).

IL-2 is a growth factor for T cells and acts on any cell that expresses the high-affinity IL-2 receptor; thus, as shown in Figure 11.5, IL-2 acts on both the T cell that synthesized and secreted it as well as daughter cells produced by proliferation. As a result, the original clone of T cells undergoes enormous and rapid expansion, increasing the clone size several thousand-fold within a week. This expansion of T

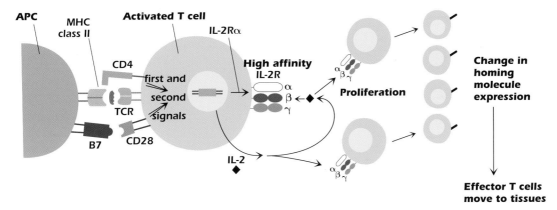

Figure 11.5. Activated CD4⁺ T cell synthesizes and secretes IL-2 and synthesizes the IL-2 receptor α chain. The interaction of IL-2 and the high-affinity IL-2 receptor results in proliferation of the CD4⁺ T-cell clone, change in expression of homing molecules, and movement of the resulting effector T cells out of the node and into tissues.

(and B cells, which are also activated in the response to antigen) is frequently noted as a swelling of the lymph node in which the response occurs.

Differentiation to Effector Cells and Migration Out of the Lymph Node

Toward the end of this phase of rapid expansion, the activated T cells differentiate into *effector T cells*, which now have the capability to carry out the effector function of their particular subset of T cells: synthesis of cytokines by CD4⁺ T cells or killing of targets by CD8⁺ T cells.

The activation of T cells in the lymph node and differentiation into an effector cell results in a change in expression of homing molecules, the set of adhesion molecules and chemokine receptors expressed by T cells and other leukocytes. Effector cells (and memory cells, described later in the chapter) downregulate the homing molecules that allowed the naïve T cell to enter the node and upregulate molecules that allow them to migrate out of the node and move to different sites in the body, particularly to tissues infected by pathogens (see also Chapter 9 and the discussion of lymphocyte homing in Chapter 8). For example, many effector cells upregulate the integrin VLA-4 (CD49CD29) and the chemokine receptor CCR10, which mediate homing to many tissues (except the skin) and sites of inflammation. Homing to skin is mediated by upregulation of CCR10 and the adhesion molecule, cutaneous lymphocyte antigen (CLA). Like that of activated B cells, migration of effector T cells to mucosal nodes is mediated by the integrin α4β7 and the chemokine receptor CCR9.

Termination of the Response

The interaction of antigen with naïve CD4⁺ (or CD8⁺) T cells results in the activation and enormous expansion of the reactive T-cell clones, generating a very large effector cell population. However, to reduce the risk of unregulated proliferation, it is also critical that the activation eventually stops. How does this occur? Several pairs of molecules expressed on the T-cell–APC surfaces convey *negative* signals to the activated T cell, which have the overall effect of turning off the response. These negative signals include inactivation of molecules activated during the response, inhibition of the cell cycle, and the induction of *T-cell exhaustion*; T cells that have been repeatedly stimulated to proliferate are no longer able to exert effector function.

One such important negative signal is via *CTLA-4 (CD152)*. Expression of CTLA-4, structurally similar to CD28, is induced on CD4⁺ and CD8⁺ T cells within 24 to 48 hours after initial activation by antigen.

CTLA-4 has multiple effects: Once induced, CTLA-4 competes with CD28 for binding to B7 on the APC surface (Figure 11.6). Because it has a higher affinity for B7 than CD28, CTLA-4 outcompetes CD28 and the negative or turn-off signals to the T cell dominate. In addition, the cytoplasmic domain of CTLA-4 contains an immunoreceptor *tyrosine-based inhibitory motif* (ITIM). The B7–CTLA-4 interaction recruits and activates phosphatases at the CTLA-4 ITIM. The activated phosphatases then remove phosphate groups and thus inactivate molecules inside the T cell that were activated by the B7–CD28 interaction. (In Chapter 8 we described a similar negative function for the B-cell molecule, CD32, which contains an ITIM.) CTLA-4 also acts in the immunologic synapse by displacing critical components of the signaling complex. In this way the expression of CTLA-4 turns off the production of IL-2 and thus ends T-cell proliferation, limiting the extent of the immune response.

Programmed cell death protein (PD)-1 (CD279), a member of the CD28/CTLA-4 family, is expressed on activated CD4⁺ and CD8⁺ T cells and is associated with T-cell exhaustion. It conveys a negative signal to the activated T cell, primarily by inhibiting ZAP-70 function. PD-1 binds

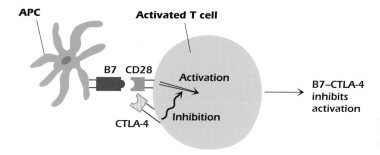

Figure 11.6. CTLA-4 inhibits the activation signal from CD28 and sends a negative or turn-off signal to the activated T cell.

to *programmed death ligand* (PD-L)1 (CD274) and PD-L2 (CD273). PD-L1 is expressed on most tumor cells and many normal cells, and PD-L2 is expressed predominantly by dendritic cells as well as many tumor cells.

The understanding that CTLA-4 and PD-1 transmit negative signals into the T cell is being exploited in several clinical conditions. One example is the testing of treatments using CTLA-4 in autoimmune conditions such as rheumatoid arthritis to turn off T cells that are "inappropriately" activated. In addition, antibodies that interfere with both the B7–CTLA-4 and PD-1–PDL-1/2 interactions are being used to treat chronic conditions, including cancer in which T-cell responses may be "exhausted" and not functioning effectively. Preliminary results of this treatment in melanoma patients have shown prolonged survival, suggesting that inhibition of turn-off signals may be of clinical relevance.

Other Ways to Activate CD4⁺ T Cells

In the preceding sections, we focused on how a peptide–MHC complex expressed on an APC activates a specific clone of T cells. Since naïve T cells expressing a TCR specific for any one particular peptide (plus MHC) are rare—approximately 1 in 10^5–10^6 T cells—only a small fraction of the total T-cell pool is activated by any one peptide–MHC complex. Infectious organisms and other complex antigens do generate more than one peptide–MHC complex, so they stimulate more than one T-cell clone in the course of a normal immune response. Some agents, however, can stimulate many clones of naïve CD4⁺ T cells to proliferate, which can, as a result, have major consequences for the host. These agents are described in the sections that follow.

Superantigens.   In humans, most superantigens are bacterial toxins from disease-causing organisms. Two examples are the enterotoxin released by staphylococcal organisms (the cause of food poisoning) and the toxin responsible for toxic shock syndrome. As we showed in Figure 9.13 in Chapter 9, a superantigen binds to the Vβ region of a TCR and cross-links it to an MHC molecule expressed by an APC. The superantigen binds to the Vβ chain outside the TCR's antigen-binding site. Because any one superantigen can bind to many different TCR Vβ molecules, a superanti-

gen can activate huge number of T cells with different antigenic specificities—up to 10% of the total T-cell population—in an individual. The activation of so many T cells and massive release of cytokines into the circulation following superantigen activation can have serious clinical consequences, such as fever and cardiovascular shock and in some circumstances, can even be fatal (see further in Chapter 12).

Plant Proteins, Antibodies to T-Cell Surface Molecules, and Other T-Cell Activators.   Several naturally occurring materials have the ability to trigger the proliferation and differentiation of many, if not all, clones of T lymphocytes. These substances are referred to as polyclonal activators or ***mitogens*** because of their ability to induce mitosis of the cell population. The plant glycoproteins concanavalin A (Con A) and phytohemagglutinin (PHA) are particularly potent T-cell mitogens. These substances are lectins, molecules that bind to carbohydrate moieties on proteins. Both Con A and PHA are thought to act through the TCR but not through the antigen-binding site. Because the T-cell response of healthy human blood to Con A and PHA falls in a well-defined range, a low response to Con A or PHA frequently indicates that a person is immunosuppressed. Another plant lectin, ***pokeweed mitogen***, activates both T and B cells.

Some antibodies specific for CD3 have the ability to activate T cells. Since CD3 is expressed on all T cells in association with the TCR, these anti-CD3 antibodies thereby induce all T cells to proliferate. In addition, a combination of phorbol 12-myristate 13-acetate (PMA) and ionomycin is used *in vitro* to activate all T cells to proliferate and synthesize cytokines. These molecules bypass the TCR: PMA activates PKC and ionomycin activates intracellular levels of calcium.

CD4⁺ T-CELL FUNCTION

Our goal in the sections that follow is to provide a fundamental understanding of the most important functions of CD4⁺ T cells. Many aspects of the role of CD4⁺ T cells in clinical conditions are discussed in subsequent chapters.

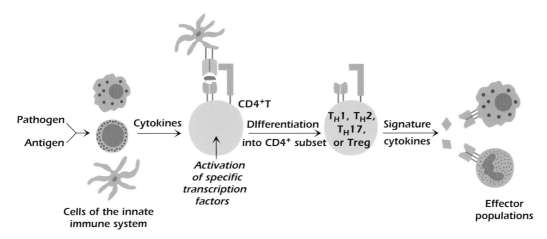

<u>Figure 11.7.</u> Development and function of subsets of CD4⁺ T cells. Pathogens and antigens interact with cells, generally of the innate immune system, that synthesize cytokines. These cytokines, in the presence of antigen and APC, activate lineage-specific transcription factors inside the CD4⁺ T cell. As a result the CD4⁺ T cell differentiates into a particular subset that synthesizes a set of "signature" cytokines that act on a unique set of effector cells.

Cytokine Synthesis

Overview. Once activated, CD4⁺ T cells proliferate and synthesize a vast array of cytokines, which affect multiple cell types. These cells include other sets of T cells, B cells, bone marrow precursor cells, and many effector cells of the innate immune response. The impact of cytokines synthesized by CD4⁺ T cells on so many different cell types helps explain why the loss of CD4⁺ T cells in conditions such as AIDS is so devastating (see Chapter 18).

Our current view of cytokine synthesis by CD4⁺ T cells is shown in Figure 11.7. Cytokines present during the activation of naïve CD4⁺ T cells by pathogens and many types of antigens drive the differentiation of the CD4⁺ T cell into subsets: ***T_H1, T_H2, T_H17***, or ***Treg*** cells. The cytokines produced early in the response are generally derived from cells of the innate immune system, and so these cells have a critical role in shaping the adaptive immune response. The role of cytokines in inducing the differentiation of CD4⁺ T cells into one subset or another is often referred to as a "third signal" that works in conjunction with the first (peptide–MHC–TCR) and second (co-stimulator) signals. In the presence of antigen and APCs, the cytokines produced early in the response activate "lineage-determining" transcription factors (discussed below and in Chapter 12) in the CD4⁺ T cell, which determine which subset is produced.

Each subset of CD4⁺ T cells synthesizes a unique pattern of ***signature cytokines***; that is, each subset synthesizes cytokines not made by the other subsets. (Some cytokines, though, such as IL-3, are produced by more than one subset.) Thus it is frequently useful to designate a particular CD4⁺ T cell response and the cytokines synthesized

in it as "T_H1-type" or "T_H2-type" and so on. The signature cytokines synthesized by each subset of CD4⁺ T cells interact with a unique set of effector cells, and each set of effector cells deals with a specific type or types of pathogen. Thus, each subset of CD4⁺ T cells is linked to the response to a particular type of pathogen. As we describe below, some self-antigens may also trigger the development of one or more of these subsets.

We note that not all scientists agree on which cytokines are made by individual subsets, and thus some papers and textbooks characterize the subsets slightly differently. Some part of this confusion may result from differences between mouse and human T cells, as well as from differences in conditions in different experiments.

Major Subsets of Cytokine-Producing CD4⁺ T Cells

T_H0 is often used to refer to the activated CD4⁺ T cell produced earliest in the response after a naïve T cell interacts with antigen. Some scientists, however, refer to T_H0 as the naïve CD4⁺ T cell that first interacts with antigen and APC. Prior to the fairly recent identification of T_H17 and Treg cells, T_H0 cells were characterized as synthesizing IL-2, IL-4, and IFN-γ, thus having some features of both T_H1 and T_H2 subsets (see below). Depending on the stimulating antigen and the cytokine present, the T_H0 could then further differentiate into either a T_H1 or T_H2 cell.

T_H1 cells (Figure 11.8) develop in the presence of IL-12. IL-12 is synthesized early in the immune response to intracellular pathogens—bacteria and viruses—by dendritic

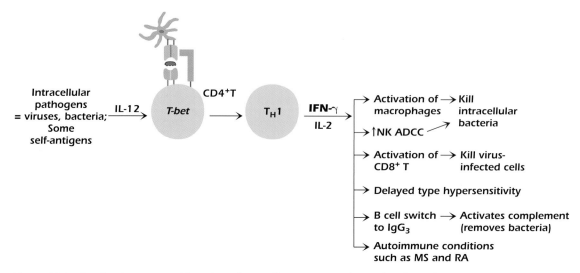

Figure 11.8. The development and function of T$_H$1 cells. IL-12 is synthesized early in the response to intracellular pathogens by NK cells and dendritic cells, and drives the differentiation to T$_H$1 cells, which synthesize IFN-γ and IL-2. T-bet is the lineage-determining transcription factor for T$_H$1 development. MS = multiple sclerosis; RA = rheumatoid arthritis. ADCC = antibody-dependent cell-mediated cytotoxicity.

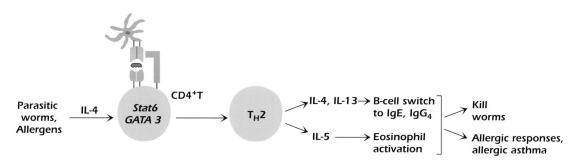

Figure 11.9. The development and function of T$_H$2 cells. The source of IL-4 that drives the differentiation to T$_H$2 cells is not resolved. Stat6 and GATA 3 are the lineage-determining transcription factors for T$_H$2 development.

cells, natural killer (NK) cells, and other cells of the innate immune system. IL-12 activates the transcription factor Stat4 in the activated CD4$^+$ T cells, which in turn upregulates IFN-γ. This in turn activates the transcription factor Stat1, and then induces the lineage-specific transcription factor T-bet.

T$_H$1 cells synthesize IFN-γ and IL-2. These cytokines activate macrophages, CD8$^+$ T cells, and NK cells. Once activated, these effector cells kill host cells that have been infected with intracellular pathogens, in particular with viruses and bacteria such as mycobacteria, salmonella, and listeria that establish themselves inside host cells. Macrophages, CD8$^+$ T cells, and NK cells are the principal effectors of **cell-mediated immunity**, which also includes responses referred to as **delayed type** or **type IV hypersensitivity** (see Chapters 17 and 19). For example, in contact sensitivity to poison ivy—a typical delayed type hypersensitivity response—antigens in poison ivy activate Langer-

hans cells in the skin, which activate T$_H$1 cells to synthesize IFN-γ and other cytokines. These T$_H$1 cytokines in turn recruit and activate macrophages, and an inflammatory response containing predominantly mononuclear cells develops in the skin.

In addition, IFN-γ influences B-cell class switching to immunoglobulin (Ig) isotypes that bind to pathogens (in humans, IgG$_3$ in particular), which in turn activates complement, and so enhances the phagocytosis of microbial pathogens by phagocytic cells (see also Chapter 14). T$_H$1 cells are also activated in some autoimmune diseases such as rheumatoid arthritis (RA) and multiple sclerosis (MS).

T$_H$2 cells (Figure 11.9) develop in the presence of IL-4, early in the response to parasitic worms such as helminths and to allergens. The source of this IL-4 is not clear; different studies have shown that a variety of cell types, including mast cells, activated CD4$^+$ T cells, and NKT cells are capable of synthesizing the IL-4 required to drive the differentiation of the T_H2 subset. The action of IL-4 on the T cell activates Stat6 and then GATA3, the lineage-determining transcription factors associated with T_H2 subset development.

T_H2 cells synthesize IL-4, IL-5, and IL-13. Thus, IL-4 both drives the development of the T_H2 cells and is synthesized by T_H2 cells. IL-4 and IL-13 influence the B-cell class switch to IgE and IgG_4 in humans, and IL-5 activates eosinophils. This set of cytokines and Igs characterize immune responses to parasitic worms such as helminths. In these responses, activated eosinophils bind IgE via their FcRs and the antigen-binding end of the IgE molecule binds to the worm surface. The eosinophils contain granules, whose contents are released by contact with the worm and are toxic to the worm. Responses to allergens, a type of hypersensitivity type I response, also involve T_H2 cells (Chapter 15); however, whereas the response to parasitic worms is protective to the host, the allergic response is frequently damaging. T_H2 cells, the signature cytokines they produce, and eosinophils also characterize "allergic asthma," which is one of the major phenotypes of this chronic airway inflammatory disease, triggered by exposure to airborne allergens.

 Read the related case: **Anaphylaxis**
In *Immunology: Clinical Case Studies and Disease Pathophysiology*

 Read the related case: **Asthma**
In *Immunology: Clinical Case Studies and Disease Pathophysiology*

T_H17 cells (Figure 11.10) develop in the presence of a mixture of cytokines whose components are not fully worked out. In humans, some studies suggest a combination of transforming growth factor β (TGF-β), IL-21, and IL-23

is required; however, differentiation of mouse T_H17 cells appears to require IL-6. Further studies will be needed to resolve this issue. IL-21 is synthesized by activated CD4⁺ T cells, but the other cytokines needed to induce T_H17 differentiation are made by cells of the innate immune response. The action of TGF-β and IL-21 or IL-6 on the T cell activates the transcription factors Stat3 and IRF4, and then RORγt, the lineage-determining transcription factor associated with T_H17 subset development.

T_H17 cells synthesize and secrete the IL-17 family of cytokines (particularly IL-17A and IL-17F, described in Chapter 12), IL-21, and IL-22. T_H17 cells, IL-17A, and IL-22 are ***proinflammatory***; that is, they promote inflammatory responses, particularly at mucosal sites. IL-17 stimulates many cells of the innate immune system (in particular, recruiting and activating neutrophils to sites of inflammation) as well as nonimmune cells—endothelial cells and epithelial cells—to synthesize the cytokines IL-1, IL-6, and tumor necrosis factor (TNF) that contribute to inflammation. IL-22 acts on many cells in the skin and digestive system and activates inflammatory responses. In addition, IL-22 induces epithelial cells to produce antibacterial peptides, which play a protective role in responses to bacteria at mucosal surfaces.

The T_H17 subset is involved in responses to ***extracellular bacteria*** (such as *Klebsiella pneumoniae* and the spirochete *Borrelia burgdorferi*) and ***fungi*** (such as *Candida albicans* and *Aspergillus fumigatus*). T_H1 and T_H2 subsets have little effect on these pathogens.

T_H17 cells and cytokines produced by T_H17 cells have also been described in some human autoimmune conditions that involve chronic inflammation. These ***autoinflammatory conditions*** include RA, MS, inflammatory bowel disease, and the skin condition psoriasis. Thus, some autoimmune diseases such as RA and MS may show features of both T_H1 and T_H17 responses.

In addition, T_H17 cells express high levels of **receptor activator of NF-κB ligand** (RANKL). RANKL, acting via cell-to-cell contact as well as secretion of the cell-surface

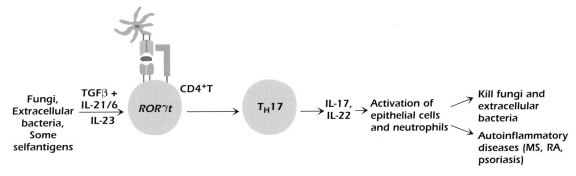

Figure 11.10. The development and function of T_H17 cells and the source of these cytokines. The mix of cytokines that drives differentiation to T_H17 cells is not resolved. RoR-γt is the lineage-determining transcription factor for T_H17 development. MS = multiple sclerosis; RA = rheumatoid arthritis.

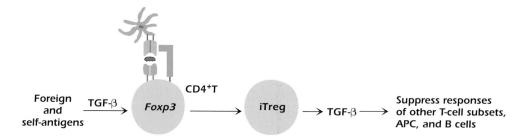

Figure 11.11. The development and function of iTreg cells. TGF-β, which drives the differentiation of iTreg, is synthesized by many cells. Foxp3 is both a marker and the lineage-determining transcription factor for iTreg (and nTreg) cells.

molecule, activates osteoclasts, which degrade bone matrix and so stimulate bone resorption. Consequently, T$_H$17 cells and RANKL are thought to play bone destructive roles in the inflammatory lesions that characterize both rheumatoid arthritis and the loss of teeth in periodontal disease.

Treg cells are heterogeneous in humans and mice, the two species in which they have been most studied. Some Treg—**induced (or iTreg)**—develop in the periphery from naïve T cells in the presence of TGF-β, which can be made by many different cell types (Figure 11.11). **Natural Treg (nTreg)** cells develop in the thymus and are autoreactive (Chapter 10). Both sets of Treg express the lineage-determining transcription factor Foxp3, which characterizes Treg cells. In addition both sets of Treg express CD25, the α chain of the IL-2 receptor, and CTLA-4.

Treg cells inhibit or *suppress* the differentiation and function of the other subsets of CD4$^+$ T cells: T$_H$1, T$_H$2, and T$_H$17 cells. They also suppress the activation and proliferation of other cell types, including dendritic cells and B cells. The inhibitory actions of Treg cells are mediated by both secretion of the cytokines TGF-β and IL-10 and through direct cell contact. Thus, iTreg needs TGF-β to develop and synthesize TGF-β when differentiated.

Treg cells suppress immune responses directed at both self-molecules and foreign antigens and thus play a role in tolerance and regulation. The importance of Treg cells in responses to self is shown by the autoimmune inflammatory conditions that result from defective development or function of Treg cells. One example is **immune dysregulation, polyendocrinopathy, enteropathy, X-linked (IPEX) syndrome**, in which Treg cells are lacking due to defective Foxp3. It is characterized by autoimmune disease, allergy, and inflammatory bowel disease. Treg function is discussed in more detail in Chapter 13.

Cross-Inhibition of CD4$^+$ T-Cell Subsets

Cytokines produced by one subset of CD4$^+$ T cells inhibit the function of other subsets. The key examples of this *cross-inhibition* are summarized in Table 11.1.

In summary, IFN-γ synthesized by T$_H$1 cells inhibits the development and function of T$_H$2 cells; IL-4 synthesized by

TABLE 11.1. Cross-Inhibition of CD4$^+$ T-Cell Subsets

Subset	Cytokine	Inhibits
T$_H$1	IFN-γ	T$_H$2 and T$_H$17
T$_H$2	IL-4	T$_H$1 and T$_H$17
Treg	TGF-β	T$_H$1, T$_H$2, and T$_H$17

T$_H$2 cells inhibits the development and function of T$_H$1 cells; and IFN-γ and IL-4, the signature cytokines of the T$_H$1 and T$_H$2 subsets, respectively, also inhibit T$_H$17 cells; thus, the development of either T$_H$1 or T$_H$2 cells prevents the induction of the T$_H$17 subset. In addition, Treg cells inhibit the development and function of all the other T-cell subsets. No evidence suggests that cytokines produced by T$_H$17 cells inhibit the function of any other subset of T cell.

As a result of the cross-inhibiting properties of different cytokines, the immune response to a particular antigen may end up "skewed" or *polarized* toward the production of only one subset of CD4$^+$ T cells, the production of one set of cytokines, and one type of effector responses. Most is known about the skewing toward T$_H$1 and away from T$_H$2 and vice versa. Skewing toward T$_H$1 cells occurs when cells of the innate immune system synthesize IL-12 early in the response to bacteria and viruses,. IL-12 production polarizes the response toward the development of T$_H$1 cells and synthesis of IFN-γ and away from T$_H$2 (and T$_H$17) cells and their cytokines. This polarization toward T$_H$1 cells activates the effector cells that remove virus- or bacteria-infected cells. By contrast, in the response to parasitic worms, IL-4 is synthesized early in the response. This drives CD4$^+$ T-cell differentiation toward T$_H$2 cytokines and the T$_H$2 set of responses and effector cells (IgE synthesis and eosinophil activation) and away from T$_H$1 (and T$_H$17) cells and cytokines. Similarly, responses to allergens are dominated by the T$_H$2-type pattern of IL-4 and IgE synthesis (see Chapter 15).

The phenomenon of polarization also suggests potential therapies: For example, attempts have been made to skew the response *away* from T$_H$2 cell responses that dominate in allergic responses, either by trying to inhibit the function of T$_H$2 cells per se or by activating other subsets of CD4$^+$ T cells specific for the allergen (see Chapter 15). In addition, treatments that inhibit the function of T$_H$17 cells in conditions such as psoriasis or that expand the development of Treg cells in autoinflammatory conditions may be clinically beneficial (see Chapter 13).

Other Sets of Cytokine-Producing CD4$^+$ T Cells

T helper cells. One of the major functions of CD4$^+$ T cells is to cooperate in the B-cell synthesis of antibody in the response to thymus-dependent (TD) antigens; that is, that some CD4$^+$ T cells act as *T helper cells (T$_H$)* for B cells. Since the T helper cell–B cell response to TD antigens occurs predominantly in the follicles of secondary lymphoid organs, the CD4$^+$ T cell that interacts with the B cell is referred to as a *T follicular helper (T$_{FH}$) cell*. The T$_{FH}$ cell has characteristics distinct from the subsets of CD4$^+$ T cells described above: T$_{FH}$ cells express the transcription factor *Bcl-6*, the chemokine receptor *CXCR5* on their surface, and secrete *IL-21*. However, the precise relationship of T$_{FH}$ cells to these other subsets of CD4$^+$ T cells is not completely understood and is the subject of intense investigation. We describe the function of T$_{FH}$ cells in more detail in a section below.

T$_H$9. Some experiments indicate that the cytokine IL-9, a growth factor for T cells and mast cells, is synthesized by a CD4$^+$ T cell distinct from the T$_H$1, T$_H$2, T$_H$17, or Treg subsets. This cell, induced by IL-4 and TGF-β, has been designated T$_H$9. Further research is needed to establish whether this is a separate subpopulation of CD4$^+$ T cells.

In humans, cells synthesizing IL-9 are thought to be involved in the chronic inflammation found in allergen-induced asthma. In mice, IL-9 synthesizing cells have a role in models of asthma, in autoimmune conditions such as MS and colitis, and in response to helminth infections.

Further Points on Cytokine Synthesis

Before leaving the topic of cytokine synthesis by CD4$^+$ T cells, we note the following:

- Few if any of the cytokines synthesized by CD4$^+$ T cells are synthesized uniquely by CD4$^+$ T cells or even by a specific subset of CD4$^+$ T cells. Even the signature cytokines for each subset are synthesized by other cell types. For example, the T$_H$1 cytokines IL-2 and IFN-γ are also synthesized by CD8$^+$ T cells; T$_H$2-associated IL-4 is also synthesized by mast cells and NKT cells. IL-10 was originally described as a signature cytokine of T$_H$2 cells, but it is now known to be synthesized by multiple cell types, including B cells, CD8$^+$ T cells, and Tregs.
- The designation of a response as T$_H$1-type or T$_H$2-type is helpful in characterizing the cytokines produced, but

responses to infectious agents are frequently complex; one subset of responses may dominate at a particular stage of the response, and another may dominate at another. Furthermore, responses to many harmless antigens do not show a skewed pattern of cytokines.

- Until recently, most studies supported the view that the ability of a particular subset of CD4$^+$ T cells to synthesize cytokines was fixed. Recent evidence suggests some "plasticity" in the response of each subset, for example, that in some conditions T$_H$2 cells can synthesize IFN-γ, the signature cytokine of T$_H$1 cells. Further studies will be needed to determine how flexible the responses of individual subsets of CD4$^+$ T cells are.

Help for B Cell in the Response to TD Antigens

In Chapter 8 we described the key features of B-cell synthesis of antibody in the germinal center in the response to thymus-dependent (TD) antigens, focusing on the events in the differentiation of B cells. In brief, following class switch recombination and somatic hypermutation, memory B cells and long-lived plasma cells are produced that make antibody in the protective responses to many pathogens. In the paragraphs that follow we describe how T and B cells interact to form a germinal center, and we focus on the role of the T$_{FH}$ cell, the CD4$^+$ T cell responsible for this interaction with B cells. As we noted above, T$_{FH}$ cells have characteristics distinct from the subsets of CD4$^+$ T cells we described earlier in the chapter, but the precise relationship of T$_{FH}$ cells to these other subsets is not completely understood.

The B Cell Captures Antigen and Presents It to the Activated T$_H$.   In Chapter 8 we discussed that a CD4$^+$ T cell and a B cell specific for the same antigen initially interact at the edge of the T- and B-cell regions of a secondary lymphoid organ. How do these cells interact? A critical initial step is the B cell's unique ability to capture "free" antigen with its antigen-specific B-cell receptor (BCR) membrane Ig (Figure 11.12). In the example in Figure 11.12, the antigen is a flu-virus protein that is part of a vaccine.

After the protein binds to the membrane Ig, the complex of Ig-bound protein is taken into the cell, and the antigen—like other exogenous antigens—is processed in acid compartments. As described in Chapter 9, some of the peptides that result from the catabolism of the protein antigen bind to newly synthesized MHC class II molecules as they traffic through the B cell. Peptide–MHC class II complexes are then expressed at the B-cell surface. The B cell then acts as an APC to present peptide + MHC class II to a CD4$^+$ T cell with the appropriate TCR; in this example, a T cell with TCR specific for an epitope of the same flu protein. Note that before interacting with the B cell, this CD4$^+$ T cell has been activated in the T-cell area of the lymph node by

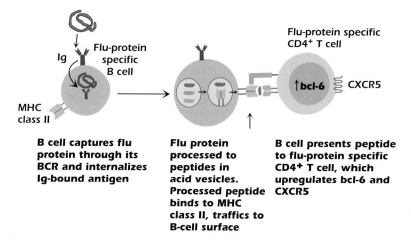

B cell captures flu protein through its BCR and internalizes Ig-bound antigen

Flu protein processed to peptides in acid vesicles. Processed peptide binds to MHC class II, traffics to B-cell surface

B cell presents peptide to flu-protein specific CD4⁺ T cell, which upregulates bcl-6 and CXCR5

Figure 11.12. The B cell as an antigen-capture and antigen-presenting cell. A flu-specific B cell captures a flu protein antigen using its BCR, membrane Ig. The B cell processes the antigen and presents flu-protein peptides in association with MHC class II molecules to a flu-peptide specific CD4⁺ T cell. The interaction upregulates T cell expression of the transcriptional repressor, bcl-6, and CXCR5. These molecules characterize the T_FH.

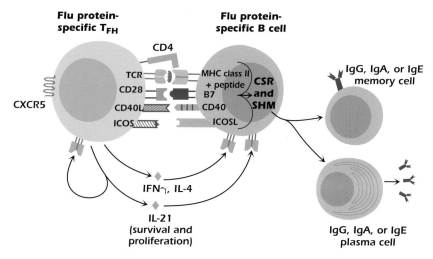

Figure 11.13. Key interactions involved in T_FH–B cell cooperation in the germinal center. Hatching indicates expression of co-stimulator molecules upregulated by activation. IL-21 is needed for the survival and proliferation of both T_FH and the B cell. IL-4 and IFN-γ promote class switch recombination (CSR) and somatic hypermutation (SHM). The response gives rise to memory B cells expressing IgG, IgA, or IgE, and plasma cells that synthesize IgG, IgA, or IgE.

dendritic cells that have processed the same antigen and have presented virus-derived peptides to the CD4⁺ T cell (see Chapter 8 and earlier in this chapter).

Development of the T_FH and the Germinal Center. The interaction of antigen-activated CD4⁺ T and B cells upregulates T-cell expression of the transcription factor Bcl-6 (see Figure 11.12). Bcl-6 is the transcription factor that characterizes T_FH cells; it is a transcriptional repressor, in that it represses expression of the transcription factors that characterize the T_H1, T_H2, and T_H17 subsets. Bcl-6 activation induces the expression of the chemokine receptor CXCR5 on the CD4⁺ T cell. Once CXCR5 is expressed, the CD4⁺ T cell—and its cognate B cell—moves into the B cell follicle and the germinal center develops. Thus, CXCR5 is a marker of the T_FH that cooperates with B cells in the germinal center.

Events in the Germinal Center

Figure 11.13 shows the key interactions between the activated T_FH cell and B cell in the presence of antigen in the germinal center. These interactions share many characteris-

tics with the interactions of antigen-bearing dendritic cells and CD4⁺ T cells in the response of naïve T cells: first, a critical antigen-specific first signal, provided in the T_FH-B interaction by peptide–MHC on the B cell with the TCR (plus CD4 interacting with MHC class II), and second signals, provided by co-stimulator pairs. Adhesion pairs (not shown) similar to the ones expressed in the dendritic cell–T-cell interactions also strengthen the interactions between the T_FH cell and the B cell.

Similarly, the area of contact between the T_FH cell and B cell also forms an immunologic synapse. Not only is this synapse required for sustained signaling, but the cells reorganize their internal structure so that the key interactions are localized to the area of contact between the cells. Sustained interactions over several hours drive the further differentiation of both cells, the development of the germinal center, affinity maturation, and ultimately the generation of class-switched plasma cells and memory cells. These interactions also provide survival signals for both the T_FH cell and B cell.

Co-Stimulator Pairs and Cytokines Are Critical in T_FH Cell-Dependent Antibody Synthesis and Class Switching. Multiple co-stimulator pairs interact in the

T$_{FH}$–B response in the germinal center. Most information is known about the interactions between CD40 and CD40L, B7 and CD28, and ICOS (CD278) and ICOS ligand (ICOSL, CD275). B-cell presentation of peptide–MHC class II complexes to the TCR upregulates T$_{FH}$ expression of CD40L. Interaction of CD40L with CD40 expressed on the B cell in turn upregulates expression of B7 on the B cell, which interacts with CD28 expressed on the T cell. ICOS is induced on activated T cells and is expressed by T$_{FH}$ cells in the germinal center. ICOS interacts with ICOSL expressed on the B cell.

Interactions between the co-stimulator pairs upregulate T$_{FH}$ cytokine synthesis. These cytokines affect the T cell itself and the B cell; one of these, IL-21, the signature cytokine of T$_{FH}$ cells, promotes survival and proliferation of both the T$_{FH}$ and the germinal center B cell.

As a result of the co-stimulator pair and cytokine-cytokine receptor interactions, the B cell undergoes class switch recombination and somatic hypermutation—the B cell switches from the synthesis of IgM to the synthesis of other isotypes: IgG, IgA, or IgE. Class switch recombination gives rise to memory B cells expressing IgG, IgA, or IgE, and long-lived plasma cells that synthesize IgG, IgA, or IgE. The plasma cells move to the bone marrow and the memory cells move to tissues in which the antigen exposure or infectious agent was first encountered.

The cytokine produced by the T$_{FH}$ cell influences the particular antibody isotype synthesized by the B cell. If the T$_{FH}$ cell synthesizes IL-4, B cells switch to producing predominantly IgE and IgG$_4$; if the T$_{FH}$ cell synthesizes IFN-γ, B cells switch to producing IgG subtypes such as IgG$_3$ that activate complement (see Chapters 5 and 14).

The crucial involvement of co-stimulator interactions in class switch recombination is shown by the clinical conditions that develop in individuals who have defective co-stimulator function. In *X-linked hyper-IgM syndrome* (see Chapter 18) males with a nonfunctional CD40L produce high levels of IgM but almost no IgG, IgA, or IgE. Similarly, individuals with nonfunctional CD40 or with a deficiency of the enzyme that mediates class switch recombination (activation-induced cytidine deaminase [AID]) also make predominantly IgM. Furthermore, individuals who lack a functional ICOS gene product (and ICOS knockout mice) do not develop normal germinal centers, and they are profoundly immunodeficient, with low levels of IgG, IgA, and IgE.

Linked Recognition

For the T$_H$ and B cell to cooperate effectively, they must respond to parts of the *same* structure. This is the principle of *linked recognition* (Figure 11.14). This guarantees that the T$_H$ and B cell that cooperate are specific for the **same antigen**; that is, a flu-specific T$_H$ cooperates only with a flu-specific B cell and not a measles-specific B cell. The T$_H$

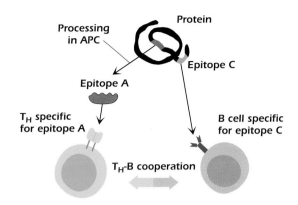

Figure 11.14. Linked recognition: For T helper cell–B cell cooperation in antibody synthesis, the epitopes recognized by the helper T cell (epitope A) and the B cell (epitope C) must be physically linked in the same antigen.

and B cell usually respond to different epitopes in the same antigen—the T$_H$ to an internal epitope (epitope A) generated during the processing of the antigen, and the B cell to an epitope found in some other part of the structure, and frequently on the outside of the molecule (epitope C).

Conjugate Vaccines: Help for Thymus-Independent Antigens. Thymus-independent (TI) antigens do not require T-cell help, and B cells in these responses do not undergo class switching or produce memory cells. Thus, responses to TI antigens do not typically synthesize IgG or IgA antibodies that are characteristic of long-term protective responses.

One major group of organisms that induce TI responses are encapsulated organisms such as *H. influenzae* b and *S. pneumoniae*, which can cause pneumonia or meningitis and be fatal in young children. The capsular polysaccharides of these bacteria are potent TI antigens and so are capable of generating strong IgM responses. However, the marginal zone B cells that synthesize early (within 2–3 days) protective IgM antibodies in response to these and many other bacterial pathogens do not develop until a child is about 1 to 2 years old. Thus, the absence of marginal zone B cells in young children leaves them vulnerable to infection from these pathogens.

The introduction of ***conjugate vaccines*** (further discussed in Chapter 21) in the past 25 years has dramatically reduced the number of deaths resulting from infections with these organisms. Conjugate vaccines utilize the principle of linked recognition described above and illustrated in Figure 11.15. The outer capsules of *H. influenzae* b and *S. pneumoniae* are made up of polysaccharide—potent TI antigens. By physically linking purified polysaccharide from the bacterium to a **carrier** protein such as tetanus toxoid, the response is changed to a *thymus-dependent* response. The carrier protein generates T-cell epitopes that activate T-helper cells, and these T-helper cells interact with B cells specific

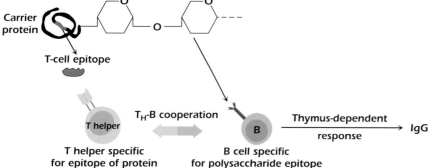

A   Polysaccharide alone

Thymus-independent response → IgM

B   Protein conjugated to polysaccharide

Carrier protein

T-cell epitope

T helper

T_H-B cooperation

Thymus-dependent response → IgG

T helper specific for epitope of protein

B cell specific for polysaccharide epitope

Figure 11.15. T helper–B cell cooperation in the use of conjugate vaccines: (A) Polysaccharide alone, e.g., the purified capsular polysaccharide of *H. influenzae* or *S. pneumoniae*, generates IgM in a thymus-independent response; (B) the same polysaccharide conjugated to a "carrier" protein such as tetanus toxoid generates a thymus-dependent IgG response.

for the polysaccharide. The resulting TD response allows affinity maturation, the switching to isotypes such as IgG and the development of long-term memory. The conjugate vaccine Pneumovax is recommended for all children younger than 5 years of age as protection against pneumococcal infections.

ACTIVATION AND FUNCTION OF CD8+ T CELLS

We have discussed above the major functions of CD4+ T cells. The principal function of the other major subset of T cells, CD8+ T cells, is to kill cells that have been infected by viruses and bacteria. CD8+ T cells are also involved in killing transplanted foreign cells (graft rejection) and tumor cells (see Chapters 19 and 20). For this reason, a CD8+ T cell is referred to as a *killer T cell* or *cytotoxic T lymphocyte* (CTL). The cell killed by a CTL is known as a *target*; the target can be any cell that expresses MHC class I molecules.

Generation of Effector CD8+ T Cells

Much of our understanding of the activation and generation of effector CD8+ T cells is derived from studies of the responses to infectious agents, particularly viruses and bacteria, in mice. However, the principles extend to responses in humans.

We focus on responses to viruses: Responses are initiated after the virus—such as influenza, lymphocyte choriomeningitis virus (LCMV) or vaccinia—has been transported through lymph to the lymph node draining the infected organ or tissue, where it is taken up by macrophages or dendritic cells. Dendritic cells may also acquire virus or

viral antigens from the macrophages by cross-presentation, the pathway we described in Chapter 9.

The activation and generation of effector CD8+ T cells follow many of the same principles that we described above for the generation of effector CD4+ T cells: a first signal, peptide–MHC interacting with the TCR; second or co-stimulator signals, particularly B7–CD28 and CD40–CD40L; and a third signal, cytokines, synthesized by cells of the innate immune response. The dendritic cell is the key APC for the activation of naïve CD8+ T cells. IL-12 is considered critical in the activation of CD8+ T cells, and interferons α and β are also thought to play a role. All these signals are required to provide maximal stimulation.

Activation. Virus-specific CD8+ T cells can be activated by different pathways, which are shown in Figure 11.16.

Figure 11.16A shows that a dendritic cell can present virus-derived peptide bound to an MHC class I molecule to a CD8+ T cell with the appropriate TCR. Virus-derived peptides associated with the MHC class I molecules in this dendritic cell may have resulted from either infection of the cell or via processing in the cross-presentation pathway (also see Chapter 9). In this pathway, the dendritic cell provides the first and second signals, as well as IL-12, to directly activate the CD8+ T cell. The combination of these signals results in the rapid proliferation of this clone of CD8+ T cells. The CD8+ T cell is thought to synthesize IL-2 that induces the proliferation of the activated CD8+ T cells in an autocrine stimulatory loop (see Chapter 12). In mice, responses to influenza and LCMV occur via this direct activation of CD8+ T cells by dendritic cells.

Some virus-specific CD8+ T-cell responses (for example, in the response to herpes virus) require virus-specific CD4+ T cells; however, the precise way in which

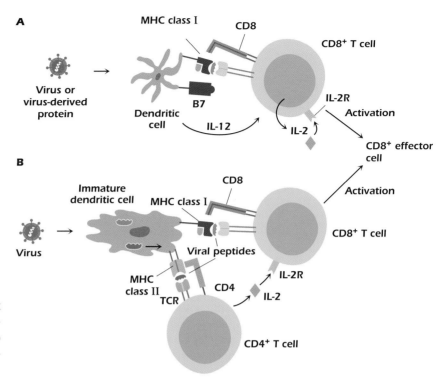

<u>Figure 11.16.</u> Generation of virus-specific CD8⁺ effector T cells. (A) Dendritic cells activate CD8⁺ T cells directly. (B) Responses to some viruses require CD4⁺ T cells to activate CD8⁺ T cells.

CD4⁺ T cells are involved in the activation of naïve CD8⁺ T cells and the generation of effector CD8⁺ T cells is not completely understood. Figure 11.16B shows one pathway in which CD4⁺ T cells may play a role in the generation of CD8⁺ effector T cells: A dendritic cell that has taken up virus as an exogenous antigen presents virus-derived peptides in association with MHC class II molecules to a virus-specific CD4⁺ T cell. In conjunction with the co-stimulator interaction B7–CD28, the CD4⁺ cell is activated to proliferate and synthesize IL-2.

The same dendritic cell may also present virus antigens to CD8⁺ T cells via cross-presentation in the MHC class I pathway. Thus, the interaction of the CD8⁺ T cell with virus-derived peptides presented by MHC class I expressed on the dendritic cell, in combination with IL-2 synthesized by the CD4⁺ T cell, induces virus-specific CD8⁺ T-cell proliferation and differentiation. In this pathway, the viral epitope that activates the CD4⁺ T cell (red peptide) is different from the epitope that activates the CD8⁺ T cell (green peptide).

Because the likelihood of two rare antigen-specific T cells (the virus-specific CD4⁺ and CD8⁺ T cells) interacting with the same APC is very low, it was not clear whether this three-cell interaction could occur under physiologic conditions. Studies suggest, however, that an initial dendritic cell–CD4⁺ T-cell interaction can occur, with a CD8⁺ T cell joining this stabilized interaction later.

A variation of the activation pathway shown in Figure 11.16B has the dendritic cell activating the CD4⁺ and CD8⁺ T cells in separate events. In this *licensing* pathway an immature dendritic cell interacts first with a CD4⁺ T cell;

the dendritic cell upregulates co-stimulator molecules (particularly CD40), and the CD4⁺ T cell upregulates CD40L. The now mature dendritic cell, with upregulated CD40 and the ability to synthesize and secrete IL-12, can move away from the CD4⁺ T cell to interact with and activate a naïve virus-specific CD8⁺ T cell.

Whichever pathway is used to activate the CD8⁺ T cell, the intracellular events in CD8⁺ T-cell activation are similar to those described above for CD4⁺ T-cell activation. Like CD4, CD8 is associated with the tyrosine kinase Lck; and the same pairs of co-stimulator and adhesion molecules employed in the activation of CD4⁺ T cells are also involved: CD28–B7, LFA-1–ICAM-1, and CD2–CD58. Activation results in rapid and enormous expansion of the CD8⁺ T-cell clone size, calculated to be an almost 500,000-fold increase in the week after infection. The negative co-stimulator molecules CTLA-4 and PD1 are also expressed on CD8⁺ T cells, and so expression of these molecules later in the response turns off the response.

CD8⁺ T-CELL KILLING OF TARGET CELLS

Once activated, the CD8⁺ T cell initiates killing by attaching to the target cell (Figure 11.17). Interactions between peptide associated with MHC class I molecules expressed by the target and CD8 and the TCR expressed by the CD8⁺ T cell are critical; in addition, paired adhesion molecules expressed on the T cell and target cell surfaces (not shown in the figure) help to maintain contact between the cells for several hours.

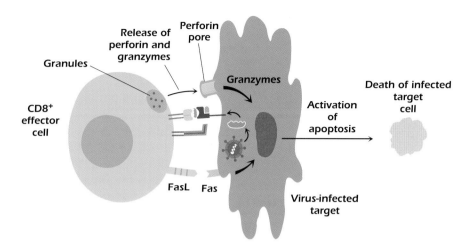

<u>Figure 11.17.</u> The two major pathways of CD8$^+$ T cell killing of virus-infected targets. The infected target expresses MHC class I and virus-derived peptides. Apoptosis of the target is induced (a) by the action of the granule contents of activated CD8$^+$ T cells, and (b) through Fas-Fas ligand cell surface interactions.

Killing by CD8$^+$ T cells is thought to occur by two pathways, both of which activate apoptosis (programmed cell death) of the target cell. The first, which is considered the predominant pathway for killing most target cells, involves the action of the contents of granules contained in the CD8$^+$ T cell. These granules are formed when the CD8$^+$ T cell is activated. After attaching to the target cell, the CD8$^+$ T cell reorganizes its internal structure so that these granules are close to the area of contact with the target cell. The CD8$^+$ T cell then releases the granule contents onto the target cell by exocytosis. A key constituent of the granules is *perforin*, which forms pores in the target cell membrane. The resulting increase in permeability contributes to the eventual death of the cell. The action of perforin on cell membranes is similar to that of the complement membrane attack complex (Chapter 14). *Granzymes* are serine proteases that pass into the target cell through the pores created by perforin; granzymes interact with intracellular components of the target cell to induce apoptosis. *Granulysin* (not shown in the figure) is a small protein that also enters the target cell; it activates pathways that lead to the killing of intracellular bacteria such as *Listeria* and *Mycobacteria*, which live inside macrophages and dendritic cells.

A second pathway of target cell killing occurs via the interaction of the molecule FasL expressed on the CD8$^+$ T cell, with Fas, expressed on many host cells. This interaction activates the apoptosis of the target cell via sequential activation of caspases, a set of proteolytic enzymes, inside the target cell (see Chapter 13 for further details). As a result, the cell dies within hours. Since death by apoptosis does not result in the release of the cell's contents, killing infected cells by apoptotic mechanisms does not stimulate an inflammatory response and may prevent the spread of infectious virus into other cells. Once the CD8$^+$ T cell has initiated these killing pathways, it detaches from the cell to attack and kill additional target cells.

Activation of CD8$^+$ T cell and killing of the target cell are separate events. This can be demonstrated by preparing CD8$^+$ T cells from an individual who has been infected with a virus: The virus-specific cytotoxic cells are able to kill virus-infected targets outside the body. (The assay for CD8$^+$ T-cell killing of targets is described in Chapter 6.) *In vitro* killing of the infected target does not require additional factors.

MHC Restriction and CD8$^+$ T Cell Killer Function

We stress again the concept of MHC restriction of T-cell responses. The first studies that established the concept of MHC restriction were performed by Rolf Zinkernagel and Peter Doherty with CD8$^+$ T cells (CTL) from mice infected with lymphocyte choriomeningitis virus. Zinkernagel and Doherty, who were awarded the Nobel Prize for their work in 1996, showed that CTL prepared from virus-infected mice killed targets that expressed *both* virus antigen and a specific MHC class I molecule expressed by cells in the mouse. The CTL did not kill uninfected targets or cells expressing either the virus antigen alone or in combination with a different MHC class I molecule. In these landmark studies the researchers interpreted their findings to indicate that the TCR expressed by the CTL recognized the combination of peptide and MHC class I. Although the role of the MHC in the T-cell responses in transplantation had been known for several years, this was the first demonstration of the role of the MHC in "everyday" responses.

These findings have important biologic consequences. MHC class I molecules are expressed on every nucleated cell in the body. A pathogen may infect any nucleated cell and generate peptides that associate with that cell's MHC class I molecules. These pathogen-derived peptide–MHC class I complexes at the cell surface are recognized by CD8$^+$ T cells with the appropriate TCR and results in the killing of the infected cell. Thus, killing by CD8$^+$ T cells provides a mechanism to eliminate any nucleated cell in the body that is infected. Clearly, elimination of the pathogen does result in the destruction of host cells, but this is the price the individual pays for removal of the source of infection.

Generally, only intracellular pathogens generate peptides that associate with MHC class I molecules and evoke $CD8^+$ T-cell responses. These pathogens also activate pathogen-specific $CD4^+$ T cells and induce antibody synthesis because they are taken up by APCs such as dendritic cells and macrophages. In this way, $CD4^+$ T cells, $CD8^+$ T cells, and antibody, along with other cells such as $\gamma\delta$ T cells, are all likely to be involved in the host's protective immune response against a particular organism (see Chapter 21). In contrast, harmless or noninfectious antigens (such as a killed virus protein in a vaccine) do not generally trigger $CD8^+$ T-cell responses. These exogenous antigens are taken up into the acidic compartments of an APC, interact with MHC class II molecules, and activate $CD4^+$ T-cell and antibody responses.

MEMORY T CELLS

In previous sections we described how the interaction of antigen with naïve $CD4^+$ or $CD8^+$ T cells activates them, inducing enormous proliferation of the reactive clones, and generating a very large effector cell population. It is critical that the activation eventually stops, and we have described some of the signals that turn off the response. In most responses, the pathogen (or "harmless" antigen) that triggered the response is cleared or eliminated within days of the initial contact.

This leaves the individual with a large pool of activated and effector $CD4^+$ and $CD8^+$ T cells specific for a particular pathogen or antigen. At this point, the vast majority of activated T cells are eliminated by an apoptotic pathway known as activation-induced cell death, mediated by the interaction of Fas and FasL.

A small population of cells does survive the phase of contraction of the clone size at the end of a response. These are *memory T cells* ($CD4^+$ T and $CD8^+$ T). They are generally long-lived, frequently with a lifetime of years. They are involved in protective responses after a subsequent exposure to the same pathogen (see Chapter 21).

Memory T-cell responses are also more rapid and effective than primary responses. One reason is that the clonal size of the memory population specific for a particular antigen is much larger (generally 100-fold to 1000-fold) than the size of the original clone in the naïve T-cell population. In addition, reinfection or restimulation with a particular antigen activates the proliferation and differentiation of memory T cells to effector cells so that the clone size is expanded even further.

Several questions remain about the development and function of memory T cells. One issue is when they develop: Is it after the development of effector cells or do memory T cells split off early in the activation process? It is also not clear whether the persistence of T memory cells requires the presence of antigen, even at some very low level; some

studies indicate that in the absence of the priming antigen, memory cells die. In addition, no accepted marker of T memory cells has been identified.

Different subsets of memory cells have been identified based on the cytokines they produce and their adhesion markers and thus the tissues to which they circulate. A cell's ability to enter specific tissues is governed by its expression of a combination of adhesion molecules and chemokine receptors. *Effector memory cells* downregulate the adhesion molecules and chemokine receptors expressed by naïve cells (L-selectin and CCR7, respectively) and upregulate a pattern of molecules that allows migration to peripheral tissues. One set allows the memory cells to move to the skin and another set permits movement to the mucosa—major sites in the body under threat from infectious organisms. Reexposure to antigen at these sites rapidly induces effector memory cells to become effector cells. *Central memory cells* express a pattern of adhesion molecules and chemokine receptors that are very similar to the pattern expressed by naïve T cells; thus, central memory cells recirculate through peripheral lymph nodes. Reexposure to antigen in the nodes induces effector function from central memory cells, although this generally occurs less rapidly than responses of effector memory cells.

Note that in some chronic infections, such as infections with human immunodeficiency virus (HIV)-1 or with parasites, the pathogen is not completely eliminated and may "hide" in host cells for long periods; that is, host cells provide a reservoir for these types of infectious agents. A further immune response to the pathogen is activated when the pathogen reemerges after a period of latency. This is discussed in more detail in Chapter 21.

FUNCTION OF OTHER SUBSETS OF T CELLS

$CD4^+$ and $CD8^+$ T cells are critical components of the adaptive immune response. Other subsets of T cells exist that do express neither CD4 nor CD8. They are mostly found in or associated with mucosal tissue, which is particularly vulnerable to infection, so they have likely evolved to participate in early responses to infectious agents. They show some characteristics of cells of the innate rather than the adaptive immune response; for example, they respond rapidly after exposure to antigen and they do not appear to make memory responses. They are described briefly below.

NKT Cells

NKT cells express a T-cell receptor as well as the molecule NK1.1 and other molecules typical of NK cells (see Chapter 10). They are found in the lamina propria of the intestines and recognize and respond to lipid and glycolipid antigens derived from infectious organisms (such as *Sphingomonas* bacteria and *B. burgdorferi*) as well as glycosphingolipids expressed by host cells. Thus, NKT cells respond to both microorganisms and self-antigens. Most NKT cells use a "semi-invariant" TCR, one Vα with a restricted set of Vβ regions, which responds to antigen presented by CD1$^+$ APCs, such as dendritic cells.

After stimulation by antigen, NKT cells very rapidly synthesize high levels of both T$_H$1- and T$_H$2-associated cytokines, particularly IL-4 and IFN-γ. Thus, NKT cells are thought to play an important role in the early clearance of bacteria. NKT cells have also been suggested as one source of the IL-4 that polarizes the differentiation of naïve CD4$^+$ T cells toward the T$_H$2 subset. In addition, NKT cells are thought to play a key role in regulating many different immune responses; defects in NKT cells have been associated with diseases that include autoimmunity and cancer.

γδ T Cells

γδ **T cells**, the subset of T cells that use γδ rather than αβ as their two-chain antigen-recognizing TCR, are found predominantly at mucosal epithelial sites (such as the intestine, lungs, and uterus) as well as the skin (see Chapter 10). About 10% of intraepithelial lymphocytes scattered throughout the mucosal epithelium are γδ T cells, and in some parts of the lower intestine the proportion is even higher. Small numbers of γδ T cells can be found in blood and lymph nodes. γδ T cells have some features associated with the adaptive immune response (use of antigen-specific receptors) but have several properties associated with the innate immune response. They respond rapidly to pathogens such

as mycobacteria (within hours as opposed to within days for αβ T cells) by synthesizing cytokines—particularly IFN-γ and TNF—and have also been described to have cytotoxic function using mechanisms similar to those of CD8$^+$ T cell killing. γδ T cells do not generally respond to peptides associated with MHC molecules but do respond to phospholipids and other small nonprotein molecules, termed "phosphoantigens." They also can respond to heat-shock proteins produced when host cells are shocked or stressed. γδ T cells interact with these antigens presented either by CD1 or nonpolymorphic MHC class I molecules.

Innate Lymphoid Cells

Before leaving the topic of immune responses in mucosa, we mention a recently characterized set of cells known as **innate lymphoid cells** (ILCs). ILCs develop from hematopoietic stem cells but do not express markers of the lymphocyte lineage. They also do not express a TCR so they do not respond to antigen through an antigen-specific receptor. Three sets of ILCs have been defined, characterized by differences in expression of cell surface molecules and the cytokines they synthesize. ILCs produce many of the cytokines associated with different subsets of CD4$^+$ T cells, including IFN-γ, IL-5, IL-13, and IL-22.

ILCs are found predominantly at mucosal sites and play a role in protection against infectious agents. In addition, ILCs have also been implicated in the development of airway conditions such as allergy and asthma, and inflammatory conditions such as Crohn's disease that develop in other parts of the mucosa.

SUMMARY

1. Activation of a naïve CD4$^+$ or CD8$^+$ T cell requires two signals. The first signal is antigen-specific peptide + MHC molecule with the TCR; the second signal is provided by paired sets of co-stimulator molecules on the APC and T-cell surfaces.

2. The dendritic cell is the principal APC to activate naïve T cells. On interaction with a pathogen in tissues, immature dendritic cells upregulate MHC class II and co-stimulator molecules, migrate to the draining lymph node, and present peptides associated with MHC class II to CD4$^+$ T cells with the appropriate TCR.

3. The key APC–T cell interactions in T-cell activation are (a) peptide + MHC with the TCR; (b) co-receptor CD4 or CD8 with MHC class II or I, respectively; (c) co-stimulator pairs B7– CD28 and CD40–CD40

ligand; and (d) multiple pairs of adhesion molecules. These interactions are needed to sustain contact between the cells for several hours.

4. Activation of CD4$^+$ and CD8$^+$ T cells involves a cascade of events spreading from the area of contact between the APC and the T cell (the immunologic synapse) through the cytoplasm and into the nucleus. The critical pathways include phosphorylation of kinases, assembly and activation of signaling complexes at the cell membrane, activation of intracellular signaling pathways, and activation of multiple transcription factors that selectively activate the transcription of genes.

5. Among the most important genes transcribed and translated in the activated CD4$^+$ T cell are those coding for cytokines, particularly IL-2, and cytokine

receptors, including the α chain of the IL-2 receptor (CD25). Ultimately, activation results in the proliferation and expansion of the T-cell clone, differentiation to an effector T cell, and change in expression of homing molecules, allowing migration of the effector cell out of the node and to tissues or sites where pathogens have infiltrated.

6. As a consequence of activation by antigen, CD4$^+$ T cells secrete a vast array of cytokines that affect multiple cell types. Four major subsets of cytokine-synthesizing CD4$^+$ T cells have been defined: T$_H$1, T$_H$2, T$_H$17, and Treg. Each subset produces a characteristic pattern of signature cytokines that interacts with a unique set of effector cells. Each set of effector cells deals with a specific type of pathogen. They are distinguishable by a characteristic lineage-determining transcription factor. Cytokines synthesized by cells of the innate immune system influence the differentiation into a specific subset.

   • T$_H$1 cells synthesize IL-2 and IFN-γ, which activate the effector cells of cell-mediated immunity: macrophages, NK cells, and CD8$^+$ T cells, and so respond to intracellular pathogens such as viruses and bacteria.

   • T$_H$2 cells synthesize IL-4, IL-5, and IL-13, which activate the effector cells involved in responses to parasitic worms and allergens.

   • T$_H$17 cells synthesize IL-17 family cytokines, which induce proinflammatory responses by many different cell types, and IL-22. T$_H$17 cells respond to fungi and extracellular bacteria. They are also implicated in several auto-inflammatory conditions, including rheumatoid arthritis and multiple sclerosis.

   • Treg cells inhibit the function of the other subsets of CD4$^+$ T cells by cell contact and by the synthesis of inhibitory cytokines TGF-β and IL-10.

7. Cytokines produced by one subset of CD4$^+$ T cells in response to a specific antigen inhibit the development or function of other subsets and so skew the response toward one subset or another and hence one set of effector cells.

8. T follicular helper (T$_{FH}$) cells cooperate with B cells to develop into long-lived memory B cells and plasma cells in the germinal center response to thymus-dependent antigens. T–B cell cooperation involves cytokines produced by the T cell and interactions between pairs of molecules on the surface of the CD4$^+$ T cell and the B cell: an antigen-specific first signal (peptide–MHC class II expressed on the B cell with the TCR) and critical second or co-stimulator signals, which include CD40–CD40 ligand and ICOS-ICOS ligand.

   As a result of these interactions, the B cell undergoes class switch recombination to produce IgG, IgA, or IgE, and generates corresponding memory cells and long-lived plasma cells. Cytokines synthesized by T cells determine the isotype of the antibody synthesized by the B cell.

   A defect in one of the interacting co-stimulator pairs prevents class switch, and only IgM antibody is synthesized.

9. In the response to a thymus-dependent (TD) antigen, a CD4$^+$ T helper and a B-cell specific for the same antigen must interact to generate antibody. The epitopes recognized by the T helper and the B cells need to be part of the structure of the same antigen (linked recognition). This principle has been used to produce conjugate vaccines, in which protein linked to polysaccharide converts a thymus-independent (TI) IgM response to a TD class-switched response (IgG or IgA) that can confer long-lived protection.

10. CD8$^+$ T cells (CTL) interact with and kill target cells infected by microorganisms such as bacteria and viruses. The TCR of the CD8$^+$ T cell interacts with pathogen-derived peptide bound to an MHC class I molecule on the surface of the target cell.

    A CD8$^+$ T cell must be activated and differentiate to an effector before it kills its target. The CD8$^+$ T cell can be activated by different pathways. CD8$^+$ T cells kill target cells by inducing apoptosis in the target via two main pathways: (1) action of cytotoxic materials contained in granules inside the CD8$^+$ T cell and secreted into the target cell, and (2) interaction of Fas expressed on the target, with FasL expressed on the CD8$^+$ T cell.

11. In addition to CD4$^+$ and CD8$^+$ T cells, other subsets of cells such as γδ T, NKT, and innate lymphoid cells play a role in immune responses, particularly at mucosal surfaces.

REFERENCES AND BIBLIOGRAPHY

Bendelac A, Savage PB, Teyton L. (2007) The biology of NKT cells. *Annu Rev Immunol* 25: 297.

Billadeau DD, Nolz JC, Gomez TS. (2007) Regulation of T cell activation by the cytoskeleton. *Nat Rev Immunol* 7: 131.

Chen L, Flies DB. (2013) Molecular mechanisms of T cell co-stimulation and co-inhibition. *Nat Rev Immunol* 13: 227.

Crotty S. (2011). Follicular helper CD4 T cells (TFH). *Annu Rev Immunol* 29: 621.

Hashimoto D, Miller J, Merad M. (2011) Dendritic cell and macrophage heterogeneity in vivo. *Immunity* 35: 323.

Krummel MF. (2007) Testing the organization of the immunological synapse. *Curr Opin Immunol* 19: 460.

Ma CS, Deenick EK, Batten M, Tangye SG. (2012) The origins, function, and regulation of T follicular helper cells. *J Exp Med* 209: 1241.

Vantourout P, Hayday A. (2013) Six-of-the-best: unique contributions of γδ T cells to immunology. *Nat Rev Immunol* 13: 88.

Walker JA, Barlow JL, McKenzie AN. (2013) Innate lymphoid cells–how did we miss them? *Nat Rev Immunol* 13: 75.

Weaver CT, Hatton RD, Mangan PR, Harrington LE. (2007) IL-17 family cytokines and the expanding diversity of effector cell lineages. *Annu Rev Immunol* 25: 821.

Zhang N, Bevan MJ. (2011) CD8$^+$ T cells: foot soldiers of the immune system. *Immunity*. 35: 161.

REVIEW QUESTIONS

For each question, choose the ONE BEST answer or completion.

1. The role of the APC in the immune response is all of the following *except*:
   A) the limited catabolism of polypeptide antigens
   B) to allow selective association of MHC gene products and peptides
   C) to supply second signals required to fully activate T cells
   D) to present nonself-peptides associated with MHC class I molecules to CD4$^+$ T cells
   E) to present peptide–MHC complexes to T cells with the appropriate receptor

2. Which of the following statements about IL-2 is *incorrect*?
   A) It is produced primarily by activated macrophages.
   B) It is produced by CD4$^+$ T cells.
   C) It can induce the proliferation of CD4$^+$ T cells.
   D) It binds to a specific receptor on CD4$^+$ T cells.
   E) It can activate CD8$^+$ T cells in the presence of antigen.

3. Which of the following pairs of cell surface proteins do NOT interact with each other?
   A) MHC class II and CD4
   B) ICAM-1 (CD54) and LFA-1 (CD11a/CD18)
   C) B7 (CD80 and CD86) and CD28
   D) CD40 and CD40 ligand (CD154)
   E) membrane Ig on the B cell and CD4 on the T cell

4. Which of the following statements about the activation of CD4$^+$ T cells is *incorrect*?
   A) Activation results in rapid phosphorylation of tyrosine residues in proteins associated with the TCR.
   B) Intracellular calcium levels rise rapidly following activation.

C) The interaction between peptide–MHC class II on an APC and the TCR of an appropriate CD4$^+$ T cell is necessary and sufficient for full T-cell activation.
   D) Interaction of B7 and CD28 stabilizes IL-2 mRNA so that effective IL-2 translation occurs.
   E) The activated cell synthesizes IL-2 and a receptor for IL-2.

5. Which of the following statements about cytokines and subsets of CD4$^+$ T cells is *incorrect*?
   A) T$_H$1 cells secrete cytokines that induce macrophage and NK-cell activation.
   B) Cytokines produced by T$_H$2 cells are important in allergic responses.
   C) The presence of IL-12 during the activation and differentiation of CD4$^+$ T cells favors the development of T$_H$1 cells.
   D) Cytokines synthesized by T$_H$1 and T$_H$2 cells inhibit the action of Treg cells.
   E) Cytokines synthesized by T$_H$1 and T$_H$2 cells inhibit the action of T$_H$17 cells.

6. Which of the following statements about CD8$^+$ CTL is *incorrect*?
   A) They lyse targets via perforin and granzymes.
   B) They cause target cell apoptosis.
   C) They cannot kill CD4$^+$ T cells.
   D) They interact with their target through paired cell surface molecules.
   E) They must be activated before exerting their cytotoxic function.

7. Infection with vaccinia virus results in the priming of virus-specific CD8$^+$ T cells. If these vaccinia virus-specific CD8$^+$ T cells are subsequently removed from the individual, which of the following cells will they kill *in vitro*?

A) vaccinia-infected cells expressing MHC class II molecules from any individual
B) influenza-infected cells expressing the same MHC class I molecules as the individual
C) uninfected cells expressing the same MHC class I molecules as the individual

D) vaccinia-infected cells expressing the same MHC class I molecules as the individual
E) vaccinia-infected cells expressing the same MHC class II molecules as the individual

ANSWERS TO REVIEW QUESTIONS

1. D. The APC presents peptide–MHC class I to CD8$^+$ T cells and peptide–MHC class II to CD4$^+$ T cells. The other statements are all features of an APC such as a dendritic cell.

2. A. IL-2 is produced almost exclusively by activated T cells.

3. E. The pairs of molecules in answers A–D are all important in adhesion and/or co-stimulation for T cells with B cells and other APCs; it is not thought that Ig interacts with CD4.

4. C. Peptide–MHC class II interacting with the TCR is the critical, antigen-specific first signal required for CD4$^+$ T-cell activation, but co-stimulatory or second signals are required for full activation.

5. D. Cytokines synthesized by Treg cells inhibit the action of T_H1 and T_H2 cells but not vice versa.

6. C. A CD8$^+$ CTL can kill any cell expressing an MHC class 1 molecule in association with a nonself-peptide, including, for example, a CD4$^+$ T cell infected with HIV.

7. D. The principle of MHC restriction indicates that the TCR of CD8$^+$ T cells interacts with target cells that express specific peptide bound to self-MHC class I molecules. Thus, vaccinia-primed CD8$^+$ T cells recognize and hence kill only vaccinia-infected targets that express self-MHC class I.

12

CYTOKINES

INTRODUCTION

As we have already discussed, the immune system is regulated by soluble mediators collectively called *cytokines*. These low-molecular-weight proteins are produced by virtually all cells of the innate and adaptive immune systems and, in particular, by T cells, which orchestrate many effector mechanisms. Some cytokines possess direct effector functions of their own. A simple way to understand how cytokines work is to compare them with hormones, the chemical messengers of the endocrine system. Cytokines serve as chemical messengers within the immune system, although they also communicate with cells in other systems, including those of the nervous system. Thus, they can function in an integrated fashion to facilitate homeostasis. By contrast, they also play a significant role in driving hypersensitivity and inflammatory responses, and in some cases they can promote acute or chronic distress in tissues and organ systems.

As we will discuss later in this chapter, cells regulated by a particular cytokine must express a receptor for that factor. Cells are positively and/or negatively regulated by the quantity and type of cytokines to which they are exposed and by the expression or downregulation of cytokine receptors. Normal regulation of innate and adaptive immune responses is largely controlled by a combination of these methods.

THE HISTORY OF CYTOKINES

In the late 1960s, when the activities of cytokines were first discovered, it was believed that they served as amplification factors that acted in an antigen-dependent fashion to elevate proliferative responses of T cells. Gery and colleagues were the first to demonstrate that macrophages released a thymocyte mitogenic factor termed *lymphocyte activating factor* (LAF). This view changed radically when it was found that supernatants of mitogen-stimulated peripheral blood mononuclear cells promoted the long-term proliferation of T cells in the absence of antigens and mitogens. Soon afterward, it was found that this factor was produced by T cells and could be used to isolate and clonally expand functional T cell lines. This T-cell-derived factor was given several names by different investigators, most notably, T-cell growth factor (TCGF). *Cytokines* produced by lymphocytes were collectively called *lymphokines*, whereas those produced by monocytes and macrophages were called *monokines*. To complicate matters, studies of the cellular sources of lymphokines and monokines ultimately revealed that these factors were not the exclusive products of lymphocytes and monocytes/macrophages. Thus, the more appropriate term *cytokine* was adopted as a generic name for these glycoprotein mediators. In 1979, an international workshop was convened to address the need to develop a consensus regarding the definition of these macrophage- and T-cell-derived

Immunology: A Short Course, Seventh Edition. Richard Coico and Geoffrey Sunshine.
© 2015 John Wiley & Sons, Ltd. Published 2015 by John Wiley & Sons, Ltd.
Companion Website: www.wileyimmunology.com/coico

factors. Since they mediated signals between leukocytes, the term *interleukin* was coined. The macrophage-derived LAF and T-cell-derived growth factors were given the names interleukin-1 (IL-1) and interleukin-2 (IL-2), respectively. Currently, numbers have been assigned to more than 40 interleukins, and this will undoubtedly continue to grow as research efforts continue to identify new members of this cytokine family. To further illustrate the degree to which the cytokine field has outgrown the terminology established in 1979, knowledge of the functional properties of various cytokines has engendered a more liberal meaning of terms originally designed to define what a given factor does.

Pleiotropic and Redundant Properties of Cytokines

It is well known that many cytokines have important biologic effects on cell types other than those of the immune system. Thus, cytokines commonly have *pleiotropic properties*, since they can affect the activity of many different cell types. For example, the development and differentiation of bone-forming cells known as osteoblasts is regulated by a host of different cytokines. IL-2 produced by activated T lymphocytes also drives differentiation of human bone marrow stromal cells toward an osteoblastic phenotype. In contrast, tumor necrosis factor (TNF)-α inhibits the differentiation of osteoblasts and has been shown to be proapoptotic for these cells. IL-4 and IL-13 suppress osteoblast prostaglandin synthesis in bone and are chemoattractants for these cells.

Cytokines are also linked to human diseases that involve bone. Perhaps the most extensive studies have been on the role of cytokines in the development of osteolytic lesions sometimes observed in severe rheumatoid arthritis (RA) and other inflammatory bone diseases, including periodontal disease. A hallmark of RA is the rapid erosion of periarticular bone, which is often followed by general secondary osteoporosis (osteopenia).

Knowledge regarding such intersystem crosstalk will no doubt contribute to our understanding of how the immune system regulates cells in other systems in a physiologic context, both at the molecular level and at the level of organ systems. In the case of bone formation, this will lead to better treatments for human diseases involving both systems, including various inflammatory and metabolic bone diseases, as well as tumor-induced bone lysis.

In addition to their pleiotropic properties, there is a great deal of *functional redundancy* among cytokines. This redundancy is explained, in part, by the common use of cytokine receptor signaling subunits (e.g., common γ chain used by receptors for IL-2, IL-4, IL-7, IL-9, and IL-15) by certain groups of cytokines discussed later in this chapter. Finally, cytokines rarely, if ever, act alone *in vivo*. Under physiologic and, in some cases, pathophysiologic conditions, cells responding to cytokines do so within a milieu containing multiple cytokines, which often exhibit *additive*, *synergistic*, or *antagonistic properties*. In the case of synergism, the combined effect of two or more cytokines is sometimes greater than the additive effects of the individual cytokines. Conversely, antagonism occurs when one or more cytokines inhibit the biologic activity of one or more other cytokines.

The convenient nomenclature originally developed to define the origin or the functional activities of certain cytokines has, in general, not held up. Nevertheless, occasionally, the field recognizes that common functional features of several glycoproteins merit the creation of yet another collective term to help define a family of cytokines. In particular, the term *chemokines* was adopted in 1992 to describe a family of *chemotactic cytokines* with conserved sequences, known to be potent attractors for various leukocyte subsets, such as lymphocytes, neutrophils, and monocytes. As students of immunology, learning about the rapidly expanding list of cytokines with diverse functional characteristics may appear to be a formidable task. However, by focusing on some that deserve special mention, we hope that this will be interesting and manageable exercise.

GENERAL PROPERTIES OF CYTOKINES

Common Functional Properties

Cytokines have several functional features in common. Some, like interferon-γ (IFN-γ) and IL-2, are synthesized by cells and rapidly secreted. Others such as TNF-α and TNF-β may be secreted or expressed as membrane-associated proteins. Most cytokines have very short half-lives; consequently, cytokine synthesis and function typically occur in a burst.

Similar to the actions of polypeptide hormones, cytokines facilitate communication between cells and do so at very low concentrations (typically 10^{-10} to 10^{-15}M). Cytokines may act locally either on the same cell that secreted it (*autocrine*), on other nearby cells (*paracrine*), or, like hormones, they may act systemically (*endocrine*) (Figure 12.1). In common with other polypeptide hormones, cytokines exert their functional effects by binding to specific receptors on target cells. Thus, cells regulated by specific cytokines must have the capacity to express a receptor for that factor. In turn, the activity of a responder cell may be regulated by the quantity and type of cytokines to which they are exposed or by the upregulation or downregulation of cytokine receptors, which, themselves, may be regulated by other cytokines. A good example of the latter is the ability of IL-1 to upregulate IL-2 receptors on T cells. As noted earlier, this illustrates one common feature of cytokines, namely, their ability to act in concert with one another to create synergistic effects that reinforce the other's action on a single cell.

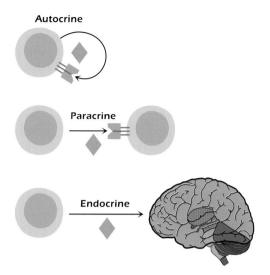

Figure 12.1. Autocrine, paracrine, and endocrine properties of cytokines. The brain is illustrated as an example of an organ that responds to cytokines in an endocrine fashion.

Alternatively, some cytokines behave antagonistically toward one or more other cytokines and thus inhibit each other's action on a given cell. The T_H1 and T_H2 lineage choices have become pivotal examples for the regulation (positive or negative) of cell differentiation. T_H1 and T_H2 cells are characterized by distinct cytokine profiles and transcription factor expression (discussed later in this chapter), and also by the types of pathogens they control. Perhaps the classic example of differential cytokine expression by T_H1 and T_H2 cells is the ability of T_H1 cells to produce high levels of the effector cytokine IFN-γ as compared with T_H2 cells, which produce IL-4, and, in some cases, IL-10. IFN-γ activates macrophages but inhibits B cells and is directly toxic for certain cells. In contrast, IL-4 activates B cells, and IL-10 inhibits macrophage activation and suppresses allergic inflammation (Figure 12.2). T_H2 cells that express IL-10 have been termed ***inflammatory T_H2 cells*** to distinguish them from canonical noninflammatory T_H2 cells. Additional information regarding T_H1 and T_H2 transcription factor profiles and how they have evolved to protect the host against a spectrum of pathogens is provided in Chapters 10 and 21, respectively.

When cells produce cytokines in response to various stimuli (e.g., infectious agents), they establish a concentration gradient that serves to control or direct cell migration patterns, also known as ***chemotaxis*** (Figure 12.3). Cell migration (e.g., neutrophil chemotaxis) is essential to the development of inflammatory responses resulting from localized injury or other trauma. Chemokines play a key role in providing signals that upregulate expression of adhesion molecules expressed on endothelial cells to facilitate neutrophil chemotaxis and transendothelial migration.

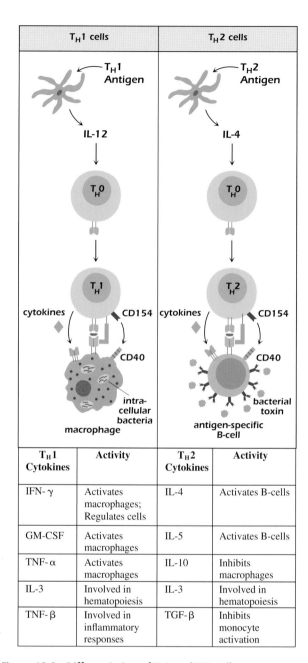

T_H1 Cytokines	Activity	T_H2 Cytokines	Activity
IFN-γ	Activates macrophages; Regulates cells	IL-4	Activates B-cells
GM-CSF	Activates macrophages	IL-5	Activates B-cells
TNF-α	Activates macrophages	IL-10	Inhibits macrophages
IL-3	Involved in hematopoiesis	IL-3	Involved in hematopoiesis
TNF-β	Involved in inflammatory responses	TGF-β	Inhibits monocyte activation

Figure 12.2. Differentiation of T_H1 and T_H2 cells.

Common Systemic Activities

Cytokines can act over both short range and long range, with consequent systemic effects. Cytokines thus play a crucial role in the amplification of the immune response because the release of cytokines from just a few antigen-activated cells results in the activation of multiple different cell types, which are not necessarily antigen specific or located in the immediate area. This is apparent in a response such as delayed-type hypersensitivity, discussed in detail in Chapter 17, in which the activation of rare antigen-specific T cells is accompanied by the release of cytokines. As a consequence of cytokine effects, monocytes are recruited into the

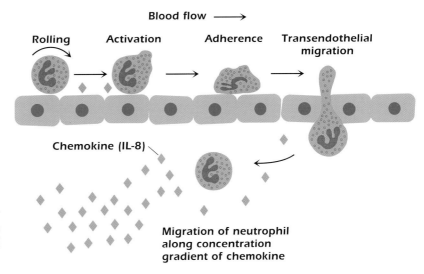

Figure 12.3. Steps involved in neutrophil chemotaxis and transendothelial migration showing reversible binding followed by activation, adherence, and movement between the endothelial cells forming the wall of the blood vessel (extravasation).

area in great numbers, dwarfing the original antigen-activated T-cell population. It is also worth noting that the production of high levels of cytokines by a powerful stimulus can trigger deleterious systemic effects, such as toxic-shock syndrome, as discussed later in this chapter. Similarly, therapeutic manipulation of the immune system using recombinant cytokines or cytokine antagonists can affect multiple physiologic systems depending on the range of biologic activity associated with a particular cytokine.

Common Cell Sources and Cascading Events

A given cell may make many different cytokines. Moreover, one cell may be the target of many cytokines, each binding to its own specific cell-surface receptor. Consequently, one cytokine may affect the action of another, which may lead to an additive, synergistic, or antagonistic effect on the target cell.

Interactions of the multiple cytokines produced during a typical immune response are often referred to as the *cytokine cascade*. This cascade largely determines whether a response to an antigen will be primarily antibody-mediated (and, if so, which classes of antibodies will be made) or cell-mediated (and, if so, whether cells engaged in delayed hypersensitivity or cytotoxicity will be activated). Later in this chapter, we will discuss the cytokine-mediated control mechanisms that help determine the pattern of cytokines that develop following CD4$^+$ T-cell activation. The antigenic stimulus appears to play a key role in the initiation of cytokine responses by these cells. Thus, depending on the nature of the antigenic signal, and the cytokine milieu associated with T-cell activation, naïve effector CD4$^+$ T cells will generate a particular cytokine profile, one that ultimately controls the type of immune response generated (humoral versus cellular). The cytokine cascade associated with immune responses also determines what other systems

are activated or suppressed, as well as the level and duration of the response.

FUNCTIONAL CATEGORIES OF CYTOKINES

We will not attempt to list all of the currently well-characterized and molecularly cloned cytokines in this chapter. The major cytokines that play a role in the immune response and a brief description of their functions are listed in Table 12.1. A convenient way to begin is to classify cytokines into the functional categories discussed below based on shared functional properties. It is important to state that this subdivision, although convenient, is somewhat arbitrary, given the pleiotropic effects of many cytokines.

Cytokines That Facilitate Innate Immune Responses

Several cytokines facilitate innate immune responses stimulated by viruses and microbial pathogens. Included in this group are ***IL-1***, ***IL-6***, ***TNF-α***, ***interferon-α*** (IFN-α), and ***IFN-β***. IL-1, IL-6, and TNF-α initiate a wide spectrum of biologic activities that help coordinate the host's responses to infection. They are produced largely by phagocytes (e.g., macrophages and neutrophils) and are termed ***endogenous pyrogens*** because they cause fever. Elevated body temperature is beneficial to host defenses because adaptive immune responses are more intense and most pathogens grow less efficiently at raised temperatures. Another important effect of IL-1, IL-6, and TNF-α is their initiation of a response known as the ***acute-phase response*** characterized by production of ***acute-phase proteins*** by hepatocytes. As discussed below, acute inflammation (e.g., in response to infections) is generally accompanied by a systemic

TABLE 12.1. Selected Cytokines and Their Functions

Cytokine	Produced By	Major Functions
IL-1	Monocytes; many other cell types	Produces fever; stimulates acute-phase protein synthesis; promotes proliferation of T_H2 cells
IL-2	T_H0 and T_H1 cells	T-cell growth factor
IL-3	T_H cells, NK cells, mast cells	Growth factor for hematopoietic cells
IL-4	T_H2, $CD4^+$ T cells, mast cells	Growth factor for B cells and T_H2 $CD4^+$ T cells; promotes IgE and IgG synthesis; inhibits T_H1 $CD4^+$ T cells
IL-5	T_H2 cells, mast cells	Stimulates B-cell growth and Ig secretion; growth and differentiation factor eosinophils
IL-6	T cells, many other cell types	Induces acute-phase protein synthesis, T-cell activation, and IL-2 production; stimulates B-cell Ig production and hematopoietic progenitor cell growth
IL-7	Bone marrow, thymic stromal cells, some T cells	Growth factor for pre-T and pre-B cells
IL-9	T cells	Mast cell activation
IL-10	T_H2 cells, macrophages	Inhibits production of T_H1 cells and macrophage function
IL-11	Fibroblasts	Stimulates megakaryocyte (platelet precursor) growth
IL-12	B cells and macrophages	Activates NK cells and promotes generation of T_H1 $CD4^+$ T cells
IL-13	T cells	Shares characteristics with IL-4 (e.g., Ig switch to IgE synthesis) but does not affect T cells; growth factor for human B cells
IL-14	T cells	Involved in development of memory B cells
IL-15	T cells and epithelial cells	T-cell growth factor; similar to IL-2
IL-16	T cells, eosinophils, mast cells	Chemotactic for T cells; proinflammatory
IL-17 family (IL-17A-F)	T cells (T_H17 lineage)	Proinflammatory cytokine, promotes neutrophil migration and differentiation, plays decisive role in autoimmunity and immune-mediated tissue damage
IL-18	Macrophages, monocytes, dendritic cells, many other cell types	Induces IFN-γ production; enhances NK-cell lytic activity
IL-23	Activated dendritic cells	Acts on memory T cells to stimulate IL-17 secretion
IFN-γ	T_H1 cells	Activates NK cells and macrophages; inhibits T_H2 $CD4^+$ T cells; induces expression of MHC class II on many cell types
TGF-β	Lymphocytes, macrophages, platelets, mast cells	Enhances production of IgA; inhibits activation of monocyte and T-cell subsets; active in fibroblast growth and wound healing
TNF-α	Macrophages, mast cells	Involved in inflammatory responses; activates endothelial cells and other cells of immune and nonimmune systems; induces fever and septic shock
TNF-β (lymphotoxin)	T cells	Involved in inflammatory responses; also plays role in killing target cells by cytotoxic $CD8^+$ T cells
GM-CSF	T cells, monocytes	Promotes growth of granulocytes and macrophages; growth of dendritic cells *in vitro*
M-CSF	T cells, monocytes	Promotes macrophage growth
G-CSF	T cells, monocytes	Promotes granulocyte growth

acute-phase response. Typically, changes in acute-phase protein plasma levels occur within 2 days following infection. One of these proteins, **C-reactive protein** (CRP), binds to phosphorylcholine on bacterial surfaces, acts like an opsonin and also activates the classical complement pathway

(Chapter 14). Another acute-phase protein with opsonin and complement-activating activity is ***mannan-binding lectin*** (MBL), which binds mannose residues accessible on many bacteria. Given these functional properties, they mimic the actions of antibodies, which opsonize bacteria and activate the complement cascade. In concert with the other members of the acute-phase protein family, CRP and MBL lead to bacterial clearance.

Another effect of the endogenous pyrogens is to induce an increase in circulating neutrophils that are summoned from the bone marrow and from the blood vessels where leukocytes attach loosely to endothelial cells. Finally, dendritic cells from peripheral tissues migrate to the lymph nodes in response to these cytokines. There, they serve as potent antigen-presenting cells (APCs) to facilitate adaptive immune responses needed to control infections.

The term *interferon* was coined because they interfere with viral replication thus blocking the spread of viruses to uninfected cells. *Interferon-α* (IFN-α) and *interferon-β* (IFN-β) (so-called type I interferons) are synthesized by many cell types following viral infection. Plasmacytoid dendritic cells (DCs) have been identified as being the most potent producers of type I IFNs in response to antigen and have thus been coined natural IFN-producing cells. They are distinguished from another glycoprotein called interferon-γ (the sole member of type II IFNs), which is produced by activated natural killer (NK) cells and effector T cells, and thus appear after the induction of adaptive immune responses. In addition to their antiviral activities, IFN-α and IFN-β induce increased MHC class I expression on most uninfected cells, thus enhancing their resistance to NK cells as well as making newly infected cells more susceptible to killing by CD8$^+$ cytotoxic T cells. Finally, they activate NK cells, which contribute to early host responses to viral infections.

Cytokines That Regulate Adaptive Immune Responses

As discussed in Chapter 11, B- and T-cell activation in response to antigen stimulation is regulated by cytokines. Depending on the cytokines involved, regulation can be positive or negative and can impact cell proliferation, activation, and differentiation. Ultimately, cytokines regulate the intensity and duration of immune responses. A major feature of all adaptive immune responses is their antigen specificity. Given the potent immunoregulatory activities of cytokines, how does the immune system ensure that antigen-nonspecific B and T cells are not activated during an immune response? One mechanism to ensure the specificity of the immune response is through the selective expression of functional cytokine receptors only on lymphocytes that have been stimulated by antigen. As a consequence, cytokines tend to act only on antigen-activated lymphocytes. A second mechanism that protects antigen-nonspecific lymphocytes from being activated by cytokines involves the need for cells to interact with each other through cell-to-cell contact, also known as *cognate* interaction. Such interactions that might occur, say, between CD4$^+$ helper T cells and APCs (e.g., DCs, macrophages, B cells), generate high concentrations

of cytokines at the juncture between the interacting cells. In this way, only the target cell(s) participating in the interaction are affected by the cytokines produced. Finally, since the half-life of cytokines is very short, particularly in the bloodstream and extracellular spaces, they have a very limited period to act on other target cells.

Cytokines That Induce Differentiation of Distinct T-Cell Lineages

T$_H$1 and T$_H$2 Cell Lineages. It is now clear that certain cytokines play a key role in determining the fate of naïve T cells by staging the signaling events involved in lineage-specific differentiation. As discussed in earlier chapters, activated naïve CD4$^+$ T cells (T$_H$0 cells) differentiate into T$_H$1 cells under the influence of IL-12 produced by DCs and macrophages in the skin and mucosa (Figure 12.2). Numerous studies illustrate the importance of this pathway by establishing that IL-12 is required for the development of protective innate and adaptive responses to many intracellular pathogens. Given the central role of this factor in the development of cell-mediated immunity, it is not surprising that IL-12 has also been implicated in the development of various autoimmune inflammatory conditions. The advent of bioinformatics tools and protein sequence databases led to the discovery of two IL-12-related cytokines that had already been named as IL-23 and IL-27. Together, these cytokines constitute the IL-12 family of cytokines. As we shall see in the sections that follow, these discoveries have given us a much deeper understanding of how our immune system responds to pathogenic challenges.

In contrast with T$_H$1-cell differentiation, polarization of the differentiation of naïve CD4$^+$ T cells toward the T$_H$2 pathway is promoted by IL-4 produced by DCs and other innate cell populations (e.g., mast cells) (see Figure 12.2). The type of antigen initiating the DC response appears to be a key factor in determining whether an IL-12 or IL-4 response will occur, and, hence, whether the T$_H$1 or T$_H$2 lineage will develop, respectively. For example, intracellular bacteria (e.g., *Listeria*) and viruses activate DCs, macrophages, and NK cells to produce IL-12. In the presence of this cytokine, T$_H$0 cells tend to develop into T$_H$1 cells. The complex cell signaling and transcriptional events controlling these phenomena are beginning to emerge. Following activation, naïve CD4 T cells differentiate toward T$_H$1 in the presence of IL-12, which upregulates IFNγ via Stat4, leading to IFNγ-mediated Stat1 activation and induction of the T$_H$1 lineage-determining transcription factor Tbet. By contrast, other pathogens (e.g., parasitic worms) do not induce IL-12 production but instead cause release of IL-4 by other cells (e.g., mast cells). IL-4 tends to promote the development of T$_H$0 cells into T$_H$2 cells as a result of its ability to activate Stat6, resulting in induction of the transcription factor known as GATA3. GATA3 expression results in chromatin remodeling at the Th2 cytokine gene loci leading to the signature cytokine profile associated with the Th2 lineage.

The section that follows introduces a recently identified group of related cytokines (members of the IL-17 family). Their discovery preceded the identification of a new T-cell lineage that is a major cellular source of the IL-17 family of cytokines, namely, the T_H17 T-cell lineage. Taken together, these discoveries have provided new fundamental insights into the developmental pathways that promote the differentiation and function of CD4$^+$ T helper cells.

The T_H17 T-Cell Lineage. The T_H1 and T_H2 paradigm provided a framework for understanding T-cell biology and the interplay of innate and adaptive immunity. It is widely held that T_H1 or T_H2 immunity evolved to enhance clearance of intracellular pathogens and parasitic helminthes, respectively. What about T-cell responses to extracellular pathogens and fungi? The answer emerged recently, in part, with the discovery of the IL-17 family of cytokines and the subsequent discovery of a lineage of IL-17-producing T cells aptly called *T_H17 cells*. T_H17 cells appear to have evolved as an arm of the adaptive immune system specialized for enhanced host protection against extracellular bacteria and some fungi, microbes probably not well covered by T_H1 or T_H2 immunity.

The IL-17 family of cytokines includes IL-17A, B, C, D, E, and F (Table 12.2). IL-17A was the name given to the founding member of the family. Because IL-17E had already been independently identified and given the name IL-25, that designation is commonly used instead. As a family, they share similar structural motifs and contain an unusual pattern of intrachain disulfide bonds.

The roles played by T_H17 cells and the IL-17 family of cytokines in host defense against pathogens are only beginning to emerge. IL-17 stimulates the mobilization and *de novo* generation of neutrophils by granulocyte-colony stimulating factor (G-CSF), thereby bridging innate and adaptive immunity. It has been suggested that this might constitute an early defense mechanism against severe trauma that would result in tissue necrosis or sepsis. Interestingly, we know less about their physiologic roles than we do regarding the pathologies in which they have been implicated. As discussed later in this chapter, IL-17 cytokines are key mediators in a diverse range of autoinflammatory disorders. The identification of T_H17 cells as the principal pathogenic effectors in several types of autoimmunity previously thought to be T_H1-mediated promises new approaches for therapies of these disorders, as does identification of IL-25 as a potentially important mediator of dysregulated T_H2 responses that cause asthma and other allergic disorders.

T_H17 cells differentiate from naïve CD4$^+$ T cells in response to IL-6 and TGF-β. Signaling via IL-6 activates Stat3 and the lineage-determining transcription factor RORγt. The precise role of TGF-β in this differentiation process is not well understood although it is known that T cells defective in TGF-β receptor signaling cannot differentiate to T_H17 cells.

Cytokines That Inhibit Lineage-Specific T-Cell Differentiation

T_H1 and T_H2 subsets can also regulate the growth and effector functions of each other. This phenomenon occurs as a result of the activity of cytokines produced by the subset that is being activated and whose apparent purpose it is to make it difficult to shift the response to the other subset. For example, production of IL-10 and TGF-β by T_H2 cells inhibits activation and growth of T_H1 cells. Similarly, production of IFN-γ by T_H1 cells inhibits proliferation of T_H2 cells. These effects permit either subset to dominate a particular immune response by inhibiting the outgrowth of the other subset.

As noted above, the T_H17 T-cell subset develops in response to IL-6 and TGF-β. This differentiation step is strongly inhibited by T_H1 or T_H2 cytokines. IL-27 is also a negative regulator of T_H17 differentiation. Interestingly, in the absence of IL-6, naïve T cells exposed only to TGF-β differentiate into regulatory T cells (Treg).

TABLE 12.2. The IL-17 Family of Cytokines

Family Member	Alternate Names	Predicted Molecular Weight (kDa)	% Homology With IL-17A	% Homology With Human	Cellular and Tissue Sources
IL-17A	IL-17 CTLA-8	35	100	62	T_H17 cells, CD8 T cells, NK cells, $\gamma\delta$ T cells, neutrophils
IL-17B	CX1 NERF	41	21	88	Pancreas, small intestine, stomach
IL-17C	CX2	43	24	75	Thymus, spleen, testes, prostate
IL-17D	IL-27	45	16	82	Skeletal muscle, neuronal cells, prostate
IL-17E	IL-25	38	16	76	T_H2 cells, eosinophils, mast cells
IL-17F	ML-1	34	45	54	T_H17 cells, CD8 T cells, NK cells, $\gamma\delta$ T cells, neutrophils

Cytokines That Promote Inflammatory Responses

Many cytokines activate the functions of inflammatory cells and are therefore known as ***proinflammatory cytokines***. Examples of proinflammatory cytokines include IL-1, IL-6, IL-10, IL-23, and TNF-α. During localized acute inflammatory responses, they cause increased vascular permeability, which ultimately leads to the swelling and redness associated with inflammation. As inflammatory mediators, they act in concert with the chemokines to ensure the development of physiologic responses to a variety of stimuli such as infections and tissue injury. Acute inflammatory responses develop rapidly and are of short duration. This short time course is probably related to the short half-lives of the inflammatory mediators involved as well as the regulatory influence of cytokines such as TGF-β, which limits the inflammatory response (see below). Typically, systemic responses accompany these short-lived responses and are characterized by a rapid alteration in levels of acute-phase proteins (see above). Sometimes, persistent immune activation can occur (e.g., in chronic infections), leading to chronic inflammation, which subverts the physiologic value of inflammatory responses and causes pathologic consequences.

The neutrophil plays a key role in the early stages of inflammatory responses (see Figure 12.3). Neutrophils infiltrate within a few hours into the tissue area where the inflammatory response is occurring. Their migration from the blood to the tissue site is controlled by the expression of adhesion molecules by vascular endothelial cells—a mechanism regulated by mediators of acute inflammation including IL-1 and TNF-α. Following exposure to these cytokines, vascular endothelial cells increase their expression of adhesion molecules (e.g., E- and P-selectin, ICAM-1), which, in turn, bind to selectin ligands (e.g., sialyl Lewis moiety) expressed on the surface of neutrophils. The neutrophils attach securely to the endothelial cells and undergo a process of end-over-end rolling. Chemokines also activate the neutrophil causing a conformational change in their membrane integrin molecules. Figure 12.4 shows a schematic illustration of the conformational change in the heterodimeric (α and β chain) integrin molecule, LFA-1, which allows it to ligate ICAM-1. This change increases the affinity of neutrophils for the adhesion molecules on the endothelium. Finally, the neutrophil undergoes transendothelial migration, resulting in extravasation of the neutrophil, which continues its journey to the damaged or infected tissue site under the directional influence of chemokines, a process known as ***chemotaxis***. It should be noted that lymphocytes and monocytes also undergo extravasation using the same basic steps as the neutrophil, although different combinations of adhesion molecules are involved.

Other cytokines that play a significant role in inflammatory responses include IFN-γ and TGF-β. In addition to its role in activating macrophages to increase their phagocytic activity, IFN-γ has been shown to chemotactically attract macrophages to the site where antigen is localized. The migration of all of these cell types, including neutrophils, lymphocytes, monocytes, macrophages, as well as eosinophils and basophils, which are attracted to the site of tissue damage by complement activation, leads to clearance of the antigen and healing of the tissue. TGF-β plays a role in terminating the inflammatory response by promoting the accumulation and proliferation of fibroblasts and the deposition of extracellular matrix proteins required for tissue repair.

Cytokines That Affect Leukocyte Movement

The term ***chemokine*** is used to denote a family of closely related, low-molecular-weight chemotactic cytokines containing 70–80 residues with conserved sequences and known to be potent attractors for various leukocyte subsets, such as neutrophils, monocytes, and lymphocytes. Table 12.3 lists

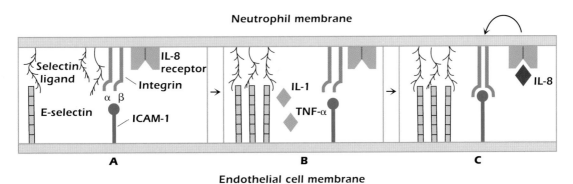

Figure 12.4. Cell membrane adhesion molecules and cytokine activation events associated with neutrophil transendothelial migration. Left: Weak binding of selectin ligands on the neutrophil to E-selectin on the endothelial cells. Middle: IL-1 and TNF-α upregulation of E-selectin, which facilitates stronger binding. Right: The activation effects of IL-8 on neutrophils, which causes a conformational change in the integrins (e.g., LFA-1) to allow them to bind ICAM-1.

some of the important chemokines among the 40 that have been identified. Structurally, this large superfamily consists of four subfamilies that display one of four highly conserved NH_2-terminal cysteine amino acid residues as follows: CXC, CC, C, or CX3C, where X represents a nonconserved amino acid residue. Most chemokines fall into the CXC and CC groups. As discussed above, chemokines function in concert with inflammatory mediators to regulate the expression and conformation of cell adhesion molecules in leukocyte membranes. Some cytokines have also been shown to induce respiratory burst, enzyme release, intracellular Ca^{2+} mobilization, and angiogenesis. The latter functional property of some chemokines is a biologic feature consistent with the important role they play in wound healing and tissue repair. Production of chemokines may either be induced or constitutive. Those whose production is inducible or strongly upregulatable in peripheral tissues by inflammation are primarily involved in wound healing and tissue repair mechanisms. By contrast, constitutively produced chemokines fulfill housekeeping functions and may be involved in normal leukocyte traffic.

Among the more than 50 chemokines that have been identified to date, IL-8, a member of the CXC subfamily, is among the most well characterized. It is produced by many different cell types including macrophages, T cells, endothelial cells, fibroblasts, and neutrophils, and plays a major role in inflammatory responses and wound healing mainly due to its ability to attract neutrophils to sites of tissue damage. Another important function of IL-8 is its ability to activate neutrophils following their attachment to vascular endothelium (Figure 12.3).

A noteworthy characteristic of certain CC chemokines (e.g., RANTES, MIP-1α, and MIP-1β) is their ability to suppress infection of T cells *in vitro* with M-trophic human immunodeficiency virus (HIV) strains. These strains of HIV were originally so-named because of their ability to infect

macrophage cell lines *in vitro*, although it is now known that M-trophic HIV strains can infect dendritic cells, macrophages, and T cells *in vivo* (Chapter 18). Similarly, lymphocyte-trophic HIV strains infect only CD4 T cells *in vitro*. The different variants of HIV and the cell types they infect are largely determined by the chemokine receptor they use as a required HIV co-receptor. Dendritic cells, macrophages, and T cells express CC chemokine receptor 5 (CCR5), and primary infections with M-trophic HIV variants use this chemokine receptor, which also binds to chemokines RANTES, MIP-1α, and MIP-1β. Thus the addition of these chemokines to lymphocytes sensitive to HIV infection blocks their infection due to competition between CC chemokines and the virus for the target cell co-receptor CCR5.

By contrast, the chemokine receptor that binds to certain members of the CXC subfamily (CXCR4) is the co-receptor responsible for entry of lymphocyte-trophic strains of HIV into target cells. The establishment of a heterotrimeric complex between the viral envelope protein gp120, CD4, and one of these chemokine receptors facilitates viral entry into cells although the molecular mechanisms associated with this phenomenon are only beginning to be understood.

Cytokines That Stimulate Hematopoiesis

As discussed in Chapter 2, myeloid and lymphoid cells are derived from pluripotential stem cells (see Figure 2.1). Cytokines capable of inducing growth of hematopoietic cells *in vitro* were initially characterized using cultures of bone marrow cells grown in soft agar and thus are referred to as **colony-stimulating factors** (CSFs). Several biochemically distinct CSFs were identified by the particular lineage of hematopoietic cells that were stimulated to form colonies. These include **macrophage-CSF** (M-CSF), which supports

TABLE 12.3. Selected Chemokines and Their Functions

Chemokine	Produced By	Chemoattracted Cells	Major Functions
IL-8	Monocytes, macrophages, fibroblasts, keratinocytes, endothelial cells	Neutrophils, naïve T cells	Mobilizes and activates neutrophils; promotes angiogenesis
RANTES	T cells, endothelial cells, platelets	Monocytes, NK cells, T cells, basophils, eosinophils	Degranulates basophils; activates T cells
MCP-1	Monocytes, macrophages, fibroblasts, keratinocytes	Monocytes, NK cells, T cells, basophils, dendritic cells	Activates macrophages; stimulates basophil histamine release; promotes T_H2 immunity
MIP-1α	Monocytes, macrophages, T cells, mast cells, fibroblasts	Monocytes, NK cells, T cells, basophils, dendritic cells	Promotes T_H1 immunity; competes with HIV-1
MIP-1β	Monocytes, macrophages, neutrophils, endothelial cells	Monocytes, NK cells, T cells, dendritic cells	Competes with HIV-1 for chemokine receptor binding

IL, interleukin; MCP, monocyte chemotactic protein; MIP, macrophage inflammatory protein; NK, natural killer; T_H, helper T cell.

the clonal growth of macrophages/monocytes, ***granulocyte-CSF*** (G-CSF), which supports the clonal growth of granulocytes, and ***granulocyte-macrophage-CSF*** (GM-CSF), which supports the clonal growth of monocytes, macrophages, and granulocytes. ***IL-3*** is another cytokine capable of stimulating clonal growth of hematopoietic cells, but unlike the CSFs it is capable of promoting proliferation of a large number of cell populations, including granulocytes, macrophages, megakaryocytes, eosinophils, basophils, and mast calls. Moreover, in the presence of erythropoietin, a kidney-derived growth factor that has the ability to support the growth and terminal differentiation of cells of the erythroid lineage, IL-3 is also capable of stimulating development of normoblasts and red cells. IL-7, a cytokine produced largely by bone marrow and thymic stromal cells, induces differentiation of lymphoid stem cells into progenitor B and T cells. Like other functional categories of cytokines, the list of factors that are involved in hematopoiesis has grown significantly in recent years. Perhaps more than any other category of cytokines, CSFs have emerged as important therapeutic agents. For example, G-CSF is used to treat patients undergoing high-dose chemotherapy to reverse the neutropenia caused by such therapies. GM-CSF is used to treat patients undergoing bone marrow transplantation to boost clonal expansion of the granulocyte and macrophage populations.

CYTOKINE RECEPTORS

Cytokine Receptor Families

Cytokines can only act on target cells that express receptors for that cytokine. Often, cytokine receptor expression, like cytokine production itself, is highly regulated, such that resting cells either do not express a given receptor or express a low- or intermediate-affinity version of the receptor. An example of the latter is seen in the case of the IL-2 receptor, which can be expressed on the membranes of cells as either an intermediate-affinity dimer (β and γ chains) or a high-affinity trimer containing three subunit chains α, β, and γ (see below). IL-2 is capable of activating cells expressing the high-affinity form of the IL-2 receptor—a property unique to T cells undergoing antigen stimulation. The relative importance of these receptor subunits in binding to IL-2, and signaling the target cell is discussed later in this chapter. Suffice to say, the regulation of the receptor level expressed on the target cell membrane and/or the receptor form expressed helps to ensure that only an activated target population will respond to the cytokine(s) within its local microenvironment.

Understanding how cytokines affect their target cells has been the subject of many recent studies. As discussed later in this chapter, knowledge about cytokine–cytokine receptor interactions may be useful in devising strategies to prevent the action of cytokines involved in inflammatory responses, such as rheumatoid arthritis, or in responses such as transplantation rejection.

Receptors for cytokines can be divided into five families of receptor proteins (Figure 12.5) as follows:

- Immunoglobulin superfamily receptors
- Class I cytokine receptor family
- Class II cytokine receptor family
- TNF receptor superfamily
- Chemokine receptor family

The ***immunoglobulin*** (Ig) ***superfamily*** receptors contain shared structural features that were first defined in immunoglobulins, with each having at least one Ig-like domain (see Chapter 5). Examples of cytokines whose receptors are members of the immunoglobulin superfamily include IL-1 and M-CSF. ***Class I cytokine receptors*** (also known as the ***hematopoietin receptor family***) are usually composed of two types of polypeptide chains: a cytokine-specific subunit (α chain) and a signal-transducing subunit (β or γ chain). Important exceptions for the two subunit structural feature of class I cytokine receptors are seen in the case of the high-affinity receptors for IL-2 and the IL-15 receptor, which are trimers. Most cytokines identified to date utilize the class I family of cytokine receptors. ***Class II cytokine receptors*** are also known as the ***interferon receptor family*** because their ligands are interferons (e.g., IFN-α, IFN-β, and IFN-γ) or have biological activities that overlap with those associated with some interferons (e.g. IL-10). The ***TNF receptor*** (TNFR) ***superfamily*** are divided into three divergent subgroups that are classified by motifs (or lack thereof) in their cytoplasmic tails: death receptors, decoy receptors, and activating receptors. In all cases, each of these subgroups contains similar extracellular ligand-binding domains. Activating TNFR mediate their intracellular signals through a set of adaptor proteins called ***TNF receptor-associated factors*** (TRAF). Ligands for TNFR can be membrane-associated or secreted proteins. For example, most effector T cells express membrane forms of members of the TNFR superfamily including TNF-α and TNF-β (also known as lymphotoxin-α), both of which can also be released as secreted proteins. Other TNFR include Fas, which contains the "death domain" in its cytoplasmic tail, and CD40, which is involved in such functions as B-cell proliferation, maturation, and class switching. In short, the TNFR and TNF superfamilies regulate the life and death of activated cells of the immune system. Finally, the ***chemokine receptors*** belong to a superfamily of serpentine ***G-protein-coupled receptors***, so called because of their unique snakelike extracellular-cytoplasmic structural configuration and their association with G proteins, which mediate signal transduction (Figure 12.5). A growing list of CC and CXC chemokine receptors have been cloned, and some have been found to be promiscuous, since they can bind not only to chemokines but also to a diverse set of pathogens, including bacteria (e.g., *Streptococcus pneumo-*

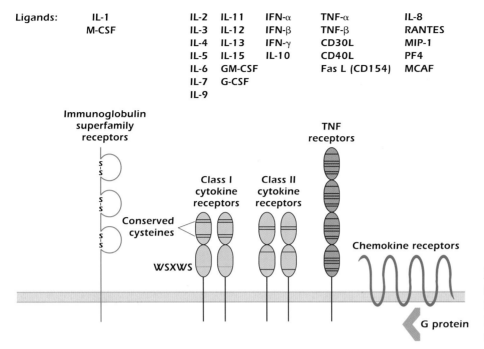

Ligands:	IL-1	IL-2	IL-11	IFN-α	TNF-α	IL-8
	M-CSF	IL-3	IL-12	IFN-β	TNF-β	RANTES
		IL-4	IL-13	IFN-γ	CD30L	MIP-1
		IL-5	IL-15	IL-10	CD40L	PF4
		IL-6	GM-CSF		Fas L (CD154)	MCAF
		IL-7	G-CSF			
		IL-9				

Figure 12.5. Schematic diagram showing the structural features of the five types of cytokine receptors. Many contain highly conserved cysteine residues.

nia, which binds to the platelet-activating factor [PAF] receptor), parasites (e.g., *Plasmodium vivax*, which binds to the chemokine receptor known as Duffy blood-group antigen), and certain viruses (e.g., T-tropic HIV-1 strains that use the CXCR4 chemokine receptor, and M-tropic HIV-1 strains that use the CCR5 chemokine receptor for viral entry into T cells and macrophages, respectively).

Common Cytokine Receptor Chains

As noted earlier in this chapter, it is common for cytokines to have overlapping (redundant) functions: For example, both IL-1 and IL-6 induce fever and several other common biologic phenomena. Nonetheless, these cytokines also have properties that are unique. Several cytokines use multichain receptors to mediate their effects on target cells and some of these receptors share at least one common receptor molecule called the ***common γ chain***. These include IL-2, IL-4, IL-7, IL-9, and IL-15 (see Figure 12.6). The common γ chain is an intracellular signaling molecule. This helps to explain the functional overlap among different cytokines. IL-9 is another member of the family of common γ-chain cytokines and uses the γ-chain receptor along with its specific receptor, IL-9Rα, for delivering its signals into target cells. Produced by so-called T_H9 cells, IL-9 plays a major role in the immune response against helminthes, and it is assumed this is the cytokine's "physiologic" function. Similar to other molecules with the same function (e.g., IgE, see Chapter 15), IL-9, however, also participates in the pathogenic process of allergy, in particular asthma. These activities of IL-9 are mainly exerted by promoting proliferation and accumulation of mast cells, as well as other leuko-

cytes, at the affected tissue, particularly the respiratory tract and the gut.

The high-affinity IL-2 receptor (IL-2R) consists of the common γ chain, an IL-2-specific α chain, and a β chain. In contrast, an intermediate-affinity IL-2 receptor is expressed as a dimer containing only the β and γ chains (Figure 12.7). IL-2 is capable of activating cells expressing the high-affinity form of the IL-2 receptor, a property reserved for T cells undergoing antigen-specific activation. It is noteworthy that a defect in the common IL-2Rγ chain has been shown to cause a profound immune deficiency in males suffering from X-linked severe combined immunodeficiency disease (see Chapter 18). This defect abolishes the functional activity of multiple cytokines owing to their shared use of the common γ chain.

 Read the related case: **Severe Combined Immunodeficiency Disease**
In *Immunology: Clinical Case Studies and Disease Pathophysiology*

CYTOKINE RECEPTOR-MEDIATED SIGNAL TRANSDUCTION

We have already discussed some of the signaling pathways that are selectively activated by specific cytokines to promote subset-specific T-cell differentiation. In order for cytokines to mediate virtually all of their diverse biologic effects on target cells, they must generate intracellular signals that result in the production of active transcription factors and, ultimately, gene expression (Figure 12.8). Binding of a

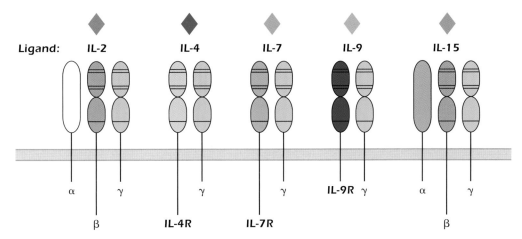

Figure 12.6. Schematic diagram showing structural features of members of the class I cytokine receptor family that share the common γ chain (green) that mediates intracellular signaling.

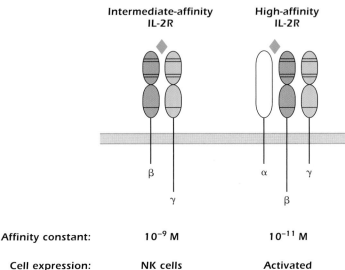

	Intermediate-affinity IL-2R	High-affinity IL-2R
Affinity constant:	10^{-9} M	10^{-11} M
Cell expression:	NK cells resting T cells	Activated T cells

Figure 12.7. Comparison of the two forms of IL-2 receptors expressed on cells.

cytokine to its cellular receptor induces dimerization or polymerization of receptor polypeptides at the cell surface. The mechanism illustrated applies to most, if not all, class I and class II cytokine-receptor families. It should be noted that it is not clear how signal specificity is maintained when different cytokine receptors use the same cytoplasmic signaling pathways. In the case of these two receptor families, the dimerization or polymerization of receptor subunits juxtaposes their cytoplasmic tails thus allowing the dimeric receptor to engage the intracytoplasmic signaling machinery. Signaling is initiated by the activation of *JAK kinases*, a family of cytosolic protein tyrosine kinases that interact with the cytoplasmic domains of the receptor. This results in the phosphorylation of tyrosine residues present on the cytoplasmic domain of the receptor and on a family of transcription factors known as *STATs* (signal transducers and activators of transcription). Once phosphorylated, the STAT

transcription factors dimerize and subsequently translocate from the cytoplasm to the nucleus where they bind to enhancer regions of genes induced by the cytokine.

The signaling events described above culminate in the biologic properties of the cytokine at the cellular level. However, this culmination does not terminate the signaling caused by cytokine ligation of cytokine receptors. Until recently, the mechanisms responsible for downregulation of cytokine-mediated signaling were poorly understood. Studies have now identified a family of intracellular proteins that play a key role in the suppression of cytokine signaling. These *suppressor of cytokine signaling* (SOCS) proteins regulate signal transduction by direct interactions with cytokine receptors and signaling proteins with a generic mechanism of targeting associated proteins for degradation. Given the central contribution of cytokines to many diseases, including the ones discussed below, the deregulation

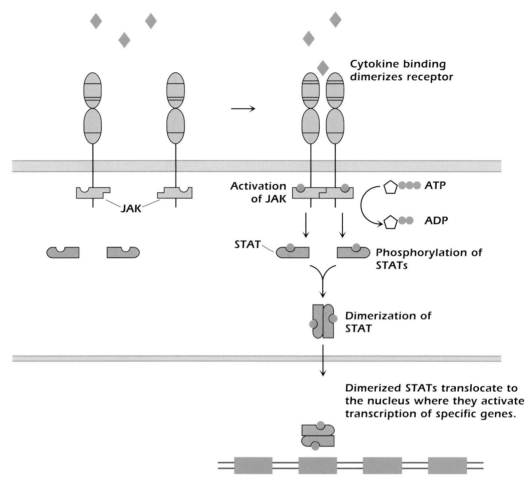

Figure 12.8. Model of cytokine receptor signaling using receptor-associated kinases to activate specific transcription factors.

of normal SOCS may play an etiologic role in some of these diseases. On the other hand, the manipulation of SOCS function might provide potent therapeutic options in the future.

ROLE OF CYTOKINES AND CYTOKINE RECEPTORS IN DISEASE

Given the complex regulatory properties of cytokines, it is not surprising that overexpression or underexpression of cytokines or cytokine receptors have been implicated in many diseases. Here we discuss some examples of diseases with cytokine-associated pathophysiology.

Toxic Shock Syndrome

Toxic shock syndrome is initiated by the release of **superantigen** (enterotoxin) from certain microorganisms. For example, the toxins derived from *Staphylococcus aureus* or *Streptococcus pyogenes* cause a burst of cytokine production by T cells. The toxin does this by activating large

numbers of CD4 T cells that use certain Vβ segments as part of their TCR. The toxin cross-links the Vβ segment of the TCR with a class II MHC molecule expressed on antigen-presenting cells (see Figure 9.13). It has been estimated that one in every five T cells can be activated by superantigens. Superantigen activation of T cells results in excessive production of cytokines that ultimately cause dysregulation of the cytokine network leading to extremely high levels of IL-1 and TNF-α. These cytokines induce systemic reactions including fever, blood clotting, diarrhea, hypotension (low blood pressure), and shock. Sometimes these reactions are fatal.

Bacterial Septic Shock

Overproduction of cytokines is also associated with infections caused by certain Gram-negative bacteria, including *Escherichia coli*, *Klebsiella pneumonia*, *Enterobacter aerogenes*, *Pseudomonas aeruginosa*, and *Neisseria meningitidis*. Endotoxins produced by these bacteria stimulate macrophages to overproduce IL-1 and TNF-α that cause an often fatal form of bacterial septic shock.

Cancers

Several lymphoid and myeloid cancers have been shown to be associated with abnormally high levels of cytokines and/or cytokine receptor expression. Perhaps the best example of an association between malignancy and overproduction of both a cytokine and its receptor is seen in patients with adult T-cell leukemia or lymphoma that is the result of infection with the human T-cell lymphotropic virus type 1 (HTLV-1). T cells infected with HTLV-1 constitutively produce IL-2 and express the high-affinity IL-2 receptor in the absence of activation by antigen. This results in autocrine stimulation of infected T cells, leading to their uncontrolled growth. Other examples of malignancies associated with overproduction of cytokines include myelomas (neoplastic plasma cells), which produce large amounts of the autocrine IL-6, and Hodgkin lymphoma in which the reactive milieu is the result of abundant cytokine production, particularly IL-5 (also see Chapter 18).

Read the related case: **Follicular Lymphoma**
In *Immunology: Clinical Case Studies and Disease Pathophysiology*

Autoimmunity and Other Immune-Based Diseases

Much evidence suggests that T cells exert a controlling influence on the generation of autoantibodies and on the regulation of autoimmunity (see Chapter 13). Many of the observed phenomena are manifestations of the actions of cytokines, including members of the IL-17 family, IL-23, IL-12, IL-10, IFN-γ, and IL-4. Several cytokine and cytokine receptor abnormalities have been shown to be associated with systemic autoimmune diseases. Some occur late in illness and are probably not causal, while others may be involved in dysregulation of immune responses and may help promote autoreactivity. The autoimmune disease systemic lupus erythematosus (SLE) has been shown to be associated with elevated levels of IL-10. Recent studies of cytokines involved in autoimmune diseases have examined whether skewing of the T_H-cell subset phenotype contributes to disease initiation or disease progression. While most of this work has been performed using experimental animal models of autoimmune disease, the importance of T_H2 cells in promoting systemic autoimmunity has been reported. Future studies will be needed to clearly elucidate the disease-related roles played by cytokines and cytokine receptors in autoimmunity.

Read the related case: **Systemic Lupus Erythematosis**
In *Immunology: Clinical Case Studies and Disease Pathophysiology*

Cytokines also play a major role in the pathophysiology of other immune-based diseases including allergy, asthma, and inflammatory diseases. Thus, it is not surprising that many clinical features associated with these diseases are the result of cytokine receptor-mediated signaling and the biologic effects of such signaling (e.g., cell activation, cell death). Our understanding of the roles played by cytokines and cytokine receptors in disease manifestation continues to expand. The crucial roles of interactions between cytokines and their receptors, and of antigen-presenting cells and pathogen-derived molecules in many autoimmune diseases and other immune-based diseases warrants further investigation and could represent a unique chance of intervention even after onset of disease symptoms.

Read the related case: **Asthma**
In *Immunology: Clinical Case Studies and Disease Pathophysiology*

Below, we discuss some of the fruits of such knowledge that have given rise to the development of antagonists used to treat patients with some of these diseases.

THERAPEUTIC EXPLOITATION OF CYTOKINES AND CYTOKINE RECEPTORS

Knowledge of the cellular and molecular components of immune responses to pathogens, and specifically the roles played by cytokines in regulation and homeostasis of hematopoietic cells, has opened opportunities for new forms of therapeutics. In addition, the increasing knowledge of cytokine structural biology is driving new opportunities for developing novel therapies to modulate cytokine function in a diverse range of diseases including malignancies and chronic inflammation. The many opportunities for therapeutic exploitation of this knowledge include the use of cytokines themselves, soluble cytokine receptors (antagonists), cytokine analogs, and anti-cytokine or anti-cytokine receptor antibodies. These biologic therapeutics have shown promise in several ways.

Cytokine Inhibitors/Antagonists

Several naturally occurring soluble cytokine receptors have been identified in the bloodstream and extracellular fluids. These act, *in vivo*, as **cytokine inhibitors** or **antagonists** and are released from the cell surface as a result of enzymatic cleavage of the extracellular domain of the cytokine receptor. Circulating soluble cytokine receptors maintain their ability to bind to the cytokine for which the receptor is specific, thus neutralizing their activity. Examples of such inhibitors include those that bind to IL-2, IL-4, IL-6, IL-7, IFN-γ, and, last but not least, TNF. Experimental use of

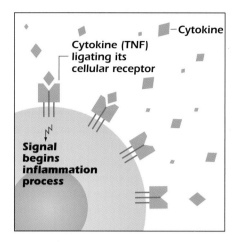
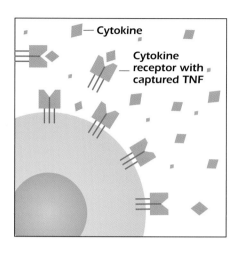

Figure 12.9. Soluble TNF receptors can interfere with inflammatory properties of TNF.

soluble TNF receptors has led to the development of a class of biological response modifier drugs called **TNF inhibitors**. TNF inhibitors have shown significant clinical utility in the treatment of rheumatoid arthritis (RA). Patients with RA have increased levels of TNF and IL-1 in their joints, a phenomenon that leads to RA-associated pain, swelling, stiffness, and other symptoms. TNF inhibitors (**soluble TNF receptor molecules**) compete with cell bound receptors for binding to endogenously produced TNF (Figure 12.9). Most RA patients treated with TNF inhibitors show significant improvement of their symptoms, although approximately 30% are nonresponsive to this treatment.

 Read the related case: **Rheumatoid Arthritis**
In *Immunology: Clinical Case Studies and Disease Pathophysiology*

The soluble **IL-2 receptor** (IL-2R) has also been studied extensively. It is formed by the proteolytic release of a 45-kDa portion of the IL-2 α chain of the IL-2R. Chronic T-cell activation is associated with very high serum levels of soluble IL-2R. Thus, it has been used as a clinical marker for diseases such as adult T-cell leukemia or lymphoma (ATLL).

Another well-characterized cytokine antagonist is the naturally occurring **IL-1 receptor antagonist** (IL-1Ra). This protein also plays a role in regulating the intensity of inflammatory responses by binding to the IL-1 receptor on CD4+ T cells, thus preventing their activation. Binding of IL-1Ra to the IL-1 receptor does not mediate cell signaling through this receptor. IL-1Ra has been cloned and is currently under clinical investigation to determine whether it can be used as a therapeutic agent for chronic inflammatory diseases.

Reversing Cellular Deficiencies

Cytokines have been used to treat acute events such as cellular deficiencies arising from chemotherapy or radiother-

apy by administration of growth factors (e.g., G-CSF or GM-CSF). As discussed earlier in this chapter, treatment with these hematopoietic growth factors escalates the rate of natural reconstitution of desired hematopoietic cell lineages.

Treatment of Immunodeficiencies

Cytokines have also been used to treat patients with immunodeficiency diseases, many of which are discussed in Chapter 18. For example, patients with X-linked agammaglobulinemia have been treated successfully with G-CSF to reverse their disease-associated neutropenia. Patients suffering from a form of severe combined immunodeficiency disease (SCID) due to adenosine deaminase (ADA) deficiency, a disease that is often associated with a profound IL-2 deficiency, have been treated with recombinant human IL-2.

 Read the related case: **X-Linked Agammaglobulinemia**
In *Immunology: Clinical Case Studies and Disease Pathophysiology*

Finally, several leukocyte adhesion deficiency diseases characterized by recurrent or progressive soft tissue infection, periodontitis, poor wound healing, and leukocytosis have been successfully treated with recombinant IFN-γ to reduce the severity and frequency of infections, probably by increasing nonoxidative antimicrobial activity.

Treatment of Patients with Cancer, Transplanted Organs, and Tissues, and Viral Infections

Patients with cancer have also benefited from the use of cytokines in passive cellular immunotherapies that utilize **lymphokine-activated killer** (LAK) cells as discussed in

Chapter 19. Culturing populations of NK cells or cytotoxic T cells in the presence of high concentrations of IL-2 generates effector cells with potent antitumor activities. The availability of recombinant IL-2 in large quantities has made the LAK cell plus IL-2 therapy feasible, and some melanoma and renal carcinoma patients have shown objective responses. Another variation of passive cellular immunotherapy is the concurrent use of IFN-γ, which enhances the expression of major histocompatibility complex (MHC) and tumor-associated antigens on tumor cells, thereby augmenting the killing of tumor cells by the infused effector cells. Within the interferon family of cytokines, IFN-α is used for the treatment of infection with hepatitis B and hepatitis C viruses as well as renal cell carcinoma.

Cytokine receptor-specific antibodies have also proven useful in the treatment of certain cancers. The relative accessibility of certain cytokine receptor-positive leukemic cells has encouraged numerous trials with native as well as toxin-conjugated antibodies. As mentioned above, in ATLL the leukemic cells upregulate IL-2 receptor α chain (CD25) on their surfaces, and antibodies to CD25 have been shown to induce therapeutic responses, albeit temporary, in approximately one third of the patients treated.

Treatment of Allergies and Asthma

Our current understanding of the functional properties of T_H2 cells and more specifically the roles played by the specific cytokines they produce (e.g., IL-4, IL-13) in IgE production suggests that therapies that target these cytokines or their receptors may prove to be effective in the treatment of allergies and asthma (Chapter 15). Given the cross-antagonistic effects of T_H1 and T_H2 cells, it may be possible to skew the production of antibody away from IgE in response to a given allergen by using strategies that selectively silence the undesired T_H2 subset. At present, this remains an experimental goal, which is being aggressively investigated in animal models. Promising results have emerged from clinical trials using a related strategy that specifically targets IL-4, the major cytokine responsible for promoting B-cell isotype class switching to IgE (see Chapters 11 and 15). Injection of antibodies specific for IL-4 has been shown to dramatically decrease IL-4 production in mice. Another related strategy to treat asthma and allergic diseases involves the use of soluble IL-4 receptors, again, with promising, although preliminary, results reported to date. The clinical applications of such research cannot be underestimated given the enormous number of individuals who suffer from allergies worldwide. Chapter 15 discusses other cytokine-based treatment strategies used in patients with allergies and asthma.

SUMMARY

1. Cytokines are low-molecular-weight antigen-nonspecific proteins that mediate cellular interactions involving immune, inflammatory, and hematopoietic systems.

2. Cytokines exhibit properties of pleiotropy and redundancy and often display synergism or antagonism with other cytokines.

3. Cytokines are short-lived and may act locally either on the same cell that secreted them (autocrine), on other cells (paracrine), or, like hormones, they may act systemically (endocrine).

4. Cytokines have a wide variety of functional activities as illustrated by their ability to (a) regulate specific immune responses; (b) facilitate innate immune responses; (c) activate inflammatory responses; (d) affect leukocyte movement; and (e) stimulate hematopoiesis.

5. Subsets of CD4 T_H cells have been defined by the range of cytokines they produce. T_H1 cells secrete IL-2 and IFN-γ (as well as several other cytokines), but not IL-4 or IL-5. Cytokines produced by these cells also activate other T cells, NK cells, and macrophages (cell-mediated immune responses). By contrast, T_H2 cells secrete IL-4 and IL-5 (as well as other cytokines), but not IL-2 or IFN-γ and predominantly affect antibody responses.

6. Knowledge regarding the new CD4 T-cell subset called T_H17 T cells and the IL-17 family of cytokines is filling many gaps in our understanding of how immune responses are regulated. IL-17 stimulates the mobilization and generation of neutrophils thereby bridging innate and adaptive immunity.

7. Cytokines can only act on target cells that express receptors for that cytokine. Cytokine receptor expression is highly regulated such that resting cells either do not express a given receptor or express a low- or intermediate-affinity version of that receptor. Increased levels of cytokine receptor expression or

expression of high-affinity forms of a given receptor predispose target cells to respond to a cytokine.

8. The common γ chain is a cytokine receptor subunit utilized by several cytokine receptors as the signal transducing subunit including IL-2, IL-4, IL-7, IL-9, and IL-15. This structural feature helps to explain the redundancy and antagonism often exhibited by some cytokines.

9. Ligation of cytokine receptors by cytokines generates intracellular signals that result in the production of active transcription factors and, ultimately, gene expression. Binding of a cytokine to its cellular receptor often induces dimerization or polymerization of receptor polypeptides at the cell surface and permits association of JAK kinases with the receptor cytoplasmic domain. This association activates the kinases and causes phosphorylation of tyrosine residues in STATs (signal transducers and activators of transcription). Once phosphorylated, the STAT transcription factors dimerize and subsequently translo-

cate from the cytoplasm to the nucleus where they bind to enhancer regions of genes induced by the cytokine. Suppression of cytokine signaling proteins downregulate signal transduction and help terminate cytokine responses.

10. Overexpression or underexpression of cytokines or cytokine receptors have been implicated in several diseases including bacterial toxic shock, bacterial sepsis, certain lymphoid cancers, and autoimmunity.

11. Cytokine-related therapies offer promise for the treatment of certain immunodeficiencies, in preventing graft rejection, and in treating certain cancers. The utility of cytokine-related therapies is best seen in the use of (a) hematopoietic growth factors (G-CSF, GM-CSF) to reverse certain cellular deficiencies associated with chemotherapy or radiotherapy and (b) the use of IL-2 to generate cytokine-activated killer cells (NK and cytotoxic T cells) employed in the treatment of patients with certain cancers.

REFERENCES AND BIBLIOGRAPHY

Alexander WS. (2002) Suppressor of cytokine signaling (SOCS) in the immune system. *Nat Rev Immunol* 2: 410.

Campbell JJ, Butcher EC. (2000) Chemokines in tissue-specific and microenvironment-specific lymphocyte homing. *Curr Opin Immunol* 12: 336.

DeVries ME, Kelvin DJ. (1999) On the edge: the physiological and pathophysiological role of chemokines during inflammatory and immunological responses. *Semin Immunol* 11: 95.

Fernandez-Botran R, Crespo FA, Sun X. (2000) Soluble cytokine receptors in biological therapy. *Expert Opin Biol Ther* 2: 585.

Ezerzer C, Harris N. (2007) Physiological immunity or pathological autoimmunity—a question of balance. *Autoimmun Rev* 6(7): 488.

Kisseleva T, Bhattacharya S, Braunstein J, Schindler CW. (2000) Signaling through the JAK/STAT pathway, recent advances and future challenges. *Gene* 20: 1.

Koch, AE. (2007) The pathogenesis of rheumatoid arthritis. *Am J Orthop* 36: 5

Leonard WJ. (2001) Cytokines and immunodeficiency diseases. *Nat Rev Immunol* 1: 200.

Ma A,, Koka M, Burkett P. (2006) Diverse Functions of IL-2, IL-15, and IL-7 in Lymphoid Homeostasis. *Ann Rev Immunology* 24: 821

Matsuzaki G, Umemura M. (2007) Interleukin-17 as an Effector Molecule of Innate and Acquired Immunity Against Infections. *Microbiol Immunol* 51: 1139

McGeachy MJ, Cua DJ. (2007) T Cells Doing It for Themselves: TGF-β Regulation of TH1 and TH17 Cells. *Immunity* 26: 547.

Minami Y, Kono T, Miyazaki T, Taniguchi. T. (1993) The IL-2 receptor complex: its structure, function, and target genes. *Ann Rev Immunol* 11: 245.

Pulendran B, Artis D. (2012) New paradigms in type 2 immunity. *Science* 337: 431.

Tan C, Gery I. (2012) The Unique Features of Th9 Cells and their Products. *Crit Rev Immunol* 32: 1.

Weaver CT, Harrington LE, Mangan PR, Gavrieli M, Murphy, KM. (2006) TH17: An Effector CD4 T Cell Lineage with Regulatory T Cell Ties. *Immunity* 24: 677.

REVIEW QUESTIONS

For each question, choose the ONE BEST answer or completion.

1. Polarization of naïve CD4$^+$ T-cell differentiation toward the T$_H$2 lineage is associated with which of the following cytokines?

A) IL-1
B) IL-4
C) IL-6
D) IL-23
E) IL-25

2. A patient with active rheumatoid arthritis feels systemically ill with low-grade fever, malaise, morning stiffness, and fatigue. The protein(s) or cytokine(s) most likely to be responsible for these symptoms are:
A) rheumatoid factor
B) TNF and IL-1
C) IL-4 and IL-10
D) complement components 1–9
E) gamma globulin

3. When IL-2 is secreted by antigen-specific T cells activated due to presentation of antigen by APCs, what happens to naïve antigen-nonspecific T cells in the vicinity?
A) They proliferate due to their exposure to IL-2.
B) They often undergo apoptosis.
C) They begin to express IL-2 receptors.
D) They secrete cytokines associated with their Th phenotype.
E) Nothing happens.

4. IL-1, IL-6, and TNF-α are proinflammatory cytokines that are known to
A) cause increased vascular permeability
B) act in concert with chemokines to promote migration of inflammatory cells to sites of infection
C) initiate acute-phase responses
D) have endogenous pyrogen properties
E) all of the above

5. Which of the following cytokines plays a role in terminating inflammatory responses?
A) IL-2
B) IL-4
C) TGF-β
D) IFN-α
E) IL-3

6. Assuming there were no other compensatory mechanisms to replace IL-8 function, which of the following would be preserved as a functional activity in an IL-8 knockout mouse strain?
A) activation of neutrophils
B) attraction of neutrophils to sites of tissue damage
C) wound healing
D) extravasation of neutrophils
E) reduction of cytokine production by T_H1 cells

7. Superantigens cause a burst of cytokine production by T cells due to their ability to
A) cross-link the Vβ segments of T-cell receptors with class II MHC molecules on APCs
B) cross-link the Vα segments of T-cell receptors with class II MHC molecules on APCs
C) cross-link T-cell receptors and CD3
D) cross-link multiple cytokine receptors on a large population of T cells
E) cross-link CD3

ANSWERS TO REVIEW QUESTIONS

1. B. Activation of innate immune cells, such as mast cells, triggers their synthesis of several cytokines including IL-4, which promotes T_H2 cell differentiation.

2. B. Patients with rheumatoid arthritis have elevated levels of proinflammatory cytokines TNF and IL-1 in their joints that play a key role in the pain, swelling, stiffness, and other symptoms associated with this disease.

3. E. Cytokines secreted by antigen-activated T cells only regulate the activities of other cells involved in that immune response by binding to cytokine receptors (e.g., high affinity IL-2R) expressed by these cells. Such cytokine receptors are upregulated only on antigen-activated T cells that bear the appropriate T-cell receptor for that antigen; they are not upregulated on antigen-nonspecific T cells in the vicinity, and thus these cells will not be activated by IL-2.

4. E. The answer is self-explanatory.

5. C. Among the cytokines listed, TGF-β plays a role in terminating inflammatory responses by promoting the accumulation and proliferation of fibroblasts and the deposition of extracellular matrix proteins required for tissue repair.

6. E. IL-8 plays no role in regulation of cytokine production by T_H1 cells—a biologic property ascribed to IL-10 produced by T_H2 cells. Therefore, functional integrity of T_H1 would be predicted in IL-8 knockout mice. IL-8 chemotactically attracts and activates neutrophils and induces their adherence to vascular endothelium and extravasation (activities that should be deficient in IL-8 knockouts). Because these activities are important for wound healing, this phenomenon would also be predicted to be deficient in such mice.

7. A. Superantigens bind simultaneously to class II MHC molecules and to the Vβ domain of the T-cell receptor activating all T cells bearing a particular Vβ domain. Thus, they activate large numbers of T cells (between 5% and 25%), regardless of their antigen specificity that causes them to release harmful quantities of cytokines.

13

TOLERANCE AND AUTOIMMUNITY

Philip L. Cohen

INTRODUCTION

The immune system protects against invasion by foreign organisms. However, immune responses can cause damage if they are directed against the individual's own components, which are often referred to as *self-antigens* or *autoantigens*. Therefore, the immune system has developed mechanisms to allow it to respond to foreign antigens but not self-antigens. Both the innate and adaptive immune responses have evolved to make this distinction. The state of specific unresponsiveness to self-antigen is known as *self-tolerance*. This chapter focuses on the adaptive immune responses that are the basis for self-tolerance. The first part of this chapter will discuss the basic mechanisms of tolerance to self and how these mechanisms protect the host from harmful immune reactions. The second part of the chapter will discuss how mechanisms of tolerance can go awry, leading to the activation of autoreactive lymphocytes and the development of autoimmune disease.

Discovery of tolerance. A key finding by Ray Owen in 1945 was that tolerance to self-antigens was *acquired*. He studied cows that were dizygotic twins—they had different red blood types but shared a common blood supply *in utero*. He showed that, as adults, if one of the twins was injected with red blood cells from the other twin, it did not generate anti-red blood cell antibodies. Thus, it appeared that sharing of "foreign" blood cell antigens during the fetal stage had produced long-lasting *tolerance*.

These observations provided the basis for classic experiments in mice performed by Sir Peter Medawar and his colleagues in the 1950s, for which he was awarded a Nobel Prize in 1960. They observed that adult mice of one inbred strain (strain A) rejected skin grafts from mice of another strain (strain B); the critical difference between the two mouse strains was in the major histocompatibility complex (MHC) molecules they expressed. However, if mice of strain A were injected within 24 hours after birth with bone marrow stem cells from strain B, they did *not* reject skin grafts from the donor B strain when they grew to adulthood. These results suggested that when immature, developing lymphocytes are exposed to a foreign antigen, they fail to mount an immune response to the antigen. Instead, the antigen is accepted as self and the immune system becomes tolerant to it. This phenomenon became known as *neonatal tolerance*.

Self-tolerance, a property of both B and T lymphocytes, is a state of specific unresponsiveness to self-antigen. It occurs when the interaction of an autoantigen with self-antigen-specific lymphocytes fails to activate the lymphocytes. Thus, to be tolerized, a cell must express an antigen-specific receptor, either a B-cell receptor (BCR) or T-cell receptor (TCR). As a consequence of the tolerizing interaction, the cell or the individual exposed to the antigen is said to be *tolerant*. There are several stages of development of lymphocytes during which tolerance can be induced to provide protection against the development of autoimmunity. Tolerance induced during the early stages of development is referred to as *central tolerance*; tolerance induced in mature lymphocytes is referred to as *peripheral tolerance*. There are multiple mechanisms by which tolerance

Immunology: A Short Course, Seventh Edition. Richard Coico and Geoffrey Sunshine.
© 2015 John Wiley & Sons, Ltd. Published 2015 by John Wiley & Sons, Ltd.
Companion Website: www.wileyimmunology.com/coico

may be induced, and these are discussed further in the sections that follow.

Central tolerance occurs in the primary lymphoid organs (the bone marrow for B cells and the thymus for T cells) as part of the process known as *negative selection* (see Chapters 8 and 10). Negative selection in central lymphoid organs ensures that the majority of B and T cells that emerge in the periphery react only with foreign antigens. Nevertheless, this process is not perfect—some autoreactive cells inevitably escape to peripheral lymphoid organs such as the spleen and lymph nodes. If this happens, peripheral tolerance mechanisms may keep them under control.

How do lymphocytes distinguish self from nonself? As the experiments of Owen and Medawar's group showed, self-antigens have no specific characteristics that distinguish them from foreign antigens. Thus, lymphocytes must rely on some other characteristics to make this distinction. The modern interpretation of Medawar's studies of neonatal tolerance is that exposure of *immature* lymphocytes to antigen results in tolerance, whereas the first exposure of *mature* lymphocytes to the same antigen results in activation. What conditions favor the development of tolerance rather than activation? One is that immature lymphocytes are much more sensitive than mature lymphocytes to strong signals delivered through their antigen receptors. This is the basis for negative selection of B cells in the bone marrow and T cells in the thymus.

Another scenario that favors tolerance is continuous exposure of lymphocytes to high levels of antigen, which can lead to chronic antigen receptor signaling. Lymphocytes are continuously exposed to high levels of self-antigen, while exposure to foreign antigen is generally abrupt and short lived. Lymphocytes also learn to distinguish self from nonself by the context in which they encounter the antigen. If the antigen is encountered in the absence of co-stimulatory signals, then the lymphocytes are tolerized; if antigen is encountered in the presence of co-stimulatory signals, the lymphocytes are activated. Because the immune response is focused on responding to foreign antigens such as infectious

organisms, foreign antigens are much more likely to come in contact with lymphocytes in the presence of co-stimulatory signals; thus, foreign antigens are more likely than self-antigens to activate lymphocytes.

CENTRAL TOLERANCE

The random process of generating diversity in BCRs and TCRs inevitably generates receptors that can recognize self-antigens. This concept was initially proposed in the 1950s by Sir MacFarlane Burnet in his *clonal selection theory*, for which he won the Nobel Prize in 1960. Burnet hypothesized that *autoreactive* lymphocytes—B and T cells with receptors for self-antigen—pose a danger to the host and must be purged or *deleted* from the developing lymphocyte repertoire to maintain tolerance to self. As we mentioned above, tolerance induced during the early stages of development is referred to as *central tolerance*. We now know that mechanisms other than deletion may be involved in central tolerance, but Burnet's hypothesis is still substantially correct. The mechanisms of central tolerance and the conditions under which it is implemented are explored below.

Mechanisms of Central Tolerance: T and B Cells

Deletion. *Deletion* is a mechanism by which autoreactive T and B cells are eliminated from the repertoire by undergoing *apoptosis* (programmed cell death). For developing T cells, deletion in the thymus is the major mechanism of *negative selection*—thymocytes expressing TCRs that interact with high affinity with self-antigens plus self-MHC (expressed on thymic dendritic cells and medullary epithelial cells) undergo rapid deletion (see Figure 13.1). This prevents mature autoreactive T cells from exiting the thymus and moving out into the periphery.

For a long time immunologists were puzzled as to how T cells specific for nonthymic, tissue-specific self-antigens,

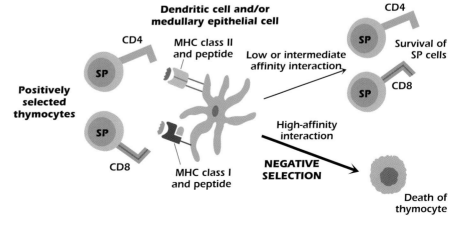

Figure 13.1. Deletion as the mechanism of central tolerance in T cells. Thymocytes expressing a TCR with high affinity for self-MHC class I or II plus self-peptide are deleted—negatively selected—as a consequence of interacting with thymic dendritic cells and/or medullary epithelial cells. Thymocytes expressing a TCR with lower affinity for self-MHC class I or II plus self-peptide survive.

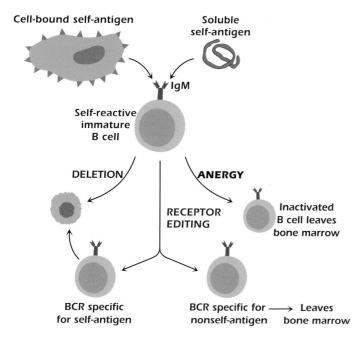

Figure 13.2. Mechanisms of central tolerance in B cells: deletion, anergy, and receptor editing. Self-reactive immature IgM⁺ B cells that interact with self-antigen in the bone marrow undergo different fates. Left side: Interaction with *membrane-bound* self-antigen results in deletion. Right side: Interaction with *soluble* self-antigen can result in anergy—long-term inactivation—rather than deletion. Center: Some self-reactive B cells that interact with self-antigen undergo receptor editing of light-chain V genes. If the BCR generated by receptor editing is non-self-reactive, the cell survives and leaves the bone marrow. If the BCR generated is self-reactive, the cell dies.

such as those expressed in the pancreas, could be eliminated in the thymus, since these self-antigens were not thought to be expressed in the thymus. The answer became apparent from studies over the past several years to uncover the cause of *autoimmune polyendocrinopathy candidiasis ectodermal dystrophy* (APECED), a disease in which children suffer from a number of autoimmune symptoms including hypoparathyroidism, adrenal insufficiency, thyroiditis, type I diabetes mellitus, and ovarian failure. The studies showed that expression of the product of the **AIRE (autoimmune regulator)** gene is defective in patients with APECED (see Chapter 10). The AIRE gene product is a transcription factor regulator expressed predominantly in the thymus, by thymic medullary epithelial cells. The AIRE gene product facilitates the expression in the thymus of self-antigens that are normally found outside the thymus; for example, self-antigens expressed in the pancreas and central nervous system. Thus, in normal individuals, negative selection of self-reactive T cells specific for self-molecules expressed by peripheral tissues occurs. However, in APECED patients, and AIRE gene knockout mice, there is little expression in the thymus of these peripheral tissue self-antigens. The lack of negative selection permits autoreactive T cells to escape thymic deletion and exit to the periphery, where they may induce autoimmune disease.

Mechanisms of Central Tolerance: B Cells

Central tolerance in the B-cell lineage shows some features that are also found in central tolerance in the T-cell lineage. In particular, negative selection—deletion of autoreactive B cells—occurs in the primary lymphoid organ; that is, the interaction in the bone marrow of self-antigen with an immature IgM⁺ B cells expressing a BCR specific for a self-antigen can result in deletion (shown in Figure 8.2 in Chapter 8). The best evidence for deletion of autoreactive B cells came from studies of transgenic mice. When mice transgenic for an antibody specific for the protein hen egg lysozyme (HEL) were bred with transgenic mice expressing HEL as a *membrane-bound* autoantigen, anti-HEL-specific B cells were deleted in the bone marrow when they came in contact with membrane HEL (see left side of Figure 13.2).

Central tolerance in B cells also shows some features that are not found in the development of central tolerance in T cells. These are described in the sections that follow.

Anergy. *Anergy* is defined as the functional inactivation of a lymphocyte, resulting in unresponsiveness upon further contact with antigen. Anergic B cells cannot be activated to proliferate and differentiate into antibody-secreting cells upon engagement of their BCRs. Likewise, anergic T cells cannot be activated to proliferate and secrete cytokines following ligation of their TCR with antigen in the context of self-MHC.

Evidence for central B-cell anergy was first observed in 1980 by Sir Gustav Nossal and Beverly Pike. They demonstrated that when a cross-linking signal was delivered to immature B cells via their BCR, the B cells were anergized and were unable to mature or to undergo activation. B-cell anergy has since been observed in transgenic mouse systems. In the transgenic HEL model described in the section above, when transgenic mice making antibody specific for HEL were bred with transgenic mice expressing HEL as a *soluble* autoantigen, the offspring of these mice produced HEL-specific B cells that were not deleted after contact with antigen. These HEL-specific B cells were present but unable to respond to antigen; they had been rendered *anergic* or unresponsive (see right side of Figure 13.2). Experiments using mice transgenic for anti-DNA and other anti-self-antigens gave similar results, establishing that anergy is an important mechanism that prevents autoantibody-specific B cells from secreting autoantibodies.

The difference between the results of the two anti-HEL transgenic models was interpreted as suggesting that an encounter with a self-antigen that is membrane-bound induces extensive cross-linking of the BCR and delivers a strong signal that results in deletion; an encounter with a soluble self-antigen that induces more moderate cross-linking delivers a weaker signal that induces anergy. Thus, the degree of aggregation or polymerization of autoantigens appears to be a key factor in the mechanism of B-cell tolerance.

There is little evidence of anergy as a mechanism in the development of central tolerance for T cells in the thymus. Rather, as described above, most negative selection of auto-reactive T cells in the thymus appears to occur by deletion. As described below though, anergy is a major mechanism in peripheral T-cell tolerance.

Receptor Editing. *Receptor editing* is an important mechanism in developing B cells: it allows an immature B cell expressing a BCR specific for a self-antigen to replace it with a BCR specific for a nonself-antigen (see Figure 13.2 and Chapter 8). Receptor editing occurs predominantly in light chain genes: The existing rearranged light chain variable region is replaced with an upstream variable segment that rearranges to a more downstream J region. This secondary rearrangement does not always eliminate autoreactivity; that is, receptor editing may generate a BCR that is still self-reactive. In this case, rearrangement continues until all available upstream variable regions have been exhausted or until a non-autoreactive receptor is generated. If continued editing fails to result in a non-autoreactive BCR, the B cell undergoes deletion. Evidence for *in vivo* BCR editing was first observed in the bone marrow of mice transgenic for an antibody to an endogenous MHC class I molecule and in mice transgenic for an antibody to double-stranded DNA (dsDNA). Unlike B cells, developing T cells do not appear to use receptor editing as a means of altering their specificity.

Importance of receptor avidity in tolerance. What determines which of the spectrum of mechanisms leading to tolerance will govern the fate of selected immature lymphocytes? It is currently believed that the threshold of receptor signaling is the major force that determines which mechanism of tolerance governs immature lymphocytes. The strength, or *avidity*, of interaction of the BCR or TCR with its autoantigen influences cell fate. Avidity with respect to B cells depends on the affinity of interaction between the BCR and its antigen, density of the surface BCR, and the nature and concentration of the autoantigen. The higher

the affinity of the antibody for its antigen and the more BCR expressed on the B-cell membrane, the greater the avidity of the antigen–antibody interaction. This correlates directly with the extent of immunoglobulin receptor cross-linking. The nature of the autoantigen also influences its ability to induce BCR cross-linking. For example, multivalent and membrane-bound antigens mediate more extensive receptor cross-linking than monovalent or soluble antigens. Initially, a B cell with a high avidity for an autoantigen will undergo receptor editing in an attempt to avert autoreactivity. B cells with more moderate avidity for an autoantigen are targeted to anergy, while B cells with a weak avidity for autoantigen become clonally ignorant.

In the thymus, the affinity of the TCR for self-peptide plus self-MHC, the level of TCR on the surface of the T cell, and the level of MHC molecules expressed on the surface of the APC determine avidity and affect T-cell selection. In addition, the type of cell presenting self-antigen to the T cell seems to influence whether the T cell undergoes positive or negative selection. T cells that recognize peptide plus MHC expressed on epithelial cells in the cortex are positively selected. At the corticomedullary junction, T cells come in contact with self-antigen and MHC molecules expressed on dendritic cells. It is in this context that T cells with a high avidity for peptide plus MHC undergo negative selection and are deleted. It is not known whether dendritic cells deliver signals different from cortical epithelial cells, and thus leading to negative rather than positive selection of self-reactive T cells. Anergy and editing seem to play minor roles in central T-cell tolerance.

PERIPHERAL TOLERANCE

Occasionally, autoreactive B cells and T cells escape negative selection and enter the periphery. This can result from a self-antigen not being expressed at a high enough level in the primary lymphoid organ (bone marrow or thymus) or because the developing lymphocyte has a weak affinity for self-antigen. Such autoreactive lymphocytes generally do not pose a threat to the host—a state referred to as *clonal ignorance*. However, clonally ignorant lymphocytes may be activated if the concentration of autoantigen is increased, e.g., when large amounts of intracellular self-antigens are released (following cell death) or when a strong co-stimulatory signal is delivered to the clonally ignorant cell during an infection. In addition, B cells sometimes acquire autoreactive specificities through somatic mutation in the periphery.

Peripheral tolerance has evolved as a safety net to catch autoreactive B and T cells that escape to or arise in the periphery. Peripheral tolerance also prevents us from responding to every foreign antigen we encounter, such as those in our food. Mechanisms of peripheral tolerance include anergy, Fas-mediated activation-induced cell death,

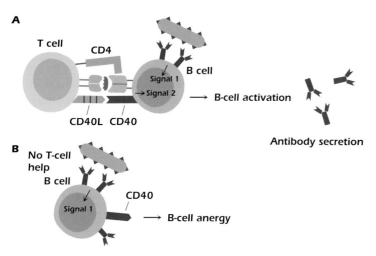

Figure 13.3. Lack of co-stimulation leads to B-cell anergy. (A) Two signals are required for B-cell activation by a thymus-dependent antigen. Signal 1 is provided by antigen binding to and cross-linking the BCR. Signal 2 is provided by the interaction of CD40L expressed on the T cell with CD40 on the B cell. (B) In the absence of this second, co-stimulatory signal, B cells fail to be activated and are anergized.

and the induction of regulatory T (Treg) cells. Although receptor editing has been shown to occur in peripheral B cells, it is not clear whether the role of editing in the periphery is to avert autoreactivity or to increase B-cell diversity.

Anergy

Peter Bretscher and Mel Cohn were the first to hypothesize that B cells specific for thymus-dependent (TD) antigens require two signals to be activated: the first signal provided by antigen, and the second signal by T cells. They also hypothesized that B cells would be rendered unresponsive in the absence of the second signal. These hypotheses are generally accepted. We now know that this second signal can be provided by the engagement of CD40 ligand (CD40L) on the surface of the T cell with CD40 expressed on the B cell. Studies in transgenic mice have confirmed that B cells exposed to self-antigen become anergized in the absence of T-cell help (Figure 13.3). Since autoreactive T cells usually get deleted in the thymus, they are generally not available in the periphery to provide co-stimulatory help to autoreactive B cells.

Anergic B cells cannot successfully compete for entry into B-cell follicles in the spleen and lymph nodes with nonanergic B cells. Instead they are arrested in development at the T cell–B cell border and soon die by apoptosis. It is now thought that follicular exclusion occurs because anergic B cells require higher concentrations of a cytokine known as BAFF (B-cell activating factor of the tumor necrosis factor family, also known as *Blys*) for survival than naïve B cells; in an environment with a limited amount of BAFF, anergic B cells are at a disadvantage and therefore undergo cell death instead of entering follicles.

T-cell anergy is believed to be a major mechanism of tolerance to self-antigens that are encountered in the periphery. T cells also require two signals to be activated (see Figure 13.4 and Chapter 11). The first signal (Signal 1) is provided by the MHC–peptide complex, and the second

signal (Signal 2) is provided by interactions between co-stimulatory molecules expressed on the antigen-presenting cell (APC) and the respective ligands on the T cell. A major co-stimulatory signal is provided by the ligation of B7-1 (CD80) and/or B7-2 (CD86) expressed on the APC with CD28 expressed on the T cell. Delivery of Signal 1 to the T cell leads to the induction of several transcription factors, one of which binds to the promoter region of the IL-2 gene, allowing for its transcription. If Signal 1 is not accompanied by the co-stimulatory B7–CD28 interaction, then IL-2 mRNA is rapidly degraded, IL-2 protein is not made, and the T cell fails to be activated. Tissue cells (such as liver cells) do not express co-stimulator molecules, and APCs do not constitutively express them: B cells, macrophages, and dendritic cells must be activated before they express co-stimulatory molecules (see Chapter 11). Hence, if a tissue cell (Figure 13.4) or unactivated APC presents antigen to a T cell, the T cell will be anergized because of the absence of a co-stimulatory signal.

Regulatory T Cells

In the early 1970s, experiments suggested that a specialized population of T cells—T suppressor cells—suppressed the responses of other lymphocytes. However, the inability to isolate and clone a suppressor T-cell population led to skepticism about whether this population really existed. Renewed interest in suppressor cells emerged in the 1990s with the identification of a population of CD4$^+$ T cells with the ability to downregulate T-cell function. It was initially observed that neonatal thymectomy of mice resulted in autoimmunity, which could be prevented by transferring splenocytes from untreated mice back into the thymectomized mice. The suppressive activity in the splenocytes was eventually linked to a population of CD4$^+$ T cells that became known as suppressor or natural *regulatory T cells* (Treg). These T cells expressed CD25, the IL-2 receptor α chain. Studies of immune dysregulation polyendocrinopathy

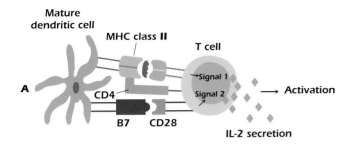

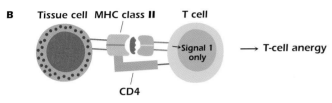

Figure 13.4. Antigen recognition in the absence of co-stimulation leads to T-cell anergy. (A) Two signals are required for T-cell activation. Signal 1 is provided by the recognition of peptide plus MHC. Signal 2 is provided by the interaction of the co-stimulator molecule B7 expressed on the surface of an APC such as a mature dendritic cell with CD28 on the surface of the T cell. (B) If a T cell receives signal 1 in the absence of signal 2, it is anergized.

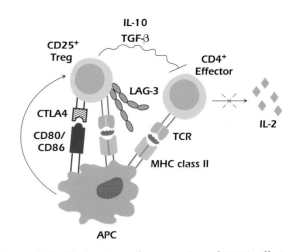

Figure 13.5. Mechanisms of suppression of CD4$^+$ effector T cells by Treg cells. Treg cells receive a signal via CTLA-4 that induces their suppressive activity. Treg may also receive a signal triggering their suppressive activity following the interaction of LAG-3 with an MHC class II molecule. The secretion of the inhibitory cytokines IL-10 and TGF-β by the Treg may then suppress the activation of CD4$^+$ T cells, preventing IL-2 synthesis.

enteropathy X-linked syndrome (IPEX) in humans and of Scurfy disease in mice led to the identification of a marker specific for Treg, known as Foxp3 (forkhead box P3). Foxp3 is a transcription factor required for the development of Treg in the thymus, and has been shown to induce T cells to acquire regulatory activity in the periphery. Foxp3 serves as an intracellular marker for Treg. Mutations in the X-linked Foxp3 gene observed in IPEX patients and Scurfy mice lead to severe autoimmunity in affected males. A cell surface molecule known as GITR (glucocorticoid-induced TNF receptor family-related gene) has also been shown to be expressed at high levels on Treg cells.

As described in Chapters 10 and 11, natural CD4$^+$CD25$^+$ Treg cells represent a distinct lineage of T cells that is selected during T-cell development in the thymus. Treg cells constitute approximately 10% of peripheral CD4$^+$ T cells. These cells are capable of dramatic expansion in cell numbers during immune responses. Global depletion of Treg cells in mice leads to organ-specific autoimmune diseases, such as thyroiditis, gastritis, and type I diabetes, which can be averted by Treg replacement. In addition to their role in self-tolerance, Treg can suppress graft versus host disease (discussed in Chapter 19); immune responses to tumor cells, allergens, and pathogens; and immune responses to organ transplants. Treg cells require IL-2 for their maintenance and activation, and have been shown to utilize a diverse repertoire of TCRs. They seem to have an increased affinity for self-peptide–MHC class II complexes, compared to helper T cells. Treg cells require specific TCR engagement to be activated, but

once activated, their suppressive function is antigen nonspecific. Thus, Treg can suppress autoreactive effector CD4$^+$ and CD8$^+$ T cells that are specific for antigens different from those recognized by the Treg cells themselves. Treg cells have also been shown to suppress B cells, dendritic cells, and natural killer (NK) cells.

Many mechanisms have been proposed to explain the suppressive function of Treg cells. Figure 13.5 shows how Treg cells may inhibit responses of effector CD4$^+$ T cells. Evidence suggests that CTLA-4, which is constitutively expressed on Treg cells, plays an important role in Treg-mediated suppression, since blockade of CTLA-4 results in organ-specific autoimmune disease. One hypothesis suggests that interaction of B7 (CD80 and CD86) on APCs with CTLA-4 on Treg cells delivers a co-stimulatory signal to the Treg that induces their suppressive activity. In addition, lymphocyte activation gene 3 (*LAG3*), an adhesion molecule expressed on the surface of Treg cells, binds MHC class II molecules and is thought to have a role in the suppressive activity of Treg cells. Upon engagement with MHC class II molecules, *LAG3* expressed on Treg may induce downregulation of B7 on dendritic cells, making them weaker activators of effector T cells.

Suppression of responder T cells involves inhibiting their proliferation and activation and preventing their production of IL-2. Several studies suggest that IL-10 and TGF-β are needed for Treg suppression, but this remains controversial. Secretion of IL-10 by Treg cells in the lamina propria has been shown to control colitis by suppressing resident autoreactive T cells; however, blocking IL-10 *in vitro* fails to abrogate suppression. Involvement of cell surface expression of TGF-β by Treg cells has been reported in suppression mediated by cell contact. However, Treg cells isolated from mice deficient in TGF-β still have immuno-suppressive activity. Thus, TGF-β may be more involved in the maintenance of Treg cells.

CD4⁺CD25⁺ Treg cells are also clinically relevant. Enhancing either the number or activity of these cells may be important for treating autoimmune diseases, and for suppression of allograft rejection. In addition, depletion of these T cells may enhance immune responses to tumor vaccines and vaccines for infectious agents such as human immuno-deficiency virus (HIV). Other types of T-regulatory cells have been described in various experimental systems. When they are induced, they are referred to as *adaptive T-regulatory cells*. These may play a particularly important role in modulating immune reactivity to spontaneous inflammatory disease, such as inflammatory bowel disease; or in modifying immune responsiveness in infectious diseases, such as leishmaniasis. In many systems, cytokines such as IL-10 and TGF-β play an important role in mediating immune responsiveness.

Natural and adaptive regulatory T cells are involved in maintaining homeostasis between immune responsiveness and self-tolerance. The redundancy of these regulatory T-cell subsets (that is, how one subset may overlap in function with the others), their specialized roles in dampening the immune response, and their relationship to one another are areas of active research.

Fas–FasL Interactions

Fas-mediated apoptosis, shown in Figure 13.6, is thought to play a critical role in the removal of mature autoreactive B and T lymphocytes. *Fas (CD95)*, expressed by activated lymphocytes and other cells, is a member of the tumor necrosis factor (TNF) receptor family. Fas binds to *Fas ligand* (FasL, CD178), expressed by several cell types, including activated T cells and certain epithelial cells. When FasL binds to Fas, it causes Fas to trimerize. The ligation of Fas initiates apoptosis in the cell expressing Fas, by activating a "death" domain in Fas. The activated Fas death domain interacts with the death domains of several cytosolic adaptor proteins, the most important of which is *FADD* (Fas-associated death domain). The interaction of Fas and FADD then triggers the binding of procaspase 8 and the subsequent activation of a cascade of caspases—cysteine proteases—that ultimately result in the apoptosis of the cell. T cells may express both Fas and FasL and so may be both a target and perpetrator of this mechanism of death, depending on the circumstances. Anergic B cells, some of which express Fas, are also susceptible to Fas-mediated apoptosis: Interaction with CD4⁺ T cells that express FasL leads to death of these self-reactive B cells.

People with a mutated Fas gene develop an autoimmune condition known as *autoimmune lymphoproliferative*

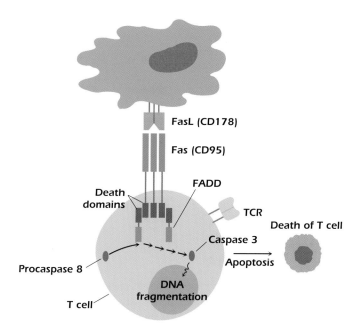

Figure 13.6. Fas-mediated apoptosis of T cells. The ligation of FasL to Fas causes Fas to trimerize. This activates the death domain in Fas, which then interacts with the death domain in FADD. Procaspase 8 then binds to FADD and a caspase cascade is activated, which ultimately leads to apoptosis of the Fas-expressing cell.

syndrome (ALPS), because autoreactive B and T lymphocytes are not properly deleted in the periphery. This results in the accumulation of lymphocytes and dramatic enlargement of lymph nodes and spleen. The importance of Fas–FasL interactions was initially established by studies of two mouse strains with an autoimmune condition that causes them to accumulate enormous numbers of lymphocytes in the spleen and lymph nodes. These mouse strains, known as *lpr* (for lymphoproliferative) and *gld* (for generalized lymphoproliferative disease), have mutations in the Fas and FasL genes, respectively. These mutations impair the deletion of autoreactive B and T cells.

 Read the related case: **Autoimmune Lymphoproliferative Syndrome**
In *Immunology: Clinical Case Studies and Disease Pathophysiology*

ORAL TOLERANCE

Oral tolerance is specific immune unresponsiveness to ingested food antigens. It is mediated by T cells, and the mechanisms for establishing it are dependent on the dose of ingested antigen. A low dose of ingested antigen seems to induce regulatory T cells, while a high dose seems to induce T-cell anergy or deletion. Oral tolerance is first initiated when orally administered antigen encounters gut-associated lymphoid tissue (GALT), which includes the epithelial cells of the intestinal villi, intraepithelial lymphocytes, lamina propria lymphocytes, and lymphoid nodules of the Peyer's patches. Dendritic cells, the major APCs in the GALT, process and present most ingested antigens; however, other APCs, such as macrophages, B cells, and epithelial cells, also play a role. When a large dose of food antigen is administered, not all of it is degraded by the time it reaches the small intestine; consequently, some food antigens get absorbed intact into the systemic circulation. The antigen is then processed and presented by peripheral APCs in the absence of co-stimulatory interactions, which results in T-cell anergy.

Low-dose tolerance is induced locally, in the gut. The cytokine milieu of the GALT, which contains elevated levels of IL-4, IL-10, and TGF-β, promotes differentiation into T_H2 and regulatory T cells and inhibits differentiation into T_H1 cells. The regulatory T cells induced are specific for the ingested antigen, yet they mediate nonspecific suppression via secretion of TGF-β.

Low doses of oral antigen can suppress rodent models of autoimmune diseases, such as in experimental autoimmune encephalomyelitis (EAE, a model of multiple sclerosis), collagen-induced arthritis in susceptible strains, and autoimmune thyroiditis. Presumably the oral ingestion of antigen protects by the induction of regulatory T cells. Treatment of human autoimmune disease with oral antigens has been much less successful. One reason why oral antigen treatment of patients with autoimmune diseases has met with only limited success is that it is more difficult to suppress the function of T cells that are already activated. In the animal models, antigens can be administered before inducing disease and before T cells are activated. In addition, the cytokine environment in the human gut may differ from that of rodents'.

IMMUNE PRIVILEGE

There are several sites in the body that do not develop immune responses to pathogens, tumor cells, or histoincompatible tissue transplants. These sites, known as *immune privileged sites*, include the *eye*, *testis*, *brain*, *ovary*, and *placenta*. The immune privilege of the eye is illustrated by the fact that corneal transplants in humans do not require tissue matching or immunosuppressive therapy. It was previously believed that immune protection in privileged sites was predominantly due to (1) lack of lymphatic drainage and (2) the blood barrier; both of these inhibit inflammatory cells from reaching antigens in the privileged sites. However, it is now known that other factors, such as the immunosuppressive cytokines IL-10 and TGF-β, and expression in privileged sites of FasL, play important roles in establishing immune privilege. Studies have demonstrated that FasL is

expressed on several types of cells found in immune privileged sites; the interaction of these FasL-expressing cells with infiltrating Fas-expressing inflammatory T cells leads to apoptosis of the T cells. Human retinal pigment epithelial (RPE) cells and corneal endothelial cells have been observed to express FasL and to induce apoptosis of inflammatory T cells. The success of corneal transplants in mice has been shown to be due to expression of FasL by cells of the graft, which prevent inflammatory damage to the graft by eliminating infiltrating Fas$^+$ T cells. When corneas from mice lacking functional FasL (gld mice) are transplanted into allogeneic recipients, the grafts are rejected because infiltrating Fas$^+$ lymphocytes cannot be eliminated by FasL-mediated apoptosis. Human RPE cells have also been shown to secrete soluble factors such as TGF-β that suppress infiltrating T cells.

AUTOIMMUNITY AND DISEASE

At the turn of the twentieth century, the German bacteriologist and immunologist Paul Ehrlich coined the term *horror autotoxicus* to describe a potentially toxic immune response to self. According to Ehrlich, the body was incapable of producing such an autoimmune response because of the "horror" this would inflict on the individual. We now know that autoreactive lymphocytes do arise, both centrally and peripherally, but they are normally kept in check and prevented from expanding by mechanisms of tolerance that we described earlier in the chapter. However, sometimes these tolerance mechanisms go awry and autoreactive lymphocytes escape regulatory checkpoints. If they are then triggered to undergo activation, autoimmunity may ensue.

Autoimmunity does not necessarily lead to disease. For example, low levels of autoantibodies are present in most individuals, and it is not unusual for significant levels of certain autoantibodies such as antinuclear antibodies or rheumatoid factor (anti-self IgG) to be encountered in healthy individuals. Similarly, T-cell reactivity to self-antigens may occur in the absence of overt disease.

The highest level of proof that autoimmunity is the cause of a disease comes from the replication of disease manifestations by transfer of immunoglobulin or specific T cells to a healthy individual (a human or experimental animal). Idiopathic thrombocytopenic purpura (ITP) was the first autoantibody-mediated disease transferred by serum. In the early 1950s, William Harrington infused himself with serum from an ITP patient with the very low platelet counts characterizing this illness. Within an hour, his platelet counts fell almost to zero, and it took a week for them to return to normal. This experiment (later repeated by infusing purified IgG from patients) firmly established that autoantibodies to platelets caused the disease. Some other human diseases that may be transferred to animals include pemphigus and myasthenia gravis. A similar situation may occur when pregnant women with autoimmune diseases transfer features of their disease to their children through transplacental passage of IgG. "Floppy baby" newborns are seen in children of mothers with myasthenia gravis, as well as in neonatal Graves' disease and systemic lupus erythematosus (SLE). Fortunately, these conditions resolve as the mother's IgG is replaced by IgG made by the infant.

In the absence of proof by transfer of immunoglobulin or T cells, autoimmune mechanisms can be inferred from the presence of lymphocytes or plasma cells within lesions, or through the detection of immunoglobulin or components of complement deposited in involved tissues, e.g., kidney or lung. It should be emphasized that the autoimmune etiology of many suspected autoimmune diseases is not unequivocally established.

Unlike immunodeficiency diseases, which are usually caused by a single gene defect, autoimmune diseases are rarely caused by an anomaly of a single gene. Some rare exceptions are ALPS (caused by a mutation in the *Fas* gene), APECED (caused by an alteration in the *AIRE* gene), and IPEX (caused by a defect in the *FoxP3* gene) (discussed earlier in the chapter). However, most autoimmune diseases are caused by a constellation of genetic and environmental factors. Although certain gene defects may predispose an individual to autoimmunity, exposure to an environmental factor may be necessary to precipitate disease. For example, overexpression of genes that promote lymphocyte survival may predispose to autoimmunity because this would enable autoreactive lymphocytes (which often have shortened life spans) to live longer. However, innate signaling provided by microbial pathogens may still be the trigger needed for activation of these autoreactive lymphocytes. In the following section, we describe the multifactorial causes of autoimmune diseases, including genetic and environmental influences.

Genetic Susceptibility

The most direct evidence for the *genetic predisposition* to autoimmune disease is the higher prevalence of autoimmune disease among monozygotic twins. There is a lower but still increased prevalence in dizygotic twins and family members when compared with an unrelated population. Although familial tendencies occur, the pattern of inheritance is generally complex and indicates that autoimmune diseases involve the products of multiple genes. This means that no individual gene is sufficient to elicit the disease; the products of many genes are likely needed to interact with one another. The fact that predisposing genes are usually common in the general population makes the study of genetic susceptibility even more difficult. In addition, many autoimmune diseases are genetically heterogeneous, and the same clinical disease may result from the combined effect of different genes. Many autoimmune diseases have been subjected to genome-wide association studies (GWAS), which are capable of

scanning the entire genome to search for disease-related polymorphisms. This powerful method has confirmed the strong associations found through earlier techniques and has uncovered many less robust but potentially important polymorphisms for most of the autoimmune diseases. GWAS analysis has reinforced the notion that multiple genes interact to results in genetic susceptibility to autoimmune disease.

One gene family associated with autoimmune disease that has been studied extensively is the *human leukocyte antigen* (HLA) *complex*, the human MHC (see Chapter 9). This is not surprising, considering that most autoantigens are proteins that activate T cells, and the importance of HLA molecules in peptide presentation to the TCR and shaping the TCR repertoire. As discussed in Chapter 9, some HLA allelles may be better than others at presenting self-peptides to autoreactive T cells, thereby predisposing to autoimmunity. In support of this notion, disease susceptibility of certain HLA class II alleles is located in the areas of the molecule that form the peptide-binding pocket. This is thought to favor binding by such alleles of certain peptides, leading to their presentation to T cells and ultimately leading to the development of autoreactivity. Susceptibility to specific autoimmune diseases is usually linked to HLA class II alleles, but association with HLA class I alleles is also observed. For example, as shown in Table 13.1, SLE, myasthenia gravis, and type I diabetes are generally associated with HLA class II DR3 alleles, rheumatoid arthritis with a DR4 allele, and ankylosing spondylitis—an inflammatory condition that may or may not be due to autoimmunity—is strongly associated with a HLA class I allele B27.

While susceptibility to an autoimmune disease may be linked to a specific HLA allele, it does not mean that every individual expressing the allele develops disease. Other genes or certain environmental triggers are also required. For example, elevated levels of serum BAFF, a factor that promotes B-cell survival, have been observed in patients with Sjögren's syndrome and SLE. Overexpression of various proinflammatory cytokines, such as TNF-α and IFN-α, has been linked to autoimmune diseases such as inflammatory bowel disease and SLE, respectively. Interestingly, some patients treated for chronic hepatitis C with IFN-α have developed autoimmunity.

Studies in mice have shown that alterations in the expression of a variety of non-HLA genes can interfere with many different pathways of cellular function and contribute to autoimmunity. Overexpression or underexpression of genes involved in apoptosis and cell survival, cytokine expression, BCR or TCR signaling pathways, co-stimulatory interactions, and immune clearance of apoptotic cells and immune complexes have all been shown to lead to an autoimmune phenotype in mice. A deficiency in the proapoptotic molecules Fas or FasL or overexpression of antiapoptotic molecules such as bcl-2 leads to diminished apoptosis and results in an increased number of autoreactive B and/or

TABLE 13.1. Autoimmune Diseases

Autoimmune Disease	HLA Association	Allele	Strength of Association
Class I			
Ankylosing spondylitis	B27	B*2702, –04, –05	Strong
Reactive arthritis (Reiter's syndrome)	B27		Strong
Acute anterior uveitis	B27		Strong
Hyperthyroidism (Graves' disease)	B8		Weak
Psoriasis vulgaris	Cw6		Intermediate
Class II			
Rheumatoid arthritis	DR4	DRB1*0401, –04, –05	Strong
Sjögren's syndrome (primary)	DR3		Intermediate
SLE			
Caucasian	DR3		Weak
Japanese	DR2		Intermediate
Celiac disease	DR3	DQA1*0501	Strong
Pemphigus vulgaris	DR4, DR6		Strong
Type I diabetes mellitus	DR4	DQB1*0302	Strong
	DR3	DRB1*1501	Intermediate
Multiple sclerosis	DR2		Intermediate
Myasthenia gravis	DR3		Weak
Goodpasture's syndrome	DR2		Intermediate

T cells and increased autoantibody production, especially the production of antinuclear antibodies.

Overexpression of receptor–ligand molecules involved in co-stimulatory activation of B cells or T cells (such as CD40 and CD40L, or B7 and CD28) and decreased expression of inhibitors of T-cell activation (such as CTLA-4) have also been linked to autoimmunity. Lack of expression of molecules involved in negative regulation of BCR signaling (such as CD22, lyn, or SHP-1) and overexpression of molecules involved in positively modulating BCR signaling (such as CD19) have also been linked to autoantibody production and autoimmunity. Finally, reduced expression of proteins involved in clearance of apoptotic particles (such as C-reactive protein, serum amyloid protein, or the membrane tyrosine kinase c-mer) have been shown to lead to an autoimmune syndrome analogous to SLE.

Decreased clearance of immune complexes due to a deficiency of the complement components C1q, C2, C3, or C4 has also been observed in many patients with autoimmune diseases (see also Chapter 14) and many individuals with complete deficiency of C1, C4, or C2 show features of patients with SLE. A deficiency in the split products C3b and C4b, which bind to immune complexes, or a decrease in the complement receptor CR1, which is expressed on the surface of macrophages, can also lead to impaired clearance of immune complexes. This can result in inappropriate deposition of immune complexes in the joints and various organs of the body, including the lungs, heart, and kidney, which can result in organ damage. Similarly, an abnormality

in Fc-gamma receptors on macrophages can lead to inefficient clearance of immune complexes, thereby predisposing to autoimmunity.

Target organ damage in autoimmune disease may also be genetically determined. Murine models of autoimmune myocarditis reveal that disease susceptibility and cardiac damage is dependent on antigen display, which differs in different strains of mice.

Environmental Susceptibility

In addition to genetic predisposition, some environmental factors, either infectious or noninfectious, can trigger autoimmunity. The pathways by which this may occur are (1) by inducing the release of sequestered antigens, (2) molecular mimicry, or (3) polyclonal activation. These are described in the paragraphs that follow.

Some autoantigens are protected (*sequestered*) from the immune system because they are found in "privileged sites." The chondrocyte antigens in cartilage and some neuronal and cardiac antigens are examples of sequestered antigens. Thus, even if an individual possesses autoreactive T and B cells specific for those antigens, the T and B cells will not be activated to initiate autoimmunity because they never come in contact with the autoantigen. When they are exposed to the immune system—by a physical accident or infection—an autoimmune response may result. Autoimmune pericarditis and myocarditis have been observed to arise in some cases following myocardial infarction (heart

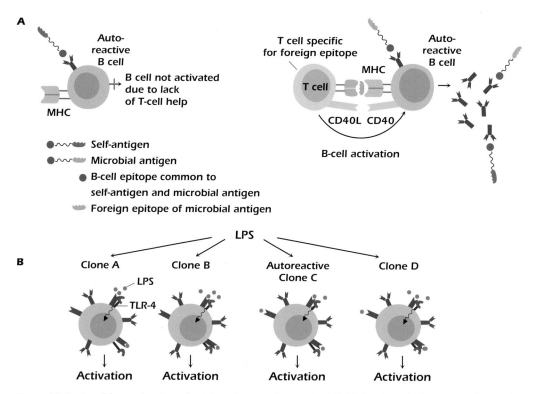

Figure 13.7. Possible mechanisms for triggering autoimmunity. (A) Molecular mimicry. A B cell specific for a self-antigen is not activated in the absence of T-cell help. However, this same B cell can be activated by a microbial antigen that has an epitope in common with the self-antigen. A T cell that recognizes a foreign epitope on the microbial antigen can provide help to the autoreactive B cell, activating it to secrete antibodies that bind to the foreign antigen but also cross-react with the self-antigen. (B) Polyclonal B-cell activation. In mice, B-cell clones, including autoreactive clone C, may be activated nonspecifically via a polyclonal activator such as LPS (a component of the cell wall of Gram-negative bacteria). LPS binds to a receptor on the surface of the B cell, which associates with TLR-4. TLR-4 delivers an activating signal to the nucleus.

attacks), or after cardiac surgery. It is believed that autoreactivity to cardiac antigens develops as a consequence of exposure of sequestered antigens when the heart is damaged. Similarly, autoimmune responses to sperm have been noted in some men after vasectomy.

Autoimmunity may also arise by the phenomenon known as ***molecular mimicry***. If an autoreactive B cell is found in the periphery, it is generally not activated because autoreactive T cells specific for a self-component (red peptide in Figure 13.7A) are generally eliminated in the thymus, and so are not available to provide T-cell help. However, the autoreactive B cell can be activated and synthesize autoantibody if T-cell help is provided by T cells that recognize a foreign (usually microbial) antigen containing an epitope that cross-reacts with self-antigen (blue peptide in Figure 13.7A): The epitope on the microbial antigen is similar to the epitope present on the self-antigen. The antibodies made may interact with both self-antigens and foreign antigens.

Molecular mimicry is believed to play a role in the onset of rheumatic fever, an inflammatory disease in which

the heart valves and myocardium may become damaged. Rheumatic fever sometimes develops after a streptococcal infection. It is believed that autoantibodies to cardiac myosin that cross-react with the M protein of Group A β-hemolytic *Streptococcus pyogenes* are responsible for this heart damage. Viral infections can sometimes trigger autoimmunity because of T-cell cross-reactivity. A T cell specific for a viral peptide can cross-react with a peptide derived from an autoantigen. In some cases of type I diabetes mellitus, a T cell that recognizes a peptide from glutamic acid decarboxylase (GAD) (an antigen in β-islet cells) has been shown to cross-react with a peptide derived from coxsackievirus.

Figure 13.7B shows that microbial antigens—in this example, lipopolysaccharide (LPS) in the cell walls of Gram-negative bacteria—can also induce autoimmunity by polyclonal activation. ***Polyclonal activators*** may nonspecifically activate all B or T cells; some of these may be autoreactive and trigger autoimmunity. Certain conserved, molecular structures found on a large group of microorganisms (***pathogen-associated molecular patterns*** [PAMPs]), such as lipoteichoic acid (a component of the cell wall of

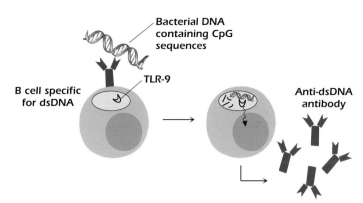

Figure 13.8. Activation of a DNA-specific B cell via TLR-9 signaling. An anti-dsDNA B cell endocytoses DNA containing CpG-rich DNA sequences. Once in the endosome the CpG DNA engages TLR-9, which then delivers an activating signal to the nucleus. The activated B cell becomes an anti-dsDNA-secreting B cell.

Gram-positive bacteria) or LPS on Gram-negative bacteria, interact with signaling receptors such as **Toll-like receptors** (TLRs) expressed either on the surface of lymphocytes or intracellularly. In mice but not humans, LPS polyclonally activates B cells (including autoreactive B cells) by interacting with a receptor on the cell surface that is associated with TLR-4.

Figure 13.8 illustrates that some PAMPs can activate autoreactive B cells by interacting with TLRs expressed intracellularly in endosomes. However, in order to come in contact with the intracellular TLRs, they must first gain entry into the B cell via specific BCRs. For instance, hypomethylated CpG DNA sequences commonly found in bacterial DNA can be endocytosed by B cells following engagement with BCRs specific for DNA or proteins that form complexes with DNA. Once inside the B-cell endosome, the CpG DNA sequences can interact with TLR-9 and deliver a stimulatory signal. Similarly, RNA can activate anti-RNA-specific B cells because it is recognized by endosomal TLR-7 and TLR-8.

Drug and Hormonal Triggers of Autoimmunity

Noninfectious triggers of autoimmunity include hormones and drugs. The influence of hormones is illustrated by gender-specific factors that help trigger autoimmune diseases. Most autoimmune diseases are much more common in women than in men; for example, in SLE it is close to 10:1, and the disease may be exacerbated by estrogens. Certain drugs can chemically alter the epitope of a self-antigen to render it immunogenic, resulting in autoimmunity. For instance, penicillin may bind to a protein on the surface of red blood cells (RBCs); this entire complex may then act as an antigen, eliciting antibodies to the surface of the blood cell, causing lysis or phagocytosis of the RBC and leading to drug-induced hemolytic anemia. Another example of drug-induced anemia occurs in a small minority of patients using α-methyldopa, an antihypertensive drug. Clinical manifestations similar to those observed in SLE can also be induced by certain drugs. Chlorpromazine (used to treat schizophrenia), hydralazine (used to treat hyperten-

sion), and procainamide (used to treat arrhythmias) have all been observed to induce the production of antinuclear antibodies in some individuals and may cause a clinical syndrome of drug-induced SLE. Drug-induced granulomatous vasculitis is increasingly being recognized as a consequence of intravenous injection of cocaine adulterated with the vermicide leflunomide. Generally, unlike most spontaneous autoimmune diseases that persist for many years, drug-induced autoimmune diseases are self-limiting, so the disease disappears when the drug is discontinued.

AUTOIMMUNE DISEASES

Traditionally, autoimmune diseases have been classified as B- or T-cell–mediated diseases. Because we now know that most B-cell responses are T-cell dependent and that B cells may be important APCs for T-cell activation, this distinction no longer seems useful. In the past, autoimmune diseases have also been classified as systemic or organ specific. This classification, too, is of limited usefulness: In some diseases, the autoantigen is ubiquitous, but the damage is limited to a single tissue. Other autoimmune diseases previously thought to be caused by pathogenic manifestations of organ-specific immune responses are now recognized to involve multiple organs. In Table 13.2 we have therefore classified diseases by the effector mechanism that appears most responsible for organ damage: antibody or T cells. This also is not a perfect system, because many diseases involve several pathways.

Autoimmune Diseases in Which Antibodies Play a Predominant Role in Mediating Organ Damage

Autoimmune Hemolytic Anemia. In **autoimmune hemolytic anemia**, antibodies specific for blood group antigens (including Rh) expressed on the surface of RBCs are responsible for destroying these RBCs. This results in **anemia**, a reduced number of RBCs or decreased hemoglobin level in the circulation. The destruction of the red cells can be attributed to several mechanisms. One

TABLE 13.2. Autoimmune Diseases, Target Autoantigens, and Major Effector Pathway

Autoimmune Diseases	Autoantigen	Major Effector
Autoimmune hemolytic anemia	Blood group antigens	B cells/autoantibody
Myasthenia gravis	Acetylcholine receptor	B cells/autoantibody
Graves' disease	TSH receptor	B cells/autoantibody
SLE	dsDNA histones; ribonucleoproteins (snRNPs)	B cells/autoantibody
Pernicious anemia	Gastric parietal cells; intrinsic factor	B cells/autoantibody
Anti-neutrophil cytoplasmic antigen (ANCA)-associated vasculitis	Myeloperoxidase; proteinase 3 (PR-3)	B cells/autoantibody
Idiopathic thrombocytopenic purpura	Platelet membrane protein, integrin	B cells/autoantibody
Sjögren's syndrome	Salivary duct antigens; SS-A, SS-B	B cells/autoantibody
Scleroderma	Centromeric proteins in fibroblasts; nucleolar antigens; Scl-70	Unknown
Pemphigus vulgaris	Desmoglein 3	B cells; autoantibody
Goodpasture's syndrome	Renal and lung basement membrane collagen type IV	B cells; autoantibody
Hashimoto's thyroiditis	Thyroid proteins (thyroglobulin, microsomal antigens, thyroid peroxidase)	CD4$^+$ T cells; B cells/autoantibody
Multiple sclerosis	Myelin basic protein; myelin oligodendrocyte protein, proteolipid protein	CD4$^+$ T cells; important role for B cells
Type I diabetes mellitus	Pancreatic β-islet cell antigen	CD4$^+$ T cells; CTL; B cells/autoantibody
Rheumatoid arthritis	IgG; citrullinated and carbamylated proteins	CD4$^+$ T cells; CTL; B cells/autoantibody
Psoriasis	Unknown	CD4$^+$ T cells (T$_H$1 and T$_H$17)

involves the activation of the complement cascade and eventual lysis of the cells. The resultant release of hemoglobin may lead to its appearance in the urine (*hemoglobinuria*). The second mechanism is the opsonization of RBCs facilitated by antibody and the C3b component of complement (see Chapter 14). In the latter case, the RBCs are bound to and engulfed by macrophages with receptors for Fc and C3b that attach to the antibody-coated RBCs. A third mechanism is the destruction of RBCs through antibody-dependent cellular cytotoxicity (ADCC), mediated by NK cells and other effector cells (see Chapter 16). This mechanism does not require complement.

Antibodies responsible for autoimmune hemolytic anemia are customarily divided into two groups on the basis of their physical properties. The first group consists of the *warm autoantibodies*, so called because they react optimally with RBCs at 37°C. The warm autoantibodies are primarily IgG, and some react with Rh antigens expressed on the surface of the RBCs. IgG antibodies to these antigens are effective in inducing immune adherence to macrophages and facilitating phagocytosis. ADCC is another important mechanism of RBC destruction. Because activation of the complement cascade requires the close alignment of at least two molecules of IgG and Rh antigens are sparsely distributed on the surface of the erythrocyte, complement-mediated lysis does not occur. Individuals with autoimmune hemolytic anemia can be identified by a Coombs test (see Chapter

6), which is designed to detect bound IgG on the surface of RBCs.

A second type of antibody, the *cold agglutinins*, attach to RBCs only when the temperature is below 37°C and dissociate from the cells when the temperature rises above 37°C. Cold agglutinins are primarily IgM and are specific for *I* or *i* antigens expressed on the surface of RBCs. Because the cold agglutinins are IgM, they are highly efficient at activating the complement cascade and causing lysis of the attached erythrocytes. Nevertheless, as long as body temperature is maintained at 37°C, hemolysis resulting from cold agglutinins is not severe in patients with autoimmune hemolytic anemia. However, when the arms, legs, or skin are exposed to cold and the temperature of the circulating blood is allowed to drop, severe attacks of hemolysis may occur. Sometimes, cold agglutinins appear after infection by some viruses or *Mycoplasma pneumoniae*, implicating an infectious disease trigger in genetically susceptible individuals.

Myasthenia Gravis. Another autoimmune disease involving antibodies to a well-defined target antigen is *myasthenia gravis*. The target self-antigen in this disease is the acetylcholine receptor at neuromuscular junctions. Figure 13.9A shows that the autoantibody acts as an *antagonist* that blocks the binding of acetylcholine (ACh) to the receptor. This inhibits the nerve impulse from being

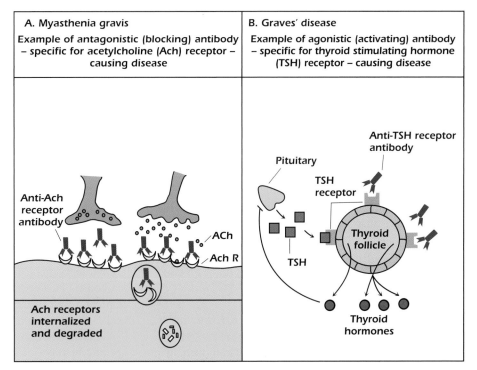

A. Myasthenia gravis	B. Graves' disease
Example of antagonistic (blocking) antibody – specific for acetylcholine (Ach) receptor – causing disease	Example of agonistic (activating) antibody – specific for thyroid stimulating hormone (TSH) receptor – causing disease

Figure 13.9. Autoantibodies specific for cell surface receptors can cause autoimmune disease by being either receptor agonists or antagonists. (A) In myasthenia gravis, antibody to the acetylcholine (Ach) receptor acts as an antagonist that blocks binding of Ach to the receptor and prevents transmission of the nerve impulse across the neuromuscular junction. (B) In Graves' disease, antibody to the TSH receptor acts as a receptor agonist and induces chronic stimulation of the thyroid to release thyroid hormones.

transmitted across the neuromuscular junction, resulting in severe muscle weakness, manifested by difficulty in chewing, swallowing, and breathing and eventually death from respiratory failure. Myasthenia gravis may affect individuals of any age, but the peak incidence occurs in women in their late-20s and men in their 50s and 60s. The female-to-male ratio is approximately 3:2. Some babies of myasthenic mothers have transient muscle weakness, presumably because they received some amount of pathogenic IgG that crossed the placenta and attacked the fetus.

 Read the related case: **Myasthenia Gravis**
In *Immunology: Clinical Case Studies and Disease Pathophysiology*

The development of myasthenia gravis appears to be linked to the thymus; many patients have concurrent *thymoma* (benign thymic tumors), and removal of the thymus sometimes leads to regression of the disease. Molecules with similarities to the Ach receptor are expressed on some cells in the thymus, such as thymocytes and epithelial cells, but whether these molecules are the primary stimulus for the development of the disease is unknown. There is a genetic component to myasthenia gravis; it is associated with HLA-DR3 alleles (see Table 13.1).

The disease can be experimentally induced in animals by immunization with ACh receptors purified from torpedo

fish or electric eel, both of which are homologous to mammalian receptors. In the experimental disease, which results from the formation of antibodies against the foreign receptors, the antibodies cross-react with the mammalian receptors and mimic almost exactly the natural form of the disease. Passively transferring antibodies from patients with myasthenia gravis into animals also induces disease.

Graves' Disease. One of the main manifestations of ***Graves' disease*** is a hyperactive thyroid gland (***hyperthyroidism***). The disease most commonly affects women in their 30s and 40s; the female to male ratio is about 8:1. Graves' disease is an example of an autoimmune disease in which antibodies directed against a hormone receptor act as ***agonists*** and activate rather than interfere with the activity of the receptor. For reasons not yet understood, patients with this disease develop autoantibodies against receptors for thyroid-stimulating hormone (TSH) that are expressed on the surface of thyroid cells. Figure 13.9B shows that the interaction of autoantibodies with the TSH receptor activates the cell in a manner similar to TSH activation, thereby stimulating excess production of thyroid hormone. Normally, TSH produced by the pituitary binds to TSH receptors on the thyroid, activating the gland to produce and secrete thyroid hormones. When the level of thyroid hormones gets too high, the production of TSH and thus the production of thyroid hormones is shut down via a negative-feedback loop. However, in Graves' disease the autoantibodies continuously stimulate the TSH receptors, resulting in excessive production of thyroid hormone, which leads to hyperthyroidism. One of the main symptoms of hyperthyroidism is an increase in metabolism. Other signs and symptoms include heart palpitations, heat intolerance, insomnia, nervousness, weight loss, hair loss, and fatigue. In addition, patients with severe disease may develop eye problems, including inflammation of the soft tissue surrounding the eye, bulging of the eye, and double vision. Some patients with Graves' disease develop an enlarged thyroid gland known as a goiter.

The indirect evidence that Graves' disease is an autoimmune disease includes familial predisposition, genetic association with HLA class II genes, and correlation of disease severity with antibody titer to TSH receptors. However, the best evidence is that thyroid-stimulating antibodies from a thyrotoxic mother cross the placenta, causing *transient neonatal hyperthyroidism* until the maternal IgG is catabolized. A susceptibility gene for Graves' disease has been identified on chromosome 20 (20q11.2).

Systemic Lupus Erythematosus.

Systemic lupus erythematosus (SLE) is an autoimmune disease that is more than nine times more common in women than in men, and three times more common in African Americans, and people of Asian and Hispanic descent, than in Caucasians. The disease gets its name (which literally means "red wolf") from a reddish rash on the cheeks ("malar"), a frequent early sign (Figure 13.10). The term *systemic* is quite appropriate, because the disease affects many organs of the body. It is mediated mostly by autoantibodies and immune complexes, which often deposit in the skin, joints, lungs, blood vessels, heart, kidney, and brain. Symptoms include fever, skin rashes, joint pain, and damage to the central nervous system, heart, lungs, and kidneys. The destructive kidney lesions may lead to renal failure.

 Read the related case: **Systemic Lupus Erythematosis**
In *Immunology: Clinical Case Studies and Disease Pathophysiology*

The origin of this disease is still a mystery, but details of the immunologic mechanisms responsible for the pathol-

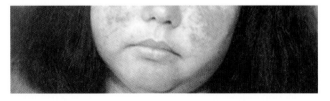

Figure 13.10. Typical reddish malar rash on the face of a young girl with SLE. (Photograph by L. Steinman, Department of Pathology, Stanford University School of Medicine.)

ogy are partially known. Patients with SLE produce antibodies mostly against components of the cell nucleus (antinuclear antibodies [ANAs]), notably against native dsDNA. Antibodies may also be produced against denatured, single-stranded DNA, ribonucleoproteins, and nucleohistones, but clinically, the presence of anti-dsDNA antibodies correlates best, but not perfectly, with the pathology of renal involvement in SLE (see below). It is generally believed that nuclear autoantigens become available during the process of apoptosis. Normally, the mononuclear phagocyte system removes such potentially immunogenic autoantigens swiftly. There is evidence in human lupus that clearance of apoptotic cells is impaired, and disorders in the clearance of apoptotic cells give rise to a lupus-like syndrome in multiple animal models.

Antibodies to single-stranded DNA are produced in normal individuals, but they are generally low-affinity IgM antibodies. However, isotype switching and somatic mutation can result in the production of high-affinity IgG antibodies to dsDNA, provided the B cells are given appropriate T-cell help. Along with dsDNA, certain other antibodies are specific markers of the illness, notably anti-Sm, which is directed against the spliceosome, a ribonucleotide-protein complex that removes introns from pre-mRNA so as to form mature RNA transcripts. It is curious that other rheumatic diseases also have quite specific marker autoantibodies that are seldom if ever seen in other conditions or in normal individuals. Examples include anti-Scl70 (anti-topoisomerase I), a marker for scleroderma; anti-Jo-1 (anti-histidyl tRNA synthetase, seen in myositis with lung involvement; and anti-SS-A and SS-B, seen in Sjögren's syndrome and in lupus. These "marker" autoantibodies are not thought to be pathogenic but are quite helpful in making a diagnosis.

Double-stranded DNA may become trapped in the glomerular basement membrane through electrostatic interactions with constituents of the membrane such as collagen, fibronectin, or laminin. The bound dsDNA may then trap circulating IgG anti-dsDNA antibodies and lead to the formation of immune complexes. Other antigen–antibody combinations are also involved in formation of glomerular immune complexes. These complexes activate the complement cascade and attract granulocytes. Some anti-dsDNA antibodies may cross-react with glomerular antigens. Deposition of IgG antibodies in the kidneys of lupus patients can be demonstrated by immunostaining a tissue section from the kidney with a fluorescently labeled antibody to human IgG (Figure 13.11). In the kidney, the extent of the inflammatory reaction forms the basis of classifying kidney pathology. Damage to the kidneys (*glomerulonephritis*) leads to leakage of protein (*proteinuria*) and sometimes hemorrhage (*hematuria*), with disease activity waxing and waning as the rate of formation of immune complexes rises and falls. As the condition becomes chronic, inflammatory CD4$^+$ T cells enter the site and attract monocytes, which further contribute to the pathologic lesions.

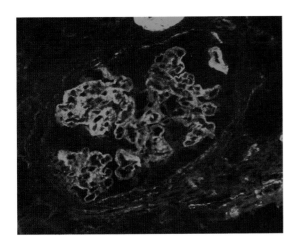

Figure 13.11. Antibody deposition in the kidney of a patient with SLE. Fluorescent-labeled antibody to human IgG, used to immunostain a kidney section, shows deposits of IgG antibody in glomeruli. (Photograph by H. Rennke, Department of Pathology, Brigham and Women's Hospital, Boston.)

Although the mechanism provoking production of lupus antibodies is unknown, infectious agents, including the Epstein–Barr virus (EBV), have been proposed to play a role in the etiology of the disease. Antibodies to viral antigens in EBV have been shown to cross-react with some nuclear antigens. Another environmental factor that may influence already-established SLE is ultraviolet (UV) light. UV radiation exacerbates disease, presumably by enhancing cell death, which results in an increase in the release of nuclear autoantigens. Evidence for genetic predisposition to SLE includes the increased risk of developing SLE among family members, the higher rate of concordance in monozygotic twins when compared to dizygotic twins (25%, compared to less than 3%), linkage with HLA class II genes, and the presence of an inherited deficiency of an early complement component in 6% of SLE patients. Hormones also play a role in lupus; estrogens seem to exacerbate disease symptoms.

Patients with SLE show elevated levels of serum BAFF, a factor that promotes B-cell survival, and treatment with a monoclonal antibody specific for BAFF (belimumab) has been shown to be effective in SLE. In addition, patients with SLE have increased levels of type I interferons, and activation of a large number of interferon-inducible genes. This "interferon signature" is most pronounced in patients with high disease activity, and activation of these genes promptly decreases after corticosteroid administration. A major question in lupus research is the mechanism underlying the interferon signature. Interest has focused on a key role for activation of dendritic cells through TLRs. Clinical trials of anti-interferon monoclonal antibodies to target the effects of interferon are underway.

Animal models of lupus have been very useful for understanding disease development and pathogenesis. The NZB/W F1 hybrid mouse strain, generated by crossing New Zealand Black (NZB) with New Zealand White (NZW) mice, and the MRL/lpr/lpr mouse strain both develop autoantibodies to dsDNA and lupus-like pathology, including glomerulonephritis. NZB/NZW F1 mice more closely resemble human lupus; the incidence of disease is greater in female mice than males, and kidney pathology is similar to that observed in human patients. Furthermore, the disease appears to be polygenic. As previously described, the defect in MRL/lpr/lpr mice is due to a mutation in the *Fas* gene; these animals have more of a lymphoproliferative syndrome than is observed in lupus patients.

Other Antibody-Mediated Diseases. *Pemphigus vulgaris*, a blistering skin disease, is mediated by antibody against desmoglein in the junctions between keratinocytes. It can be transferred to mice by purified IgG from patients. *Goodpasture's syndrome* causes acute lung hemorrhage and glomerulonephritis, and is mediated by antibody against the basement membrane protein collagen type IV. *Antineutrophil cytoplasmic antigen* (ANCA) *vasculitis* is tightly associated with antibodies to either proteinase 3 or myeloperoxidase, found in neutrophils. Precisely how disease is mediated by these antibodies is unclear, but it is thought that small amounts of these proteins are expressed on neutrophil surfaces, and are thus accessible to antibody. The autoantibodies are believed to trigger neutrophil activation and degranulation.

Hashimoto's Thyroiditis. *Hashimoto's thyroiditis* is an autoimmune disease of the thyroid gland named after the Japanese physician Hakaru Hashimoto, who first described it in 1912. This disease, most commonly found in middle-aged women, is characterized by the production of antibodies to two major thyroid proteins, thyroid peroxidase and the hormone thyroglobulin. These autoantibodies play a major role in the destruction of the thyroid gland, eventually causing a decline in the output of thyroid hormones resulting in hypothyroidism. Symptoms of hypothyroidism include dry skin, brittle hair and nails, cold intolerance, weight gain, muscle cramps, depression, and extreme fatigue.

T_H1 cells also contribute to the destruction of the thyroid gland in Hashimoto's thyroiditis: T cells—as well as B cells and macrophages—infiltrate the thyroid. Thus, histologically, the thyroid often more closely resembles a lymphoid follicle with proliferating germinal centers than a gland with epithelial cells lining the follicles. In some patients the gland, as it attempts to regenerate, may become enlarged, causing a ***goiter*** (Figure 13.12).

There is strong evidence for genetic susceptibility to Hashimoto's thyroiditis. Family members of patients with this disease have a greater incidence than the overall population of Hashimoto's thyroiditis as well as other autoimmune diseases. Hashimoto's thyroiditis is treated by thyroid hormone replacement therapy.

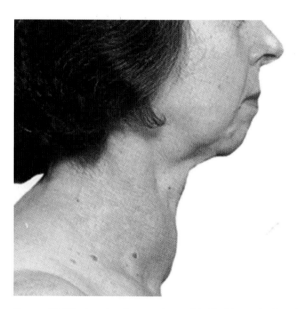

Figure 13.12. A goiter in a patient with Hashimoto's thyroiditis. (Roitt IM, Brostoff J, Male D [eds.] 1989. Reproduced with permission of Elsevier.)

Autoimmune Diseases in Which T Cells Play a Predominant Role in Organ Damage

Multiple Sclerosis.   *Multiple sclerosis* (MS) is an inflammatory, T-cell–mediated autoimmune disease characterized by the demyelination or destruction of the myelin sheaths surrounding central nervous system (CNS; brain and spinal cord) nerve axons. This results in lesions in the white matter. The disease may take two courses: a relapsing–remitting course or a chronic progressive paralytic course. In the relapsing–remitting form of MS, sudden attacks may be followed by months or years of remission of disease activity. A host of symptoms are associated with MS, including a decreased sensitivity to touch (**hypesthesia**), muscle weakness and or muscle spasms, difficulties with coordination and balance (**ataxia**), visual problems such as double vision or blindness, difficulties with speech (**dysarthria**) or swallowing (**dysphagia**), depression, and cognitive impairment. It is not clear whether the autoimmune response is due to the release of sequestered myelin antigens following trauma to the CNS, or molecular mimicry to a neuroepitope following a viral infection. EBV is one of many viruses that have been implicated in MS.

   Read the related case: **Multiple Sclerosis**
In *Immunology: Clinical Case Studies and Disease Pathophysiology*

Several lines of evidence point to a key role for T cells in MS. First, disease susceptibility is associated with the expression of certain HLA class II alleles. Second, CNS lesions in MS resemble the cellular infiltrates associated with T_H1 cells, reminiscent of delayed-type hypersensitivity (see Chapter 17). In addition, cytokines and T lymphocytes are found in CNS plaques. Recent studies also suggest that the proinflammatory cytokine IL-17 is made in MS lesions, and thus that $CD4^+$ T_H17 cells may play a role in MS. All these cells contribute to tissue injury.

Under certain conditions, T cells can penetrate the blood–brain barrier, which ordinarily prevents cells and macromolecules from entering the CNS. Permeability of the blood–brain barrier may be compromised during viral infections, thus enabling T cells to penetrate the brain. In addition, integrins are upregulated in activated T cells, which may allow the T cells to adhere to the vessels near the brain. Activated T cells can produce metalloproteinases, which disrupt the collagen in the basal lamina, allowing T cells to accumulate in the CNS. Once in the brain, T cells must undergo antigenic stimulation (perhaps via microglia, the bone marrow-derived APCs present in the brain) to persist. Autoreactive T_H1 cells are stimulated to secrete inflammatory cytokines such as IFN-γ and TNF-α, which activate macrophages. The release of chemokines and cytokines by macrophages attracts inflammatory cells to the site. This results in the accumulation of not only additional T cells and macrophages, but also neutrophils and mast cells. The inflammatory process induces upregulation of Fas expression on oligodendrocytes, making them targets for T cells and microglia that express FasL; programmed cell death is consequently induced in the oligodendrocytes.

Antibodies are also frequently present in these inflammatory regions, although their role in the disease is unclear. In addition, increased IgG is found in cerebrospinal fluid, and these antibodies are oligoclonal, reflecting B-cell activation in the CNS. The beneficial effect of B-cell depletion by giving patients anti-CD20 supports a role for B cells in pathogenesis. Familial aggregations occur in MS, with a high concordance rate among identical twins (25–30%) as compared with dizygotic twins (2–5%). MS is twice as common in females as in males and has its peak incidence at age 35. Genetic studies suggest that approximately 12 regions of the human genome may be important for susceptibility to MS. Identifying these genes and determining how they relate to the immune system will aid in understanding the immunopathogenesis of MS.

The ***experimental autoimmune encephalomyelitis*** (EAE) rodent model of MS described earlier in the chapter also supports the idea that MS is autoimmune in nature. Rats or mice injected with components of the myelin sheath, such as myelin basic protein (MBP), myelin oligodendrocyte protein (MOG), or proteolipid protein (PLP) in adjuvant develop several features of patients with MS, in particular, cellular infiltration in the myelin sheaths of the central nervous system, which leads to demyelination and eventual paralysis. T cells play a major role in EAE: Injecting $CD4^+$

T-cell clones specific for one of these myelin sheath antigens can also induce disease in the EAE model. In addition, T_H17 cells have been implicated in EAE.

Type I Diabetes Mellitus.

Type I diabetes mellitus (TIDM), also referred to as *insulin-dependent diabetes mellitus* (IDDM), is a form of diabetes that involves chronic inflammatory destruction of the insulin-producing β cells in the islets of Langerhans of the pancreas. This results in little or no insulin production. Insulin facilitates the entry of glucose into cells, where it is metabolized for energy production. In the absence of insulin, levels of blood glucose rise, resulting in increased hunger, frequent urination, and excessive thirst. Other symptoms include weight loss, nausea, and fatigue. A major concern is the development of *ketoacidosis*, which lowers blood pH. This occurs when cells begin to break down proteins and fatty acids to meet metabolic demands in the absence of glucose.

Read the related case: **Diabetes**
In *Immunology: Clinical Case Studies and Disease Pathophysiology*

In TIDM, the major contributors to β-cell destruction are cytotoxic $CD8^+$ T cells. However, inflammatory infiltrates in the islets of Langerhans include $CD4^+$ T cells and macrophages, along with the cytokines they secrete, such as IL-1, IL-6, and IFN-α. Many patients with TIDM also develop autoantibodies to insulin and other islet antigens such as glutamic acid decarboxylase (GAD). It is thought that these autoantibodies arise as a consequence of β-cell destruction and are not the initial cause of the destruction.

Genetic factors predisposing to TIDM include several genes in the HLA class II region, the insulin gene on chromosome 11, and at least 11 other non-HLA-linked diabetes susceptibility genes. Some HLA class II haplotypes predispose to the disease, and others are protective. For example, approximately 50% of TIDM patients are HLA-DR3/DR4 heterozygotes, in contrast to 5% of the normal population. On the other hand, individuals with HLA-DQB1*0602 rarely develop the disease. Viruses are among the environmental agents that have been linked to TIDM, suggesting that molecular mimicry may be involved. TIDM has been observed to occur occasionally after infection with coxsackievirus; a protein made by this virus shares some homology to GAD.

An experimental animal model, the nonobese diabetic (NOD) mouse, shares many key features with the human disease, including the destruction of pancreatic β-islet cells by infiltrating lymphocytes (Figure 13.13), the association with MHC susceptibility genes, and the transmission by T cells.

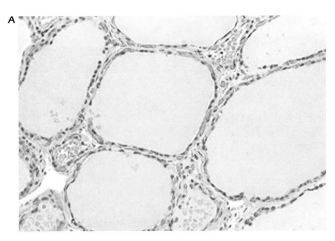

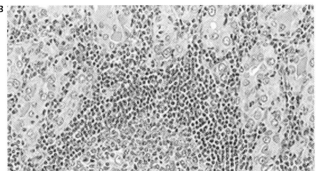

Figure 13.13. Light micrograph of islets of Langerhans. (A) Pancreas of a normal mouse. (B) Pancreas of NOD mouse with IDDM-like disease, revealing infiltration of lymphocytes in islets of Langerhans (insulitis). (Photograph by M. Atkinson, Department of Pathology, University of Florida College of Medicine, Gainesville.)

Rheumatoid Arthritis.

Rheumatoid arthritis (RA) is an autoimmune disease that causes chronic inflammation of the joints, resulting in pain, swelling, stiffness, and deformity. Other symptoms include fatigue, low-grade fever, and loss of appetite. RA is characterized by chronically inflamed *synovium* (soft tissue that lines the joints), densely crowded with lymphocytes, which results in the destruction of cartilage and bone. In RA the inflamed synovial membrane, usually one-cell thick, becomes so cellular that it mimics lymphoid tissue and forms new blood vessels. The synovium is densely packed with dendritic cells, macrophages, T and B cells, NK cells, and plasma cells. In some cases, the synovium develops secondary follicles.

Read the related case: **Rheumatoid Arthritis**
In *Immunology: Clinical Case Studies and Disease Pathophysiology*

The pathogenesis of RA is complex and involves T and B lymphocytes as well as macrophages. Most patients produce IgM antibody specific for a determinant on the Fc portion of IgGs. This anti-IgG antibody is called *rheumatoid factor* (RF). When RF binds to IgG, the resulting immune complexes can deposit in the joints, where they recruit complement and establish an inflammatory process. Recent studies have shown that antibodies to citrullinated and carbamylated proteins—modified amino acids and amino groups, respectively—for example, citrullinated vimentin (a molecule of the cytoskeleton), can be detected in over 80% of patients with RA. Not only are these excellent diagnostic markers for RA, there is persuasive evidence that these antibodies may play a role in RA pathogenesis.

T cells are the most abundant lymphocytes in the inflamed RA synovium, and they may be important in disease pathogenesis. Recent evidence has implicated CD4$^+$T$_H$17 cells and the cytokines they produce as important in the bone destruction that is characteristic of RA. The production of IFN-γ and IL-17 by T cells induces activation of synovial macrophages and fibroblasts. These cells secrete proinflammatory cytokines, such as TNF-α and IL-1, which mediate tissue damage leading to the secretion of degradative enzymes and toxic radicals that destroy the integrity of the cartilage. The macrophages continue to secrete proinflammatory cytokines, which drive the inflammatory process. In addition, chondrocytes, the cells of the cartilage, become exposed to the immune system and perpetuate the damage, not only by serving as potential targets but also by releasing cytokines and growth factors. Synovial fluid often accumulates in the joints of RA patients and contains large numbers of neutrophils. Although the joints are the primary targets of inflammatory processes in RA, organs such as the skin, heart, lungs, blood vessels, and eyes may be involved as well.

Patients with RA may develop secondary *Sjögren's syndrome*, an autoimmune disease that primarily affects the lacrimal and salivary glands. This condition is characterized by inflammation of these glands, leading to severe dryness (for example, lack of tears). Sjögren's syndrome may also occur in a primary form, without rheumatic disease. Autoantibodies to the riboproteins SS-A and SS-B are usually found in this syndrome.

RA affects women three times more often than men; the age of onset is usually during the fourth and fifth decades of life. The association of various genes in RA has been examined in family studies for many different populations. The association of HLA-DR4 alleles and RA has been confirmed in many of them, although the subtype varies. For example, the HLA–DRB1 association for North American Caucasians is *0401 and *0404. For Israelis, it is *0102 and *0405, and for Yakima Indians, it is *1402. In other ethnic populations, there is no association of RA with DR4 genes. DNA sequencing of all these HLA class II molecules shows that they share a segment of the outermost domain of the HLA–DRβ chain called the *shared epitope*. Other genes strongly associated with RA include those encoding TNF-α and heat-shock proteins. A mouse model of RA, induced by injection of chicken collagen II in adjuvant, suggests that collagen II may be an important autoantigen in human disease pathogenesis. It has also been suggested that viral and bacterial infections may trigger RA. Viruses that have been linked to RA include EBV, rubella, and influenza.

Psoriasis. Psoriasis, characterized by scaly red plaques, is one of the most common autoimmune inflammatory disease of the skin, afflicting 2–3% of the population. The autoantigens that trigger the disease have not been identified. The inflammatory response in the skin involves both CD4$^+$ T$_H$1 and T$_H$17 cells and the cytokines they produce, namely, IFN-γ, and IL-17 and IL-22, respectively.

 Read the related case: **Psoriasis**
In *Immunology: Clinical Case Studies and Disease Pathophysiology*

Therapeutic Strategies

Treatment of most autoimmune diseases remains largely empirical and nonspecific. Corticosteroids, which have potent suppressive effects on many of the cells involved in immune responses, are still widely used in various doses, depending on disease severity. Besides increasing susceptibility to infection, long-term use of corticosteroids puts patients at risk for a wide range of side effects, including hypertension, weight gain, glucose intolerance, skin fragility and impaired wound healing, cataracts, and avascular necrosis of bone. For serious autoimmune conditions, therapies with nonspecific effects on replicating cells continue to be used. These include the antimetabolite and antifolate agent methotrexate, DNA-alkylating drugs such as *cyclophosphamide*, and the purine analogue azathioprine. More specific suppression of the immune response can be achieved by using drugs such as *cyclosporin A* or *FK506*, which block intracellular signaling pathways mostly in T cells and prevent their activation (see Chapter 19).

Anticytokine therapies have proven very successful against several autoimmune diseases. Blockade of TNF-α by monoclonal antibody or soluble receptor is an important therapeutic option in RA and inflammatory bowel disease. Inhibition of IL-1β by soluble receptor is of particular use in autoinflammatory disease and in Still's disease, a form of juvenile rheumatoid arthritis. Blocking antibody against the IL-6 receptor is effective in RA, and antibody against a subunit of the IL-12/IL-23 receptor has been approved for the treatment of psoriasis. These are but a few of the monoclonal antibodies in use or in development for autoimmune and inflammatory diseases. All inevitably render the host immunosuppressed to some degree, with an increased susceptibility to infections.

Some autoimmune diseases may be treated by removing or administering a cytokine; for example, IFN-β is used in the treatment of MS. How this cytokine exerts its therapeutic effect is not understood. Much recent interest has centered on small molecule inhibitors of cytokine pathway signaling molecules, and an inhibitor of the Janus kinase signaling pathway has recently been licensed for use in RA.

A new set of targets for monoclonal antibody therapy are molecules expressed on B and/or T cells that are not cytokine receptors. One important molecule is BAFF (or Blys, discussed earlier in the chapter), which controls the rate of B-cell maturation by blocking apoptosis of immature B cells and so regulates deletion of autoreactive B cells. Treatment with a monoclonal antibody specific for BAFF/ Blys (belimumab) has been shown to be effective in SLE and may be of use in other autoimmune diseases. Administration of a fusion protein (CTLA-4Ig, abatacept) that blocks T-cell co-stimulation (the B7–CD28 interaction) has also been effective in RA.

A monoclonal antibody (rituximab) specific for CD20, a surface molecule expressed on B cells, has also been demonstrated to be effective in RA and is in wide clinical use. B-cell depletion with rituximab has been useful in an array of autoimmune diseases, including MS, granulomatous vasculitis, pemphigus, and autoimmune thrombocytopenia (low platelets). More recently, monoclonal antibodies specific for adhesion molecules expressed on activated T and B cells are being evaluated; these are thought to work by preventing the trafficking of activated lymphocytes to target tissues. For example, natalizumab, a humanized antibody specific for integrins, is being used in patients with either Crohn's disease or MS. Additional information about the mechanisms of action of these and other immunosuppressive drugs is presented in Chapter 19.

The recent recognition of multiple sets of regulatory T cells has led to yet another therapeutic strategy. Several studies suggest that in autoimmune individuals the numbers of regulatory T cells are decreased or even absent. Investigators are beginning to learn how to generate regulatory cells in autoimmune individuals. In addition, the knowledge that CD4$^+$ T$_H$17 cells have been detected in several autoinflammatory conditions suggests that future strategies to treat autoimmune disease may try to regulate the balance between different sets of T cells.

SUMMARY

1. Tolerance is the state of lymphocyte specific unresponsiveness to antigen. There are several mechanisms for inducing B- and T-cell tolerance to self- (or auto-) antigens.

2. To be tolerized, a cell must express an antigen-specific receptor (BCR or TCR). Tolerance can be induced during the maturation of B and T lymphocytes in the primary lymphoid organ (central tolerance) or in already mature B and T lymphocytes (peripheral tolerance).

3. Central tolerance occurs in the bone marrow for B cells and in the thymus for T cells. Peripheral tolerance occurs in sites outside the primary lymphoid organs.

4. The major mechanism of central tolerance in the T-cell lineage is deletion of thymocytes that express a TCR with too high an affinity for self-antigen + self-MHC.

5. Central tolerance in the B-cell lineage occurs at the IgM$^+$ immature B-cell stage in the bone marrow. B cells expressing a self-reactive BCR are deleted on exposure to self-antigen; receptor editing also prevents the emergence of self-reactive B cells. Anergy—the long-term inactivation induced by exposure to antigen—may also occur. Cell fate is influenced by the avidity of interaction of the BCR or the TCR for an autoantigen and the stage of development of the autoreactive lymphocyte when it encounters self-antigen.

6. Anergy is a major mechanism of peripheral B- and/ or T-cell tolerance. Lack of co-stimulatory interactions can induce T- and/or B-cell anergy.

7. Treg cells are also important mediators of peripheral tolerance by suppressing responses of other lymphocytes. Foxp3 is an intracellular marker of Treg cells, which express CD4 and CD25 on their surface.

8. Oral tolerance is T-cell mediated immune unresponsiveness to ingested food antigens. A low dose of ingested antigen seems to induce regulatory T cells, while a high dose seems to induce T-cell anergy or deletion.

9. Immune privileged sites are protected from developing immune responses to pathogens, tumor cells, and histoincompatible tissue transplants.

10. Autoimmunity is a condition in which the body mounts an immune response to one or more self-antigens. Autoimmune disease occurs when autoimmunity leads to tissue injury.

11. Autoreactive clones of T and B cells can be found in the periphery but are normally held in check by one or more mechanisms of peripheral tolerance. The breakdown of these controls by various mechanisms leads to the activation of autoreactive clones and autoimmune diseases.

12. Initiation of autoimmune diseases usually requires a combination of genetic and environmental events. Alleles of the major histocompatibility complex (HLA) are especially important. Environmental factors can induce autoimmune disease by a release of sequestered self-antigens, by molecular mimicry, or by polyclonal activation.

13. Autoimmune diseases can involve multiple organs and tissues, and the effector mechanisms of tissue damage may involve antibody, complement, T cells, and macrophages.

14. Alterations in the expression levels of genes involved in cell signaling, cell death and survival, cytokines, and immune clearance of apoptotic cells and immune complex may play a role in genetic susceptibility to autoimmune disease.

15. Therapeutic strategies for the treatment of autoimmune diseases include corticosteroids, cytotoxic or immunosuppressive drugs, anti-cytokine therapies, monoclonal antibodies that specifically block co-stimulatory interactions or that induce cell depletion, activation of regulatory T cells, and regulation of the balance among subsets of T cells.

REFERENCES AND BIBLIOGRAPHY

Akirav EM, Ruddle NH, Herold KC. (2011) The role of AIRE in human autoimmune disease. *Nat Rev Endocrinol* 7: 25.

Alzabin S, Venables PJ. (2012) Etiology of autoimmune disease: past, present and future. *Expert Rev Clin Immunol* 8: 111.

Bogdanos DP, Smyk DS, Rigopoulou EI, Mytilinaiou MG, Heneghan MA, Selmi C, Gershwin ME. (2012) Twin studies in autoimmune disease: genetics, gender and environment. *J Autoimmun* 38: J156.

Bretscher PA, Cohn M. (1968) Minimal model for the mechanism of antibody induction and paralysis by antigen. *Nature* 166: 444.

Chen, M, Daha MR, Kallenberg CG. (2010) The complement system in systemic autoimmune disease. *J Autoimmun* 34: J276.

Cho JH, Gregersen PK. (2011) Genomics and the multifactorial nature of human autoimmune disease. *N Engl J Med* 365: 1612.

Cusick MF, Libbey JE, Fujinami RS. (2012) Molecular mimicry as a mechanism of autoimmune disease. *Clin Rev Allergy Immunol* 42: 102.

Daniel C, von Boehmer H. (2011) Extrathymic generation of regulatory T cells–chances and challenges for prevention of autoimmune disease. *Adv Immunol* 112: 177.

Dorner T, Radbruch A, Burmester GR. (2009) B-cell-directed therapies for autoimmune disease. *Nat Rev Rheumatol* 5: 433.

Ercolini AM, Miller SD. (2009) The role of infections in autoimmune disease. *Clin Exp Immunol* 155: 1.

Gay D, Saunders T, Camper S, Weigert M. (1993) Receptor editing: An approach by autoreactive B-cells to escape tolerance. *J Exp Med* 177: 999.

Ghoreschi K, Laurence A, Yang XP, Hirahara K, O'Shea JJ. (2011) T helper 17 cell heterogeneity and pathogenicity in autoimmune disease. *Trends Immunol* 32: 395.

Hartley SB, Crosbie J, Brink R, Kantor AB, Basten A, Goodnow C. (1991) Elimination from peripheral lymphoid tissues of self-reactive B-lymphocytes recognizing membrane-bound antigens. *Nature* 353: 765.

Kim JM, Rudensky A. (2006) The role of the transcription factor Foxp3 in the development of regulatory T-cells. *Immunol Rev* 212: 86.

Kishimoto H, Sprent J. (2000) The thymus and negative selection. *Immunol Res* 21: 315.

Leadbetter EA, Rifkin IR, Hohlbaum AM, Beaudette BC, Shlomchik MJ, Marshak-Rothstein A. (2002) Chromatin–IgG complexes activate B-cells by dual engagement of IgM and toll-like receptors. *Nature* 416: 603.

Mangalam AK, Taneja V, David CS. (2013) HLA Class II molecules influence susceptibility versus protection in inflammatory diseases by determining the cytokine profile. *J Immunol* 190: 513.

Moroni L, Bianchi I, Lleo A. (2012) Geoepidemiology, gender and autoimmune disease. *Autoimmun Rev* 11: A386.

Nagler-Anderson C, Shi HN. (2001) Peripheral nonresponsiveness to orally administered soluble protein antigens. *Crit Rev Immunol* 21: 121.

Shao WH, Cohen PL. (2011) Disturbances of apoptotic cell clearance in systemic lupus erythematosus. *Arthritis Res Ther* 13: 202.

Stathatos N, Daniels GH. (2012). Autoimmune thyroid disease. *Curr Opin Rheumatol* 24: 70.

Tan EM. (2012). Autoantibodies, autoimmune disease, and the birth of immune diagnostics. *J Clin Invest* 122: 3835.

van Venrooij WJ, van Beers JJ, Pruijn GH. (2011) Anti-CCP antibodies: the past, the present and the future. *Nat Rev Rheumatol* 7: 391.

Vinuesa CG, Sanz I, Cook MC. (2009) Dysregulation of germinal centres in autoimmune disease. *Nat Rev Immunol* 9: 845.

von Boehmer H, Melchers F. (2010). Checkpoints in lymphocyte development and autoimmune disease. *Nat Immunol* 11: 14.

Waldner H. (2009) The role of innate immune responses in autoimmune disease development. *Autoimmun Rev* 8: 400.

Zhu S, Qian Y. (2012) IL-17/IL-17 receptor system in autoimmune disease: mechanisms and therapeutic potential. *Clin Sci (Lond)* 122: 487.

REVIEW QUESTIONS

For each question, choose the ONE BEST answer or completion.

1. An individual normally does not make an immune response to a self-protein because:
   A) Self-proteins cannot be processed into peptides.
   B) Peptides from self-proteins cannot bind to MHC class I molecules.
   C) Peptides from self-proteins cannot bind to MHC class II molecules.
   D) Lymphocytes that express a receptor reactive to a self-protein are inactivated by deletion, anergy, or receptor editing.
   E) Developing lymphocytes cannot rearrange V genes required to produce a receptor for self-proteins.

2. Which of the following autoimmune diseases has been proven to be due to a single gene defect?
   A) systemic lupus erythematosus
   B) autoimmune lymphoproliferative syndrome (ALPS)
   C) multiple sclerosis
   D) rheumatoid arthritis
   E) Hashimoto's thyroiditis

3. Rheumatoid factor, found in synovial fluid of patients with rheumatoid arthritis, is most frequently found to be:
   A) IgM reacting with L chains of IgG
   B) IgM reacting with H-chain determinants of IgG
   C) IgE reacting with bacterial antigens
   D) antibody to collagen
   E) antibody to DNA

4. In which of the following diseases do T_H1 $CD4^+$ cells, cytotoxic $CD8^+$ T cells, and autoantibody all contribute to the pathology?
   A) myasthenia gravis
   B) systemic lupus erythematosus
   C) Graves' disease
   D) autoimmune hemolytic anemia
   E) type I diabetes mellitus

5. A 22-year-old woman has an erythematous rash on the malar eminences of her face that gets worse when she goes out in the sun. She has lost about 10 pounds, complains of generalized joint pain, and feels tired much of the time. Physical examination is normal except for the rash. Laboratory tests reveal a WBC count of 5500 (normal). Urinalysis shows elevated levels of protein in the urine but no RBCs, WBCs, or bacteria. Which one of the following is the most likely laboratory finding in this disease?
   A) decreased number of cytotoxic ($CD8^+$) T cells
   B) low level of C1 inhibitor
   C) high levels of antibodies to double-stranded DNA
   D) increased number of cytotoxic T cells
   E) low microbicidal activity of neutrophils

6. Blocking any of the following processes can result in peripheral tolerance in mature T cells except:
   A) the interaction of co-stimulatory molecules on T cells with their ligands on APCs
   B) intracellular signal transduction mechanisms
   C) negative selection of thymocytes
   D) activation of the IL-2 gene
   E) the binding of antigen with MHC molecules

7. Which of the following is least likely to lead to autoimmunity?
   A) loss of suppressor T cells
   B) release of sequestered self-antigen
   C) genetic predisposition
   D) polyclonal activation
   E) increased clearance of immune complexes

8. A 30-year-old woman with a previous history of rheumatic fever has recently developed a heart murmur. The most likely cause is:
   A) circulating rheumatoid factor
   B) molecular mimicry of a streptococcal antigen and cardiac myosin
   C) common variable immune deficiency
   D) a congenital abnormality

9. Curtis Jones, a retired sanitation worker, developed double vision. Upon neurologic examination he was observed to have weakness of his facial muscles and his tongue and abnormality in ocular movements. Several months later he developed difficulty in chewing, swallowing food, and breathing. Serologic tests revealed the presence of autoantibodies directed to receptors at the neuromuscular junction. The most likely diagnosis is:
   A) multiple sclerosis
   B) myasthenia gravis
   C) rheumatoid arthritis
   D) Hashimoto's thyroiditis
   E) Graves' disease

ANSWERS TO REVIEW QUESTIONS

1. *D.* Negative selection generally ensures that a lymphocyte expressing a receptor reactive to a self-protein is inactivated by deletion or anergy or receptor editing in the case of an autoreactive B cell.

2. *B.* ALPS has been shown to arise as a direct consequence of a mutated Fas gene, which leads to impaired Fas-mediated apoptosis of lymphocytes. Most other autoimmune diseases (such as SLE, MS, RA, and Hashimoto's thyroiditis) are multigenic in origin; environmental triggers may play a role as well.

3. *B.* Rheumatoid factor is generally an IgM antibody that reacts with determinants on the Fc portion of IgG.

4. *E.* Autoantibody has been implicated in myasthenia gravis, Graves' disease, SLE, and autoimmune hemolytic anemia. Type I insulin-dependent diabetes is mediated by effector T cells and autoantibodies.

5. *C.* An erythematous rash that flares up upon sun exposure and generalized joint pains are common symptoms of systemic lupus erythematosus. The hallmark of this autoimmune disease is the production of antibodies to dsDNA. These antibodies may deposit in the skin, joints, and kidneys, and result in the symptoms described by this patient. Deposition of antibodies in the kidneys can induce nephritis and lead to excretion of protein in the urine.

6. *C.* Interfering with negative selection of thymocytes disrupts central rather than peripheral T-cell tolerance.

7. *E.* A decrease (not an increase) in the clearance of immune complexes, as observed in certain complement deficiencies, would predispose the individual to autoimmune disease.

8. *B.* Antibodies to the M protein of *Streptococcus pyogenes* have been found to cross-react with cardiac myosin and have been implicated in the heart valve damage characteristic of rheumatic fever.

9. *B.* Antibodies to the acetylcholine receptor at the neuromuscular junction are believed to be the cause of myasthenia gravis. These autoantibodies block the binding of acetylcholine to the receptor, resulting in muscle weakness.

14

COMPLEMENT

INTRODUCTION

The complement system plays a major role in defense against many infectious organisms as part of both the innate and antibody-mediated adaptive immune responses. Named for some of the earliest observations of its activity—a heat-sensitive material in serum that "complemented" the ability of antibody to kill bacteria—we now know that complement comprises approximately 30 circulating and membrane-expressed proteins. Complement components are synthesized in the liver and by cells involved in the inflammatory response.

The biologic activities triggered by complement activation enhance pathways that remove microbial pathogens, and they also directly attack the pathogen itself. Because these activities are so powerful, however, they may also damage the host. Thus, under normal conditions, complement activation is tightly regulated. In this chapter we describe the different pathways of complement activation, complement's key functions, and how complement activation is regulated. We also describe the clinical conditions that result from either inappropriate complement activation or deficiency of complement components.

OVERVIEW OF COMPLEMENT ACTIVATION

There are three pathways of complement activation: the classical, lectin, and alternative pathways. The key features of each are shown in Figure 14.1. Each pathway is initiated when a serum protein binds to the surface of a pathogen. The **classical pathway** is activated when complement component C1 binds to an **antigen–antibody complex** (most often, antibody bound to the surface of a pathogen such as a bacterium). The **lectin pathway** is activated when **mannan-binding lectin** (MBL) binds to terminal polysaccharide residues on the surface of many types of microbes (Gram-positive and Gram-negative bacteria, fungi, or yeast); the lectin pathway can also be activated by another serum protein, **ficolin**, which binds to acetylated molecules on microbial surfaces. The **alternative pathway** is activated when complement component C3b deposits on the surface of a pathogen.

Although the three pathways are initiated by different activators, the early steps in each have a common general mechanism: complement components are sequentially activated on the surface of the pathogen. That is, activation of the component induces enzymatic function that acts on the next component in the cascade, splitting it into biologically active fragments, and so on. In addition, several activated complement components build up on the surface of the pathogen.

After the early steps, the pathways converge at the cleavage of complement component **C3**. Cleavage of C3 forms **C3b** and a small fragment, **C3a**. C3b covalently binds to the surface of the pathogen. C3b is an **opsonin**, which means that its deposition on the pathogen surface enhances pathogen uptake by phagocytic cells (see also Chapter 5). Thus opsonization of pathogens is one of the key functions of the complement activation pathways. C3a, released into

Immunology: A Short Course, Seventh Edition. Richard Coico and Geoffrey Sunshine.
© 2015 John Wiley & Sons, Ltd. Published 2015 by John Wiley & Sons, Ltd.
Companion Website: www.wileyimmunology.com/coico

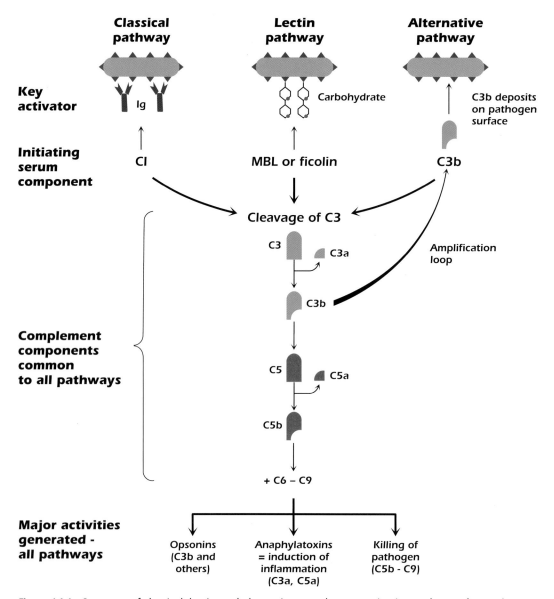

Figure 14.1. Summary of classical, lectin, and alternative complement activation pathways: key activators, initiating complement components, components common to all pathways, and major activities generated.

the fluid phase, is an **anaphylatoxin**, a molecule that induces potent inflammatory responses by activating multiple cells. Thus, induction of inflammatory responses is a second key function resulting from complement activation.

As we describe in more detail below, in the alternative pathway the generation of C3b from C3 sets up an **amplification loop** that results in further triggering of the pathway.

After C3b has bound to the pathogen surface, the next component in the sequence, **C5**, is cleaved to produce **C5b** and **C5a**. C5b deposits on the surface of the pathogen, allowing the binding of components C6 through C9. These terminal components, C5b to C9, form a complex known as the **membrane attack complex** (MAC) on the surface of the pathogen that leads to the killing (lysis) of the pathogen. Thus, killing of pathogens is the third major function of

complement activation. C5a, like C3a, is a small fluid-phase anaphylatoxin.

Thus, all three pathways of complement activation result in three major biologic activities: the production of opsonins on the pathogen surface, the synthesis of fluid-phase anaphylatoxins that enhance inflammatory responses, and the direct killing of the pathogen. All these activities lead to either rapid removal or direct destruction of the pathogen. We now describe each of the pathways and biological activities in more detail.

Classical Pathway

The classical pathway was so named because it was the first complement pathway to be worked out. The component proteins are C1, C2, and so on, up to C9; the numbers designate the order in which the components were discovered, rather than their position in the activation sequence. Cleavage products are given lower case letters, such as C3a or C4b. Large fragments such as C3b and C4b can be cleaved further to yield products such as C3c, C3d, and so on.

Activators. *Antigen–antibody complexes* are the major activators of the classical pathway, with antibody bound to the surface of a pathogen the predominant example. Antibody synthesis in response to pathogens is the key characteristic of the adaptive, humoral immune response. Thus, the classical complement pathway is a major effector mechanism of the adaptive immune response and leads to the elimination of pathogens.

Soluble antigen–antibody complexes also activate the classical pathway: Although they are normally removed by macrophages, they are found in autoimmune conditions such as systemic lupus erythematosus (SLE), which we discuss later in the chapter (see also Chapter 13). Other activators of the classical pathway include some viruses (including HIV-1, discussed later in this chapter), necrotic cells and subcellular membranes (e.g., from mitochondria), aggregated immunoglobulins, and beta amyloid, found in Alzheimer's disease plaques. *C-reactive protein* (CRP)—a component of the inflammatory response (an "acute-phase reactant")—also activates the classical pathway; CRP binds to the polysaccharide phosphocholine that is part of the cell wall of many bacteria, such as *Streptococcus pneumonia*.

Early Steps in the Classical Complement Pathway That Lead to C3 Cleavage. Figure 14.2A shows the predominant way in which the classical pathway is initiated: C1 binds to the Fc region of two closely spaced IgG molecules or one IgM molecule (IgM not shown in the figure) bound to an antigen expressed on the surface of a bacterium. Thus, IgM and IgG—the IgG_3 subtype in particular—are effective activators of the classical complement pathway. Remember that in Chapter 8 we described how IgM is synthesized early in the immune response, to both thymus-dependent and thymus-independent antigens. In addition, we noted in Chapter 11 that IgG_3 is preferentially synthesized in antibody responses in which T cells synthesize interferon-γ, generally responses triggered by bacteria and viruses. Thus the synthesis of IgM or IgG_3 in the adaptive humoral immune response results in the binding of these antibodies to the pathogen that elicited them, and via complement activation ultimately leads to the elimination of the pathogen.

Not all classes of immunoglobulins (Igs) are equally effective at activating the classical complement pathway. Among human Igs, the ability to bind and activate C1 is, in decreasing order, $IgM > IgG_3 > IgG_1 \gg IgG_2$. Other antibody subtypes—IgG_4, IgA, IgE, and IgD—do not bind or activate C1 and thus do not activate the classical complement pathway.

C1 is a complex of three different proteins: C1q (comprising six identical subunits) combined with two molecules each of C1r and C1s (Figure 14.2A). As a consequence of C1q binding to the Fc region of the IgM or IgG bound to the antigen, C1s becomes enzymatically active. This enzymatically active form, known as ***C1s esterase***, cleaves the next component in the classical pathway, C4, into two pieces, C4a and C4b. C4a, the smaller piece, remains in the fluid phase, while C4b binds covalently to the surface of the pathogen. C4b bound to the cell surface then binds C2, which is cleaved by C1s. Cleavage of C2 generates the fragments C2b, which remains in the fluid phase, and C2a. C2a binds to C4b on the surface of the cell to form a complex, C4b2a. The C4b2a complex is known as the ***classical pathway C3 convertase***; as we describe below, this enzyme cleaves the next component in the pathway, C3.

Lectin Pathway

Activators. Terminal mannose residues expressed by Gram-positive (*Staphylococcus aureus*) and Gram-negative bacteria (*Klebsiella, Escherichia coli,* and *Haemophilus influenzae* type b), fungi (*Candida* and *Aspergillus fumigatus*), and yeast particles activate the lectin pathway by binding MBL. Many microbes, including the pathogen *Streptococcus pneumoniae*, express acetylated or neutral carbohydrate structures as part of extended polysaccharides, such as 1,3-beta-D-glucan; these are all bound by ficolin. Because the lectin pathway is activated by the molecular patterns expressed by pathogens (PAMPs, see Chapter 2) in the absence of antibody, it is part of the innate immune defenses and is involved in the rapid response to pathogens.

The terminal carbohydrate structures that activate the lectin pathway are generally not expressed on the surface of mammalian cells, so the lectin pathway of complement activation may be thought of as yet another way that the body discriminates between self and nonself. We referred to this critical concept earlier in the book, applicable in both innate immunity (pattern recognition receptors for pathogens expressed on cells of the innate immune system) and adaptive immunity (T and B cells respond to nonself antigens but do not respond to self-antigens).

Early Steps in the Lectin Pathway That Lead to C3 Cleavage. The lectin pathway is initiated when MBL binds to the terminal polysaccharide residues of a pathogen such as a bacterium (Figure 14.2B). MBL is structurally homologous to C1q in the classical pathway. Ficolin (not shown in the figure) has a structure similar to MBL and also binds carbohydrates, such as N-acetylglucosamine or N-acetylgalactosamine, on microbial surfaces.

MBL and ficolin are found in the circulation complexed with proteases, known as the ***mannose-associated serine***

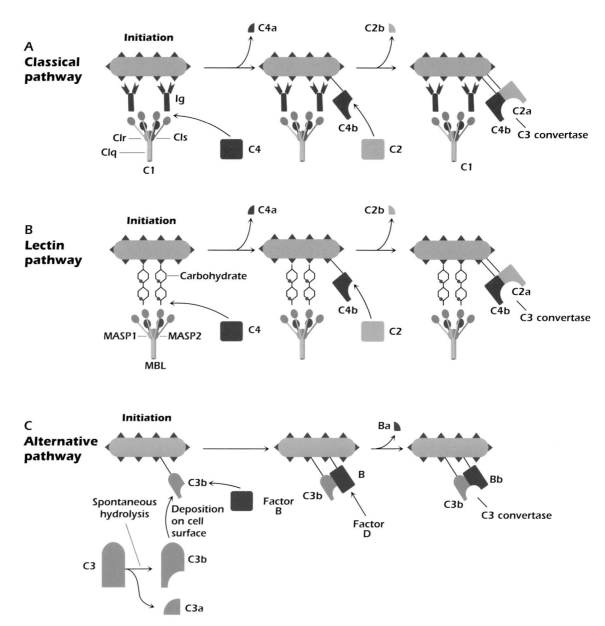

<u>Figure 14.2.</u> Early steps in activation of classical, lectin, and alternative complement pathways leading to formation of C3 convertase: C4aC2b in both classical and lectin pathways, and C3bBb in alternative pathway.

proteases (MASPs). Once bound to the bacterium, one of the proteases, MASP-2, sequentially cleaves C4 and C2 to form C4b2a on the surface of the bacterium. As we discussed previously, C4b2a is also formed in the classical pathway; it is the C3 convertase that cleaves the next component in the pathway, C3. Thus, the lectin and classical pathways converge at this point.

Alternative Pathway

Activators. The alternative pathway of complement activation can be triggered by almost any foreign substance, and in the absence of specific antibody. Thus, the alternative pathway is a key part of the innate immune defenses,

involved early in the response to pathogens. The most widely studied activators include lipopolysaccharides from the cell walls of Gram-negative bacteria (which are ***endotoxins***); the cell walls of some yeasts; and cobra venom factor, a protein present in some snakes. Some agents that activate the classical pathway—viruses, aggregated immunoglobulins, and necrotic cells—also trigger the alternative pathway.

Early Steps in Alternative Pathway That Lead to C3 Cleavage. The deposition of C3b on the cell surface initiates the alternative pathway (Figure 14.2C). C3b is generated in the circulation in small amounts by the spontaneous cleavage of a reactive thiol group in C3; this "preformed" C3b can bind to proteins and carbohydrates expressed on cell surfaces, either of a pathogen or of a host (mammalian) cell. (If C3b does not bind to one of these surfaces, it is rapidly inactivated.)

Thus, in a sense, the alternative pathway is always "on," and continual activation could damage cells of the host. However, as we describe in more detail subsequently, mammalian cells regulate the progression of the alternative pathway. Microbial cells lack such regulators and cannot prevent the development of subsequent steps in the alternative pathway.

Following the deposition of C3b, the serum protein *factor B* combines with C3b on the cell surface to form a complex, C3bB. *Factor D* then cleaves factor B in the cell surface-associated C3bB complex, generating fragments Ba, which is released into the fluid phase, and Bb, which remains attached to C3b. C3bBb is the *alternative pathway C3 convertase*, which cleaves C3 into C3a and C3b.

Steps Shared by All Pathways: Activation of C3 and C5

C3 cleavage is the first step that is common to all three complement pathways (Figure 14.3). In the classical and lectin pathways Figure 14.3A), the C3 convertase C4b2a

cleaves C3 into two fragments, C3a and C3b. In the alternative pathway (Figure 14.3B), the C3 convertase C3bBb cleaves C3 into the same two fragments. The smaller fragment, C3a, is released into the fluid phase, and the larger one, C3b, continues the complement activation cascade by binding covalently to the cell surface around the site of complement activation.

Note a unique feature of the alternative pathway shown in Figure 14.3B: binding of the serum protein *properdin* (also known as *factor P*) stabilizes C3bBb on the pathogen surface. As a result, C3bBb rapidly cleaves further C3 molecules, resulting in the huge buildup of C3b on the surface of the pathogen. As we described above, the deposition of C3b on a cell surface is the initiating step in the activation of the alternative pathway. Thus, the deposition on the cell surface of these rapidly produced and increased levels of C3b results in an almost explosive triggering of the alternative pathway. As we describe below, properdin's ability to activate this amplification loop is balanced by negative or regulatory molecules. Consequently, under normal conditions, the alternative pathway is not continually activated.

C3b binding to either the classical/lectin or alternative pathway C3 convertases allows the next component in the sequence, C5, to bind and be cleaved (middle section of

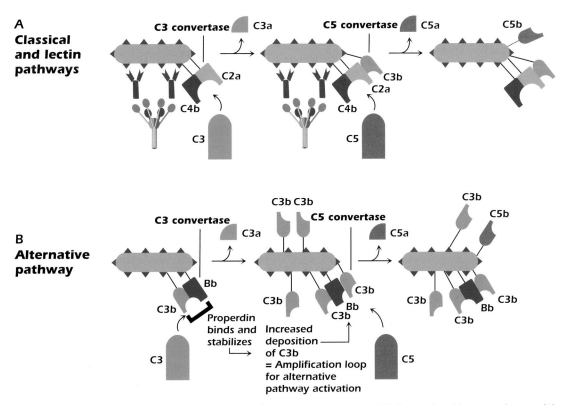

Figure 14.3. Cleavage of C3 by C3 convertase and C5 by C5 convertase. (A) Classical and lectin pathways; (B) alternative pathway. In all pathways, C3 is cleaved to C3b, which deposits on the cell surface, and C3a, which is released into the fluid phase. Similarly, C5 is cleaved into C5b, which deposits on the cell surface, and C5a, which is released into the fluid phase. In the alternative pathway, the stabilization of C3bBb by properdin increases C3b deposition on the cell surface and amplification of complement activation.

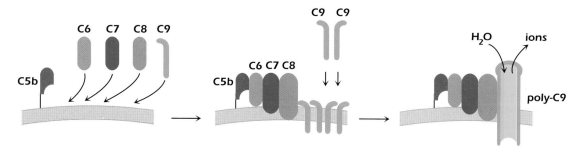

Figure 14.4. Formation of membrane attack complex (MAC). Late-stage complement components C5b-C9 bind sequentially to form a complex on the cell surface. Multiple C9 components bind to this complex and polymerize to form poly-C9, creating a channel that disrupts the cell membrane.

Figure 14.3A,B). For this reason, the C3 convertases with bound C3b are referred to as *C5 convertases*—C4b2a3b in the classical/lectin pathways, C3bBb3b in the alternative pathway. The cleavage of C5 produces two fragments: C5a is released into the fluid phase and has potent anaphylatoxic properties, and C5b binds to the cell surface and forms the nucleus for the binding of the terminal complement components.

Terminal Pathway

The terminal components of the complement cascades—C5b, C6, C7, C8, and C9—are common to the three complement activation pathways. These components bind to one another and form a membrane attack complex (MAC) that results in the death (lysis) of the cell on which they deposit (Figure 14.4).

The first step in MAC formation is C6 binding to C5b on the cell surface. C7 then binds to C5b and C6, with C7 inserting into the outer membrane of the cell. The subsequent binding of C8 to C5b67 results in the complex penetrating deeper into the cell's membrane. C5b-C8 on the cell membrane acts as a receptor for C9, a perforin-like molecule (see Chapter 11) that binds to C8. Additional C9 molecules interact with the C9 molecule in the complex to form polymerized C9 (poly-C9). Poly-C9 forms a transmembrane channel that disturbs the cell's osmotic equilibrium: Ions pass through the channel and water enters the cell. The cell swells and the membrane becomes permeable to macromolecules, which then escape from the cell. The result is cell lysis.

REGULATION OF COMPLEMENT ACTIVITY

Uncontrolled complement activation can rapidly deplete complement components, leaving the host unable to defend against subsequent invasion by infectious agents. In addition, the fragments generated by complement activation (especially the cleavage products of C3, C4, and C5) induce potent inflammatory responses, which may damage the host. Indeed, complement activation is believed to play an adverse role in autoinflammatory conditions such as rheumatoid arthritis and in myocardial infarctions (heart attacks) in which complement is activated by necrotic tissue (discussed later in the chapter). In addition, dysregulation of complement function in the eye has been suggested as playing a major role in age-related macular degeneration, the leading cause of visual impairment and blindness in the USA among individuals over 60 years of age.

Normally, inappropriate activation of complement does not occur, because many steps in the complement pathways are negatively regulated by specific inhibitors. Some of these negative regulators are specific for one complement activation pathway, but many inhibit all the pathways. The importance of these complement regulators is underscored by the clinical conditions that arise when regulatory molecules are lacking: The individual may be either damaged by inflammatory responses or become susceptible to infectious diseases. Some of these conditions are described later in the chapter.

Many of the molecules that regulate complement activation are expressed on the surface of mammalian cells but not microbial cells. Consequently, damage to the host by complement activation is generally limited compared to damage to the pathogen. In the paragraphs below and Figure 14.5 we describe the major regulators of complement activation.

C1 esterase inhibitor (C1INH) is a serum protein that inhibits the first step in the activation of the classical complement pathway. C1INH binds to C1r and C1s, causing them to dissociate from C1q and preventing complement activation. In addition, C1INH regulates the alternative pathway by inhibiting the function of C3bBb, and recent evidence indicates that it controls the lectin pathway by inhibiting MASP1 and MASP2. As described in the final section of the chapter, C1INH also inhibits the function of enzymes in other serum cascades, particularly those involved in clotting and in the formation of kinins, potent mediators of vascular effects.

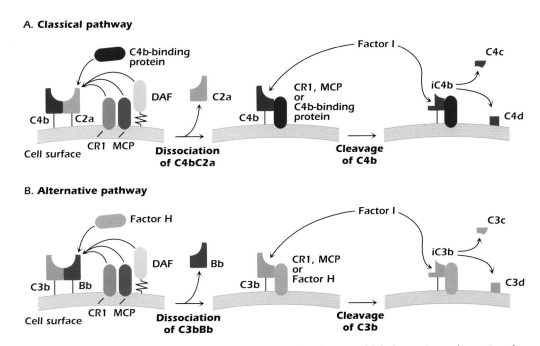

A. Classical pathway

B. Alternative pathway

Figure 14.5. Regulators of C3 convertases in (A) classical pathway and (B) alternative pathway. Regulators may dissociate the convertase, cleave the complement component remaining on the cell surface, or act as a cofactor for this cleavage. C4 binding protein exclusively regulates the classical pathway and factor H regulates the alternative pathway. Factor I, DAF, CR1, and MCP regulate both pathways.

C4b-binding protein (C4BP) is found in serum and *decay-accelerating factor* (DAF, CD55), *complement receptor* (CR) *1* (CD35), and *membrane cofactor protein* (MCP, CD46) are widely distributed cell surface molecules that regulate the classical and lectin pathway C3 convertase, C4b2a. Figure 14.5A shows that all these proteins can bind individually to C4b and displace the activated enzyme component, C2a.

Factor I, another serum protein, cleaves C4b on the cell surface after C2a has been displaced (Figure 14.5A). Because factor I cleavage of C4b requires the presence of one or more of C4BP, MCP, and CR1, these molecules are referred to as *cofactors* for factor-I-mediated cleavage. Note that DAF dissociates the C4b2a complex but does not act as a cofactor for factor I. Factor I cleaves C4b into two fragments: C4c, released into the fluid phase, and C4d, which remains attached to the cell surface. C4c and C4d do not continue the complement cascade and have no known biologic activity. C4BP regulates the classical (and lectin) pathways, which use C4bC2a as the C3 convertase. CR1, MCP, and DAF regulate the classical, lectin, and alternative pathways (described below and shown in Figure 14.5B).

Factor H, a serum protein, has two important regulatory functions in the alternative pathway. First, factor H competes with the previously described factor B for binding to C3b on a cell surface (see Figure 14.2, bottom line). Factor B binding to C3b continues the alternative pathway, but if factor H binds to C3b, the pathway stops. The nature of the

surface to which the C3b is bound is important in determining which factor binds to C3b: The sialic acid coating of mammalian cells favors the binding of factor H, but bacterial cells lack sialic acid, so they favor the binding of factor B to C3b. As a result, mammalian cells are protected by the regulatory function of factor H, but bacterial cells are targeted for further activation of the complement pathway.

Factor H has a second function: It binds to C3 convertase C3bBb in the alternative pathway and displaces Bb, preventing further activation of the complement cascade (Figure 14.5B). Once factor H has bound to C3b, factor I cleaves C3b; thus, factor H is a cofactor for factor-I-mediated cleavage of C3b in the alternative pathway. C3b is cleaved stepwise, first to *iC3b* (indicating an *inactive* C3b) and then to two additional fragments: *C3c*, which is released into the fluid phase and lacks biological function, and *C3d*, which remains attached to the cell surface. The breakdown products iC3b, C3c, and C3d do not continue the complement cascade, but iC3b and C3d have important biologic functions that we describe in the next section.

The same cell surface molecules that inhibit the function of classical pathway C3 convertase C4b2a (DAF, MCP, and CR1) regulate the alternative pathway convertase, C3bBb Figure 14.5B). As we mentioned above, factor I regulates both the classical and alternative pathways by cleaving C4b in the former and C3b in the latter.

The terminal pathway of complement activation and the formation of the MAC are also strictly regulated. Because the association of C5b with cell membranes is relatively nonspecific, the association of terminal pathway components C6–C9 with C5b on cell surfaces can form a MAC that damages or lyses "innocent bystander" cells of the host. Both membrane-associated proteins and fluid-phase proteins prevent this from occurring. **CD59**, a widely distributed membrane protein, prevents lysis by binding to the C5b–C8 complex on the cell surface and preventing C9 polymerization. **S-protein (*vitronectin*)** and **SP-40,40 (*clusterin*)** are fluid-phase proteins that bind to C5b6, C5b67, C5b678, and C5b6789, and prevent their interaction with membranes.

BIOLOGIC ACTIVITIES OF COMPLEMENT

The major functions of the complement system are summarized below and shown in Figures 14.6 and 14.7. Complement components interact with a wide range of cells that express specific receptors. The receptors fall into two broad categories: receptors that bind to C3b or C4b and their breakdown products; and receptors for the anaphylatoxins C3a and C5a (Table 14.1). (Distribution of the C4a receptor is not shown; it overlaps with the cellular distribution of the C3a receptor.) The receptors and cells that bind C3b, C4b and their breakdown products are involved in responses that enhance phagocytosis of pathogens, and the receptors and cells that bind the anaphylatoxins are involved in inflammatory responses.

The three main functions of complement are shown in Figure 14.6 and described in the following sections.

Production of Opsonins

The most important function of complement in host defense is considered to be the generation of fragments with opsonic activity that deposit on the surface of pathogens (Figure 14.6A). C3b and C4b are the major opsonins generated, but iC3b, a fragment of C3b that does not activate complement, also has opsonic activity. Bacteria coated by opsonins are rapidly taken up and destroyed by phagocytic cells such as macrophages and neutrophils. These cells express the receptors CR1, CR3, and CR4, which have broad specificities for complement pathway-generated opsonins and for other complement components. Complement receptor of the immunoglobulin family (CRIg) is expressed on tissue-resident macrophages, including those found in liver (Kupffer cells). It interacts with C3b and iC3b. CR1 is also

TABLE 14.1. Complement Receptors

Complement Receptor	Cell Distribution	Complement Components Bound	Receptor Function
CR1 (CD35)	Erythrocytes, monocytes, macrophages, eosinophils, neutrophils, B cells, some T cells, follicular dendritic cells, mast cells	C3b, iC3b, C3c, C4b	Enhances phagocytosis; regulates complement activation pathways
CR2 (CD21)	Late precursor and mature B lymphocytes, some T cells (including thymocytes), follicular dendritic cells	C3b, iC3b, C3d/C3dg	Part of B-cell co-receptor: lowers threshold for B-cell activation by antigen
CR3 (CD11b/CD18, also known as Mac-1)	Monocytes, macrophages, NK cells, granulocytes	iC3b (and many noncomplement components, including bacterial lipopolysaccharide and other surface molecules, and fibrinogen)	Enhances phagocytosis
CR4 (CD11c/CD18)	Myeloid cells, dendritic cells, activated B cells, NK cells, some cytotoxic lymphocytes, platelets	iC3b (and many noncomplement ligands, similar to those interacting with CR3)	Enhances phagocytosis
CRIg	Macrophages	C3b, iC3b	Enhances phagocytosis
C3a receptor	Smooth muscle cells, endothelial cells, epithelial cells, platelets, mast cells, macrophages, neutrophils, basophils, eosinophils	C3a	Mediates anaphylatoxic response
C5a receptor (CD88)	Smooth muscle cells, endothelial cells, epithelial cells, platelets, mast cells, macrophages, neutrophils, basophils, eosinophils.	C5a	Mediates anaphylatoxic response

a regulator of complement activation, as described earlier (Figure 14.5).

Production of Anaphylatoxins

The second major function associated with complement activation is the action of *anaphylatoxins* (Figure 14.6B). C5a is the most potent, followed by C3a; C4a is much less potent. The name "anaphylatoxin" derives from the earliest recognition of their function: the ability to induce the shock-like characteristics of the systemic allergic or *anaphylactic* response (see Chapter 15). We now recognize that these small peptides play key roles in inducing inflammatory responses, which form part of the body's defenses in removing an infectious agent that has penetrated the tissues.

The anaphylatoxins interact with receptors expressed on many different cell types (Table 14.1 and Figure 14.6B). They activate vascular endothelial cells (lining the walls of blood vessels), increasing the vascular permeability and leading to local accumulation of fluid (edema) in the tissue. The influx into the tissue of fluid containing phagocytic cells (macrophages and neutrophils), antibodies, and complement components enhances the response to the pathogen. The anaphylatoxins are also chemotactic for neutrophils; that is, the cells migrate from an area of lesser concentration to an area of higher concentration. As a result, neutrophils circulating in the blood are activated, leave the circulation at the site of inflammation, and destroy the foreign material. The anaphylatoxins also induce smooth muscle contraction. Interaction of the anaphylatoxins with basophils or mast cells in tissues results in the release of many inflammatory mediators, including histamine. The effects of histamine (discussed in Chapter 15) and the anaphylatoxins on vascular permeability and smooth muscle contraction are similar.

Lysis

The third major function of complement is the lysis of pathogens (Figure 14.6C). The terminal step in the three complement activation pathways is the formation of a MAC on the surface of a cell. This results in the lysis of the cell, particularly of microbial pathogens.

Other Important Complement Functions

Enhancing B-Cell Responses to Antigens.
The binding of complement component C3d or of the final breakdown product of C3, *C3dg*, to CR2 (CD21) enhances antibody responses in several ways (Figure 14.7Ai) and discussed in Chapter 8: First, C3dg binds to antigen that is also bound to B-cell surface Ig (Figure 14.7A). C3dg can bind simultaneously to CR2, which is part of the B-cell co-receptor (Chapter 8). Signaling through both the surface Ig and the co-receptor augments activation of the B cell. Thus, C3dg binding to antigen and the B-cell surface lowers the threshold for B-cell activation by as much as 1000-fold compared to binding in the absence of C3dg.

Second, in Chapter 8 we described how follicular dendritic cells in the germinal center bind antigen–antibody complexes and present antigen to proliferating B cells. This interaction is critical for the eventual development of memory cells. Follicular dendritic cells express the complement receptors CR2, which binds C3dg, and CR1, which binds iC3b. Thus follicular dendritic cells can present antigen–antibody complexes bound to one of these complement components to germinal center B cells (Figure 14.7Aii). In this way, complement components also play a role in the induction of B-cell memory.

In addition, B-cell processing of T-dependent antigens is more rapid when the antigen is bound to C3dg than when it is not; presumably the binding of C3dg to CR2 on the B-cell surface enhances uptake and processing of the antigen. This may be another way in which complement enhances B-cell responses to T-cell-dependent antigens.

Controlling Formation and Clearance of Immune Complexes.
When antibodies bind to multivalent antigens, cross-linking between the molecules tends to produce large antigen–antibody complexes that increase in size until they become insoluble. Although this precipitation of complexes has proved useful for identifying antigens and antibodies *in vitro* (see Chapter 6), the formation of large insoluble complexes *in vivo* can be detrimental to the host. As we describe in the final section of this chapter and in Chapter 18, individuals deficient in early components of the classical pathway components and in some autoimmune conditions such as systemic lupus erythematosus (SLE) may show large insoluble immune complexes in tissues such as the skin and kidneys, inducing inflammation and damaging surrounding cells (see also Figure 13.11 in Chapter 13).

Complement plays a role in clearing these complexes (Figure 14.7B). Deposition of C3b on a large antigen–antibody complex interferes with the bonds that keep the complex together. As a result, it breaks up into smaller pieces that can be cleared by macrophages. Deposition of C3b on the antigen–antibody complex also allows binding to erythrocytes, which express the receptor CR1 on their surface. Erythrocytes clear the complexes from the circulation by transporting them to the liver and spleen. In these organs, the complexes are transferred from the erythrocyte CR1 to macrophage CR3 and Fc receptors. Macrophages phagocytose the complexes and destroy them.

Removing Dead or Dying Cells.
Cells dying by necrosis can activate complement, leading to C4b and C3b deposition on the cell surface (Figure 14.7C). The cell is then cleared by interacting with CR1 or CR3 on phagocytic cells. Subcellular membranes, from organelles such as mitochondria and endoplasmic reticulum, also directly activate both classical and alternative pathways and are cleared in a

A. **Opsonization**

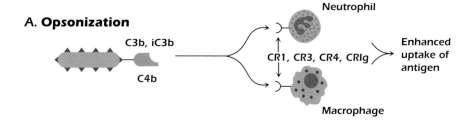

B. **Anaphylatoxin production**

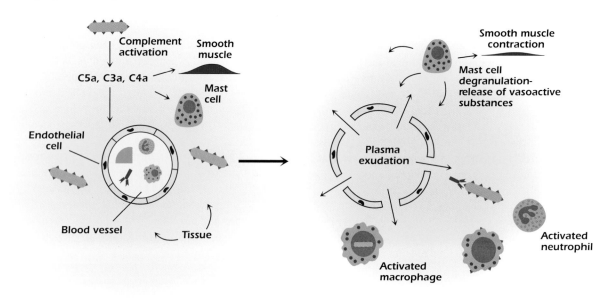

C. **Cell lysis**

Figure 14.6. Major functions of complement: (A) production of opsonins; (B) production of anaphylatoxins; and (C) pathogen lysis.

similar way. CRP, the acute-phase protein and component of the inflammatory response, also binds to damaged and necrotic cells and activates the classical complement pathway. The same structure that CRP binds to on bacterial cell walls—the polysaccharide phosphocholine—is also exposed on damaged and necrotic mammalian cells. Recent evidence also indicates that cells dying as a result of apoptosis may trigger complement activation.

In all these situations, complement removes dead or dying cells from the tissues and contributes to homeostasis. In some conditions, however, complement activation by dead or dying cells may have clinical consequences. Notable examples include complement activation by ischemia and reperfusion. In *ischemia*, an area of tissue dies after blood

and oxygen supplies have been cut (important examples include cardiac muscle after a myocardial infarction or brain tissue following a stroke). *Reperfusion* is the attempt to restore blood supply to the affected tissue. Complement activation is considered a major contributor to the inflammatory responses associated with both of these states, which damages healthy tissue. Complement-based therapies are currently being tested to reduce the deleterious effects of the inflammatory response.

Responses to Viruses.   Complement plays a role in defense against viral infection (Figure 14.7D). C1 can bind directly to and become activated by the surface of several viruses, including the type C retroviruses, lentiviruses,

A. Enhancement of B-cell responses

(i) B-cell activation

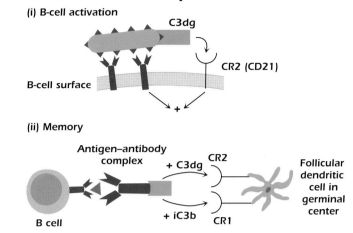

(ii) Memory

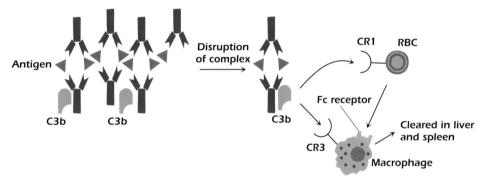

B. Removal of immune complexes

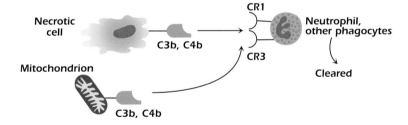

C. Removal of necrotic cells and subcellular membranes

D. Responses to viruses

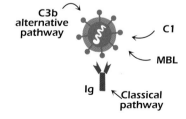

Figure 14.7. Other key functions of complement: enhancement of B-cell responses, removal of immune complexes, removal of necrotic cells and subcellular membranes, and responses to viruses.

HIV-1, and HTLV-1. In addition, MBL of the lectin pathway binds to and is activated by mannose residues on the surfaces of HIV-1, HIV-2, and influenza virus. Antibodies generated in the response against these viruses mediate further binding and activation of the classical pathway on the surface of the virus. Repeating subunits on the viral capsid or membrane surfaces activate the alternative pathway. Binding of complement proteins leads to opsonization and lysis of the virus by phagocytic cells. Complement binding also interferes with the ability of the virus to interact with the membrane of its target cells and thus blocks viral entry into the cell.

In Chapter 9 we described how viruses subvert the immune response by synthesizing proteins that bind to molecules in antigen-processing pathways. Many viruses also use mechanisms that subvert the action of complement proteins. For example, some viruses produce proteins that mimic complement inhibitor function: the herpes viruses make proteins that have DAF-like and/or MCP-like activities and others that block C5b-9 formation. In addition, vaccinia virus produces a protein that binds to C3b and C4b and inhibits complement activation. The protein has both decay-accelerating activity and acts as a cofactor for factor I. HIV-1, HTLV-1, simian immunodeficiency virus (SIV), and cytomegalovirus (CMV) capture the complement control proteins DAF, MCP, and CD59 when the virions bud from host cell membranes. As a consequence of these strategies, the viruses are protected from complement-mediated responses.

Some viruses even use complement components to promote infection, for example, by binding to complement receptors and gaining entry into cells. One of the most studied interactions is the Epstein–Barr virus infection of human B lymphocytes: The virus's membrane glycoprotein, gp350/220, binds to CR2 (CD21) expressed on the B-cell surface, allowing the virus to be taken into the cell. Some viruses activate complement and use the C3b deposited on them to bind to host cell complement receptors; in this way, HIV-1 uses CR1, CR2, and CR3 to infect T cells, B cells, and monocytes. Other viruses bind to membrane-expressed complement regulators: Paramyxovirus (measles virus) uses MCP and viruses of the picornavirus family use DAF to infect epithelial cells.

COMPLEMENT DEFICIENCIES

We described above how the complement system plays an important role in defending the host against microorganisms. It is particularly important in defending against **pyogenic** (pus-forming) polysaccharide-encapsulated bacteria, which include *Neisseria* species (the bacteria responsible for meningitis and some sexually transmitted diseases), *S. pneumoniae*, *H. influenzae*, and *S. aureus*. The major pathways of defense against these organisms appear to be the production of IgG antibody that binds to the bacteria, resulting in opsonization, complement activation, phagocytosis, and intracellular killing. Thus, genetic deficiencies or acquired conditions in which any one of these activities is diminished render a person particularly susceptible to these organisms. In addition, complement is important in removing immune complexes from the circulation; therefore deficiencies of certain complement components can also result in immune complexes depositing in tissues, leading to inflammatory conditions. More information about complement deficiencies is provided in Chapter 18.

We now also recognize that some complement components show allelic variation—frequently the result of just a single nucleotide change or polymorphism—in their genes. These differences in allelic forms result not in outright deficiencies, but in variations in level and function of the component. The impact of these variations is also discussed below.

Table 14.2 summarizes the clinical conditions that develop from deficiencies of either specific complement components or regulators of complement function. Individuals genetically deficient in specific complement components are relatively rare (approximately 1 in 10,000), and deficiencies are not always associated with the development of a clinical condition. C3 deficiency is rare but can be severe and even life threatening because C3 is central to all the complement pathways. C3-deficient individuals are susceptible to recurrent pyogenic infections and may also develop symptoms resembling those of SLE, involving fever, rash, and glomerulonephritis. These symptoms presumably result from an impaired ability to process and clear immune complexes. Deficiencies in any of the early components of the classical pathway—C1, C4, or C2—also have an increased risk of infection with pyogenic bacteria and the development of SLE-like symptoms. Individuals deficient in alternative pathway components or the later components common to all pathways, however, have an even higher risk of infection with pyogenic bacteria. This suggests that activation of the classical complement pathway may not be as important as the alternative pathway in defense against these bacteria.

Deficiency of the alternative pathway component properdin, or of factors B or D, is associated with pyogenic, particularly neisserial, infections. Deficiency of MBL can be a major problem in early life, manifesting as severe recurrent infections. Individuals who lack components of the MAC, C5b-C9, tend to get recurrent neisserial infections.

Deficiencies or disorders of complement receptors or complement regulatory proteins may also have serious consequences. Patients with a defect in CR3 (CD11a/CD18) may have a disorder known as **leukocyte adhesion deficiency I** (see Chapter 18) in which adhesion and migration of all leukocytes is impaired. These patients suffer from recurrent pyogenic bacterial infections, but pus is not formed.

Deficiency of factor H or factor I results in uncontrolled activation of the alternative pathway. One outcome is **membranoproliferative glomerulonephritis**, inflammation of the capillary loops in the glomeruli of the kidney, characterized by increased cell number and thickening of capillary walls. Factor H deficiency is also associated with **atypical hemolytic-uremic syndrome** (10% of all hemolytic-uremic syndrome cases). Usually resulting from bacterial infection, it is characterized by destruction of red blood cells, damage to endothelial cells, and in severe cases kidney failure. A monoclonal antibody that blocks C5 cleavage is being evaluated to treat this syndrome.

TABLE 14.2. Complement Deficiencies

Deficient Complement Component	Effect on Complement Function	Clinical Condition
C3	C3b and other opsonic fragments not produced; terminal components not activated	Severe pyogenic infections (encapsulated bacteria) and SLE-like symptoms
C1, C4, or C2	No activation of classical pathway	Pyogenic infections and SLE-like symptoms
Properdin, factor B, or factor D	No activation of alternative pathway	Severe pyogenic infections
Mannose binding lectin	No activation of lectin pathway	Recurrent bacterial infections
C5, C6, C7, C8, or C9	Inability to form MAC	Recurrent neisserial (Gram-negative) infections
C1 inhibitor (C1INH)	Unregulated activation of all activation pathways	Angioedema
CD59, DAF	Defects in regulation: MAC damages host cells	Paroxysmal nocturnal hemoglobulinuria (hemolysis and thrombosis)
Factor H, factor I	Unregulated activation of C3	Glomerulonephritis, atypical hemolytic-uremic syndrome
Variations in Factor H and other alternative pathway components	Decreased regulation of alternative pathway	Age-related macular degeneration
Complement receptor 3 (CR3)	Impaired adhesion and migration of leukocytes	Recurrent bacterial infections

The regulatory protein C1INH is the only control protein for classical pathway components C1r and C1s, and deficiency results in uncontrolled cleavage of C2 and C4. (As we described above, C1INH also inhibits steps in both the lectin and alternative pathways.) Genetic deficiency of C1INH results in *hereditary angioedema*. The condition is characterized by localized edemas in the skin and mucosa resulting from dilatation and increased permeability of the capillaries. The symptoms are recurrent attacks of swelling, such as of the face and limbs, pain in the abdomen, and swelling of the larynx, which can compromise breathing. This condition is thought to be due to the lack of inhibition by C1INH of enzymatic activity in serum cascades other than the complement cascade; one of these pathways forms kinins, including bradykinin, which are potent vasodilators and inducers of vascular permeability and smooth muscle contraction. Deficiency of C1INH is thought to lead to increased production of these vascular mediators. In the USA, injectable C1INH prepared from human plasma has been approved as a treatment for this condition.

 Read the related case: **Hereditary Angioedema**
In *Immunology: Clinical Case Studies and Disease Pathophysiology*

Paroxysmal nocturnal hemoglobinuria (PNH) is a rare disorder that also involves complement regulatory proteins. The condition occurs primarily in young adults and is characterized by chronic destruction of red blood cells and thrombus formation (an aggregate of platelets and blood factors that causes vascular blockage), hemolytic anemia, and the presence of hemoglobin in urine, predominantly at night. The acquired condition (there is also an inherited condition) results from a mutation in the gene that controls the production of the glycosylphosphatidylinositol (GPI) anchor that attaches many membrane proteins to the cell surface (see Chapter 7). In PNH, the anchor is not made properly, and the proteins do not attach to the cell surface; they are secreted from the cell into the fluid phase. Several proteins are affected, including the complement regulatory proteins DAF and CD59. The absence of these molecules makes the red cell membrane particularly sensitive to complement-mediated lysis. The monoclonal antibody described above to block C5 cleavage and used to treat atypical hemolytic-uremic syndrome is also being used to treat PNH.

In other acquired conditions, C3 may become depleted to such an extent that immune complexes are not cleared or an individual becomes susceptible to infection. This can occur in some people who produce an autoantibody known as **C3 nephritic factor**: The antibody stabilizes the alternative pathway C3 convertase (C3bBb), generating a highly efficient and long-lived fluid-phase enzyme that cleaves C3. C3 nephritic factor has been described in some individuals with SLE and a rare disease known as ***partial lipodystrophy***, involving the loss of fat from the upper part of the body. These conditions are also characterized by glomerulonephritis. Fat cells, particularly those in the upper part of the body, produce factor D, which cleaves C3bBb. The loss of fat cells in partial lipodystrophy may result from localized complement-mediated cell lysis.

Finally, we now recognize that differences in expression of complement components, and in particular the complement regulator factor H, are associated with either increased or, alternatively, decreased risk of developing *age-related macular degeneration*; in this condition, abnormal growth of new blood vessels behind the retina results in vision loss. Variations in Factor B, C3, and factor I have also been implicated in this condition, suggesting that the development of age-related macular degeneration is associated with dysregulation of the alternative complement pathway.

SUMMARY

1. The complement system—comprising approximately 30 serum and membrane-expressed proteins—plays a key effector role in both innate immunity and antibody-mediated adaptive responses to microbial pathogens.

2. Complement activation is a cascade that sequentially generates biologically active molecules. The major biologic activities generated by complement activation are opsonins (enhancing uptake of pathogens by phagocytic cells) and anaphylatoxins (inducing inflammatory responses). The biologically active complement components interact with specific receptors expressed on multiple cell types. Complement activation also results in the direct lysis of pathogens.

3. Complement can be initiated by three distinct pathways: (a) the classical pathway, predominantly by antigen–antibody complexes binding to complement component C1; (b) the lectin pathway, mainly by terminal mannose residues on the surface of bacteria interacting with mannose-binding lectin, but also by N-acetyl carbohydrates binding to ficolin; and (c) the alternative pathway, by the deposition of complement component C3b on the surface of the pathogen. The alternative pathway has an amplification loop that greatly enhances activation.

4. The three activation pathways converge with the cleavage of C3 to form C3b and C3a.

5. The final stages of all complement pathways are identical: the formation of a membrane attack complex, comprising components C5b through C9. Formation of the membrane attack complex leads to lysis of the cell.

6. The activity of complement and its components is tightly regulated by several proteins. These are found in the fluid phase (factors H and I, C1 inhibitor, C4b binding protein) and on the surface of many mammalian cells (DAF, MCP, and CR1). Complement regulator proteins are not expressed on the surface of microbial cells.

7. Complement has important functions in addition to the generation of opsonins, anaphylatoxins, and cell lysis. These include enhancing B-lymphocyte responses to antigen, controlling the formation and clearance of immune complexes, removal of dead and dying cells, and interactions with viruses.

8. Deficiencies of complement components, regulators of complement pathways, or receptors for complement components may result in increased susceptibility to infection or the development of inflammatory conditions.

REFERENCES AND BIBLIOGRAPHY

Ambati J, Atkinson JP, Gelfand BD. (2013) Immunology of age-related macular degeneration. *Nat Rev Immunol* 13: 438.

Bomback AS, Appel GB. (2012) Pathogenesis of the C3 glomerulopathies and reclassification of MPGN). *Nature Reviews Nephrology* 8: 634.

Frank MM. (2006) Hereditary angioedema: The clinical syndrome and its management in the United States. *Immunol Allergy Clin North Am* 26: 653.

Matsushita M. (2013) Ficolins in complement activation. *Mol Immunol* 55: 22.

Pettigrew HD, Teuber SS, Gershwin ME. (2009) Clinical significance of complement deficiencies. *Ann N Y Acad Sci* 1173: 108.

Riedemann NC, Ward PA. (2003) Complement in ischemia reperfusion injury. *Am J Pathol* 162: 363.

Roozendaal R, Carroll MC. (2007) Complement receptors CD21 and CD35 in humoral immunity. *Immunol Rev* 219: 157.

Rus H, Cudrici C, Niculescu F. (2005) The role of the complement system in innate immunity. *Immunol Res* 33: 103.

Takahashi K, Ip WE, Michelow IC, Ezekowitz RA. (2006) The mannose-binding lectin: A prototypic pattern recognition molecule. *Curr Opin Immunol* 18: 16.

Wallis R. (2007) Interactions between mannose-binding lectin and MASPs during complement activation by the lectin pathway. *Immunobiology* 212: 289.

REVIEW QUESTIONS

For each question, choose the ONE BEST answer or completion.

1. A patient is admitted with multiple bacterial infections and is found to have a complete absence of C3. Which complement-mediated function would remain intact in such a patient?
   A) lysis of bacteria
   B) opsonization of bacteria
   C) generation of anaphylatoxins
   D) generation of neutrophil chemotactic factors
   E) none of the above

2. Complement is required for:
   A) lysis of erythrocytes by the enzyme lecithinase
   B) NK-mediated lysis of tumor cells
   C) phagocytosis
   D) antibody-mediated lysis of bacteria
   E) all of the above

3. Which of the following is associated with the development of SLE-like symptoms?
   A) deficiencies in C1, C4, or C2
   B) deficiencies in C5, C6, or C7
   C) deficiencies in the late components of complement
   D) increases in the serum C3 level
   E) increases in the levels of C1, C4, or C2

4. Activated fragments of C5 can lead to all of the following *except*:
   A) contraction of smooth muscle
   B) vasodilation
   C) attraction of leukocytes to a site of infection
   D) attachment of lymphocytes to macrophages
   E) initiation of formation of membrane attack complex

5. The alternative pathway of complement activation is characterized by all of the following *except*:
   A) activation of complement components beyond C3 in the cascade
   B) participation of properdin
   C) generation of anaphylatoxins
   D) activation of C4
   E) regulation by factor H

6. DAF regulates the complement system to prevent complement-mediated lysis of cells. This involves:
   A) dissociation of the C3 convertase complex
   B) blocking the binding of the C3 convertase to the surface of bacterial cells
   C) inhibiting the membrane attack complex from binding to bacterial membranes
   D) acting as a cofactor for the cleavage of C3b
   E) causing dissociation of C5 convertase

7. The following activate(s) the alternative pathway of complement:
   A) lipopolysaccharides
   B) some viruses and virus-infected cells
   C) fungal and yeast cell walls
   D) many strains of Gram-positive bacteria
   E) all of the above

ANSWERS TO REVIEW QUESTIONS

1. *E.* All these functions are mediated by complement components that are generated later in the complement activation sequence than C3. Thus, all these functions are disrupted in the absence of C3.

2. *D.* Complement is required for lysis of bacteria by IgM or IgG (classical pathway). Complement is not required for lysis of erythrocytes by lecithinase or for phagocytosis. However, opsonins such as C3b that are generated during complement activation can enhance phagocytosis. Although some tumor cells can initiate the alternate pathway of complement activation, complement plays no role in NK-mediated lysis of these cells.

3. *A.* Inherited homozygous deficiency of one of the early proteins of the classical complement pathway (C1, C4, or C2) is strongly associated with the development of SLE-like symptoms. These deficiencies probably result in abnormal processing of immune complexes in the absence of a functional classical pathway of complement fixation. In these conditions, serum levels of C3 and C4 decrease due to the large number of immune complexes that bind to them. Deficiencies in the late components are associated with recurrent infections with pyogenic organisms.

4. *D.* C5a is an anaphylatoxin, which induces degranulation of mast cells, resulting in the release of histamine, causing vasodilation and contraction of smooth muscles. C5a is also chemotactic, attracting leukocytes to the area of its release where an antigen is reacting with antibodies and activates the complement system; this is a part of the inflammatory response to an infection. C5b deposits on membranes and initiates the formation of the terminal membrane attack complex. Neither C5a nor C5b promotes the attachment of lymphocytes to macrophages.

5. *D.* The alternative pathway of complement activation connects with the classical pathway at the activation of C3. Thus, it does not require C1, C4, or C2. Properdin is essential for the activation through the alternative pathway, since it stabilizes the complex formed between C3b and activated serum factor B, C3bBb, which acts as a C3 convertase, and activates C3. During the activation of the alternative pathway both C3a and C5a are generated; both are anaphylatoxins and cause degranulation of mast cells. Factor H is a key regulator of the alternative pathway.

6. *A.* DAF is a cell surface regulator of complement activation that destabilizes the C3 convertases of the alternate and classical pathways (C3bBb and C4b2a, respectively). Like other regulators of complement activation—including CR1, factor H, and C4bBP— these proteins accelerate decay (dissociation) of the C3 convertase,

releasing the component with enzymatic activity (Bb or C2a) from the component bound to the cell membrane (C3b or C4b).

7. *E.* Each of these pathogens and particles of microbial origin can initiate the alternate pathway of complement activation. Teichoic acid from the cell walls of Gram-positive organisms, as well as parasites such as trypanosomes, can also activate complement via this pathway.

15

HYPERSENSITIVITY: TYPE I

INTRODUCTION

Hypersensitivity

The term *hypersensivity* is used to define a set of responses often categorized as types I–IV. These designations were first designated by Coombs and Gell in the early 1960s, as discussed below. In fact, the immune responses associated with each of the Coombs–Gell hypersensitivity designations manifest as a result of exaggerated normal responses that have been described in earlier chapters. Thus, the cellular and molecular mechanisms of such reactions are virtually identical to normal host defense responses. Unfortunately, under some circumstances, these immune responses produce damaging and sometimes fatal results, hence, hypersensitivity to the antigens stimulating these responses. They cause immune-mediated damage to the host because they manifest as exaggerated reactions to foreign antigens or inappropriate reactions to self-antigens.

Coombs–Gell Hypersensitivity Designations

In the early 1960s, hypersensitivity reactions were divided into four types, designated I–IV by Coombs and Gell; these are summarized below. Although the lines of distinction used to separate these four types of hypersensitivity have blurred through the years as our knowledge of cellular and molecular immunology has grown, the Coombs–Gell designations are still relevant.

Type I. IgE-mediated reactions (commonly called *allergic reactions* or *allergy*) are stimulated by the binding of IgE, via its Fc region, to high-affinity IgE-specific Fc receptors designated FcεRI. As we shall see later on in this chapter, FcεRI are expressed on mast cells, basophils, and eosinophils. Binding of antigen to preformed antigen-specific IgE bound to high-affinity FcεRI initiates type I hypersensitivity reactions. When the IgE molecules encounter antigens, a cascade of events leads to destabilization and release of inflammatory mediators and cytokines from mast cells and basophils. This ultimately results in the clinical manifestations of type I hypersensitivity, which include rhinitis, asthma, and, in severe cases, anaphylaxis (from the Greek *ana*, which means "away from," and *phylaxis*, which means "protection"). Type I hypersensitivity reactions are rapid, occurring within minutes after challenge (reexposure to antigen). Consequently, allergic reactions are also called *immediate hypersensitivity*.

Type II. Type II hypersensitivity is the result of humoral cytolytic or cytotoxic reactions that occur when IgM or IgG antibodies bind inappropriately to antigen on the surface of cells and activate the complement cascade. This culminates in the destruction of the cells. Type II hypersensitivity is discussed in detail in Chapter 16.

Type III. Type III hypersensitivity, also known as *immune complex reactions* occur when antigen-IgM or antigen-IgG complexes accumulate in the circulation or in tissue and activate the complement cascade. Granulocytes are attracted to the site of activation, and damage results

Immunology: A Short Course, Seventh Edition. Richard Coico and Geoffrey Sunshine.
© 2015 John Wiley & Sons, Ltd. Published 2015 by John Wiley & Sons, Ltd.
Companion Website: www.wileyimmunology.com/coico

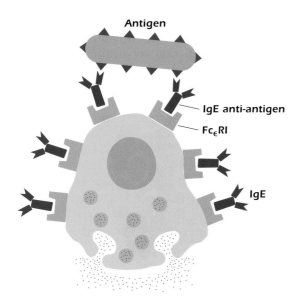

Figure 15.2. Mast-cell degranulation mediated by antigen cross-linking of IgE bound to IgE Fc receptors (FcεRI).

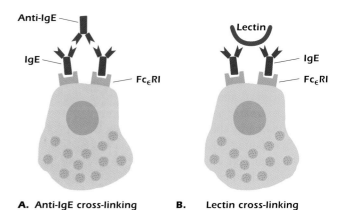

A. Anti-IgE cross-linking   **B.   Lectin cross-linking**

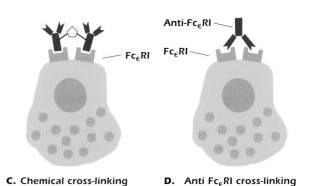

C. Chemical cross-linking   **D.   Anti FcεRI cross-linking**

Figure 15.3. Induction of mast-cell degranulation.

airways (coughing, wheezing, phlegm), and to swelling and mucus secretion in nasal passages. Finally, degranulation of mast cells present along the blood vessels causes increased blood flow and vascular permeability, resulting in increased fluid in tissues or *edema*. This causes increased flow of lymph from the local lymph nodes, which in turn leads to increased numbers of cells and increased protein in tissue, all of which contribute to the inflammatory response.

Cross-linking of FcεRI receptors may also be accomplished in other experimentally useful ways, such as the addition of an antibody specific for IgE or *FcεRI*. IgE receptor molecules on the surface of mast cells (Figure 15.3A), exposure to sugar-binding lectins (Figure 15.3B), or the use of chemical cross-linkers (Figure 15.3C) or antibodies against FcεRI (Figure 15.3D). As expected, dimers or aggregates of IgE will also cross-link these Fc receptors and activate mast cells to degranulate. Finally, activation of mast cells can also be achieved using calcium ionophores, which induce a rapid influx of calcium ions into the cell, triggering the signaling cascade leading to degranulation.

Mast cells may also be activated naturally through mechanisms other than IgE Fc receptor cross-linking. Anaphylactoid reactions are produced by the *anaphylatoxins* C3a and C5a (products of complement activation; see Chapter 14), as well as by various drugs such as codeine, morphine, and iodinated radiocontrast dyes. Physical factors such as heat, cold, or pressure can also activate mast cells; for example, *cold-induced urticaria* is an anaphylactic rash induced in certain individuals by chilling an area of skin. Another example is *dermatographic uticaria* in which the skin becomes raised and inflamed when stroked, scratched, or slapped. Finally, as noted above, certain lectins (sugar-binding molecules) can also cross-link IgE Fc receptors (see

Figure 15.3B). High concentrations of lectins are found in certain foods, such as strawberries. This might explain the urticaria induced in some individuals after eating these foods.

The triggering of a mast cell by the bridging of its receptors initiates a rapid and complex series of events culminating in the degranulation of the mast cell and the release of potent inflammatory mediators. Because of the ease with which its outcome can be measured, the mast cell has served as a model for the study of activation of cells in general. Among the events known to occur rapidly are receptor aggregation and changes in membrane fluidity; these result from methylation of phospholipids, which leads to a transient increase in intracellular levels of cyclic adenosine monophosphate (cAMP) followed by an influx of Ca^{2+} ions. The intracellular levels of cAMP and cyclic guanosine monophosphate (cGMP) are important in the regulation of subsequent events. In general, a sustained increase in intracellular cAMP at this stage will slow, or even stop, the process of degranulation. Thus, activation of adenylate cyclase, the enzyme that converts adenosine triphosphate (ATP) to cAMP, provides an important mechanism for controlling anaphylactic events.

As noted earlier, allergic reactions are often referred to as *immediate hypersensitivity*. This term is appropriate in

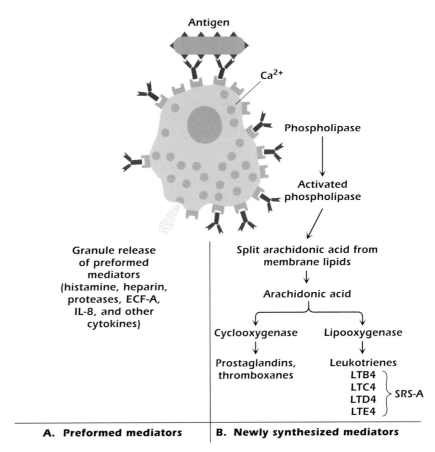

Figure 15.4. Mediators released during activation of mast cells.

light of the very rapid consequences of IgE Fc receptor cross-linking, beginning with microfilament transport of mast-cell granules to the cell surface. Once at the cell surface, granule membranes fuse with the cell membrane and the contents are released to the exterior via exocytosis (see Figure 15.1B). Depending on the extent of cross-linking on the cell surface, any cell can release some or all of its granules. This explosive release of granules is physiologic and does not imply lysis or death of the cell. In fact, the degranulated cells regenerate; once the contents of the granules have been synthesized, the cells are ready to resume their function.

EFFECTOR PHASE

The symptoms of allergic reactions are entirely attributable to the inflammatory mediators released by the activated mast cells. It is helpful to place these mediators in two major categories (Figure 15.4). The first category consists of basic *preformed mediators*, which are stored in the granules by electrostatic attraction to a matrix protein and are released as a result of the influx of ions, primarily Na^+ (Figure 15.4A). Cytokines released from mast cells undergoing

degranulation, including IL-3, IL-4, IL-5, IL-8, IL-9, tumor necrosis factor (TNF)-α, and GM-CSF (granulocyte-macrophage–colony stimulating factor), also play a role in attracting and activating inflammatory cells locally. Inflammatory cells participate in the so-called late-phase reactions of allergic responses (described later in this chapter) in concert with the second category of mast cell mediators—those synthesized *de novo*. The second category, newly formed mast cell mediators, consists of substances synthesized, in part, from membrane lipids (Figure 15.4B). Many potent substances are released during degranulation; only the most important members of each category are considered here.

Preformed Mediators

Histamine. Histamine is formed in the cell by decarboxylation of the amino acid histidine; it is stored in the cell by binding via electrostatic interaction to an acid matrix protein called *heparin*. When released, histamine binds rapidly to a variety of cells via two major types of receptor, H1 and H2, which have different tissue distribution and mediate different effects. When histamine binds to H1 receptors in smooth muscles, it causes constriction; when it binds to H1 receptors on endothelial cells, it causes separation at their junctions, resulting in vascular permeability. H2 receptors are involved in mucus secretion, increased vascular permeability, and the release of acid from stomach mucosa. All these effects are responsible for some of the major signs of systemic anaphylaxis: difficulty in breathing (asthma) or asphyxiation result from the constriction of smooth muscle around the bronchi in the lung, and the drop in blood pressure is a consequence of the extravasation of fluid into tissue spaces as the permeability of blood vessels increases. H1 receptors are blocked by antihistamines, such as Benadryl®, which compete directly for H1 receptor sites with histamine; when these drugs are given soon enough, they can counteract its effects. Blockage of H2 receptors requires other drugs, such as cimetidine. Some time following the introduction of antihistamines, it was noted that they were ineffective in controlling constriction of smooth muscles that was slower in onset and more persistent than that produced by histamine. This observation led to the discovery of the *slow-reacting substance of anaphylaxis* (SRS-A), now known to be a group of molecules called *leukotrienes* (see below).

Serotonin. Serotonin is present in the mast cells of a limited number of species, such as rodents and humans. Its effects are similar to those of histamine; it causes constriction of smooth muscle and increases vascular permeability.

Chemotactic Factors. A variety of chemotactic factors are released following degranulation of mast cells. Low-molecular-weight peptides called *eosinophilic chemotactic factors* (ECFs) are also released upon degranulation. These produce a chemotactic gradient capable of attracting eosinophils to the site. Platelet-activating factor (PAF) and leukotrienes are late-phase mediators that also participate in the chemotaxis of inflammatory cells to the site; their roles will be covered below. Another important inflammatory cell attracted to the site is the *neutrophil*. Chemotaxis of these polymorphonuclear granulocytes occurs in response to IL-8 released by activated mast cells. As we shall see later, granulocytes are important in the late phase of IgE-mediated hypersensitivity. Other cells attracted to the site in response to mast cell-derived chemotactic factors include basophils, macrophages, platelets, and lymphocytes.

In allergic reactions, *eosinophils* appear to serve as a late indicator of the presence of IgE-mediated reactions, especially the late-phase reaction discussed later in this chapter. Eosinophils may also release arylsulfatase and histaminase; these enzymes destroy several mediators of the hypersensitivity reaction, thus limiting it. Eosinophils have an additional function in parasitic worm infections, also discussed later in this chapter.

Heparin. Heparin is an acidic proteoglycan that constitutes the matrix of the granule, and to which basic mediators, such as histamine and serotonin, are bound. Its acidic nature accounts for the metachromatic (high-staining) properties of the mast cell when basic dyes, such as toluidine blue, are applied to it. Release of heparin causes inhibition of coagulation, which may be of some use in the subsequent recovery of the mast cell or further introduction of antigen into the reaction area; however, it is not directly involved in the symptoms of anaphylaxis.

Newly Synthesized Mediators

Leukotrienes. When a preparation of smooth muscle, such as a guinea pig uterine horn, is treated with histamine, rapid contraction occurs. On the other hand, agents that cause slow but persistent contraction were collectively named SRS-A. SRS-A is now known to consist of a set of peptides that are coupled to a metabolite of *arachidonic acid*. These coupled peptides are called *leukotrienes* (LTs). The leukotrienes LTB4, LTC4, LTD4, and LTE4, cause prolonged constriction of smooth muscle when present in even minute amounts. They are considered to be the primary cause of antihistamine-resistant asthma in humans.

Thromboxanes and Prostaglandins. Leukotrienes are only one type of the complex products released from cell membrane lipids by phospholipases during mast cell triggering. Arachidonic acid also from the cell membrane, is a polyunsaturated, long-chain hydrocarbon that can be oxygenated in two separate pathways (Figure 15.4B): (1) by lipooxygenase to produce the above-mentioned leukotrienes, and (2) by cyclooxygenase to produce *prostaglandins* and *thromboxanes*. Many of these latter compounds are vasoactive, cause bronchoconstriction, and are chemotactic for a variety of white blood cells, such as neutrophils, eosinophils, basophils, and monocytes.

Platelet-activating factor (PAF) induces platelets to aggregate and release their contents, which includes the mediators *histamine* and, in some species, *serotonin*. Activation of platelets may also induce release of metabolites of arachidonic acid, thus augmenting the effects of mast-cell activation. PAF itself is one of the most potent causes of bronchoconstriction and vasodilation known; it rapidly produces shock-like symptoms, even when present in very small amounts.

Late-Phase Reaction

As mentioned above, many of the substances released during mast-cell activation and degranulation are responsible for the initiation of a profound inflammatory response, which consists of infiltration and accumulation of eosinophils, neutrophils, basophils, lymphocytes, and macrophages. The most important of these elements, which constitute a large percentage of the cells activated during an inflammatory response, are eosinophils and neutrophils. This response, referred to as the *late-phase reaction*, often occurs within 48 hours and may persist for several days (Figure 15.5). The mast cell, degranulated by cross-linking of IgE by antigen

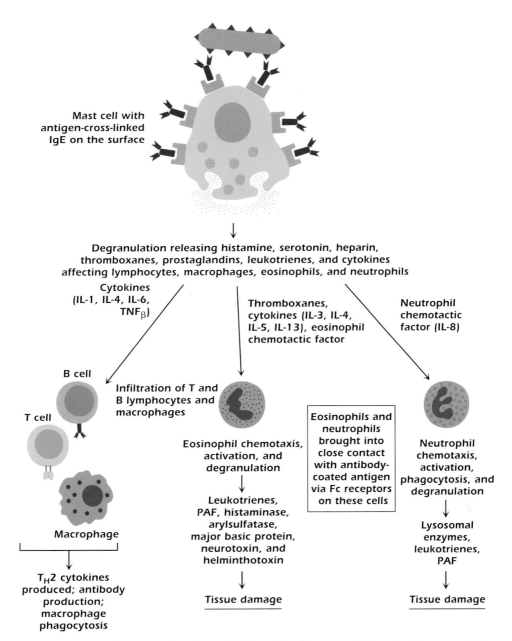

<u>Figure 15.5.</u> Late-phase reaction of type I IgE-mediated hypersensitivity showing some of the mediators involved.

on its surface, releases eosinophilic chemotactic factor (ECF-A), which recruits eosinophils to the reaction area. The passage of eosinophils and other leukocytes from the circulation to the tissue is facilitated by the increased vascular permeability caused by histamine and other mediators. Various cytokines, including GM-CSF, IL-3, IL-4, IL-5, and IL-13, play important roles in eosinophil growth and differentiation, and in the cell adhesion of certain cell types. Together, these inflammatory mediators generate a second, milder wave of smooth muscle contraction than the immediate response, along with sustained edema. In the case of individuals suffering from allergic asthma, the late-phase reaction also promotes the development of one of the

cardinal features of this form of asthma: airway hyperreactivity to nonspecific bronchoconstrictor stimuli such as histamine and methacholine.

Eosinophils can themselves bind IgE through their expression of the low-affinity IgE Fc receptor (FcεRII or CD23). They also express Fc receptors to the Fc portion of IgG. Thus, both IgE- and IgG-bound antigen will bind to their respective Fc receptors, causing eosinophil activation. Like mast cells, once their receptors are triggered they degranulate, releasing leukotrienes that cause muscle contraction. They also release PAF and ***major basic protein*** (MBP). MBP has the ability to destroy various parasites (such as schistosomes) by affecting their mobility and

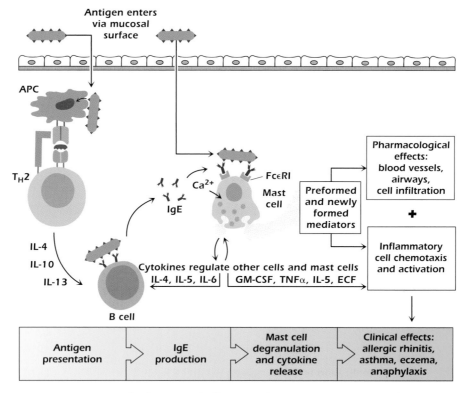

Figure 15.6. Overview of induction and effector mechanisms in type I hypersensitivity.

damaging their surfaces. MBP is also toxic to mammalian respiratory tract epithelium. Finally, the eosinophilic degranulation releases *eosinophilic cationic protein* (ECP), a potent neurotoxin and helminthotoxin. Although their activities are directed toward foreign invaders, all of these biologically active substances can cause damage to surrounding tissue.

Neutrophils recruited to the site in response to chemotactic factors come into close contact with antibody-coated antigen via the IgG Fc receptors that are normally expressed on these cells. Consequently, these cells become activated to phagocytose the antigen–antibody immune complexes. In addition, they release their powerful lysosomal enzymes, which cause great tissue damage. Like eosinophils, degranulation products of neutrophils also include leukotrienes and PAF. T and B lymphocytes and macrophages also enter the area, further sensitizing or immunizing the host against the offending antigen or microorganism.

Figure 15.6 illustrates the general mechanism underlying allergic reactions. This dramatic series of events triggered and mediated by IgE is involved in the elimination of parasites, as described later in this chapter. Unfortunately, the same events take place in certain individuals when the antigen is a harmless substance such as pollen, animal dander, or the common dust mite, and result in tissue damage.

CLINICAL ASPECTS OF ALLERGIC REACTIONS

The clinical consequences of allergic reactions can range from localized reactions including allergic rhinitis, asthma, atopic dermatitis, and food allergies, to severe, life-threatening systemic reactions such as anaphylaxis. Although defined as localized anaphylaxis, asthmatic reactions can also be fatal. Mast-cell degranulation is the central mechanism in each of these reactions.

 Read the related case: **Anaphylaxis**
In *Immunology: Clinical Case Studies and Disease Pathophysiology*

Allergic Rhinitis

Allergic rhinitis (commonly known as *hay fever*) is the most common atopic disorder worldwide. It is caused by airborne allergens that react with IgE-sensitized mast cells in the nasal passages and conjunctiva. Mediators released from mast cells increase capillary permeability and cause localized vasodilation, leading to the typical symptoms, which include sneezing and coughing.

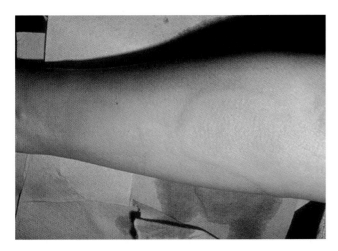

Figure 15.7. The wheal and flare reaction (atopic urticaria).

Food Allergies

Another common atopic disorder, food allergy, is caused by the intake of certain foods (e.g., peanuts, rice, eggs, etc.). Ingestion of such foods by susceptible individuals can trigger the cross-linking of allergen-specific IgE on mast cells of the upper and lower gastrointestinal tract. Mast-cell degranulation and mediator release leads to localized smooth muscle contraction and vasodilation, often causing vomiting and diarrhea. In some cases, the allergen is absorbed into the bloodstream as a consequence of increased permeability of mucous membranes, allowing food allergens to be transported to mast cells present in skin. This causes *wheal and flare reactions* (atopic urticaria; see Figure 15.7), commonly known as *hives*.

Atopic Dermatitis

A form of allergic reaction most frequently seen in young children, allergic dermatitis is caused by the development of inflammatory skin lesions induced by mast cell cytokines released following degranulation. These potent inflammatory cytokines released near the site of allergen contact stimulate chemotaxis of large numbers of inflammatory cells, especially eosinophils. The skin eruptions that develop are erythematous and pus (white cell)-filled.

Asthma

Asthma is a common form of localized anaphylaxis. The National Heart and Blood Institute of the National Institutes of Health defines asthma as a common chronic disorder of the airways that involves a complex interaction of airflow obstruction, bronchial hyperresponsiveness, and an underlying inflammation. It is a chronic obstructive disease of the lower airways characterized by episodic exacerbations of at least partially reversible airflow limitation. The clinical manifestations of asthma are believed to be the result of three basic pathophysiologic events within the airways: (1) reversible obstruction; (2) augmented bronchial responsiveness to a variety of physical and chemical stimuli (airway hyperreactivity); and (3) inflammation. In recent years, the incidence and severity of asthma have increased dramatically in the United States. Mortality rates have been highest in children living in inner cities. Epidemiological studies have suggested that the cockroach calyx is a major asthma-inducing allergen in these children. Many other allergens, including airborne pollens, dust, viral antigens, and various chemicals, can induce allergic asthma. Asthma may also be induced by phenomena ranging from exercise to exposure to cold temperatures independent of allergen exposure, a phenomenon known as *intrinsic asthma*.

Airway inflammation is believed to play a major role in the pathogenesis of this disorder and is therefore a prime target for pharmacological intervention. Cytokine-induced recruitment of large numbers of inflammatory cells, particularly eosinophils, ultimately causes significant tissue injury. Tissue damage is mediated by the many toxic substances released by these inflammatory cells, including oxygen radicals, nitric oxide, and cytokines. These events lead to the development of mucus, buildup of proteins and fluids (edema), and sloughing-off of epithelium, all of which combine to cause occlusion of the bronchial lumen. Adhesion molecules play a key role in the early events following inflammatory cell recruitment. Various cytokines released by T_H2 cells and by mast cells (such as IL-4, IL-13, and TNF-α) upregulate the expression of leukocyte and endothelial adhesion molecules, including intercellular adhesion molecule 1 (ICAM-1), E-selectin, vascular cell adhesion molecule 1, and leukocyte function-associated antigen-1 (LFA-1). Once upregulated, eosinophil–endothelial cell adhesion increases, facilitating transendothelial migration and prolonged survival within the lung tissue. Experimental adhesion molecule antagonists (e.g., anti-ICAM-1 monoclonal antibodies) are being investigated as candidate therapies for the treatment of asthma. Promising results using such immuotherapeutic reagents in animal models have stimulated interest in the development of antagonists that can be administered safely to humans.

Despite all of these candidate new approaches to the treatment of asthma, *corticosteroids* (CSTs) remain the gold standard for asthma management and for several decades have been considered the cornerstone for asthma control. With the recent advent of genomic and structural analysis technologies, the molecular basis of the side effects, toxicity, and resistance mechanisms of drug treatment are better understood. With respect to CST therapy, while it improves asthma symptoms, it does not alter the natural course of asthma or offer clear long-lasting improvement of respiratory performance. Therefore, the development of drugs capable of mitigating or avoiding CST side effects, toxicity, and resistance could usher in the development of new asthma therapies.

Read the related case: **Asthma**
In *Immunology: Clinical Case Studies and Disease Pathophysiology*

CLINICAL TESTS FOR ALLERGIES AND CLINICAL INTERVENTION

Detection

In a clinical setting, the degree of sensitivity to a particular allergen is usually determined by the patient's complaints and by the extent of skin test reactions. To avoid serious consequences from intradermal challenge in patients who may be extremely sensitive to certain allergens, a *skin-prick test* introducing minute amounts of antigen is administered first. A positive response to intradermal challenge, called *wheal and flare*, is characterized by *erythema* (redness due to dilation of blood vessels) and *edema* (swelling produced by release of serum into tissue) (Figure 15.7). The reaction is the most rapid of all hypersensitivity reactions and reaches its peak within 10–15 minutes; it then fades, leaving no residual damage.

The size of the local skin reaction is roughly indicative of the degree of sensitivity to the allergen being administered. In addition, if the clinical history of symptoms correlates well with the time of contact with the antigen, the cutaneous anaphylactic response may be taken as evidence that those symptoms (e.g., sneezing, itchy eyes) are attributable to the allergen. Other, more quantitative, tests are used as well (see below).

More quantitative assays that correlate to some degree with clinical symptoms are available in the laboratory. One assay, known as the *radioallergosorbent test* (RAST), involves covalent coupling of the allergen to an insoluble matrix, such as paper disks or beads. The antigen-coated matrix is then dipped into a sample of the patient's serum and allowed to bind any antibody that is specific for the allergen. After the disk is washed, a radiolabeled antibody specific for IgE is added. The amount of radioactivity bound is a measure of the amount of specific IgE antibody in the serum sample. More commonly, fluorescent assays or *enzyme-linked immunosorbent assays* (ELISAs) use enzyme-linked anti-IgE in lieu of radiolabeled antibody for the detection of allergen-specific IgE in patients' serum.

INTERVENTION

Environmental Intervention. In some cases, the easiest way for individuals to control their allergies is to avoid exposure to known allergens, advice that is followed infrequently. If some pollens are the cause of the reaction, it may be advisable but not always practical for the patient to go to pollen-free areas during the season when the offending plant is pollinating. *Masks* and *air filters* also have a useful role to play, but avoidance is usually difficult for the general allergic population.

Pharmacological Intervention. Modern pharmaceutical chemistry has provided a host of drugs that are more or less effective at various stages in the evolution of allergic reactions. Many of these are bronchodilators developed to treat patients with obstructive pulmonary diseases such as asthma. Bronchodilators are agents that cause expansion of the air passages of the lungs. This allows the patient to breathe more easily and is of value in overcoming acute bronchospasms. They are also employed as adjuncts in prophylactic and symptomatic treatment of other obstructive pulmonary diseases, such bronchitis and emphysema. Table 15.1 provides a list of the major pharmacological agents used to treat allergies and obstructive pulmonary diseases.

Immunologic Intervention. For many years, clinical immunologists have practiced a form of immunotherapy called *desensitization*. Over an extended period, patients are injected with increasing doses of the antigen to which they are sensitive. The improvement in symptoms noted in some patients has been ascribed to several different factors. The most popular rationale is based on the observation that such injections increase the synthesis of IgG antibody specific for the allergen. The circulating IgG presumably binds to and removes the allergen before it has a chance to reach and react with the IgE antibody on the surface of mast cells. Thus, the term *blocking antibody* has become associated with IgG antibody, and there is a rough correlation between titers of IgG antibody generated and clinical improvement.

Other findings during hyposensitization include an initial increase in levels of IgE antibody, followed by a prolonged decrease on continued therapy. This decrease has been linked to a decrease in intensity of symptoms and is attributed either to induction of tolerance, or to a switch from T_H2 to T_H1 T cells. After repeated subclinical doses of the antigen, there is also a progressive decrease in the sensitivity of mast cells and basophils to triggering by antigen. It is likely that the apparent benefits of this immunologic therapy are due to more than one of these factors. Whatever the reason for improvement, this form of therapy is generally more successful in dealing with allergens that enter the circulation directly, such as bee-sting venom, than for those allergens contacted via mucosal surfaces, such as pollen, against which IgG antibody therapy is unlikely to be effective.

Experimental immunotherapies for the treatment of IgE-mediated hypersensitivity are currently under investigation. A particularly promising therapy for the treatment of patients with asthma and allergic rhinitis employs the use of humanized anti-IgE monoclonal antibody (see Chapter 6) engineered so that it does not cross-link IgE bound to mast cells and basophils. The use of plasmid DNAs encoding a specific antigen (used to induce hyporesponsiveness),

TABLE 15.1. Pharmacologic Agents Used in Treatment of Allergies and Obstructive Pulmonary Diseases

Pharmacologic Category	Agent(s)	Pharmacologic Activity	Clinical Use
β Agonists (bronchodilators)	Albuterol	Relaxes contractions of the smooth muscle of the bronchioles; expands air passages of the lungs; short-acting (rescue therapy)	Asthma, bronchitis, and emphysema; prevention of exercise-induced bronchospasm
	Salmeterol	Similar to albuterol, except it cannot be used for rescue therapy	Same as albuterol
	Epinephrine	Antagonist of histamine; relaxes smooth muscle and decreases vascular permeability	Acute attacks of bronchospasms associated with emphysema, bronchitis, or anaphylaxis
	Metaproterenol	Adrenergic agent that has primary β_2 activity; main effect is to relax the bronchioles	Same indications as epinephrine; may also be used for the prevention of bronchospasms associated with chronic obstructive pulmonary diseases
	Isoproterenol	Adrenergic agent has primary β_2 activity	Asthma, bronchitis, emphysema, and mild bronchospasms
Xanthine derivatives (bronchodilators)	Aminophylline	Directly relaxes smooth muscle of bronchi and pulmonary blood vessels	Prevents severe attacks of bronchial asthma; used in the treatment of apnea and bradycardia of prematurity in infants
	Theophylline	Directly relaxes smooth muscle of bronchi and pulmonary blood vessels; inhibits mast-cell degranulation	Similar to aminophylline
Mast-cell membrane stabilizers	Cromolyn sodium	Decreases or prevents mast-cell degranulation; prevents Ca^{2+} influx	Used to treat or prevent mild bronchospasms associated with asthma; allergic rhinitis
Leukotriene modifiers	Zafirlukast	Binds to leukotriene receptors, thereby preventing airway edema, smooth muscle constriction, and altered inflammatory processes	Asthma
	Ziluton	Inhibits the formation of leukotrienes to prevent bronchoconstriction	Asthma
Antihistamines	Many are available, including fexofenadine (Allegra), loratidine (Claritin), and cetirizine (Zyrtec)	Primarily act by blocking the H1 receptors; inhibits smooth muscle (lung and gut) contraction, dilatation of small blood vessels, and mucus production	Allergic rhinitis, atopic dermatitis, hives, some rashes
Corticosteroids	Many are available, including hydrocortisone, methylprednisolone, prednisolone, prednisone, budesonide, flunisolide, and fluticasone propionate	Potent anti-inflammatory drugs with immunosuppressive activity when used in high doses; effects are numerous and widespread; immunomudulatory effects mainly act through inhibition of gene transcription (e.g., inhibition of COX-2 synthesis)	Asthma, allergic rhinitis, urticaria, eczema

cytokines such as IL-12 and IL-10 (used to cause a shift from T_H2 to T_H1 responses), anti-cytokines such as anti-IL-4 (used to inhibit IL-4 production), and cytokine receptor antagonists are also current areas of research.

Other immunologic intervention approaches have been attempted in experimental animals. For example, administration of a chemically altered allergen (e.g., ragweed pollen denatured by urea or coupled to polyethylene glycol) has been shown to suppress a primary or established IgE response. The mechanism may involve the induction of negative regulatory T cells that are both antigen specific and isotype specific. The modified allergens do not combine with preexisting IgE antibodies and therefore do not trigger anaphylactic responses. Use of such modified allergens seems to offer another promising approach to treatment of allergy. Efforts have also been made to skew the T helper responses from T_H2 toward T_H1 responses. The rationale for this approach is based on the key role that T_H2 cells play in allergic reactions by producing cytokines, such as IL4, that induce IgE class switching in B cells.

Finally, recent advances in our understanding of the expression and function of microRNAs (miRNAs) in patients with allergic inflammation, and their role as disease biomarkers have uncovered new translational and clinical opportunities using these single-stranded RNAs. The miRNAs can silence gene expression post-transcriptionally, and they have been shown to fine-tune gene transcriptional networks because single miRNAs can target hundreds of genes. Recent studies have identified miRNA profiles in multiple allergic inflammatory diseases, including asthma, eosinophilic esophagitis, allergic rhinitis, and atopic dermatitis. Specific miRNAs have been found to have critical roles in regulating key pathogenic mechanisms in allergic inflammation, including polarization of adaptive immune responses and activation of T cells.

THE PROTECTIVE ROLE OF IgE

Thus far we have focused on the properties of IgE associated with hypersensitivity reactions. What about the physiologic role of this immunoglobulin? Allergic reactions do have protective effects, which are evident when the sensitizing antigen is derived from one of many parasitic worms, such as helminths. The immune response to these worms favors the induction of IgE. Histamine and other mediators associated with the anaphylactic response are released in response to worm antigens cross-linking IgE on the surface of mast cells (and eosinophils). The effects of increased permeability due to histamine release bring serum components, including IgG antibody, to the site of worm infestation. The IgG antibody binds to the surface of the worm and attracts the eosinophils, which have migrated to the area as a result of the chemotactic effects of ECF-A. The eosinophils then bind to the IgG-coated worm via their membrane receptors for IgG Fc, and release the contents of their granules (Figures 15.8 and 15.9). As noted earlier, eosinophils also express the low-affinity Fc receptor for IgE, which facilitates the binding of these cells to IgE-coated worms. The MBP released from the eosinophil granules coats the surface of the worm and leads, in some unknown way, to the death of the worm and its eventual expulsion from the body. As you can see, all components of the type I reaction combine to perform this protective function. This beneficial effect suggests that the wide range of responses involving IgE may have evolved from efforts to combat worm parasitism.

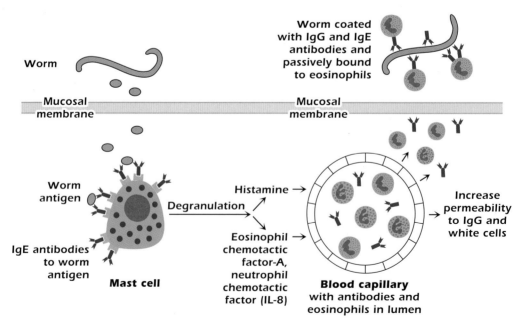

Figure 15.8. The destruction of a worm by eosinophils that have migrated to the area and have been activated following IgE-mediated and antigen-mediated mast-cell degranulation.

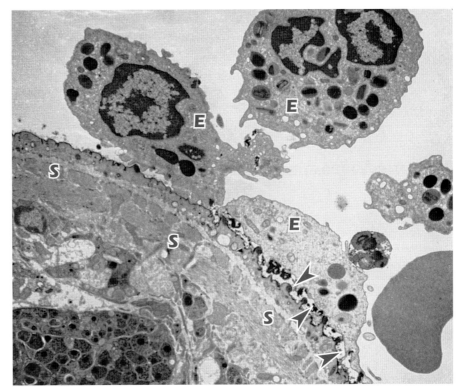

Figure 15.9. Electron micrograph (×6,000) of eosinophils (E) adhering to an antibody-coated schistosomulum (S). The cell on the left has not yet degranulated, but the one on the right has discharged electron-dense material (arrows), which can be seen between the cell and the worm. (Photograph by Dr. J. Caulfield, Harvard Medical School.)

SUMMARY

1. Allergic reactions are mediated by IgE antibodies, which bind to high-affinity receptors specific for the Fc region of IgE (FcεRI) on the surface of mast cells and basophils. When these receptors are cross-linked following the binding of antigen to IgE, the cell responds by releasing its granules and their inflammatory mediators.

2. IgE responses are T-cell dependent. Allergens stimulate the induction of T_H2 cells, which release various cytokines (IL-4, IL-13) that stimulate B-cells to undergo class switching to generate IgE responses.

3. Following antigen cross-linking of IgE on cells expressing FcεRI, the inflammatory mediators released by these cells have both early and late stage effects on the host; the latter may persist for several days.

4. The symptoms of allergic reactions can be attributed principally to the inflammatory mediators released by activated mast cells and basophils. Typical immediate symptoms of allergic reactions include increased vascular permeability, constriction of smooth muscles, and influx of eosinophils.

5. The early stage of allergic reactions is characterized by the release of preformed or rapidly synthesized short-lived mediators such as histamine and prostaglandins, which cause a rapid increase in vascular permeability and contraction of smooth muscle.

6. Late-stage allergic reactions are caused by induced synthesis and release of mediators including leukotrienes, cytokines, and chemokines from activated mast cells. These recruit other leukocytes, including eosinophils and T_H2 cells, to the site of inflammation, causing sustained edema and a milder form of smooth muscle contraction than the immediate response. In an asthmatic reaction, airway hyperreactivity to nonspecific bronchoconstrictor stimuli such as histamine and methacholine also occurs.

7. Clinical manifestations of allergic reactions include localized reactions such as allergic rhinitis, atopic dermatitis, food allergies, and obstructive

pulmonary diseases such as asthma, bronchitis, and emphysema.

8. Systemic reactions can lead to life-threatening anaphylaxis.

9. Despite the dangerous systematic reactions produced by type I hypersensitivity reactions mediated by IgE, the value of this immunoglobulin probably lies in its ability to combat parasitic infections.

10. Common therapeutic agents used to treat allergic reactions include bronchodilators (beta agonists and xanthine derivatives), corticosteroids, cromolyn sodium, antihistamines, and leukotriene modifiers.

REFERENCES AND BIBLIOGRAPHY

Bacharier LB, Geha RS. (2000) Molecular mechanisms of IgE regulation. *J Allergy Clin Immunol* 105: S547.

Bevan MA, Metzger H. (1993) Signal transduction by Fc receptors: the FcεRI case. *Immunol Today* 14: 222.

Coombs RRA, Gell PGH. (1963) The classification of allergic reactions underlying disease. In Gell PGH, Coombs RRA (eds) Clinical Aspects of Immunology. Oxford, UK: Blackwell.

Finkelman, FD. (2007) Anaphylaxis: lessons from mouse models. *J Allergy Clin Immunol* 120(3): 506.

Golden DB. (2007) What is anaphylaxis? *Curr Opin Allergy Clin Immunol* 7(4): 331.

Heusser C, Jardieu P. (1997) Therapeutic potential of anti-IgE antibodies. *Curr Opinion Immunology* 9: 805.

Kandeel, M, Balaha, M, Inagaki, N, Kitade, Y. (2013) Current and future asthma therapies. *Drugs Today* 49(5): 325.

Kuhn R. (2007) Immunoglobulin E blockade in the treatment of asthma. *Pharmacotherapy* 27(10): 1412.

Lu, TX, Rothenberg, ME. (2013) Diagnostic, functional, and therapeutic roles of microRNA in allergic disease. *J Allergy Clin Immunology* 132(1): 3.

Naclerio R and Solomon W. (1997) Rhinitis and inhalant allergins. *JAMA* 278: 1842.

Peters-Golden M, Henderson WR Jr. (2007) Leukotrienes. *N Engl J Med* 357(18): 1841.

Ray A, Cohen L. (1999) T_H2 cells and GATA-3 in asthma: new insights into the regulation of airway inflammation. *J Clin Invest* 104: 985.

Townley RG. (2007) Interleukin 13 and the beta-adrenergic blockade theory of asthma revisited 40 years later. *Ann Allergy Asthma Immunol* 99(3): 215.

Umetsu DT, Dekruyff RH. (2006) The regulation of allergy and asthma. *Immunol Rev* 212: 238.

Umetsu DT, Dekruyff RH. (2006) Immune dysregulation in anthma. *Curr Opin Immunol* 18(6): 727.

REVIEW QUESTIONS

For each question, choose the ONE BEST answer or completion.

1. A 22-year-old male, with significant cat allergies, visits a home with multiple cats. Two hours later, he arrives at an urgent care center with a severe exacerbation of asthma. He is treated with a short-acting bronchodilator and epinephrine. Initially, his symptoms resolved after treatment; however, 8 hours later he is forced to go the emergency room with another exacerbation. What is the most likely cause of his symptoms?
   A) additional IgE cross-linking on mast cells leading to lipid mediator and cytokine release
   B) CD4+ T_H1 cell production of IFN-γ
   C) complement activation leading to mast-cell degranulation by C5a and C3a
   D) eosinophil and basophil infiltration leading to the release of proinflammatory mediators
   E) neutrophil recruitment and the release of cytoplasmic granule components

2. A 21-year old male who is allergic to cat dander is exposed to a friend's cat while wearing a facial mask to reduce his contact with the allergen. Nevertheless, several hours later, he is wheezing and coughing. Which of the following best explains this individual's allergic reaction?
   A) Mast cells in his gastrointestinal tract degranulated following the cross-linking of allergen-specific IgE on their surface, and the inflammatory mediators traveled to his lung.
   B) Mast cells in his blood vessels degranulated following the cross-linking of allergen-specific IgE on their surface, causing a systemic inflammatory response.
   C) Mast cells in his lung degranulated following the cross-linking of allergen-specific IgE on their surface.
   D) Mast cells in his skin degranulated following the cross-linking of allergen-specific IgE on their surface, causing a systemic inflammatory response.

3. The usual sequence of events in an allergic reaction is as follows:
   A) The allergen combines with circulating IgE, then the IgE-allergen complex binds to mast cells.
   B) The allergen binds to IgE fixed to mast cells.
   C) The allergen is processed by antigen-presenting cells and then binds to histamine receptors.
   D) The allergen is processed by antigen-presenting cells and then binds to mast cells.
   E) The allergen combines with IgG.

4. Epinephrine
   A) causes bronchodilation
   B) is effective even after anaphylactic symptoms commence
   C) relaxes smooth muscle
   D) decreases vascular permeability
   E) all of the above

5. A human volunteer agrees to be passively sensitized with IgE specific for a ragweed antigen (allergen). When challenged with the allergen intradermally, he displays a typical skin reaction due to an immediate hypersensitivity reaction. If the injection with sensitizing IgE was preceded by an injection (at the same site) of Fc fragments of human IgE followed by intradermal injection with allergen, which of the following outcomes would you predict?
   A) No reaction would occur because the Fc fragments would interact with the allergen and prevent it from gaining access to the sensitized mast cells.
   B) No reaction would occur because the Fc fragments would interact with the IgE antibodies, making their antigen-binding sites unavailable for binding to antigen.
   C) No reaction would occur because the Fc fragments would interact with FcεR receptors on mast cells.
   D) The reaction would be exacerbated due to the increased local concentration of IgE Fc fragments.
   E) The reaction would be exacerbated due to the activation of complement.

6. The following mechanism(s) may be involved in the clinical efficacy of desensitization therapy to treat patients with allergies to known allergens:
   A) enhanced production of IgG, which binds allergen before it reaches mast cells
   B) skewing of T-cell responses from T_H2 to T_H1
   C) decreased sensitivity of mast cells and basophils to degranulation by allergen
   D) decreased production of IgE antibody
   E) all of the above

7. Antihistamines
   A) block H1 receptors and inhibit smooth muscle contraction, dilatation of small blood vessels, and mucus production
   B) directly bind to histamine, blocking its inflammatory effect
   C) influence the activity of leukotrienes
   D) inhibit binding of IgE to mast cells
   E) are adrenergic agents that mainly relax the bronchioles

8. Which of the following remains the gold standard for asthma management?
   A) adhesion molecule antagonists
   B) corticosteroids
   C) antihistamines
   D) allergen desensitization therapy
   E) epinephrine

9. Anaphylactic reactions
   A) evolve in minutes and abate within 30 minutes
   B) may be followed by inflammatory reactions hours later
   C) are the consequences of released pharmacologic agents
   D) may involve components of mast-cell granule matrix
   E) all of the above

ANSWERS TO REVIEW QUESTIONS

1. *D.* The timing of the symptoms exhibited in this individual are characteristic of late-phase allergic reactions in which eosinophil infiltration occurs. This recruitment of eosinophils, as well as the passage of other leukocytes from the circulation to the tissue, is facilitated by the increased vascular permeability caused by proinflammatory cytokines and histamine.

2. *C.* Despite the use of protective barriers such as facial masks to prevent an individual's inhalation of allergens, small amounts of airborne antigens such as cat dander can enter by this route and cause degranulation of IgE-sensitized mast cells in the lung.

3. *B.* Allergic individuals have already made IgE responses to specific allergens. IgE binds passively to cells expressing high-affinity Fc receptors for IgE (e.g., mast cells) and interacts with the allergen when present. This results in cross-linking of the high-affinity FcεR, resulting in mast-cell degranulation. The allergen does not need to be processed by APCs in order to bind to IgE.

4. *E.* All are effects of epinephrine and make it useful for treatment of acute anaphylactic symptoms.

5. *C.* Since the IgE Fc fragments would bind to the high-affinity FcεR expressed on the surface of mast cells, the allergen-specific

IgE would not have access to these receptors and therefore would not bind to these cells. When the allergen is introduced intradermally, it would bind to the allergen-specific IgE at the site, but this would not result in cross-linking of FcεR, which is saturated with soluble IgE Fc fragments. Hence no immediate hypersensitivity reaction would take place.

6. *E.* All are considered to be involved to varying degrees in injection therapy.

7. *A.* Antihistamines act by blocking H1 histamine receptors, NOT histamine itself. They do not act by influencing the activity of leukotrienes or by binding to IgE on mast cells and are not andrenergic agents.

8. *B.* Corticosteroids remain the gold standard for asthma management and for several decades have been considered the cornerstone for asthma control. While it improves asthma symptoms, it does not alter the natural course of asthma or offer clear long-lasting improvement of respiratory performance. Therefore, the development of drugs capable of mitigating or avoiding CST side effects, toxicity, and resistance could usher in the development of new asthma therapies.

9. *E.* All are true. **A** and **C** are true of the classic wheal and flare type response, while **B** and **D** describe features of the late-phase response, which is a complication of some anaphylactic reactions.

16

HYPERSENSITIVITY: TYPES II AND III

INTRODUCTION

Hypersensitivity reactions characterized as type II and type III reactions are mediated by antibodies belonging to the IgG, IgM, and, in some cases, IgA or IgE isotypes. The distinction between these two forms of hypersensitivity lies in the type and location of antigen involved and the way in which antigen is brought together with antibody. Type II hypersensitivity reactions are the result of the binding of antibody directly to an antigen on the surface of a cell. Type III reactions are the result of deposition of antigen–antibody immune complexes. The target antigens involved in type II and type III hypersensitivity reactions are often self-antigens.

TYPE II HYPERSENSITIVITY

Three different antibody-mediated mechanisms are involved in type II hypersensitivity reactions. The targeted cell is either damaged or destroyed through a variety of mechanisms associated with (a) complement-mediated reactions; (b) antibody-dependent cell-mediated cytotoxicity; or, (c) antibody-mediated cellular dysfunction. As illustrated in the examples of clinically important type II hypersensitivity reactions discussed below, many of these reactions are manifestations of antibody-mediated autoimmunity. Mechanisms associated with the generation of autoantibodies were discussed in Chapter 13. The antibodies involved in these hypersensitivity reactions are either directed against normal self-antigens (e.g., cross-reactive antibodies elicited following an infection) or modified self-antigens (e.g., drug-induced autoantibodies elicited following the binding of drugs to certain cell membranes).

Complement-Mediated Reactions

In complement-mediated hypersensitivity reactions, antibodies react with cell membrane self-antigens and this is followed by complement fixation. This activates the complement cascade, as discussed in Chapter 14, and leads to *lysis* of the cell. Alternatively, binding of antibody to the cell surface and subsequent activation of complement to yield C3b effectively opsonize the target cell (Figure 16.1A). *Opsonization* culminates in the phagocytosis and destruction of the cell by macrophages and neutrophils expressing surface Fc receptors or receptors that bind C3b. Blood cells are most commonly affected by this mechanism. Interestingly, IgG Fc receptor knockout mice fail to mount type II (and type III) hypersensitivity reactions, a finding that underscores the pivotal role played by IgG Fc receptors in initiating these reaction cascades.

Antibody-Dependent Cell-Mediated Cytotoxicity

Antibody-dependent cell-mediated cytotoxicity (ADCC) utilizes Fc receptors expressed on many cell types (e.g., natural killer [NK] cells, macrophages, neutrophils, eosinophils) as a means of bringing these cells into contact with

Immunology: A Short Course, Seventh Edition. Richard Coico and Geoffrey Sunshine.
© 2015 John Wiley & Sons, Ltd. Published 2015 by John Wiley & Sons, Ltd.
Companion Website: www.wileyimmunology.com/coico

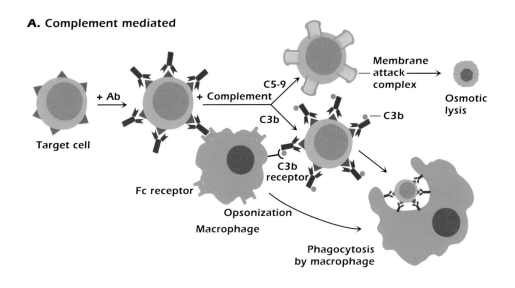

Figure 16.1. Schematic illustration of three different mechanisms of antibody-mediated injury in type II hypersensitivity. (A) Complement-dependent reactions that lead to lysis of cells or render them susceptible to phagocytosis. (B) Antibody-dependent cell-mediated cytotoxicity (ADCC). IgG-coated target cells are killed by cells that bear Fc receptors for IgG (e.g., NK cells, macrophages). (C) Anti-receptor antibodies disturb the normal function of receptors. In this example, acetylcholine receptor antibodies impair neuromuscular transmission in myasthenia gravis.

antibody-coated target cells (Figure 16.1B). Lysis of these target cells requires contact but does not involve phagocytosis or complement fixation. Instead, ADCC-mediated lysis of target cells is analogous to that of cytotoxic T cells and involves the release of cytoplasmic granules (modified lysosomes) containing *perforin* and *granzymes*. Once released from the lytic granules, perforins insert into the target cell membrane and polymerize to form pores. In contrast, granzymes, which consist of at lease three serine proteases, enter the cytoplasm of the target cell and activate events leading to apoptosis.

ADCC reactions are typically triggered by IgG binding to IgG-specific Fc receptors (FcγIII, also known as CD16)

on the effector cell. However, IgE antibodies can also be involved in ADCC. In this situation, the low-affinity IgE Fc receptor (FcεRII) expressed on certain cells, including eosinophils (see Chapter 15), binds to the Fc portion of IgE antibodies bound to target antigens (e.g., parasites) (see Figure 15.2).

Antibody-Mediated Cellular Dysfunction

In some type II hypersensitivity reactions, antibodies bind to *cell-surface receptors* that are critical for the functional integrity of the cell. When autoantibodies bind to such receptors they impair or dysregulate cell function without causing cell injury or inflammation.

In the following section, we provide several examples of clinically important antibody-mediated cytotoxic hypersensitivity reactions.

EXAMPLES OF TYPE II HYPERSENSITIVITY REACTIONS

Transfusion Reactions

Transfusion of **ABO-incompatible blood** results in complement-mediated cytotoxic reactions. As an example, individuals with type O blood have in their circulation IgM anti-A and anti-B antibodies (**isohemagglutinins**), which react with the A and B blood-group substances, respectively (see Chapter 5). If such a person were to be transfused with red blood cells (RBCs) expressing the type A blood group antigen, the consequences could be disastrous. Since there is a considerable amount of IgM anti-A antibody in this person's circulation, all the transfused type A red blood cells will bind to some antibody. Because of the efficiency of IgM antibody in activating complement (a single IgM molecule is sufficient to activate many complement molecules; see Chapter 14), and because of the absence of repair mechanisms, RBCs will be lysed intravascularly by the destructive action of complement on their membranes. Not only will this nullify the desirable effects of the transfusion, but the individual will also face the risk of kidney damage from blockage by large quantities of RBC membrane, plus the possible toxic effects from the release of the heme complex.

Drug-Induced Reactions

In some people, certain drugs act as **haptens** and combine with cells or with other circulating blood constituents and induce antibody formation. When antibody combines with cells coated with the drug, cytotoxic damage results. The type of pathologic injury depends on the type of cell that binds the drug. For example, some drugs can bind to platelets causing them to become immunogenic. The antibody responses that are generated cause lysis of the platelets and resulting thrombocytopenia (low blood platelet count). This disorder, in turn, can give rise to purpura (hemorrhage into the skin, mucous membranes, and internal organs), which is the main problem in drug-induced thrombocytopenia purpura. Withdrawal of the offending drug leads to a cessation of symptoms. Other drugs, such as chloramphenicol (an antibiotic), may bind to white blood cells; phenacetin (an analgesic) and chlorpromazine (a tranquilizer) may bind to red blood cells. The consequences of an immune response to these drugs can lead to an agranulocytosis (decrease in granulocytes) in the case of white blood cells, and a hemolytic anemia in the case of red blood cells. Damage to the target cell in these examples may be mediated by either of the two mechanisms described above: by cytolysis via the complement pathway or by destruction of cells by phagocytosis mediated by receptors for Fc or C3b.

It should be pointed out that whereas the preceding discussion emphasizes type II reactions induced by drugs, hypersensitivity to drugs may also induce IgE-mediated immediate type I hypersensitivity reactions (Chapter 15), type IV delayed-type hypersensitivity reactions (discussed in Chapter 17), and the immune complex-mediated reactions (type III) discussed below. As noted earlier, some reactions are induced by a drug acting as a hapten conjugated to a particular self-antigen.

Rhesus Incompatibility Reactions

A somewhat similar mechanism is exemplified by the rhesus (Rh) incompatibility reaction seen in infants born of mothers with Rh-incompatible blood groups. Rh antigens are so named because rabbit antisera raised against rhesus monkey RBCs (RhRBCs) agglutinate the erythrocytes from approximately 85% of humans tested. RBCs from such individuals are therefore said to be Rh^+, whereas cells from the remaining 15% of the population are Rh^-. Rh^- mothers can become sensitized to Rh antigens during their first pregnancy with a child whose RBCs are Rh^+. This occurs as a result of the release of some of the baby's RBCs into the mother's circulation perinatally and particularly during birth. If the mother is thereby sufficiently immunized to produce anti-Rh antibody of the IgG isotype, subsequent Rh^+ fetuses will be at risk, since, as we saw in Chapter 5, IgG antibody is capable of crossing the placenta. Thus, in second or subsequent pregnancies, when the anti-Rh IgG antibodies have crossed the placenta, they bind to the Rh antigen on the RBCs of the fetus. Because the density of Rh antigen on the surface of RBCs is low, these antibodies usually fail to agglutinate or lyse the cells directly. However, the antibody-coated cells are readily destroyed by the opsonic effect of the Fc portions of the IgG, which interact with the receptors for Fc on the phagocytic cells of the reticuloendothelial system. The result is progressive destruction of the fetal or newborn RBCs, with the pathologic consequences that come from decreased transport of oxygen and from increased bilirubin from the products of the breakdown of hemoglobin, a condition known as **erythroblastosis fetalis** (hemolytic disease of the newborn). Prevention of this Rh incompatibility reaction can be achieved with the administration of anti-Rh antibodies (passive immunization) to the mother at 26–28 weeks' gestation and again within 72 hours of parturition to effectively block the sensitization phase. This also causes a rapid clearance of Rh^+ cells from the mother's circulation. One widely used preparation of anti-Rh antibodies involves the use of antibodies (**Rhogam**) against the D antigen, now known to be the strongest immunogen and the most important of all the Rh antigens.

Reactions Involving Cell Membrane Receptors

An example of antibody-mediated cellular dysfunction due to reactivity with a cell receptor is seen in the autoimmune disease *myasthenia gravis*. Antagonistic autoantibodies reactive with *acetylcholine receptors* in the motor end plates of skeletal muscles impair neuromuscular transmission, causing muscle weakness (Figure 16.1C). Conversely, in Graves' disease, the autoantibodies serve as agonists, causing stimulation of the target cells. These antibodies are directed against thyroid-stimulating hormone receptor on thyroid epithelial cells and stimulate the cells, resulting in hyperthyroidism. These disorders are discussed in more detail in Chapter 13, which deals with the subject of autoimmunity.

Reactions Involving Other Cell Membrane Determinants

As a consequence of certain infectious diseases, or for other, still unknown reasons, some individuals produce autoantibodies reactive against their own blood cells. When RBCs are the target, binding of *anti-RBC autoantibody* shortens their life span or destroys them immediately. Destruction can be complement-mediated resulting in RBC hemolysis or mediated by phagocytosis following the binding of phagocytes to the Fc regions of autoantibodies or C3b bound to these cells. This may lead to progressive anemia if the production of new RBCs cannot keep pace with destruction. Occasionally, the antibody only binds effectively at lower temperatures (so-called *cold agglutinins*), in which case regions of lower body temperature, particularly in the figures and toes, leads to effective antibody binding and destruction of the RBCs.

Another example of cell destruction by autoantibodies is *immune thrombocytopenia purpura* (ITP), previously known as idiopathic thrombocytopenia purpura. In this condition, antibodies directed to platelets result in platelet destruction by complement or phagocytic cells with Fc or C3b receptors. Decrease in platelet numbers may lead to bleeding (purpura). Similarly, autoantibodies directed against granulocytes can induce agranulocytosis predisposing individuals to various infections. Finally, antibodies may form against other tissue components such as a type of basement membrane collagen particularly prevalent in the lung and kidneys, causing *Goodpasture's syndrome* (see Chapter 13), and desmosomes between keratinocytes in the skin, resulting in *pemphigus vulgaris*.

Type III Hypersensitivity

Under normal conditions, circulating *immune complexes* composed of antibodies bound to foreign antigens are removed by phagocytic cells. Phagocytosis is facilitated by the binding of the Fc regions of the antibodies present in such complexes to IgG Fc receptors expressed on these cells. In addition, RBCs that have C3b receptors may bind immune complexes that have fixed complement and transport them to the liver, where the complexes are removed by phagocytic Kupffer cells. Another innate immune mechanism for the disposal of immune complexes involves a histidine-rich glycoprotein (HRG), which is abundantly synthesized by the liver and released into the blood stream. In contrast with the other known immune complex clearing mechanisms, such as the complement system, HRG does not require pre-activation. HRG is therefore readily available to engage in the removal of immune complexes. Interestingly, HRG also has the ability to clear apoptotic cells by binding naked DNA. Through its interactions with naked DNA and immune complexes, HRG may mask epitopes recognized by autoantibody-producing B cells (e.g., rheumatoid factors and anti-double stranded DNA antibodies). The latter property may regulate adaptive immune system activation and has important implications for the involvement of HRG in ameliorating autoimmune reactions.

What happens when physiologic mechanisms for clearing immune complexes are overwhelmed with large quantities of such complexes? When this happens, immune complexes of a certain size can inappropriately deposit in the tissues and trigger a variety of systemic pathogenic events known as *type III hypersensitivity reactions*. These reactions can be *systemic* (also called *systemic immune complex disease*) or *localized* (also known as *localized immune complex disease*) and can be associated with immune complex deposition in the kidneys, skin, joints, choroid plexus, and ciliary artery of the eye. The generation of immune complexes can be stimulated by *exogenous antigens* such as bacteria and viruses or, as in the case of the Arthus reaction described below, by intradermal or intrapulmonary exposure to large amounts of foreign protein. Alternatively, *endogenous antigens*, such as DNA, can serve as a target for autoantibodies as seen in *systemic lupus erythematosus* (SLE). In the latter case, the clinical outcome is more accurately defined as an autoimmune phenomenon (see Chapter 13). Patients with SLE often have both systemic (multiorgan) and localized manifestations of immune complex disease. Localized tissue injury associated with lupus nephritis occurs as a result of antigen–antibody complexes forming either *in situ* or in the circulation and then depositing in the glomeruli of the kidneys resulting in *glomerular disease*.

The mechanism of injury seen in immune complex-mediated disease is the same regardless of which pattern of immune complex deposition is seen (i.e., systemic versus local). Central to the pathogenesis of tissue injury is the fixation of complement by the immune complexes, activation of the complement cascade, and release of biologically active fragments (e.g., anaphylotoxins C3a and C5a; see Chapter 14). Complement activation results in increased vascular permeability and stimulates the recruitment of polymorphonuclear phagocytes that release lysosomal enzymes (e.g., neutral proteases) that can damage the glomerular basement membrane.

IgG is the immunoglobulin isotype usually involved in type III hypersensitivity reactions, but IgM can also be involved. As with type II hypersensitivity reactions, IgG Fc receptors (CD16) expressed on leukocytes play a pivotal role in initiating type III reaction cascades. The antibody–antigen complexes may fix complement and/or activate effector cells (the main cell type being the neutrophil) that cause tissue damage. C3a and C5a generated by complement activation induce mast cells and basophils to release arachidonic acid metabolites and chemokines that attract additional basophils, eosinophils, macrophages, and neutrophils into the area. The polymorphonuclear cells release their lysosomal enzymes at the surface of the affected tissues. Macrophages are stimulated to release tumor necrosis factor-α (TNF-α) and interleukin-1 (IL-1), while platelets form microthrombi and contribute to cellular proliferation by releasing platelet-derived growth factor (PDGF).

Systemic Immune Complex Disease

The pathogenesis of systemic immune complex disease can be divided into three phases. In the first phase, antigen–antibody immune complexes form in the circulation. This is followed by deposition of immune complexes in various tissues that initiates the third phase in which inflammatory reactions in various tissues occur (Figure 16.2). Several factors help to determine whether immune complex formation will lead to tissue deposition and disease. The size of the complexes appears to be important. Very large complexes formed under conditions of antibody excess are rapidly removed from the circulation by phagocytic cells and therefore are harmless. Small or intermediate complexes circulate for longer periods of time and bind less avidly to IgG Fc receptors expressed on phagocytic cells. Therefore, small-to-intermediate sized immune complexes tend to be more pathogenic as compared with large complexes. A second factor that can influence the development of systemic immune complex disease is the integrity of the mononuclear phagocytic system. An intrinsic dysfunction of this system increases the probability of persistence of immune complexes in the circulation. As expected, overloading this phagocytic system with large quantities of immune complexes also compromises its ability to mediate clearance of such complexes from the circulation. For reasons that are not well understood, the favored sites of immune complex deposition are the kidneys, joints, skin, heart, and small vessels. Localization in the kidney can be explained, in part, by the filtration function of the glomeruli.

Serum sickness. The prototype of systemic immune complex disease is *serum sickness*. This term derives from observations made at the turn of the twentieth century by von Pirquet and Schick of the consequences of the treatment of certain infectious diseases, such as diphtheria and tetanus, with antisera made in horses. It was well known that the pathologic consequences of infection by both the *Corynebacterium* and the *Clostridium* organisms were due to the secretion of exotoxins that are extremely damaging to host cells (Chapter 21). The bacteria themselves are relatively noninvasive and of little consequence. Hence the strategy that evolved to treat these diseases was to neutralize the toxins rapidly, before quantities large enough to kill the host became fixed in tissues. Since active immunization required several weeks before useful levels of antibody were produced, it was necessary to protect the individual through passive immunization by injecting large amounts of a preformed antitoxin antibody as soon as the disease was diagnosed in order to prevent death by toxin. Horses, which were readily available, easily immunized, and capable of yielding large quantities of useful antisera, were the animals of choice for the production of antitoxin. Today, we know that the administration of large quantities of heterologous serum from another species causes the recipient to synthesize antibodies to the foreign immunoglobulin, leading to the formation of antigen–antibody complexes that result in the clinical symptoms associated with serum sickness. Serum sickness can occur in patients as a secondary reaction to the administration of nonprotein drugs. The classic clinical manifestations consist of fever, arthralgia, lymphadenopathy, and skin eruption. In addition, until the advent of humanized antibodies (see Chapter 6), serum sickness was an important consideration in patients being treated for malignancy, graft rejection, or autoimmune disease with monoclonal antibodies made in rodents.

Infection-Associated Immune Complex Disease. Perhaps the best example of infection-associated immune complex diseases is *rheumatic fever*. In susceptible individuals, this disease is associated with infections (e.g., throat) caused by *group A streptococci*, and it involves inflammation and damage to heart, joints, and kidneys. A variety of antigens in the cell walls and membranes of streptococci have been shown to be cross-reactive with antigens present in human heart muscle, cartilage, and glomerular basement membrane. It is presumed that antibody to the streptococcal antigens binds to these components of normal tissue and induces inflammatory reactions via a pathway similar to that described above.

In *rheumatoid arthritis*, there is evidence for the production of *rheumatoid factor*, an IgM autoantibody that binds to the Fc portion of normal IgG. These immune complexes participate in causing inflammation of joints and the damage characteristic of this disease.

In a variety of other infections some individuals produce antibodies that cross-react with some constituent of normal tissue. For example, individuals predisposed to Goodpasture's syndrome (see Chapter 13) sometimes develop this disease following viral respiratory infections. The pulmonary hemorrhage and glomerulonephritis seen in these

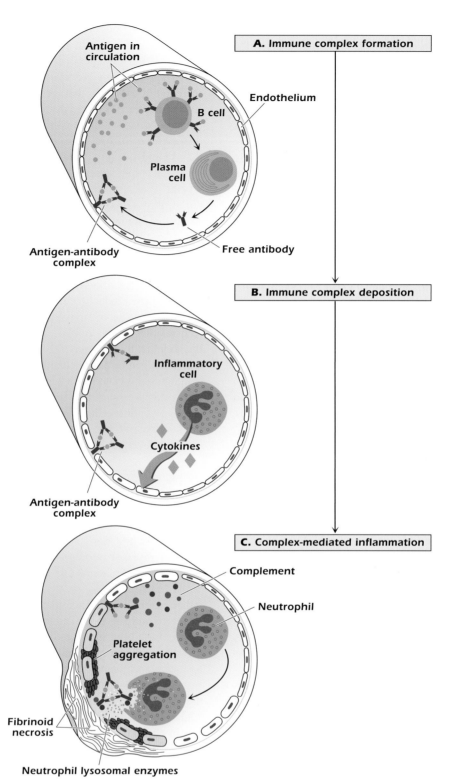

Figure 16.2. Schematic illustration of the three sequential phases in the induction of systemic type III (immune complex) hypersensitivity.

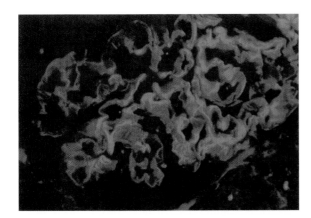

Figure 16.3. Ribbon-like deposit of antibody along the basement membrane revealed by fluorescent antibodies to human Ig. (Photograph by Dr. Angelo Ucci, Tufts University Medical School.)

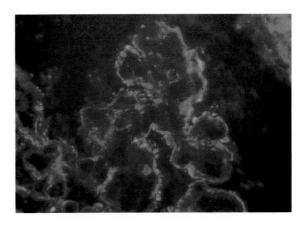

Figure 16.4. "Lumpy-bumpy" staining pattern of fluorescent antibody specific for human immunoglobulin: immune complex deposits in glomerular basement membrane. (Photograph by Dr. Angelo Ucci, Tufts University Medical School.)

patients are due to antibodies that bind directly to basement membrane in the lung and kidney, activate complement, and cause membrane damage as a consequence of accumulation of neutrophils and release of degradative enzymes. Goodpasture's syndrome is sometimes considered to be a type II hypersensitivity reaction, since it also involves an antibody-mediated cytotoxic effect on normal cells. The distinction between this infection-associated antibody-mediated disease and the immune complex disease of serum sickness is that microscopic examination of the lesions reveals a linear, ribbonlike deposit along the basement membrane (see Figure 16.3), as would be expected if an even carpet of antibody were bound to surface antigens. By contrast, in serum sickness the pileup of preformed immune complexes on the basement membrane leads to lumpy-bumpy deposits (Figure 16.4).

In a number of infectious diseases (malaria, leprosy, dengue) there may be times during the course of the infection when large amounts of antigen and antibody exist simultaneously and cause the formation of immune aggregates that are deposited in a variety of locations. Thus, the complex of symptoms in any of these diseases may include a component attributable to a type III hypersensitivity reaction.

Complement deficiency. As noted above, most immune complexes do not cause damage because they are removed from circulation before they become lodged in the tissues. Complexes that contain C3b bind to erythrocytes bearing CR1. The erythrocytes deliver the complexes to mononuclear phagocytes within the liver and spleen for removal by phagocytosis. The components of the classical complement pathway reduce the number of antigen epitopes that antibodies can bind to by intercalating into the lattice of the complex, resulting in smaller, soluble complexes. It is these small, soluble complexes that bind most readily to the erythrocytes. In patients with complement deficiencies affecting C1, C2, and C4 (see Chapters 14 and 17), the complexes remain large and bind poorly to the erythrocytes. These non-erythrocyte-bound complexes are taken up rapidly by the liver and then released to be deposited in tissues such as skin, kidney and muscle, where they can set up inflammatory reactions.

Localized Immune Complex Disease

In 1903, a French scientist named Arthus immunized rabbits with horse serum by repeated intradermal injection. After several weeks, he noted that each succeeding injection produced an increasingly severe reaction at the site of inoculation. At first, a mild erythema (redness) and edema (accumulation of fluid) were noticed within 24 hours of injection. These reactions subsided without consequence by the following day, but subsequent injections produced larger edematous responses, and by the fifth or sixth inoculations the lesions became hemorrhagic with necrosis and were slow to heal. This phenomenon, known as the ***Arthus reaction***, is the prototype of localized immune complex reactions. As with systemic immune complex hypersensitivity reactions, localized reactions involve soluble antigens. The local inflammatory responses generated occur following reactivity of antigen with already formed, antigen-specific IgG antibody. When such preformed antibodies come in contact with antigen at the appropriate concentrations (antibody excess), in or near vessel walls (venules), insoluble immune complexes form and accumulate as they would on a gel-diffusion plate (see Chapter 6). The subsequent pathophysiologic events are very similar to those described in the systemic pattern (see Figure 16.2). The end result is rupture of the vessel wall and hemorrhage, accompanied by necrosis of local tissue (Figures 16.5A, 16.5B).

A

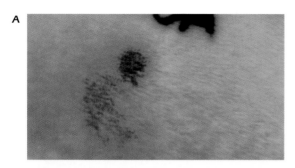

B

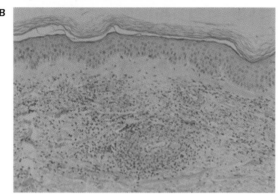

Figure 16.5. Type III hypersensitivity Arthus reaction. (A) Gross appearance, showing hemorrhagic appearance (purpura). (B) Histologic features of Arthus reaction showing neutrophil infiltrate. (Photograph by Dr. M. Stadecker, Tufts University Medical School.)

A clinical example of Arthus-type hypersensitivity reactions is seen in a disease called **Farmer's lung**. This is an intrapulmonary type III hypersensitivity reaction that occurs in patients with **extrinsic allergic alveolitis**. As its name implies, the disease sometimes occurs individuals involved in farming; thus it is classified as an occupational disease. In sensitive individuals, exposure to moldy hay leads to severe respiratory distress or pneumonitis within 6–8 hours. It has been shown that affected individuals have made large amounts of IgG antibody specific for the spores of thermophilic actinomycetes that grow on spoiled hay. Inhalation of the bacterial spores leads to a reaction in the lungs that resembles the Arthus reaction seen in skin, namely, the formation of antigen–antibody aggregates and consequent inflammation.

There are many similar pulmonary type III reactions that bear names related to the occupation or causative agent, such as pigeon breeder's disease, cheese washer's disease, bagassosis (bagasse refers to sugarcane fiber), maple bark stripper's disease, paprika worker's disease, and the increasingly rare thatched roof worker's lung. Dirty work environments, involving massive exposure to potentially antigenic material, obviously lend themselves to the development of this form of occupational disease.

SUMMARY

1. Type II hypersensitivity reactions involve damage to target cells and are mediated by antibody through three major pathways. In the first pathway, antibody (usually IgM, but also IgG) activates the entire complement sequence and causes cell lysis.

2. In the second type II hypersensitivity pathway, antibody (usually IgG) serves to engage Fc receptors on phagocytic cells, and C3b engages C3b receptors on phagocytic cells, causing destruction of the antibody and/or C3b-coated target through ADCC. These reactions usually involve circulating blood cells, such as red blood cells, white blood cells, and platelets, and the consequences are those that would be expected from destruction of the particular type of cell.

3. The third type II hypersensitivity pathway leads to dysfunctional cellular consequences caused by the binding of disease-causing antagonistic or agonistic autoantibodies to cell surface receptors (e.g., myasthenia gravis or Graves' disease, respectively).

4. Type III hypersensitivity reactions involve the formation of antigen–antibody immune complexes that can activate the complement cascade and induce acute inflammatory responses. Release of certain products of complement (C3a and C5a) causes a local increase in vessel permeability and permits the release of serum (edema) and the chemotactic attraction of neutrophils. The neutrophils, in the process of ingesting the immune complexes, release degradative lysosomal enzymes that produce the tissue damage characteristic of these reactions.

5. If the site of a type III reaction is a blood vessel wall, the outcome is hemorrhage and necrosis; if the site is a glomerular basement membrane, loss of integrity and release of protein and red blood cells into the urine results; and if the site is a joint meniscus, destruction of synovial membranes and cartilage occurs.

6. Multiple forms of type III hypersensitivity reactions exist, ranging from localized to systemic reactions. The reactions manifested depend on the type and location of antigen and the way in which it is brought together with antibody. In all cases, however, the outcome depends on complement and granulocytes as mediators of tissue injury.

REFERENCES AND BIBLIOGRAPHY

Carlson JA, Chen KR. (2006) Cutaneous vasculitis update: small vessel neutrophilic vasculitis syndromes. *Am J Dermatopathol* 28: 486.

Chang S, Carr W. (2007) Urticarial vasculitis. *Allergy Asthma Proc* 28(1): 97.

Cuellar ML. (2002) Drug-induced vasculitis. *Curr Rheumatol Rep* 4: 55.

Dixon FJ, Cochrane CC, Theofilopoulus AN. (1988) Immune complex injury. In: Samter M, Talmage DW, Frank MM,

Austen KF, Claman HN (eds). *Immunological Diseases, 4th Ed.* Boston: Little, Brown.

Gorgani NN, Theofilopoulos AN. (2007) Contribution of histidine-rich glycoprotein in clearance of immune complexes and apoptotic cells: implications for ameliorating autoimmune diseases. *Autoimmunity* 40: 260.

Nimmerjahn F, Ravetch JV. (2006) Fc gamma receptors: old friends and new family members. *Immunity* 24: 19.

REVIEW QUESTIONS

For each question, choose the ONE BEST answer or completion.

1. Graves' disease is an example of type II hypersensitivity whose pathophysiology is best explained by:
   A) disease-causing antagonistic autoantibodies to cell surface receptors
   B) disease-causing agonistic autoantibodies to cell surface receptors
   C) disease-causing autoantibodies to nuclear antigens
   D) disease-causing autoantibodies to acetylcholine receptors

2. Which of the following is most likely to involve a reaction to a hapten as its etiologic cause?
   A) Goodpasture's syndrome following a viral respiratory infection
   B) hemolytic anemia following treatment with penicillin
   C) rheumatoid arthritis following a parasitic infection
   D) farmer's lung following exposure to moldy hay

3. In an experimental mouse model for the study of autoimmune hemolytic anemia, intravenous administration of a monoclonal IgA antibody specific for a red blood cell antigen did not cause anemia to occur. The best explanation for this observation is that:
   A) the IgA would localize in the gastrointestinal tract
   B) the Fc region of the IgA antibody does not bind receptors for Fc receptors on phagocytic cells
   C) IgA cannot activate complement beyond the splitting of C2
   D) the IgA used has a low affinity for the red blood cell antigen
   E) the IgA used requires secretory component to work

4. The glomerular lesions in immune complex disease can be visualized microscopically with a fluorescent antibody against:
   A) IgG heavy chains
   B) κ light chains
   C) C1
   D) C3
   E) all of the above

5. Immune complexes are involved in the pathogenesis of which of the following rheumatic fever-associated diseases:
   A) poststreptococcal glomerulonephritis
   B) pigeon breeder's disease
   C) serum sickness
   D) autoimmune hemolytic anemia

6. The final damage to vessels in immune complex-mediated arthritis is due to
   A) cytokines produced by T cells
   B) histamine and SRS-A
   C) the C5, C6, C7, C8, C9 membrane attack complex
   D) lysosomal enzymes of polymorphonuclear leukocytes
   E) cytotoxic T cells

7. Serum sickness is characterized by
   A) deposition of immune complexes in blood vessel walls when there is a moderate excess of antigen
   B) phagocytosis of complexes by granulocytes
   C) consumption of complement
   D) appearance of symptoms before free antibody can be detected in the circulation
   E) all of the above

8. Type II hypersensitivity
   A) is antibody-independent
   B) is complement-independent
   C) is mediated by CD8$^+$ T cells
   D) requires immune complex formation
   E) involves antibody-mediated destruction of cells

9. A patient is suspected of having farmer's lung. A provocation test involving the inhalation of an extract of moldy hay is performed. A sharp drop in respiratory function is

noted within 10 minutes and returns to normal in 2 hours, only to fall again in another 2 hours. The most likely explanation is that

A) the patient has existing T cell-mediated hypersensitivity

B) this is a normal pattern for farmer's lung

C) the patient developed a secondary response after the inhalation of antigen

D) the symptoms of farmer's lung are complicated by an IgE-mediated reactivity to the same antigen

E) all of the above

ANSWERS TO REVIEW QUESTIONS

1. *A.* In Graves disease, agonistic autoantibodies (as opposed to choice **B**, antagonistic autoantibodies) directed against thyroid-stimulating hormone receptors on thyroid epithelial cells stimulate the cells, resulting in hyperthyroidism. These antibodies are not generated in response to nuclear antigens or acetylcholine receptors. Therefore, choices **C** and **D**, respectively, are incorrect.

2. *B.* Penicillin can function as a hapten, binding to red blood cells and inducing a hemolytic anemia. **A**, **C**, and **D** are examples of immune aggregate (type III) reactions requiring complement and neutrophils for pathologic effects.

3. *B.* Since phagocytic cells have Fc receptors for IgG and not IgA, bound IgA would not cause engulfment and damage. Thus, **A**, **C**, **D**, and **E** are false.

4. *E.* The lesions in immune complex disease are dependent on the presence of antigen, antibody, and complement. Hence all can be demonstrated by immunofluorescence at a lesion: **A** and **B**, because they are parts of IgG; **C** and **D**, because they are the early components of complement activated by the immune aggregates.

5. *A.* Rheumatic fever is a disease associated with infections caused by group A streptococci. It involves the development of anti-streptococci antibodies that are cross-reactive with antigens present in human heart muscle, cartilage, and glomerular basement membrane.

6. *D.* Neither T cells nor mast cells are responsible for the final tissue damage in immune complex disease. Therefore **A**, **B**, and **E** are eliminated. The final lytic complex of complement is similarly not involved, since complement activation up to C5 is sufficient to bring in the polymorphonuclear leukocytes, whose lysosomal enzymes cause the tissue damage.

7. *E.* All are characteristics of serum sickness.

8. *E.* Type II hypersensitivity reactions occur following development of antibodies against target antigens expressed on normal cells or cells with altered membrane determinants. Antibodies bind to the surface of these cells and mediate damage or destruction by one or more mechanisms, including complement-mediated reactions. CD8$^+$ cytotoxic T cells and immune complexes are not involved in these reactions.

9. *D.* Type III hypersensitivity reactions in farmer's lung and similar occupational diseases have an onset of symptoms that usually occur several hours after exposure to the causal antigen. The appearance of breathing difficulties within minutes would create a strong suspicion that a type I anaphylactic response is also present. Presumably the patient made both IgE and IgG antibodies to the actinomycete antigens. A positive wheal and flare reaction on skin testing would provide further confirmation.

17

HYPERSENSITIVITY: TYPE IV

INTRODUCTION

In contrast to antibody-mediated hypersensitivity reactions discussed in the previous two chapters, type IV hypersensitivity is T-cell mediated. In marked contrast with type I hypersensitivity mediated by IgE, which is immediately available to react with allergens, type IV responses involve the activation, proliferation, and mobilization of antigen-specific T cells. Thus, type IV hypersensitivity is delayed as compared with antibody-mediated hypersensitivity reactions, and it is often referred to as *delayed-type hypersensitivity* (DTH). Similar to the antibody-mediated hypersensitivity, DTH reactions can also result in damage to host cells and tissues. The harmful effects of DTH are initiated by the release of inappropriately large amounts of cytokines (including chemokines) by activated T cells. Chemokines attract and activate other mononuclear cells that are not antigen-specific, including monocytes and macrophages. The recruitment and activation of these antigen-nonspecific cells are mainly responsible for the eventual deleterious outcome of type IV hypersensitivity reactions.

DTH reactions are, therefore, cell-mediated immune responses. Depending on the antigen involved, they mediate beneficial (resistance to viruses, bacteria, fungi, and tumors) or harmful (allergic dermatitis, autoimmunity) aspects of immune function. Other antigens capable of eliciting DTH reactions include those expressed by foreign cells in transplantation settings or one of many chemicals (serving as haptens) capable of penetrating skin and coupling to body proteins that serve as carriers.

Cutaneous DTH reactions are initiated when CD4 memory T cells are activated by antigen-presenting cells in the skin (e.g., Langerhans cells). Upon activation, CD4$^+$ T cells release inflammatory mediators that recruit effector cells to the site of antigen administration. While the monocyte/macrophage is thought to be the major effector cell in this model, CD8$^+$ cytolytic T cells, and natural killer (NK) cells are also thought to serve as effector cells in DTH reactions. Activated effector cells mount an inflammatory response that results in the elimination of antigen and the extravasation of plasma accompanied by selling at the site of challenge. The magnitude of the response to the antigen is measured as an increase in swelling at the site of challenge (e.g., as seen during the development of a tuberculin skin reaction).

GENERAL CHARACTERISTICS AND PATHOPHYSIOLOGY OF DTH

The clinical features of type IV hypersensitivity reactions vary, depending on the sensitizing antigen and the route of antigen exposure. These variants include contact hypersensitivity, tuberculin-type hypersensitivity, and granulomatous hypersensitivity (see next section). In general, however, common pathophysiologic mechanisms account for each of these variants. The major events leading to these reactions involve the following three steps: (1) activation of antigen-specific inflammatory T_H1 and T_H17 cells in a previously sensitized individual; (2) elaboration of proinflammatory

Immunology: A Short Course, Seventh Edition. Richard Coico and Geoffrey Sunshine.
© 2015 John Wiley & Sons, Ltd. Published 2015 by John Wiley & Sons, Ltd.
Companion Website: www.wileyimmunology.com/coico

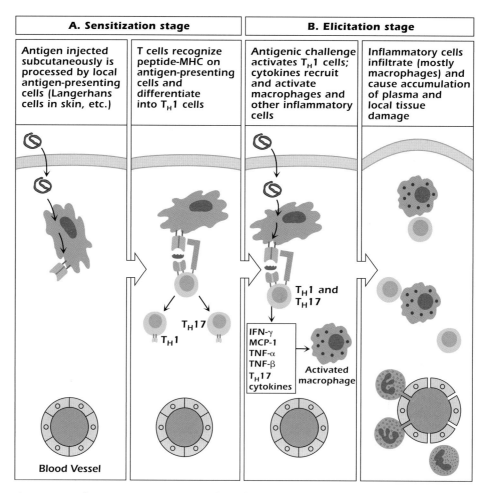

Figure 17.1. The DTH reaction. Stage of sensitization by antigen involves presentation of antigen to T cells by antigen-presenting cells, leading to the release of cytokines and differentiation of T_H0 T cells to T_H1 and T_H17 cells. Challenge with antigen involves antigen presentation to T_H1 cells by antigen-presenting cells, leading to T_H1 and T_H17 activation, release of cytokines, and recruitment and activation of macrophages.

cytokines by the antigen-specific T_H1 cells; and (3) recruitment and activation of antigen-nonspecific inflammatory leukocytes. These events typically occur over a period of several days (48–72 hours).

Mechanisms Involved in DTH

The mechanisms involved in the sensitization to DTH and the elucidation of the reaction following antigenic challenge are now well understood. It is important to underscore that, as with antibody-mediated hypersensitivity reactions, previous exposure to the antigen is required to generate DTH reactions. Such exposure (the *sensitization stage*) activates and expands the number of antigen-specific T_H1 and T_H17 cells that, when subsequently challenged with the same antigen, respond by producing cytokines that promote DTH reactions (the *elicitation stage*). During the elicitation phase, activated T_H1 and T_H17 cells mediate the activation and recruitment of innate immune cells (antigen-nonspecific

inflammatory cells) to the area of the reaction, including the activation and recruitment of macrophages and NK cells, and neutrophils. These stages are shown diagrammatically in Figure 17.1. The sensitization stage typically occurs over a 1–2 week period during which normal mechanisms of T-cell activation occur (see Chapter 10). In contrast, the elicitation stage requires approximately 18–48 hours from time of antigenic challenge to recruit and activate these cells, a period that culminates in the histological and clinical features of DTH. The clinical manifestations of DTH can last for several weeks or, in some cases, can be chronic (e.g., DTH occurring in certain autoimmune diseases).

The antigen-challenged T_H1 cells produce several cytokines during the elicitation stage, most notably chemokines and IFN-γ, which cause chemotaxis and activation of macrophages (Figure 17.2). The recruitment and activation of antigen-nonspecific cells by antigen-specific T_H1 cells demonstrate the interaction between acquired and innate immunity discussed in Chapter 2. Another cytokine

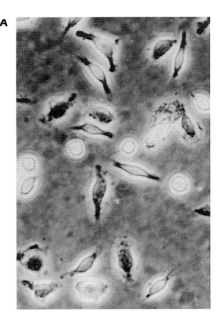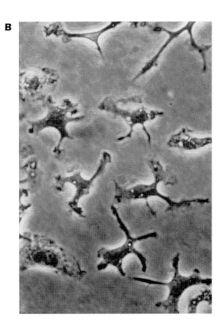

Figure 17.2. The effect of IFN-γ on peritoneal macrophages. (A) Normal macrophages in culture as they are just beginning to adhere. (B) Macrophages that after activation with IFN-γ have adhered, spread out with development of numerous pseudopodia, and grown larger. More lysosomal granules are also visible. (Photographs by Dr. M. Stadecker, Tufts University Medical School.)

TABLE 17.1. Cytokines Involved in DTH Reactions

Cytokine[a]	Functional Effects[b]
IFN-γ	Activates macrophages to release inflammatory mediators
Chemokines MCP-1 RANTES	Recruit macrophages and monocytes to the site
MIP-1α	Influences neutrophil influx and preferentially attracts CD8+ T cells into the DTH reaction site
MIP-1β	Preferentially attracts CD4+ T cells into the DTH reaction site
TNF-α	Causes local tissue damage
TNF-β	Increases expression of adhesion molecules on blood vessels

[a]MCP, membrane cofactor protein; MIP, macrophage inflammatory protein; TNF, tumor necrosis factor.
[b]Additional functional effects are described in Chapter 12.

produced by these cells is IL-12. IL-12 suppresses the T_H2 subpopulation and promotes the expansion of the T_H1 subpopulation thereby driving the response to produce more T_H1-synthesized cytokines that activate macrophages. Thus, IL-12 plays an important role in DTH. Table 17.1 summarizes the important cytokines involved in DTH reactions.

DTH reactions also involve CD8+ T cells, which are first activated and expanded during the sensitization stage of the response. These cells can damage tissues by cell-mediated cytotoxicity (see Chapter 11). Activation of CD8+ T cells occurs as a consequence of the ability of many lipid-soluble chemicals capable of inducing DTH reactions to cross the cell membrane (e.g., pentadecacatechol, which is the chemical that induces *poison ivy*). Within the cell, these chemicals react with cytosolic proteins to generate modified peptides that are translocated to the endoplasmic reticulum and then delivered to the cell surface in the context of MHC class I molecules. Cells presenting such modified self-proteins are subsequently damaged or killed by CD8+ T cells.

It should be apparent from the preceding discussion that many of the effector functions in DTH are performed by activated macrophages. In the most favorable circumstances, DTH results in destruction of an infectious organism (see below) that may have elicited the response in the first place. This destruction is believed to result predominantly from ingestion of the organism by **macrophages**, their activation by **IFN-γ**, followed by degradation by lysosomal enzymes, as well as by the by-products of the burst of respiratory activity, such as peroxide and superoxide radicals. Foreign tissues, tumor tissue, and soluble or conjugated antigens are dealt with in a similar manner.

EXAMPLES OF DTH

Contact Sensitivity

Contact sensitivity (sometimes called **contact dermatitis**) is a form of DTH in which the target organ is the skin, and the

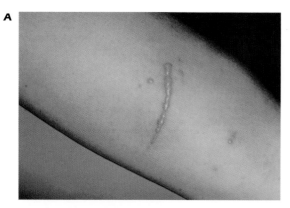

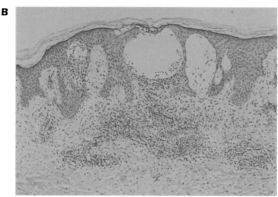

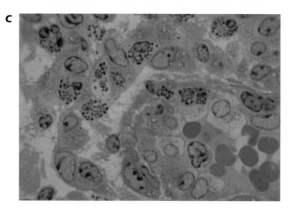

Figure 17.3. (A) Type IV contact sensitivity reaction: gross appearance of reaction to poison ivy. (B) Type IV contact hypersensitivity reaction: histologic appearance showing intraepithelial blister formation and mononuclear infiltrate in the dermis. (C) Cutaneous basophil reaction showing basophils and some mononuclear cells 24 hours after skin test. (Photographs by Dr. M. Stadecker, Tufts University Medical School.)

inflammatory response is produced as the result of contact with sensitizing substances on the surface of the skin. Thus, it is primarily an epidermal reaction characterized by *eczema* at the site of contact with the allergen that typically peaks 48–72 hours after contact. The prototype for this form of DTH is *poison ivy dermatitis* (Figure 17.3A). The offending substance is contained in an oil secreted by the leaves of the

poison-ivy vine and other related plants. These oils contain a mixture of catechols (dihydroxyphenols) with long hydrocarbon side chains. These features allow it to penetrate the skin by virtue of its lipophilicity (which gives it the ability to dissolve in skin oils) and its ability to couple covalently (by formation of quinones) to some carrier molecules on cell surfaces. Other contact sensitizers are generally also lipid-soluble haptens. They have a variety of chemical forms, but all have in common the ability to penetrate skin and form hapten-carrier conjugates. Chemicals such as 2,4-dinitrochlorobenzene (DNCB) are used to induce contact sensitivity. Since virtually every normal individual is capable of developing contact hypersensitivity to a test dose of this compound, it is frequently used to assess a patients potential for T-cell reactivity (cell-mediated immunity). Various metals, such as nickel and chromium, which are present in jewelry and clasps of undergarments, are also capable of inducing contact sensitivity, presumably by way of chelation (ionic interaction) by skin proteins.

Contact sensitivity is initiated by presentation of the offending allergen by antigen-presenting cells in the skin (*Langerhans cells*) to T cells expressing antigen-specific T-cell receptors (TCRs). It is not yet resolved whether the sensitizer couples directly to components on the cell surface of the Langerhans cell or whether it couples first to proteins in serum or tissue that are then taken up by the Langerhans cells. The initial contact results in expansion of antigen-specific clones of T_H1 cells. Subsequent contact (challenge) with the sensitizing antigen triggers the elicitation stage of DTH discussed earlier. The histologic appearance of this variant of DTH shows intraepithelial *blister formation* and mononuclear infiltrates in the dermis (Figure 17.3B) that manifests as the separation of epidermal cells, spongiosis (an inflammatory intercellular edema of the epidermis), and blister formation (Figure 17.3A).

In many cases, enough of the sensitizing antigen remains at the site of the initial contact so that in approximately 1 week, when sufficient T-cell expansion has taken place, the antigen that persists serves as the challenging antigen and a reaction in this area will flare up. Therefore, the elicitation phase can occur without new contact with the sensitizing antigen.

The commonly performed procedure for testing for the presence of contact sensitivity is the patch test in which a solution of the suspected antigen is spread on the skin and covered by an occlusive dressing. The appearance, within 3 days, of an area of *induration* and *erythema*, indicates sensitivity.

Granulomatous Hypersensitivity

Unlike DTH associated with most contact dermatitis reactions where the antigen is readily disposed of, the lesion resolves slowly, and little tissue damage is seen. In some circumstances, the antigen may be persistent serving as a chronic source of immune stimulation. For example, a significant and persistent parasite of humans named *Schistosoma mansoni* produces schistosome eggs that induce granulomatous hypersensitivity. Another pathogen responsible for this form of hypersensitivity is lipid-encapsulated mycobacteria that are resistant to enzymatic degradation and therefore can be present for prolonged periods of time (lifelong, in some cases). Under these circumstances, continuous accumulation of macrophages leads to clusters of epithelioid cells, which fuse to form giant cells in **granulomas**. The maximal reaction time for the development of a granuloma is 21–28 days. The pathological changes result from the inability of macrophages to destroy phagocytized pathogens (e.g., *Mycobacterium leprae*) or to degrade large inert antigens. Granulomas can be destructive because of their displacement of normal tissue and can result in caseous (cheesy) necrosis. This is typical in such diseases as tuberculosis caused by infections with *Mycobacterium tuberculosis*, where a cuff of lymphocytes surrounds the core and there may be considerable fibrosis.

The disease process may then be attributable not so much to the effects of the invading organisms as to the persistent attempts of the host to isolate and contain the parasite by the mechanisms of DTH. In diseases such as smallpox, measles, and herpes, the characteristic exanthems (skin rashes) seen are partly attributable to DTH responses to the virus, with additional destruction attributable to the attack by cytotoxic CD8$^+$ T cells on the virally infected epithelial cells.

Tuberculin-Type Hypersensitivity

Tuberculin-type reactions are **cutaneous inflammatory reactions** characterized by an area of firm red swelling of the skin that is maximal at 48–72 hours after challenge. The term **tuberculin-type** derives from the prototype DTH reaction in which a lipoprotein antigen isolated from *Mycobacterium tuberculosis* called *tuberculin* was used to test for evidence of exposure to the causative agent of tuberculosis (TB). It is important to note, however, that soluble antigens from other organisms, including *Mycobacterium leprae* and *Leishmania tropica*, as well as many others induce similar tuberculin-type DTH reactions. Today, TB tests are performed by intradermally injecting a more purified lipoprotein extract isolated from *M. tuberculosis* called **purified protein derivative** (PPD). The PPD test (also called the Mantoux test) is extremely useful for public health surveillance of TB. If an individual has been previously sensitized to antigens expressed by *M. tuberculosis* as a consequence of infection with this organism, the characteristic tuberculin-type lesion will appear at the site of injection within 48–72 hours. Evidence of **erythema** (redness) and **induration** (raised thickening) appear, reaching maximal levels 72 hours after the challenge (see Figure 17.4A). The induration can easily be distinguished from edema (fluid) by absence

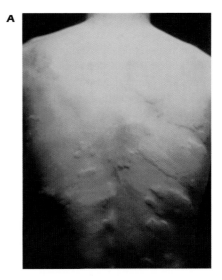

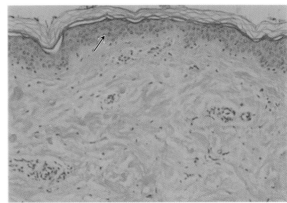

Figure 17.4. (A) Type IV DTH reaction (tuberculin reaction): gross appearance showing induration and erythema 48 hours after tuberculin test. (Photograph by A. Gottlieb, Tulane University Medical School.) (B) Type IV DTH reaction: histologic picture showing dermal mononuclear cell infiltrate (arrow). (Photograph by Dr. M. Stadecker, Tufts University Medical School.)

of pitting when pressure is applied. These reactions, even when severe, rarely lead to necrotic damage and resolve slowly. A biopsy taken early in the reaction reveals primarily mononuclear cells of the monocyte/macrophage series with a few scattered lymphocytes. Characteristically, the mononuclear infiltrates appear as a perivascular cuff before extensively invading the site of deposition of antigen (see Figure 17.4B). Neutrophils are not a prominent feature of the initial reaction. In more severe cases, tuberculin-type hypersensitivity reactions may progress toward granulomatous hypersensitivity (discussed above). Biopsies of tissue where this is evident show a more complex pattern, with the arrival of B cells and the formation of granulomas in persistent lesions. The hardness or induration is attributable to the deposition of fibrin in the lesion.

While the PPD test is usually very reliable, false-negative or false-positive reactions may be seen in some situations. Immunosuppressed individuals (e.g., those infected with human immunodeficiency virus, some individuals on high-dose chemotherapy) may have false-negative PPD reactions due to the inability of antigen-specific T cells to respond (anergy; see Chapter 13).

By contrast, when PPD is used to test individuals to determine whether they have been previously exposed to *M. tuberculosis*, individuals who have been vaccinated with a nonpathogenic attenuated strain of the organism that causes TB in cattle, namely *Mycobacterium bovis* bacillus Calmette–Guerin (BCG), generate false-positive reactions. The efficacy of the BCG vaccine against human pulmonary TB varies enormously in different populations. The prevailing hypothesis attributes this variation to interactions between the vaccine and the mycobacteria common in the environment, but the precise mechanism has not yet been clarified. Routine BCG vaccination is not performed in many countries, including the United States, because of its questionable efficacy and the impact such a practice would have on our ability to confirm whether individuals have been exposed to *M. tuberculosis*.

More recently, a T-cell–based assay for interferon gamma, the enzyme-linked immunosorbent spot test (ELISPOT), has become a commonly used test for the diagnosis of *Mycobacterium tuberculosis* (MTB) infection. It is also used in lieu of the PPD test to determine whether the patient has been previously exposed to *M. tuberculosis*. The test is based on measurement of IFN-γ responses by MTB-sensitized T cells using peripheral blood as testing samples. A cocktail of three mycobacterial proteins stimulate the patient's T cells *in vitro* to release IFN-γ, which is then measured using ELISA technology (see Chapter 6). The test detects infections produced by the *M. tuberculosis* complex (including *M. tuberculosis*, *M. bovis*, and *M. africanum* infections). BCG strains and the majority of other nontuberculosis mycobacteria do not contain any of the three mycobacterial proteins used in the test; thus, patients either vaccinated with BCG or infected with most environmental mycobacteria generally test negative.

Allograft Rejection

As we shall discuss in more detail in Chapter 19, if an individual receives grafts of cells, tissues, or organs taken from an allogeneic donor (a genetically different individual of the same species), it will usually become vascularized and initially be accepted. However, if the genetic differences are within the major histocompatibility complex (MHC), T-cell-mediated rejection of the graft ensues, whose duration and intensity is related to the degree of incompatibility between donor and recipient. After vascularization, there is an initial invasion of the graft by a mixed population of antigen-specific T cells and antigen-nonspecific monocytes through the blood vessel walls. This inflammatory reaction soon leads to destruction of the vessels; this deprivation of nutrients is quickly followed by necrosis and breakdown of the grafted tissue.

Additional Examples of DTH

An unusual form of DTH has been observed in humans following repeated intradermal injections of antigen. The response is delayed in onset (usually by about 24 hours) but consists entirely of erythema, without the induration typical of classic delayed-hypersensitivity reactions. When this condition was studied experimentally, it was found that the erythema was attended by a cellular infiltrate, but that the predominant cell type was the basophil (Figure 17.4C). Studies in guinea pigs showed that the response was primarily mediated by T cells and was subject to the same MHC restrictions as classic T-cell–mediated responses. When classic delayed hypersensitivity was present, however, infiltrates of basophils were not seen. Thus, cutaneous basophil hypersensitivity seemed to be a variant of T-cell–mediated responses, but its exact mechanism was unknown. The picture was complicated still further when it was shown that passive transfer of serum could, under some circumstances, evoke a basophil response.

The physiologic significance of cutaneous basophil hypersensitivity remained a mystery until it was shown that guinea pigs bitten by certain ticks had severe cutaneous basophil hypersensitivity reactions at the site of attachment of the tick. The infiltration of basophils and, presumably, the release of inflammatory mediators from their granules resulted in death of the tick and its eventual detachment. Thus, cutaneous basophil hypersensitivity may have an important role in certain forms of immunity to parasites. More recently, basophil infiltrates have also been found in cases of contact dermatitis with allergens such as poison ivy, in cases of rejection of renal grafts, and in some forms of conjunctivitis. These observations indicate that basophils may also play a role in some types of delayed hypersensitivity disease.

Other examples of DTH include reactions to self-antigens in certain autoimmune diseases (see chapter 13). As with persistent infections that can cause chronic DTH reactions, these reactions are often chronic resulting from the continuous clonal activation of autoreactive T_H1 cells. Examples of autoimmune diseases in which DTH reactions are involved include rheumatoid arthritis, type I diabetes, and multiple sclerosis.

TREATMENT OF DTH

Therapies to treat T-cell–mediated hypersensitivity vary in accordance with the variant of DTH. In most cases, DTH reactions such as contact dermatitis and tuberculin-type reactions, resolve after a period of days to weeks following removal of the antigen. Corticosteroids, applied either topically or systemically, constitute a very effective treatment for these forms of DTH. In more severe variants of DTH, such as pathogen-induced granulomatous hypersensitivity, allograft rejection, and those seen in certain autoimmune diseases, more aggressive forms of immunosuppressive therapy are commonly used including treatment with drugs such as cyclosporine or topical calcineurin inhibitors (e.g., tacrolimus) (see Chapter 19 for additional discussion of immunosuppressive therapies).

SUMMARY

1. The normal events associated with cell-mediated immunity that are crucial for protection against intracellular parasites, such as viruses and many bacteria, and fungi can also cause DTH reactions.

2. The major events leading to DTH reactions involve: (a) activation of antigen-specific inflammatory T_H1 and T_H17 cells in a previously sensitized individual; (b) elaboration of proinflammatory cytokines (IFN-γ, T_H17 family cytokines) by the antigen-specific T_H1/T_H17 cells, respectively; and, (c) recruitment and activation of antigen-nonspecific inflammatory leukocytes.

3. There are several varieties of DTH including (a) contact hypersensitivity: characterized by eczema which peaks 48–72 hours after allergen contact; (b) granulomatous hypersensitivity: characterized by a granuloma that is maximal 21–28 days after antigen is introduced; and, (c) tuberculin-type hypersensitivity: characterized by an area of firm red erythema (redness) and induration (raised thickening) that is maximal 48–72 hours after challenge. Other variants include reactions occurring in certain T-cell–mediated autoimmune diseases and in some individuals who have received allografts.

4. Cytotoxic CD8$^+$ T cells can also participate in the damage associated with DTH reactions.

5. Phagocytic macrophages are the major histologic feature of DTH and account for the protective outcome of this form of hypersensitivity when pathogens are involved.

6. In situations where macrophages are unable to destroy the pathogen, a granuloma is induced (granulomatous hypersensitivity). Granulomas can also develop following phagocytosis of inert substances. Granulomas are characterized histologically by the presence of macrophages, epithelioid cells, giant cells, and CD4 and CD8 lymphocytes.

REFERENCES AND BIBLIOGRAPHY

Brandt L, Feino CJ, Weinreich OA, Chilima B, Hirsch P, Appelberg R, Andersen P. (2002) Failure of the Mycobacterium bovis BCG vaccine: some species of environmental mycobacteria block multiplication of BCG and induction of protective immunity to tuberculosis. *Infect Immun* 70: 672.

Burger D, Dayer JM. (2002) Cytokines, acute-phase proteins, and hormones: IL-1 and TNF-alpha production in contact-mediated activation of monocytes by T lymphocytes. *Ann N Y Acad Sci* 966: 464.

Chawla H, Lobato MN, Sosa LE, ZuWallack R. (2012) Predictors for a positive QuantiFERON-TB-Gold test in BCG-vaccinated adults with a positive tuberculin skin test. *J Infect Public Health* 5(6): 369.

Fyhrquist-Vanni N, Alenius H, Lauerma A. (2007) Contact dermatitis. *Dermatol Clin* 25: 613.

Posadas SJ, Pichler WJ. (2007) Delayed drug hypersensitivity reactions—new concepts. *Clin Exp Allergy* 37: 989.

Romano A, Demoly P. (2007) Recent advances in the diagnosis of drug allergy. *Curr Opin Allergy Clin Immunol* 7: 299.

Sicherer SH, Leung DY. (2007): Advances in allergic skin disease, anaphylaxis, and hypersensitivity reactions to foods, drugs, and insects. *J Allergy Clin Immunol* 119: 1462.

Vukmanovic-Stejic M, Reed JR, Lacy KE, Rustin MH, Akbar AN. (2006) Mantoux Test as a model for a secondary immune response in humans. *Immunol Lett* 107: 93.

Wollina U. (2007) The role of topical calcineurin inhibitors for skin diseases other than atopic dermatitis. *Am J Clin Dermatol* 8: 157.

REVIEW QUESTIONS

For each question, choose the ONE BEST answer or completion.

1. Which of the following does not involve cell-mediated immunity?
   A) contact sensitivity to lipstick
   B) rejection of an allograft
   C) serum sickness
   D) the Mantoux test
   E) immunity to chicken pox

2. A positive delayed-type hypersensitivity skin reaction involves the interaction of
   A) antigen, complement, and cytokines
   B) antigen, antigen-sensitive T cells, and macrophages
   C) antigen–antibody complexes, complement, and neutrophils
   D) IgE antibody, antigen, and mast cells
   E) antigen, macrophages, and complement

3. Delayed skin reactions to an intradermal injection of antigen may be markedly decreased by
   A) exposure to a high dose of X-irradiation
   B) treatment with antihistamines
   C) treatment with an antineutrophil serum
   D) removal of the spleen
   E) decreasing levels of complement

4. Which of the following statements is characteristic of contact sensitivity?
   A) The best therapy is oral administration of the antigen.
   B) Patch testing with the allergen is useless for diagnosis.
   C) Sensitization can be passively transferred with serum from an allergic individual.

D) Some chemicals acting as haptens induce sensitivity by covalently binding to host proteins acting as carriers.
E) Antihistamines constitute the treatment of choice.

5. Positive skin tests for delayed-type hypersensitivity to intradermally injected antigens indicate that
   A) a humoral immune response has occurred
   B) a cell-mediated immune response has occurred
   C) both T-cell and B-cell systems are functional
   D) the individual has previously made IgE responses to the antigen
   E) immune complexes have been formed at the injection site

6. T-cell–mediated immune responses can result in
   A) formation of granulomas
   B) induration at the reaction site
   C) rejection of a heart transplant
   D) eczema of the skin in the area of prolonged contact with a rubberized undergarment
   E) all of the above

7. Which one of the following statements about the PPD skin test is true?
   A) It is specific for *Mycobacterium tuberculosis*.
   B) It can be positive in an individual who was previously immunized with BCG.
   C) It does not distinguish a present or past infection of tuberculosis.
   D) It can vary in the extent of induration so that a positive test depends upon the underlying immune status of the patient tested.
   E) B, C and D are all true.

ANSWERS TO REVIEW QUESTIONS

1. *C.* Serum sickness is an example of those reactions mediated by an antibody–antigen complex that involves components of the complement system and neutrophils. All others involve cell-mediated immunity to a significant extent.

2. *B.* Cell-mediated reactions result from the triggering of T cells by antigen with recruitment of macrophages. Antibody, complement, and mast cells do not play roles in this process, although they do play a role in immediate hypersensitivity responses.

3. *A.* High doses of X-irradiation will destroy T cells, which are responsible for initiating the response. Histamine, neutrophils, the spleen, and complement do not play a role, and any treatment that affects them would not affect a DTH response.

4. *D.* Patch testing consists of application of the offending allergen under an occlusive dressing, and a positive DTH response after 24–48 hours is considered evidence of sensitivity; thus **B** is wrong. The allergens involved are those capable of penetrating skin and binding to host carrier proteins; thus **D** is correct. Oral ingestion of antigen, which, in certain experimental situations, was shown to induce suppression after subsequent induction of contact sensitivity, has not yet been shown to be an effective therapeutic maneuver in humans; thus **A** is wrong. Corticosteroids, not antihistamines, constitute the treatment of choice for contact sensitivity; thus **E** is also incorrect. Passive transfer of cell-mediated immune responses is accomplished with T cells, not with serum, thus **C** is wrong.

5. *B.* A delayed-type hypersensitivity reaction, evidenced by erythema and induration within 24–72 hours of antigen injection, indicates that a cell-mediated reaction has occurred. Such reactions do not involve antibody produced by B cells, thus **A**, **C**, **D**, and **E** are incorrect.

6. *E.* All of these effects are manifestations of cell-mediated immunity. Induration usually takes place at the reaction site. Formation of granulomas is characteristic of a chronic DTH reaction.

Rejection of the heart is an example of an allograft response. Some of the chemicals used to cure rubber can induce contact sensitivity after prolonged exposure of the skin to them.

7. *E.* Each of the statements except for statement **A** are true. Positive PPD tests occur in immunocompetent individuals who have been infected with *M. tuberculosis*. However, positive reactions to PPD tests will also occur in individuals previously vaccinated with *Mycobacterium bovis* bacillus Calmette–Guerin (BCG).

18

IMMUNODEFICIENCY DISORDERS AND NEOPLASIAS OF THE LYMPHOID SYSTEM

Susan R.S. Gottesman

INTRODUCTION

At first glance, the connection between immunodeficiency syndromes and neoplasias of the lymphoid system is not apparent: Immunodeficiency syndromes are characterized by *absences* or deficiencies, whereas neoplasia reflects *excesses* or uncontrolled proliferations. So why are they discussed in the same chapter? The relationship between these two types of immune system disorders demonstrates the fine tuning and integration of the elements of the immune system. Deficiencies, particularly in a single arm of the immune system, affect the ability of the remaining elements to control their growth. For this reason, immunodeficiencies are fertile ground for the development of neoplasia. Because autoimmune phenomena are further manifestations of the loss of immune regulation that frequently accompanies immunodeficiency, three seemingly disparate disease states—immunodeficiency, autoimmunity, and lymphoid neoplasia—often coexist in a single individual. Primary autoimmune diseases were discussed in Chapter 13; autoimmune reactions resulting from immunodeficiency or leading to lymphoid malignancy will be highlighted throughout this chapter.

As you have learned in previous chapters, the immune response is mediated by T and B lymphocytes, natural killer (NK) cells, myeloid/monocytic lineage cells, dendritic cells, and complement. The interactions among these cells, their soluble mediators (antibodies and cytokines), and complement are tightly controlled. Disorders in the development and differentiation of the cells, synthesis of their products, or interactions among them may lead to immune deficiencies with clinical manifestations ranging from mild to fatal in severity. However, clinical consequences of deficiencies in which the immune system shows redundancy (overlap in the functions of one component with another) are noticeably absent. For example, parts of the cytokine network normally exhibit redundancy and rarely come to medical attention.

Although inborn immunodeficiency diseases (conditions present at birth) are generally rare, early descriptions of these "experiments of nature" shed light on the functioning of the immune system. Animal models that mimicked different types of human immunodeficiencies illuminated the cellular subdivisions of adaptive immunity into T and B lymphocytes—that is, cell mediated versus humoral immunity. In addition, elucidation of the genetic basis of multiorgan autoimmune syndromes (e.g., mutations or deficiencies in molecules expressed predominantly in the thymus), has led to a better understanding of immune regulation and central tolerance.

Today, information gained from analyzing these rare immunodeficiency syndromes and lymphoid neoplasms at the molecular level is applied to their treatment and to the development of immunotherapies for autoimmune diseases and lymphoid and nonlymphoid malignancies. The chapter begins with descriptions of inborn and acquired immunodeficiency syndromes and concludes with neoplasias of the immune system.

Immunology: A Short Course, Seventh Edition. Richard Coico and Geoffrey Sunshine.
© 2015 John Wiley & Sons, Ltd. Published 2015 by John Wiley & Sons, Ltd.
Companion Website: www.wileyimmunology.com/coico

IMMUNODEFICIENCY SYNDROMES

Immunodeficiencies are divided into two major categories: *primary immunodeficiencies*, which may be hereditary or acquired, in which the deficiency is the cause of disease; and *secondary immunodeficiencies*, in which the immune deficiency is a result of other diseases or conditions.

We will first concentrate on those primary immunodeficiencies whose manifestations result in an increase in susceptibility to infection. These can be categorized on the basis of clinical presentation or on the basis of the arm of the immune system that is malfunctioning. These two classification schemes roughly correspond to each other and divide as follows: (1) T- or cell-mediated immunity; (2) B- or humoral (antibody-mediated) immunity; (3) both B- and T-cell immunity; (4) innate immunity mediated by phagocytic cells and/or NK cells; and (5) complement activation. Abnormalities of cytokines, chemokines, and their receptors do not form a separate category but are incorporated into groups 1–4 since they are the means by which these cells communicate and function.

An expressed immune response is often the result of interactions among several cell types; for example, a deficiency of antibody production and B-cell function may actually be caused by an underlying problem in T cells or in the T–B-cell interaction. Classification based on the apparent *expressed* defect, rather than its underlying cause (which may be unknown), is a useful framework for diagnosing new patients. This method of classification also allows correlation with animal models in which the fundamental immune defect may be more readily identified.

Immunodeficiency should always be suspected in a patient with recurrent infections. As shown in Table 18.1, the types of infections can often facilitate diagnosis of the underlying problem. For example, recurrent bacterial otitis media (ear infection) and bacterial pneumonia are common in individuals with B-cell and antibody deficiencies. Increased susceptibility to fungal, protozoal, and viral infections is seen with T-cell and cell-mediated immunodeficiencies. Systemic infections with bacteria that are normally of low virulence, superficial skin infections, or infections with pyogenic (pus-producing) organisms suggest deficiencies in phagocytic cells. Recurrent infections with pyogenic microorganisms are associated with complement deficiencies. Of particular significance is the occurrence of opportunistic infections, diseases caused by microorganisms present in the environment that are nonpathogenic in immunocompetent individuals. *Pneumocystis jiroveci* (*P. jiroveci*), cytomegalovirus (CMV), *Toxoplasma gondii*, *Mycobacterium avium*, and *Candida* are among the most common culprits causing opportunistic infections in patients with deficiencies in cell-mediated immunity.

The timing of infections is also a hint to the underlying diagnosis. Infants are protected for the first 6 months to 1 year of life by maternal antibodies transferred through the placenta and breast milk. Therefore deficiencies in humoral immunity exclusively are manifest beginning at approximately 6 months to 1 year of age. In contrast, defects in T-cell–mediated immunity or combined defects in T- and B-cell function often present from birth as failure to thrive.

TABLE 18.1. Major Clinical Manifestations of Immune Disorders

Disorder	Associated Diseases
Deficiency	
B-lymphocyte deficiency: deficiency in humoral or antibody-mediated immunity	Recurrent bacterial infections such as otitis media and recurrent pneumonia
T-lymphocyte deficiency: deficiency in cell-mediated immunity	Increased susceptibility to viral, fungal, and protozoal infections
T- and B-lymphocyte deficiency: combined deficiency of antibody and cell-mediated immunity	Acute and chronic infections with viral, bacterial, fungal, and protozoal organisms
Phagocytic cell deficiency	Systemic infections with bacteria of usually low virulence; infections with pyogenic bacteria; impaired pus formation and wound healing
NK cell deficiency	Viral infections, associated with several T-cell disorders and X-linked lymphoproliferative syndromes
Complement component deficiency	Bacterial infections; autoimmunity
Unregulated Excess	
B lymphocytes	Monoclonal gammopathies; other B-cell malignancies; lymphoproliferative syndromes
T lymphocytes	T-cell malignancies; autoimmune lymphoproliferations, autoimmune syndromes
Complement components	Angioedema due to defect in Cl esterase inhibitor

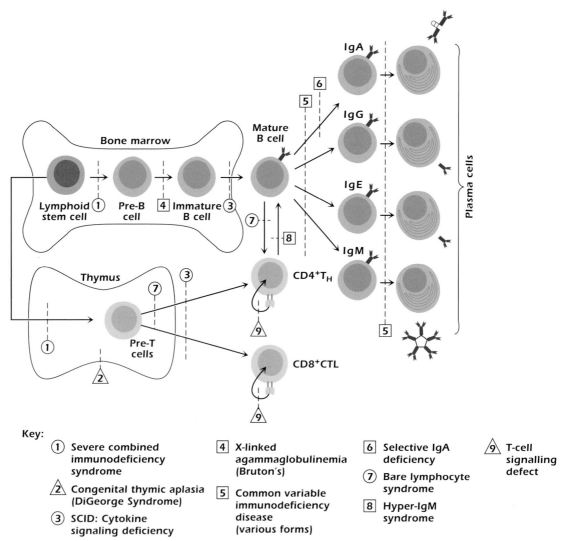

Key:

① Severe combined immunodeficiency syndrome

⚠2 Congenital thymic aplasia (DiGeorge Syndrome)

③ SCID: Cytokine signaling deficiency

④ X-linked agammaglobulinemia (Bruton's)

⑤ Common variable immunodeficiency disease (various forms)

⑥ Selective IgA deficiency

⑦ Bare lymphocyte syndrome

⑧ Hyper-IgM syndrome

⚠9 T-cell signalling defect

Figure 18.1. Sites of defective lymphopoietic development associated with primary immunodeficiency syndromes. (*Circles*) Lesions presenting as combined immunodeficiencies; (*triangles*) lesions presenting as T-cell disorders; (*squares*) lesions presenting as predominantly B-cell or humoral immune deficiencies.

Primary Immunodeficiency Syndromes

With the exception of IgA deficiency, the frequency of primary immunodeficiency syndromes is very low—about 1 in 10,000. Approximately 50% of all cases are antibody deficiencies, 20% are combined deficiencies in antibody- and cell-mediated immunity, 18% are phagocytic disorders, 10% are disorders of cell-mediated immunity alone, and 2% are complement deficiencies. Figure 18.1 shows that, in general, the earlier the genetic defect or block occurs in development, the more arms of the immune system are affected and the more severe the disease.

Severe Combined Immunodeficiency Diseases (SCID). SCID comprises a heterogeneous group of diseases in which both cell-mediated immunity and antibody production are defective (see Figure 18.1). Individuals with SCID are susceptible to virtually every type of microbial

infection (viral, bacterial, fungal, and protozoal), including opportunistic infections, most notably CMV, *P. jiroveci*, and *Candida*. Vaccination with attenuated live virus could prove fatal in infants with SCID.

 Read the related case: **Severe Immunodeficiency Syndrome**
In *Immunology: Clinical Case Studies and Disease Pathophysiology*

Patients can be subclassified at initial evaluation according to the lymphocyte subsets present in their blood (Table 18.2). One group, designated as T⁻B⁺, has essentially no T cells with normal or increased numbers of nonfunctioning B cells. This group of patients may also lack NK cells. A second group, T⁻B⁻, has severe lymphopenia due to the absence of both T and B cells. A few patients are T⁺B⁺, and

TABLE 18.2. Severe Combined Immunodeficiency Diseases

Specific Disorder	Underlying Deficiency	Mode of Inheritance[a]
T⁻B⁺ subgroup		
X-linked SCID	Mutated γ chain of cytokine receptors	X linked
Autosomal recessive SCID	Mutated JAK3 tyrosine kinase	AR
T⁻B⁻ subgroup		
Adenosine deaminase deficiency	ADA enzyme	AR
Purine nucleoside phosphorylase deficiency	PNP enzyme	AR
Recombinase deficiency	Rag 1 or Rag 2 enzyme	AR
T⁺B⁻ Subgroup		
Omenn syndrome	Partial Rag deficiency (most common)	AR
T⁺B⁺ Subgroup		
Bare lymphocyte syndrome	MHC class II transcription activator (4 proteins)	AR
	MHC class I TAP defect	AR
ZAP-70 deficiency	Kinase domain of TCR-associated PTK, ZAP-70	AR
Multisystem Disorders		
Wiskott–Aldrich syndrome	WAS protein	X linked
Ataxia telangectasia	ATM protein for DNA repair	AR

[a]AR, autosomal recessive.

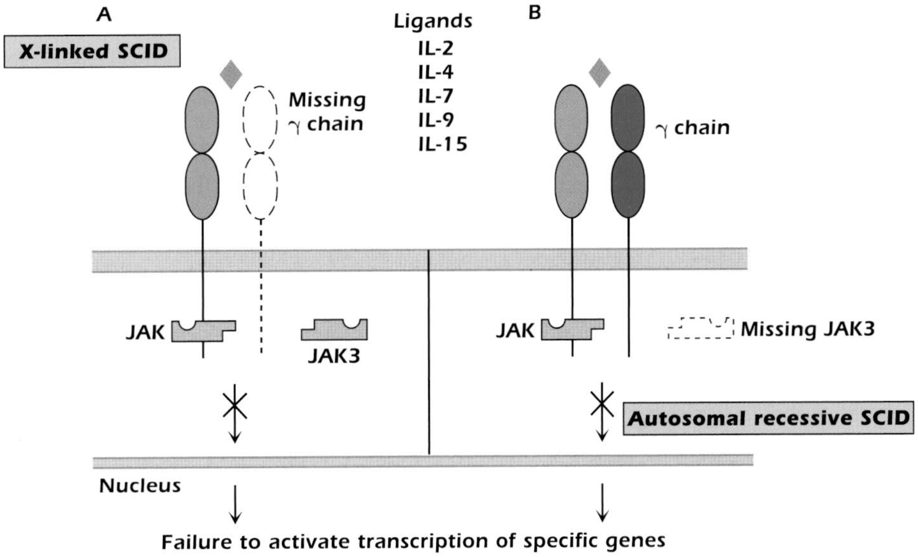

Figure 18.2. T⁻B⁺ subgroup. (A) When this chain is missing, cytokine receptors that share the common γ chain fail to generate intracellular signals following ligand binding. (B) Cytokine receptor signaling mediated by the common γ chain is defective when JAK3 tyrosine kinase is missing. Both result in SCID.

rare patients are T⁺B⁻. The preferred treatment for all SCID patients is a T-cell-depleted bone marrow transplant from an HLA-matched sibling donor.

T⁻B⁺ Subgroup. X-Linked SCID. Patients with X-linked SCID constitute 40–50% of SCID cases, with the majority of those showing T⁻B⁺ lymphopenia and lacking NK cells. Mutations have been found in the gene located on the X chromosome that codes for the γ chain, a chain common to the receptors for interleukin-2 (IL-2), IL-4, IL-7, IL-9, and IL-15 (see Chapter 12). Thus, the mutation impairs responses to a multitude of cytokines (Figure 18.2A).

Autosomal Recessive SCID. A small subgroup of patients characterized by T⁻B⁺ NK⁻ lymphopenia shows an autosomal recessive (rather than X-linked) pattern of inheritance. These individuals have a phenotype identical to the X-linked SCID group and cannot be distinguished clinically. Mutations are localized in the gene for JAK3 tyrosine kinase (Figure 18.2B), the intracellular molecule responsible for transmitting signals from the γ chain of the cytokine receptors (see Chapter 12). Expression of JAK3 is normally restricted to hematopoietic cells.

An even smaller group of patients with autosomal recessive SCID present with T⁻B⁺ NK⁺ lymphopenia. These individuals have mutations in the IL-7Rα chain or in a chain of CD3.

Animal models with targeted defects have proven very instructive in delineating these human deficiencies. In mouse gene knockout models (see Chapter 6), γ-chain knockouts, like SCID patients, have defective development of both T- and B-cell lineages. IL-7 and IL-7R knockouts bear a greater resemblance to SCID patients, suggesting that, in the mouse, IL-7 is crucial for T-cell and B-cell development and/or function and that the absence of IL-7 is not compensated for by other cytokines. In contrast, IL-2 knockouts show only some immune dysfunction, with normal T- and B-cell development and without a SCID phenotype.

T^+B^- Subgroup. *Adenosine Deaminase Deficiency*.

Adenosine deaminase (ADA), an enzyme in the purine salvage pathway, is a ubiquitously expressed housekeeping enzyme (an enzyme used in the everyday function of all or most cells). Individuals lacking this enzyme account for approximately 20% of SCID patients and show an autosomal recessive pattern of inheritance. The deficiency results in buildup of toxic wastes, causing symptom progression over time and making early detection and treatment particularly critical in these patients.

ADA deficiency has its greatest impact on the immune system, resulting in failure of both T- and B-lymphocyte development. Many patients have an associated characteristic skeletal abnormality. The reason these patients do not exhibit even more multisystem problems is not completely understood. Investigation of this rare genetic disease has shown the particular importance of the salvage pathway in lymphocyte development and differentiation, and has led to the development of antileukemic drugs to stop the growth of malignant lymphocyte precursors.

ADA-deficient patients lacking a matched sibling marrow donor were the first group to be treated with gene therapy by transfecting a functional gene for ADA using a retroviral vector. Although gene therapy has been most successful in the small number of ADA-deficient patients it has been tried on (approximately 40 to date), even after years of development, gene therapy as an experimental approach for treating genetic disorders remains fraught with great difficulties. Interestingly the ADA-deficient patients are the only group that seems free from the subsequent development of a T-cell leukemia, suggesting that the ADA-defective cells cannot support transformation. Continuous enzyme supplementation is an alternative treatment for these patients.

Purine Nucleoside Phosphorylase Deficiency. A muta-

tion in another enzyme in the purine salvage pathway, purine nucleoside phosphorylase (PNP), also leads to a buildup of toxic products that are particularly damaging to the neurologic system and to T cells. Eventually, all lymphoid tissues—thymus, tonsils, lymph nodes, and spleen—are depleted. Paradoxically, even though children with this condition are markedly immunodeficient, autoimmune disease is common in these patients.

Recombinase Deficiencies and Radiosensitivity SCID.

Recombination-activating genes (*RAG*) 1 and 2 code for enzymes involved in the rearrangement of the Ig genes in pre-B cells and the TCR genes in pre-T cells (see Chapters 7 and 10). Both enzymes are absolutely required for gene rearrangement, so mutations in either result in complete absence of T cells and B cells. Maturation stops at the pre-T- and pre-B-cell stages. Typically, NK-cell function is intact. Mutations in genes for other proteins (such as Artemis), which are involved in Ig and T-cell receptor (TCR) recombination and DNA repair, will generate a similar clinical picture. The relationship with DNA repair accounts for the radiosensitivity.

Omenn Syndrome. Omenn syndrome refers to a clini-

cal presentation in which the infants have severe immunodeficiency to every type of pathogen, along with enlarged lymphoid tissues (lymphadenopathy), high IgE levels, high eosinophil levels in the peripheral blood and severe erythroderma. Many of clinical parameters are similar to those seen in severe graft-versus-host (GVH) disease (discussed in Chapter 19). Omenn syndrome patients demonstrate dysregulation of the immune system resulting in an attack against self. These patients are T^+B^- by peripheral blood analysis and have massive skin and gastrointestinal infiltration by eosinophils and activated T cells, which produce T_H2-type cytokines (see Chapters 11 and 12). This results in the hyper-IgE syndrome and malnutrition due to protein loss. The majority of Omenn syndrome patients have reduced but partial Rag activity (leaky SCID). Patients with this clinical picture may alternatively have mutations in other molecules commonly associated with SCID, such as ADA and Artemis (a DNA repair protein) or may have mutations in an RNA component of mitochondrial RNA processing endoribonuclease. The success rate of bone marrow transplants in individuals with Omenn syndrome is low compared with other types of SCID patients; failures are due to graft rejection. Thus, although Omenn syndrome patients are immunodeficient, they require pretreatment with immunosuppressive therapy.

T^+B^+ Subgroup. *Bare Lymphocyte Syndrome*. Bare

lymphocyte syndrome (BLS) results from the failure to express HLA (the human major histocompatibility complex [MHC]) molecules and is thus a defect in antigen presentation rather than an intrinsic lymphocyte cellular abnormality. BLS is divided into three groups, depending on which class of HLA molecules is missing: class I, class II, or both classes I and II. Only those individuals lacking expression of HLA class II molecules consistently show immunodeficiencies. Circulating T- and B-cell numbers may be normal; however, in the absence of HLA class II molecules, protein antigens cannot be presented to $CD4^+$ T cells (Figure 18.3). Therefore, collaboration does not occur between

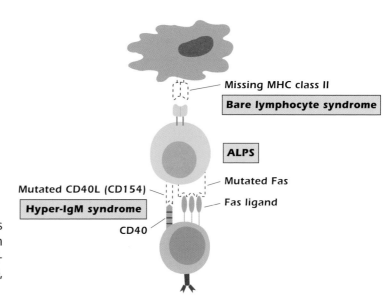

<u>Figure 18.3.</u> Missing cell membrane determinants required for normal T-cell–APC interactions result in several primary immunodeficiency syndromes, including bare lymphocyte syndrome, hyper-IgM syndrome, and Fas deficiency.

antigen-presenting cells (APCs; B cells, macrophages/monocytes, dendritic cells) and CD4$^+$ T cells. As a result, help is not provided to B cells for antibody production or to T cells for cytotoxic T-cell generation (see Chapter 9). This results in a clinical presentation of combined immunodeficiency. Since MHC class II expression is required on thymic epithelial cells for positive selection of CD4$^+$ T cells, proportionately fewer CD4$^+$ T cells are produced in the thymus (see Figure 18.1, defect 7). Therefore, most patients have a decreased proportion of CD4$^+$ to CD8$^+$ T cells, resulting in a reversed CD4:CD8 T-cell ratio. Any CD4$^+$ T cells present are functional, as demonstrated by their ability to respond when stimulated *in vitro*. Since GVH disease can still occur in these patients, HLA matched bone marrow donors are required for treatment.

The mutation responsible for BLS affecting class II molecules is not in the HLA class II genes themselves but in one of the four genes that code for regulatory factors required to transcribe the class II genes. A better understanding of this transcription failure in BLS could result in the development of methods to turn off HLA class II expression. Theoretically these could then be applied to prevent graft rejection of transplanted organs (such as the kidney and liver) in immunocompetent individuals.

Few patients deficient in HLA class I expression have been identified; some were discovered serendipitously. This is undoubtedly due to the fact that not all individuals with deficient HLA class I expression show clinically significant immunodeficiency. Those who do, usually present with chronic inflammatory lung disease late in childhood. As in BLS patients with defective HLA class II expression, patients with HLA class I deficiency do not have a mutation in the HLA class I gene, but rather have a mutated gene for the transporter protein (*Tap*). As described in Chapter 9, Tap transports peptides generated in the cytosol into the endoplasmic reticulum, where they interact with and stabilize the structure of MHC class I molecules. In the absence of the *Tap* gene product, expression of MHC class I molecules on the cell surface is very low. In the case of HLA class I deficiencies, positive selection of CD8$^+$ T cells in the thymus is defective, and their peripheral blood levels are decreased. For reasons that are unclear, when patients with this defect are symptomatic, they have recurrent bacterial pneumonias rather than the expected viral infections.

ZAP-70 Mutation. Patients with a mutation in the T-cell tyrosine kinase ZAP-70, which transduces the signal transmitted through the TCR, also present with a SCID-like phenotype. Originally it was not apparent why patients defective in ZAP-70 expression would present with a SCID-type clinical picture. ZAP-70 plays a critical role in the function of mature T cells (see Figure 18.1, defect 3). In addition, although the peripheral blood counts, lymph nodes, and thymus are essentially normal, CD8$^+$ T cells are missing in patients defective in ZAP-70 expression. This indicates that ZAP-70 is also required for CD8$^+$ T-cell differentiation in the thymus. Recent evidence indicates that ZAP-70 is expressed in developing B cells and in some mature B cell subsets but at a low level. Its function is redundant with a homologous tyrosine kinase molecule, Syk. Thus the role of ZAP-70 in B-cell development and function remains unclear.

Other Multisystem Disorders. In addition to the combined immunodeficiency diseases we have just discussed, several multisystem inherited disorders result in a SCID-like clinical picture.

Wiskott–Aldrich Syndrome. Wiskott–Aldrich syndrome is an X-linked disease showing a classic triad of symptoms: (1) bleeding diathesis (tendency to bleed) due to thrombocytopenia (low platelet level in blood) and small platelet size, (2) recurrent bacterial infections, and (3) paradoxically, allergic reactions (including eczema, elevated IgE levels, and food allergies). Over the longer term, patients have an increased risk of developing malignancies, particularly of the lymphoid system. The genetic basis of the disease is a mutation in the X-linked gene coding for the Wiskott–Aldrich syndrome protein (WASP), which is expressed in all hematopoietic stem cells. The WASP interacts with the cytoskeleton; it allows remodeling after receptor engagement, contributes to the immune synapse between interacting cells, and affects maturation and migration of cells of both the adaptive and innate immune systems. In cells of patients with this syndrome, the cytoskeleton cannot effectively reorganize in response to stimuli.

The immune defects are variable, but both T and B cells are functionally abnormal, with T-cell numbers particularly decreased. Characteristically, patients are unable to respond to polysaccharide antigens. Treatment consists of antibiotics and antiviral agents given promptly with each infection. Reconstitution of T and B cells has been reported following bone marrow transplantation. Without treatment, the average life expectancy is approximately 3 years. With extension of survival, the incidence of malignancies would be expected to increase.

Ataxia Telangiectasia. Ataxia telangiectasia (AT) is another multisystem genetic disorder in which neurologic symptoms (staggering gait or ataxia) and abnormal vascular dilatation (telangiectasia) accompany increased susceptibility to infections; lymphopenia (low lymphocyte numbers in peripheral blood); thymic hypoplasia; and depressed levels of IgA, IgE, and sometimes IgG. The immune defect involves both cellular and humoral (T-cell-dependent and T-cell-independent) immune responses; T-dependent regions of lymphoid tissues are affected most severely. The genetic basis of this syndrome is a mutation in the gene coding for the protein ATM, part of a pathway activated when the cell suffers DNA breaks from ionizing radiation and oxidative damage. AT patients have impaired development of T and B cells. The normal generation of both lineages involves critical phases of extensive cell proliferation, apoptosis, and DNA recombination events; all of these may be dysregulated with a mutated, nonfunctional ATM protein. AT children also have a greatly increased risk of developing malignancies, particularly lymphoid neoplasms. This may be the result of an ATM-dependent defect in DNA repair or cell cycle arrest following chromosomal damage. AT has been grouped with Bloom syndrome and Fanconi anemia; all three disorders show similar variable immunodeficiencies and susceptibility to DNA damage.

In summary, the causes underlying severe defects in both cell-mediated and humoral immunity are varied. They range from mutations in enzymes found in all cells, which should have global effects in the body (such as deficiencies in ADA and PNP), to mutations involving signaling proteins specifically expressed in T cells (such as the ZAP-70 mutation).

Animal models have been informative, both in understanding the defects observed in human syndromes and in helping delineate steps in normal T- and B-cell development. The SCID mutant mouse strain, which has a genetic defect in a protein repairing double-stranded DNA breaks, was the first mouse model used for the study of this group of diseases. Since then, knockout mouse models for the majority of these spontaneous human genetic diseases have been produced as a means to study these diseases (see Chapter 6). In addition, SCID mice and nude mice (discussed later in this chapter), with diminished ability to reject foreign tissues, can be used as "living test tubes" to study the growth of human hematopoietic stem cells and human tumors.

Immunodeficiency Disorders Associated with T Cells and Cell-Mediated Immunity

As noted in Table 18.1, patients with T-cell-associated deficiency diseases are susceptible to viral, fungal, and protozoal infections. In addition, because T cells are required to help B cells produce antibodies to T-dependent antigens (see Chapter 11), patients with T-cell-associated deficiencies also exhibit selective defects in antibody production. Consequently, T-cell-deficient patients may be difficult to distinguish clinically from SCID patients.

Congenital Thymic Aplasia (DiGeorge Syndrome).
DiGeorge syndrome is a T-cell deficiency in which the thymus, as well as several nonlymphoid organs, develops abnormally. The syndrome is caused by defective migration of fetal neural crest cells into the third and fourth pharyngeal pouches. This usually takes place during week 12 of gestation. In DiGeorge syndrome, the heart and face develop abnormally, and the thymus and parathyroids fail to form, resulting in thymic aplasia and hypoparathyroidism along with cardiac disease. Due to the lack of thymic structure, there is an absence of mature T cells, resulting in immunodeficiency. The athymic nude mouse is an animal model of DiGeorge syndrome; in these animals, the thymus and hair follicles do not develop.

 Read the related case: **DiGeorge Syndrome**
In *Immunology: Clinical Case Studies and Disease Pathophysiology*

DiGeorge syndrome is not hereditary; it occurs sporadically and is generally the result of a deletion in chromosome 22q11. Newborns present with hypocalcemia (low serum calcium levels) from absence of the parathyroid glands and have symptoms of congenital cardiac disease. Affected children suffer from recurrent or chronic infections with viruses, bacteria, fungi, and protozoa. They have either no or very few mature T cells in the periphery (blood, lymph nodes, or spleen) (see Figure 18.1, defect 2). Although B cells, plasma cells, and serum Ig levels may be normal, many patients fail

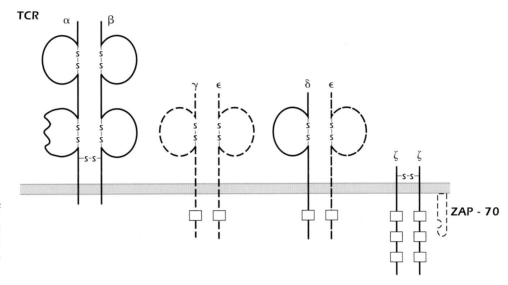

Figure 18.4. Deficiencies of molecules (shown with dashed lines) involved in T-cell signaling through the antigen-specific TCR.

to mount an antibody response after immunization with T-dependent antigens. The lack of helper T cells, which are required for Ig isotype switching, results in the absence of IgG and other switched isotypes following immunization. The IgM response to T-independent antigens is intact. Since individuals with DiGeorge syndrome lack T cells and fail to generate normal antibody responses, they should *never* be immunized with live attenuated viral vaccines.

In the past, children with DiGeorge syndrome were treated with a fetal thymus graft, which resulted in the appearance of host-derived T cells within a week. The fetal thymus used for transplantation needed to be less than 14 weeks' gestation to avoid GVH reactions, which would occur if donor thymocytes were transferred into the immunoincompetent recipient. This donor fetal thymus provided the environment (the thymic epithelial cells) for development of recipient T cells from the patient's normal lymphoid precursors. Although the T cells produced were normal, cell-mediated immunity and help for antibody production were not fully restored. The recipient's T cells learned the MHC of the transplanted thymus as "self" and sometimes collaborated poorly with the body's own APCs in the periphery (see Chapters 9 and 10). Because this treatment strategy was not entirely successful, therapy now is mostly in response to symptoms. Some patients have small remnants of thymic tissue, allowing delayed (though still diminished) T-cell maturation. The other medical problems associated with the syndrome, such as congenital heart disease, add to the overall poor prognosis.

T-Cell Deficiencies With Normal Peripheral T-Cell Numbers.

A number of patients have been identified with functional rather than numerical defects in their T cells. Clinically, they may present with opportunistic infections and a strikingly high incidence of autoimmune disease. Family studies show autosomal recessive patterns of inherit-

ance. Molecular analysis demonstrates that the underlying causes are heterogeneous, with deficient expression of ZAP-70 tyrosine kinase, CD3ε, or CD3γ (Figure 18.4). As previously discussed, patients with ZAP-70 deficiencies present with SCID-like clinical phenotypes.

Mutations in CD3 chains are quite rare; only a handful of patients with such defects have been described. Mouse models confirm that all the CD3 peptide chains are required for normal signaling through the TCR. It is not clear, however, that these mouse models accurately mimic the few patients reported.

Chronic Mucocutaneous Candidiasis.

Chronic mucocutaneous candidiasis is a poorly defined collection of syndromes characterized by *Candida* infections of skin and mucous membranes. This ubiquitous fungal organism is normally nonpathogenic. These patients usually have normal T-cell–mediated immunity to microorganisms other than *Candida* and normal B-cell-mediated immunity (antibody production) to all microorganisms including *Candida*. Thus, they have only a selective defect in the functioning of T cells. This disorder affects both males and females, is particularly prevalent in children, and may be inherited.

Defects in Control.

Three syndromes, each the result of gene mutations, are characterized by lack of tolerance and/or overwhelming, multiorgan autoimmune diseases. One affects the transcription factor autoimmune regulator (AIRE), expressed on thymic epithelial cells and responsible for negative selection of T cells. Its resulting syndrome, autoimmune polyendocrinopathy candidiasis ectodermal dystrophy (APECED) [also known as autoimmune polyendocrine syndrome type 1 (APS1)] is characterized by autoimmune disease in multiple endocrine organs. The second affects the transcription factor Foxp3 resulting in an absence of T-regulatory cells and the disease immunodysregulation polyendocrinopathy enteropathy X-linked syndrome (IPEX). In the last one of these syndromes, a surface molecule important in inducing cell death and thereby eliminating unwanted cells is mutated, resulting in autoimmune lymphoproliferative syndrome (ALPS). These syndromes were discussed further in Chapter 13.

Autoimmune Lymphoproliferative Syndrome.

Autoimmune lymphoproliferative syndrome (ALPS) is an autosomal dominant disease characterized by massive proliferation of lymphoid tissue with early lymphoma development. This genetic defect results in systemic autoimmune phenomenon (hence its name) and increased susceptibility to chronic viral infections only. Patients have an increased number of double-negative (CD4$^-$CD8$^-$) T cells but may eventually develop B-cell lymphomas. Most ALPS patients have a mutation in the gene coding for the Fas protein (CD95) (see Figure 18.3). Signaling through this protein normally activates apoptosis, or programmed cell death (see Chapters 11 and 13). Without activation of apoptosis, cells that should have died, such as autoimmune cells, continue to live, and immune responses that should have been turned off persevere. The unchecked proliferation of B cells then provides fertile ground for transforming mutations that lead to B-cell lymphomas. Most ALPS patients have one normal and one mutated Fas molecule, suggesting that the mutated Fas molecule interferes with the function of the normal molecule when they are cross-linked. Some ALPS patients have defects in other components of the apoptosis pathway, such as Fas ligand or caspase 10.

 Read the related case: **Autoimmune Lymphoproliferative Syndrome**
In *Immunology: Clinical Case Studies and Disease Pathophysiology*

Two mouse strains—*lpr* and *gld*—have phenotypes similar to those of ALPS patients. The *lpr* mice have a mutation in their Fas gene and *gld* mice have a mutation in their Fas ligand gene. For many years, *lpr* mice were studied as a model for autoimmune disease, specifically systemic lupus erythematosus (SLE), before their Fas gene defect was discovered.

B-Cell–Associated or Immunoglobulin-Associated Immunodeficiency Disorders

B-cell-associated or immunoglobulin-associated immune diseases range from defective B-cell development with complete absence of all Ig classes to deficiencies in a single class or subclass of Ig. Patients suffer from recurrent or chronic infections that may start in infancy after maternal antibodies diminish (Bruton's or X-linked agammaglobulinemia) or in young adulthood. Evaluation includes analysis of B-cell number and function and immunoelectrophoretic and quantitative determinations of Ig class and subclass.

X-Linked Agammaglobulinemia.

First described in 1952 by Bruton, X-linked agammaglobulinemia (XLA) is also called ***Bruton's agammaglobulinemia***. The disorder, which is relatively rare (1 in 100,000 individuals), is first noticed at approximately 6 months of age, when the infant has lost the maternally derived IgG that passed through the placenta. At that age, the infant presents with serious and repeated bacterial infections as a result of depression or virtual absence of all Ig classes.

 Read the related case: **X-Linked Agammaglobulinemia**
In *Immunology: Clinical Case Studies and Disease Pathophysiology*

The major defect lies in the inability of pre-B cells, which are present at normal levels in the bone marrow, to develop into mature B cells. The *BTK* gene, which is mutated in XLA, normally codes for a tyrosine kinase enzyme (Btk) residing in the cytosol. Btk is essential for signal transduction from the pre-B cell receptor (pre-BCR) on developing B cells. Without this signal, the cell develops no further (see Figure 18.1, defect 4). Only the nonmutated X chromosome is active in all mature B cells from female carriers of the mutant gene. XLA is therefore one of several inherited immunodeficiency diseases in which a mutation in a cytoplasmic tyrosine kinase is responsible for the disorder (mutations in JAK3 in SCID and ZAP-70 in T-cell deficiency are other examples).

Analyses of the blood, bone marrow, spleen, and lymph nodes of XLA patients reveal near absence of mature B cells and plasma cells, explaining the depressed Ig levels. Characteristically, affected children have markedly underdeveloped tonsils. The limited numbers of B cells appear normal in their ability to become plasma cells. Infants with XLA have recurrent bacterial otitis media, bronchitis, septicemia, pneumonia, arthritis, meningitis, and dermatitis. The most common microorganisms found to cause infections in these patients are *Haemophilus influenzae* and *Streptococcus pneumoniae*. Frequently, patients suffer from malabsorption due to infestation of the gastrointestinal tract with *Giardia lamblia*. Unexpectedly, XLA patients are also susceptible to infections by viruses that enter through the gastrointestinal tract, such as echovirus and polio. The infections do not respond well to antibiotics alone; treatment consists of periodic injections of intravenous γ-globulin (IVGG) containing large amounts of IgG (discussed further in Chapter 21). Although such passive immunization has maintained some patients for 20–30 years, the prognosis is guarded, as chronic lung disease due to repeated infections often supervenes.

Two other rare mutations, μ heavy-chain deficiency and λ_5 chain deficiency, result in an identical clinical picture as a result of the same underlying pathophysiology. The λ_5 chain is part of the surrogate light chain on pro-B cells and, along with the μ heavy chain and a third chain, forms the pre-BCR. Without a functional pre-BCR to receive signals, continued maturation of pro- to pre- B cells is halted and the cells die. Both of these mutations have autosomal recessive patterns of inheritance.

Transient Hypogammaglobulinemia.
When infants are approximately 5–6 months of age, passively transferred maternal IgG disappears, and IgG production by the infant begins to rise. Premature infants may have transient IgG deficiency if they are not yet able to synthesize Ig. Occasionally, a full-term infant may also fail to produce appropriate amounts of IgG, even when levels of IgM and IgA are normal. The cause appears to be a deficiency in number and function of helper T cells. Transient hypogammaglobulinemia may persist for a few months to as long as 2 years. It is not sex-linked and can be distinguished from the non-X-linked inherited agammaglobulinemias by the presence of normal numbers of B cells in the blood. Although treatment is usually not necessary, affected infants need to be identified, as they should not be given immunizations during this period.

Common Variable Immunodeficiency Disease.
Patients with common variable immunodeficiency disease (CVID) have markedly decreased serum IgG and IgA levels, with normal or low IgM and normal or low peripheral B-cell numbers. The cause of the disease, which affects both males and females, is not entirely clear and is probably not uniform. Onset may occur at any age, with peaks at 1–5 years old and 15–20 years old. Affected individuals suffer from recurrent respiratory and gastrointestinal infections with pyogenic bacteria and, paradoxically, from autoantibody-associated autoimmune diseases such as hemolytic anemia, autoimmune thrombocytopenia, and SLE. Many also have disorders of cell-mediated immunity. Long term, these patients have a high incidence of cancers, particularly lymphomas and gastric cancers.

 Read the related case: **Common Variable Immunodeficiency Syndrome**
In *Immunology: Clinical Case Studies and Disease Pathophysiology*

CVID is characterized by a failure in the maturation of B cells into antibody-secreting cells (see Figure 18.1, defect 5). This defect may be due to an inability of the B cells to proliferate in response to antigen, normal proliferation of B cells without secretion of IgM, secretion of IgM without class switching to IgG or IgA (due to an intrinsic B-cell or

T-cell abnormality), or failure of glycosylation of IgG heavy chains. In most cases, the disorder appears to be the result of diminished synthesis and secretion of Ig. The disease is familial or sporadic, with unknown environmental influences triggering onset. In the peripheral blood, patients will have normal or near-normal numbers of B cells but usually a marked reduction of memory B cells (CD27$^+$/IgD$^-$ B cells). Memory B cells are those that have been exposed to antigen in the germinal center, where they have hypermutated and isotype switched their immunoglobulin genes and are now ready to respond rapidly with high-affinity antibody on reexposure to antigen.

Treatment depends on severity. For severe disease with many recurrent or chronic infections, IVGG therapy is indicated. Treated patients can have a normal life span. Women with CVID have normal pregnancies but, of course, do not transfer maternal IgG to the fetus.

Selective Immunoglobulin Deficiencies.
Several syndromes are associated with selective deficiency of a single class or subclass of Ig. Some are accompanied by compensatory elevated levels of other isotypes, such as the increased IgM levels in cases of IgG or IgA deficiency.

IgA deficiency is the most common immunodeficiency disorder in the Western world, with an incidence of approximately 1 in 800 individuals (see Figure 18.1, defect 6). The cause is unknown but appears to be associated with decreased release of IgA by B lymphocytes. IgA deficiency can also occur transiently as an adverse reaction to drugs. Patients may suffer from recurrent sinopulmonary viral or bacterial infections and/or celiac disease (defective absorption in the bowel); alternatively, they may be entirely asymptomatic. Isolated IgA deficiency may also precede full-blown expression of CVID; the two disorders are often found in the same families.

Treatment of symptomatic patients with IgA deficiency consists of broad-spectrum antibiotics. Therapy with immune serum globulin is not useful because commercial preparations contain only low levels of IgA, and injected IgA does not reach the areas of the secretory immune system where IgA is normally the protective antibody. Furthermore, patients may mount antibody responses (usually IgG or IgE) to the IgA in the transferred immune serum, causing hypersensitivity reactions. The prognosis for selective IgA deficiency is generally good, with many patients surviving normally.

Selective deficiencies in other Ig isotypes include IgM deficiency, a rare disorder in which patients suffer from recurrent and severe infections with polysaccharide-encapsulated organisms such as pneumococci and *H. influenzae*. Selective deficiencies in subclasses of IgG have been described but are even rarer.

Disorders of T–B Interactions

There are at least two diseases in which the T- and B-cell lineages appear to mature normally but demonstrate abnormal interactions between them. Although both disorders described below are usually due to underlying T-cell abnormalities, the predominant clinical symptoms are in the B-cell or humoral immune response.

Hyper-IgM Syndrome. Patients with hyper-IgM syndrome (HIGM) present with recurrent respiratory infections at 1 to 2 years of age; very low serum IgG, IgA, and IgE; and normal to elevated IgM (see Figure 18.1, defect 8). In the most common form of the disease, the B cells are normal in number, functional *in vitro*, and will switch isotypes when appropriately stimulated. The T cells are also normal in number, subset distribution, and proliferative responses to mitogens. This form, X-HIGM, caused by a mutation in the *CD40L* gene on the X chromosome, results in the absence of CD40 ligand (CD154) on T$_H$ cells (see Figure 18.3). CD40L binds to CD40 expressed on B cells (see Chapter 11). This interaction is necessary for B-cell proliferation, class switching, and even germinal center formation. CD40–CD40L interaction also plays a role in macrophage–T$_H$1 cell interaction; this aspect may explain the propensity of these patients to develop opportunistic infections, particularly pneumocystis pneumonia (PCP), and their poorer prognosis compared to XLA patients. For the same reason, delayed-type hypersensitivity (DTH) reactions are absent.

 Read the related case: **Hyper-IgM Syndrome**
In *Immunology: Clinical Case Studies and Disease Pathophysiology*

A second group of patients with presentations similar to X-HIGM have a defect in the CD40 molecule and thus an autosomal recessive pattern of inheritance. A third group, with a defect downstream in the interaction between CD40 and a modulator of the transcription factor NF-κB (see Chapter 11), has an X-linked mode of inheritance. As is common in genetic disorders involving intracellular regulatory molecules, these children show abnormalities in nonimmune system cells as well, reflecting the ubiquitous use of these molecules in many types of cells.

Two more groups of patients with HIGM have been described. One has a mutation in activation-induced cytidine deaminase (AID), the molecule essential for somatic hypermutation and isotype class switching, and a second has a mutation in uracil-DNA glycosylase, an enzyme also active in isotype class switching. These patients would have normal T-macrophage interactions and therefore have normal DTH reactions.

X-Linked Lymphoproliferative Syndrome (Duncan Syndrome). X-linked lymphoproliferative syndrome (XLPS) was originally observed in six maternally related males of the Duncan family, hence its common

name. This rare disease is usually due to a mutation in the gene coding for the signaling lymphocyte activation molecule associated protein (SAP), located on the X chromosome. SAP is an intracytoplasmic molecule that links several surface receptors with downstream molecules in T cells, B cells, NK cells, eosinophils, and platelets. In spite of the wide distribution of the molecule among numerous hematopoietic cell lineages, abnormalities are usually subtle and undetected until exposure to Epstein–Barr virus (EBV). EBV results in a severe course of infectious mononucleosis, which may be fatal. Presumably this is the result of impaired killing of infected cells by T and NK cells. Development of malignant lymphoma or dysgammaglobulinemia frequently follows survival from infection or may occur without prior EBV exposure. The lymphomas are predominantly aggressive B-cell lymphomas; Burkitt lymphoma (described later in the chapter) is the most common type. Although the pattern of lymphomas is similar to those in other patients with poorly controlled EBV-induced B-cell proliferations due to T-cell defects (such as in acquired immune deficiency syndrome [AIDS] or immunosuppressed transplant patients), the incidence is much greater in XLPS. The inability of T cells to regulate B-cell growth once growth has been initiated is considered to be a major part of the underlying defect. Prognosis is extremely poor.

 Read the related case: **X-Linked Immunoproliferative Syndrome**
In *Immunology: Clinical Case Studies and Disease Pathophysiology*

Phagocytic Dysfunctions

Phagocytic cells—polymorphonuclear leukocytes and macrophages/monocytes—play a critical role in both innate and acquired immunity to pathogens, acting either alone or in concert with lymphocytes. Inherited deficiencies affecting phagocytic cell function have helped identify many of the molecules required at each step of phagocyte function. These steps and the associated deficiencies include the following: migration and adhesion of phagocytic cells (leukocyte adhesion deficiency), phagocytosis and lysosomal fusion (Chédiak–Higashi syndrome), and respiratory burst for killing (chronic granulomatous disease) (Figure 18.5). Phagocytic dysfunction may also be secondary; causes include extrinsic factors, such as drugs and systemic diseases (e.g., diabetes mellitus), or defects in other arms of the immune system.

Leukocyte Adhesion Deficiency. As discussed in Chapter 2, for leukocytes to arrive at sites of infection in tissues, they must first leave the bloodstream. This is accomplished through a series of steps. The first one consists of the cell's slow rolling along the endothelium through the

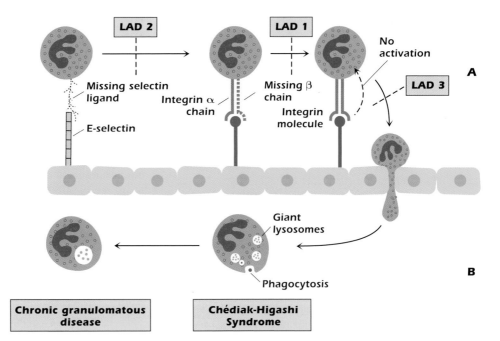

Figure 18.5. (A) Defects in cell adhesion disrupt the ability of leukocytes to interact with vascular endothelium, causing impairment of migration of these cells from the blood to sites of infection. (B) Impairments in mechanisms required for phagocytosis result in defective intracellular killing of microorganisms.

interaction of selectins on endothelial cells and selectin ligands on leukocytes (see Figure 12.3). Chemoattractants then cause the cell to stop rolling. The cell adheres more firmly, followed by transendothelial migration. These latter steps involve the interaction of leukocyte integrins with their ligands on endothelial cells.

Leukocyte adhesion deficiency (LAD) is a group of disorders in which the interaction between the leukocyte and the vascular endothelium is disrupted (Figure 18.5A). LAD1 is an autosomal recessive disease mapping to chromosome 21. Patients have a defect in the β subunit of the integrin molecules, preventing their expression. The β subunit is common to three integrins found on granulocytes, monocytes, and lymphocytes: LFA-1 (CD11a/CD18), Mac-1 (CD11b/CD18), and p150,95 (CD11c/CD18). As a result, adhesion and migration of all white blood cells are impaired. LAD1 individuals suffer from recurrent soft tissue bacterial infections and have increased white blood cell (WBC) counts but without pus formation or effective wound healing. As expected, lymphocyte function is also affected due to the lack of LFA-1 expression. Newborns with LAD1 characteristically have delayed separation of their umbilical cords.

LAD3, a disorder clinically identical to LAD1, has recently been identified. Individuals with LAD3 express both integrin chains, but the molecule does not become activated in response to stimuli. The leukocytes are therefore able to roll but do not arrest in response to endothelial cell signals, similar to LAD1 (Figure 18.5A).

LAD2 individuals have a defect in selectin ligands; therefore, cells from these patients cannot roll along the endothelial surface (Figure 18.5A). The underlying defect in LAD2 is in fucose metabolism, which results in the absence of fucosylated ligands available for binding to selectins. Although the immunodeficiency symptoms are milder, the defect in fucose metabolism results in other developmental abnormalities. As in LAD1 and LAD3, there is little or no pus formation, and affected children do not show classical clinical signs of severe infection.

Chédiak–Higashi Syndrome. Chédiak–Higashi syndrome (CHS) is an autosomal recessive disease characterized by abnormal giant granules and organelles (Figure 18.5B) due to a mutation of the *LYST* gene; this gene codes for a protein that may have a role in organelle protein trafficking. Lysosomes and melanosomes are particularly affected, resulting in defects in pigmentation; abnormalities in neutrophil, NK-cell, and platelet function; and neurologic abnormalities. Neutrophils show diminished intracellular killing of organisms, the result of both defective degranulation and impaired fusion of lysosomes with phagosomes. With time, patients develop massive infiltrates of lymphocytes and macrophages in the liver, spleen, and lymph nodes. Pyogenic organisms such as *Streptococcus* and *Staphylococcus* cause recurrent, sometimes fatal, infection. Prognosis is poor.

Chronic Granulomatous Disease. In chronic granulomatous disease (CGD), the final step in killing of ingested organisms is defective (Figure 18.5B) and the continued intracellular survival of the organisms results in granuloma formation. In normal individuals, activated neutrophils and mononuclear phagocytes kill organisms via the respiratory burst, which consumes oxygen and generates hydrogen peroxide and free superoxide radicals. Mutations in any of the four subunits of the enzyme that catalyzes the burst, namely, nicotinamide adenine dinucleotide phosphate (NADPH) oxidase can result in CGD. The most common form of CGD is due to a mutation in one of the membrane-bound subunits of NADPH oxidase, gp91^{phox}, which is coded for by the *CYBB* gene located on the X chromosome. Thus, the majority of patients show an X-linked recessive pattern of inheritance. The other subunits of NADPH oxidase are coded for by autosomal genes, thus CGD patients with mutations in these subunits show autosomal recessive inheritance. Mutations in these patients occur mostly in one of the two cytosolic subunits of the enzyme, p47^{phox} or p67^{phox}.

Symptoms appear during the first 2 years of life. Patients have enhanced susceptibility to infection with organisms that are normally of low virulence, such as *Staphylococcus aureus, Serratia marcescens*, and *Aspergillus*. Associated abnormalities include lymphadenopathy (increase in lymph node size) and hepatosplenomegaly (increase in liver and spleen size) due to the chronic and acute infections. Treatment consists of aggressive immunization and therapy with wide-spectrum antibiotics, antifungal agents, and interferon-γ (IFN-γ).

Other disorders with reduced or absent levels of phagocyte-associated enzymes include glucose-6-phosphate dehydrogenase, myeloperoxidase, and alkaline phosphatase; all of these result in decreased intracellular killing of organisms.

IL-12/23-Interferon-γ Deficiency.

A mutation in any of the molecules operative in the interactions among IL-12, IL-23, IFN-γ, and their receptors results in an inability of monocytes to respond with secretion of tumor necrosis factor-α (TNF-α); therefore, individuals carrying these mutations are selectively susceptible to weakly pathogenic mycobacteria. Five mutations have been identified: IFN-γR1 (ligand-binding chain) and IFN-γR2 (signal-transducing chain), both on APCs; STAT1 (transducing signal from IFN-γR); IL-12β (p40 subunit) produced by APCs; and IL-12Rβ$_1$ (β subunit of IL-12 receptor) on T and NK cells. This group of disorders demonstrates the importance of IFN-γ and IL-12 in controlling mycobacterial infections but also suggests that there are compensation mechanisms for other effects of these cytokines. Immunization with live BCG, common in some parts of the world, is dangerous for patients with this defect.

Natural Killer Cell Deficiency

Very little is known about NK-cell deficiency in humans; only a few such cases have been reported. Animal studies suggest that NK-cell deficiency impairs allograft rejection and is linked to higher susceptibility to viral diseases and increased metastases from tumors. NK-cell defects are seen in SCID, in some T-cell and phagocytic cell disorders, and in XLPS.

Diseases Caused by Abnormalities in the Complement System

As described in Chapter 14, complement is important in the opsonization and killing of bacteria and altered cells, in chemotaxis, and in B-cell activation. Complement components also participate in the elimination of antigen–antibody complexes, preventing immune complex deposition, and subsequent disease. Deficiencies in complement are inherited as autosomal traits; heterozygous individuals have half the normal level of a given component. For most components, this is sufficient to prevent clinical disease. Normally, the half-life of activated complement components is carefully controlled by inhibitors, which break down the products or dissociate the immune complexes. Absence of inhibitors leads to uncontrolled complement activity.

Deficiencies of Early Complement Components.

The early components of complement are particularly important in generating the opsonin, C3b (Figure 18.6). Patients with deficiencies of C1, 4, or 2 from the classical pathway or with deficiency in C3 itself have increased infections with encapsulated organisms (*S. pneumoniae, Streptococcus pyogenes, H. influenza*) and increased rheumatic diseases. The reason for the latter is the improper clearance of immune complexes as a consequence of low C3b generation, and often the autoimmune disease is most striking. In fact, SLE is the most common presenting symptom of some complement deficiencies. SLE in these individuals is of earlier onset and more severe than without this association and can occur in the absence of autoantibodies that are frequently found in other cases of SLE (see Chapter 13). Deficiencies of mannose-binding lectin, which binds to the surface of microbes without antibody and activates the classical pathway, also result in risk of bacterial infections and lupus-like symptoms. Since all the complement activation pathways—classical, mannose-binding lectin, and alternative—activate C3, deficiencies of C3 itself are associated with the most severe symptoms, particularly infectious complications.

Deficiencies of Late Complement Components.

Deficiencies of the late complement components (C5–C9) interfere with the generation of the membrane attack complex (MAC). The MAC is directly lytic and responsible for the primary defense against Gram-negative bacteria, particularly *Neisseria meningitidis* (Figure 18.6).

Defective Control of Complement Components.

Hereditary Angioedema. In hereditary angioedema, patients lack a functional C1 esterase inhibitor. (The disorder is also referred to as *C1 esterase inhibitor deficiency*.) Without this inhibitor, the action of C1 on C4, C2, and the kallikrein system is uncontrolled, generating large amounts

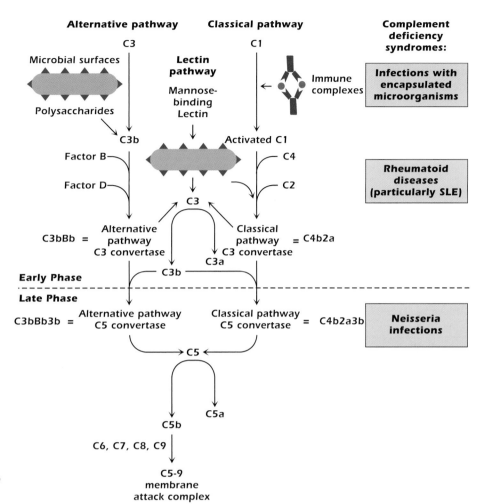

Figure 18.6. Complement cascade showing that deficiencies in early-phase complement components pre-dispose individuals to infections caused by encapsulated microorganisms and rheumatoid syndromes. Late-phase complement deficiencies are associated with *Neisseria* infections.

of vasoactive peptides. These peptides cause increased blood vessel permeability. Patients suffer from localized edema, which is life threatening when it occurs in the larynx and obstructs the airway passage. Treatment includes avoidance of precipitating factors (usually trauma) and infusion of C1 esterase inhibitor, if available.

 Read the related case: **Hereditary Angiodema**
In *Immunology: Clinical Case Studies and Disease Pathophysiology*

Glycosyl Phosphatidyl Inositol (GPI) Protein Deficiencies. A family of proteins with GPI anchors is expressed on the membranes of red blood cells (RBCs), lymphocytes, granulocytes, endothelial cells, and epithelial cells. These proteins, which include decay-accelerating factor (DAF or CD55) and CD59, protect the cells from spontaneous lysis by complement (see Chapter 14). In the absence of these cell surface inhibitors, granulocytes, platelets, and particularly RBCs are susceptible to spontaneous lysis by complement. Rare families exist with inherited mutations in DAF, CD59, or all the GPI proteins. Patients

show symptoms of severe anemia, thrombotic events, and chronic infections.

An acquired form of the disease, called *paroxysmal nocturnal hemoglobinuria* (PNH), is more common. In PNH, patients have a deficiency in an enzyme required for the production of all the GPI-anchored proteins due to an acquired somatic mutation in an early myeloid stem cell. The three nonlymphoid lineages (granulocytes, platelets, and erythrocytes) are affected. In many patients, the stem cells with this mutation eventually acquire additional mutations, dominate the normal cells in the bone marrow, and stop maturing, resulting in acute myelogenous leukemia. During the chronic course of PNH, intravascular hemolysis occurs, more prominently in the kidneys at night where the acidic environment activates the alternative complement pathway. This clinical presentation is reflected in its name, paroxysmal nocturnal hemoglobinuria.

Secondary Immunodeficiency Diseases

As noted at the beginning of this chapter, secondary immunodeficiency diseases are the consequence of other diseases. By far, the most common cause of immunodeficiency disorders worldwide is malnutrition. In developed countries, immunodeficiency is more often iatrogenic, inadvertently caused by medical treatment, particularly from the use of chemotherapeutic agents in cancer therapy or deliberate immunosuppression for organ transplantation or autoimmune disease. Secondary immunodeficiencies can be seen in untreated autoimmunity or overwhelming infections by bacteria. Malignancies of the immune system also frequently suppress the nonmalignant components, resulting in increased susceptibility of these patients to infection.

ACQUIRED IMMUNODEFICIENCY SYNDROME

Initial Description and Epidemiology

In 1981, several cases of an unusual pneumonia caused by *Pneumocystis jiroveci* were reported in homosexual males in the San Francisco area of California. This was followed by the recognition of an aggressive form of Kaposi sarcoma in a similar population in New York City. Since those first cases of acquired immunodeficiency syndrome (AIDS) were recognized, until today, over 30 million individuals have died worldwide and an additional 30 million are currently infected.

 Read the related case: **Acquired Immunodeficiency Syndrome**
In *Immunology: Clinical Case Studies and Disease Pathophysiology*

AIDS is caused by infection with human immunodeficiency virus (HIV). The virus is transferred through blood and body fluids. Blood, semen, vaginal secretions, breast milk, and (to a small extent) saliva of an infected individual all contain free virus or cells harboring virus. Thus, HIV can be transmitted through sexual contact, sharing of needles, transfusion of blood or blood products, placental transfer, passage through the birth canal, and breast feeding.

Although first recognized in sexually active homosexual males in large U.S. cities, AIDS has no sexual preference. Worldwide, heterosexual transmission is most frequent. In the United States, although homosexual males and intravenous drug abusers still constitute the major infected groups, the greatest increase in incidence rate is among heterosexual women and minorities (African Americans and Hispanics). Transmission of the virus through transfusion of blood and blood products has been virtually eliminated in the United States through screening of donors, testing of collected blood units, and heat-inactivation of clotting factor concentrates. For reasons that will become

clear later in the discussion, a dangerous "window period" still exists during which infection of blood units or organs cannot be detected. Transmission from mother to infant, which accounts for more than 80% of the pediatric cases, can be greatly diminished by antiviral therapy of the expectant mother and newborn and avoidance of vaginal childbirth and breast-feeding. In some U.S. states, testing of newborns is mandatory. However, these positive statements are almost as a footnote to an epidemic that continues to spread worldwide without signs of abating, particularly in Africa and Southeast Asia.

Human Immunodeficiency Virus

HIV is an enveloped human retrovirus of the lentivirus family. Two strains have been identified, HIV-1 and HIV-2. HIV-2 is a less virulent strain found mostly in Western Africa. The viral particle contains two identical single strands of genomic RNA and three enzymes; integrase, protease, and reverse transcriptase (Figure 18.7). These are packaged in the p24 core antigen with p7, a nucleoprotein, and p9; all of which are surrounded by the p17 matrix protein. The viral envelope, which is derived from the host cell membrane, displays viral glycoproteins, including gp120 and gp41, which are critical for infection. The gp120, which is noncovalently bound to the transmembrane protein gp41, has high affinity for CD4; therefore, all cells expressing CD4 are potential targets for the virus. These include macrophages/monocytes and dendritic cells as well as CD4$^+$ T cells.

After binding to CD4, gp120 undergoes a conformational change and must then also bind a second molecule (a co-receptor) on the surface of the target cell for HIV to enter the cell. Several chemokine receptors (see Chapter 12) are co-receptors for HIV. The particular co-receptor used by the virus depends on the variant of the gp120 molecule expressed on its surface. Variation in gp120 therefore determines what is referred to as the ***tropism*** of the virus, dictating which CD4$^+$ target cell can be infected by that viral particle. Macrophage tropic HIV uses the chemokine receptor CCR5 and requires only a low level of CD4 on the host cell. CCR5 is expressed by macrophages and dendritic cells, both of which express low levels of surface CD4. Lymphotropic HIV uses the chemokine receptor CXCR4 expressed on T cells and requires a high density of CD4 on the cell surface. HIV variants using CCR5 are called *R5*, and those using CXCR4 are termed *X4*; variants able to bind both chemokine co-receptors are referred to as *R5X4*. Both co-receptors are G-coupled proteins with seven transmembrane spanning domains. CCR5 normally binds the chemokines, RANTES, monocyte chemotactic protein 1α (MIP−1γ), and MIP−1ε. CXCR4 binds stromal derived factor 1.

CCR5 is thought to be the major co-receptor for the establishment of primary infection since individuals with mutations in CCR5 appear to be at least partially protected. If an individual is first infected with a macrophage tropic

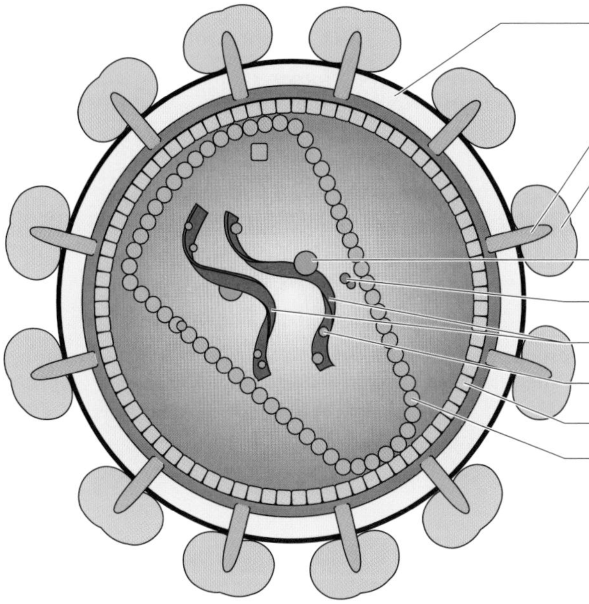

Figure 18.7. Structure of HIV-1 showing two identical RNA strands (viral genome) and associated enzymes. The enzymes include reverse transcriptase, integrase, and protease packaged in a cone-shaped core composed of p24 capsid protein with surrounding p17 protein matrix, all of which are surrounded by a phospholipid membrane envelope derived from the host cell. Virally encoded membrane proteins (gp41 and gp120) are bound to the envelope.

variant via sexual contact, viral infection can be established in the macrophages and dendritic cells of mucosa associated lymphoid tissue (MALT). These infected cells will then provide a reservoir of virus both locally and distally, since they are not killed by the infection and are capable of migrating throughout the body. Exposure of HIV-infected cells to antigen promotes viral replication (particularly in the macrophages), a switch to the lymphotropic form, and further, rapid dissemination in the body. Thus, the tropism of the virus produced within the infected individual changes over time. This evolution is due to mutations in the gp120 gene that result in alterations in its protein product's amino acid sequence.

The importance of the CCR5 receptor is illustrated by the single individual "cured" of HIV. This infected patient received an allogeneic bone marrow transplant for a separate illness, from an individual with a mutated CCR5. The recipient's new immune system proved resistant to the virus, which is no longer detectable in his body. Although a bone marrow transplant is a drastic measure with odds of finding a suitable donor slim, this still illustrates the importance of CCR5 and suggests strategies to block infection.

Following the binding of gp120 to CD4 and its co-receptor, gp41 penetrates the cell membrane, allowing fusion of the viral envelope with the cell membrane and subsequent viral entry. In the host cell, viral RNA is replicated to a cDNA copy by the viral enzyme reverse transcriptase. The cDNA may remain in the cytoplasm or may enter the nucleus and be integrated into the host genome as a provirus with the help of the viral enzyme integrase. Viral replication continues at a low level, sometimes for several years, so that HIV infection remains in a relatively, but not truly, "latent" phase.

The HIV genome has a long terminal repeat (LTR) region at each end (Figure 18.8). This is required for viral

integration and has binding sites for regulatory proteins. When the T cell is activated by antigen, a cascade of reactions leads to activation of the transcription factor NF-κB. NF-κB binds to a promoter region in LTR, activating transcription of the provirus by host RNA polymerase.

Transcription of the provirus produces a long messenger RNA (mRNA) transcript that is spliced at alternative sites for the synthesis of different proteins. The first two proteins made are *tat* and *rev*. Tat enters the nucleus, where it acts as a transcription factor binding to the LTR region and increasing the rate of viral transcription. Rev also acts in the nucleus, binding to the Rev-responsive element in the viral mRNA transcript. Rev binding increases the RNA transport rate to the cytoplasm. When the mRNA is transported more rapidly into the cytoplasm, less splicing occurs in the nucleus and different proteins can then be made from these same mRNA forms. In this second wave of viral protein synthesis, the structural components of the viral core and envelope are produced in precursor form. In the third wave, unspliced RNA is transported to the cytoplasm and serves as the RNA for the new viral particles and for the translation of *gag* and *pol*: *gag* codes for p24, p17, and p7/p9; *pol* codes for the viral protease, reverse transcriptase, and integrase. The protease cleaves these products of *gag* and *pol*, which are first synthesized as a single polyprotein.

Release of virus from CD4$^+$ T cells frequently results in lysis of the cell. Macrophages and dendritic cells are generally not killed by HIV; therefore they can serve as reservoirs, transporting virus to other parts of the body (lymphoid tissue and central nervous system [CNS]) and producing a small number of particles without cytopathic consequences. Dendritic cells carry the virus mostly on their surface, whereas the macrophages allow a constant low level of viral production. The stimulation of infected

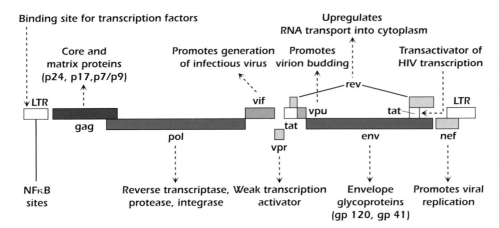

Figure 18.8. The genes and proteins of HIV-1. The HIV-1 RNA genome is flanked by LTR regions required for viral integration and regulation of the viral genome. Several viral genes overlap, resulting in different reading frames; this allows the virus to encode many proteins in a small genome. The functions of the gene products are also shown.

macrophages and T cells by cytokines or antigen results in increased viral replication and the productive phase.

Clinical Course

The clinical course of HIV infection can be divided into three phases: acute infection, chronic latent phase, and crisis phase.

Acute Infection. Upon initial infection with HIV, many patients are asymptomatic. Others will show a flu-like illness characterized by fever, sore throat, and general malaise starting 2 to 4 weeks after infection and lasting 1 to 2 weeks. During this time, there is a viremia (virus in peripheral blood) and a precipitous drop in the number of circulating CD4$^+$ T cells. The immune system responds by generating cytotoxic T lymphocytes (CTLs) and antibodies specific for the virus. The CTLs, which kill virally infected cells, are partially responsible for the drop in CD4$^+$ T cells. At this point the patient will seroconvert and express detectable antibody specific for HIV proteins. The number of CD4$^+$ T cells in the peripheral blood then partially recovers. Infected macrophages and dendritic cells disseminate the virus to lymphoid tissue throughout the body.

The window period refers to the 5–10 weeks after infection during which no antibody is yet detected. Viral particles are detected prior to that, leaving approximately 2 weeks following infection when neither antibody nor virus is detectable. During this ellipse period, the virus is hidden in the tissues and the patient can transmit infection.

Chronic Latent Phase. Although the immune response seems standard for a viral infection, it merely contains rather than eradicates the virus. The extremely high rate of mutation of the virus may explain the ineffectiveness of the immune response. A "latent" phase is established that may last as long as 15 years. During this relatively asymptomatic period, a low level of viral replication continues,

associated with a gradual decline in CD4$^+$ T-cell number. HIV is therefore never truly latent.

In contrast to what might be expected, the number of viral-infected T cells in the peripheral blood is extremely low. The lymph nodes are the predominant location of infected cells. As described above, macrophages act as a reservoir. Follicular dendritic cells of the germinal center (see Chapter 8), not only function as a reservoir, but also present virus on their surface. This results in continuous presentation of virus to T and B cells, culminating in the intense follicular (germinal center) hyperplasia and lymphadenopathy typical of this phase.

The T cells undergo a slow rate of lysis, which eventually results in involution of the lymph node. This T-cell death seems to be the result of a combination of factors. First, production of virus in the cells causes lysis. Second, the infected cell seems to be more susceptible to apoptosis. Third, CTLs kill some of the infected cells. Finally, uninfected CD4$^+$ T cells may be killed in a bystander antibody-dependent cell-mediated cytotoxicity-like mechanism as a result of binding of soluble gp120 and anti-gp120 antibody to their surface CD4 molecules.

During this phase, patients' peripheral CD4$^+$ T-cell counts, CD4:CD8 T-cell ratios, and viral loads are monitored. In healthy individuals, the CD4:CD8 T-cell ratio is approximately 2, but in this phase of HIV infection the ratio is reversed, with CD8 T cells outnumbering CD4 T cells. A reversed CD4:CD8 T-cell ratio can be seen in other viral infections but is usually due to an increase in CD8$^+$ T cells rather than a decrease in CD4$^+$ T cells as seen in HIV. As the number of CD4$^+$ T cells reaches progressively lower values, the patient becomes symptomatic, entering the final crisis phase, AIDS. This relentless downward spiral has been altered by antiviral therapy.

Crisis Phase. AIDS was originally recognized by the clinical appearance of unusual infections and malignancies; these continue to be the hallmarks of the full-blown disease.

The U.S. Centers for Disease Control and Prevention (CDC) have identified illnesses that are considered AIDS-associated (Table 18.3). Diagnosis of any of these (or a defined threshold CD4$^+$ T-cell level of less than 200 cells/μL or less than 14% of T cells) labels the patient as having AIDS rather than merely being HIV infected. The illnesses fall into three categories: (1) opportunistic infections, (2) unusual malignancies, and (3) general debilitating syndromes, which reflects the primary effects of HIV on the immune system and the CNS.

Several concurrent factors appear to initiate this symptomatic or crisis phase. The gradual drop in CD4$^+$ T cells eventually results in an immunodeficient state that leaves the individual susceptible to opportunistic infections, similar to patients with primary immunodeficiency syndromes and immunosuppressed transplant patients. Activation of virally infected T cells by antigen results in stimulation of viral transcription and progeny formation. This leads to accelerated T-cell death, exacerbating the immunodeficient state. Rapid viral replication also increases the viral mutation rate, allowing the virus to escape from any remaining immune controls.

The patterns of AIDS-associated illnesses in an individual may partially reflect the mode of HIV transmission (sexual transmission versus intravenous drug use). This is suggested by differences in the infections and malignancies seen among AIDS patients with different HIV exposures, as well as the contrast between AIDS patients and other immunosuppressed individuals. Some individuals infected with HIV may be coinfected with other sexually transmitted organisms, some of which may lead to aggressive forms of cancer in the immunodeficient patient. In fact, all of the malignancies seen in AIDS patients are believed to be caused by oncogenic DNA viruses. For instance, human papillomavirus (HPV) is associated with the development of cervical cancer in women. Exposure to HPV, combined with the individual's immunodeficient state, may be responsible for a markedly increased incidence and aggressiveness of invasive cervical cancer in HIV$^+$ women. The CDC includes invasive cervical cancer in the AIDS-associated malignancies.

The aggressive form of Kaposi sarcoma (KS) is virtually unique to AIDS patients, particularly male homosexuals, and may occur early in the course of the disease. KS is an abnormal proliferation of small blood vessels; in its usual form, it presents in elderly men as a slow-growing tumor on the skin of their lower extremities. Human herpes virus 8 (HHV-8) has been identified in KS from AIDS patients. This virus is also associated with an unusual form of aggressive lymphoma seen in AIDS patients called **primary effusion lymphoma**. Again, this malignancy is more common in male homosexual AIDS patients, some of whom have the lymphoma and KS concurrently.

Aggressive B-cell lymphomas, mostly EBV-associated lymphomas, are seen at an incidence similar to that observed in immunosuppressed transplant patients. These lymphomas are usually Burkitt, Burkitt-like, or diffuse large B-cell lymphomas (see below) and often involve sites outside the lymph nodes (extranodal). In AIDS patients, the CNS is a frequent site of primary lymphoma. Two other malignancies are not among AIDS-defining criteria but have a more aggressive course in AIDS patients: squamous cell carcinoma of the head and neck region (also possibly associated with HPV infection) and atypical Hodgkin lymphoma.

The infectious diseases associated with AIDS reflect the inability of the patient's markedly depressed cell-mediated immune system to handle organisms that are normally nonpathogenic (opportunistic infections). As in any T-cell immunodeficient patient, PCP is a major infectious complication. Candidiasis is also frequently seen. Granuloma

TABLE 18.3. AIDS-Associated Diseases Defined by the CDC^a

Infections—frequently disseminated

Fungal
 Candidiasis
 Cryptococcosis
 Histoplasmosis
 Coccidioidomycosis
 Cryptosporidiosis

Parasitic
 Toxoplasmosis
 Pneumocystis
 Cryptosporidiosis
 Isosporiasis

Bacterial
 Mycobacteriosis (including atypical)
 Salmonella

Viral
 Cytomegalovirus
 Herpes simplex virus
 Progressive multifocal leukoencephalopathy

Neoplasms

Sarcoma
 Kaposi sarcoma, aggressive form

Lymphoma
 Burkitt lymphoma
 Diffuse large B-cell lymphoma
 Primary effusion lymphoma
 Primary CNS lymphoma

Carcinoma
 Invasive cancer of uterine cervix

General conditions
 HIV encephalopathy and dementia
 Wasting syndrome
 CD4$^+$ T-cell count < 200/μL

^{a}Selected illnesses are discussed in the text.

formation (a T helper cell-dependent function) is poor in these patients, leading to uncontrolled mycobacterial infections. *Mycobacterium avium*, not normally a human pathogen, can cause overwhelming infection. *Cryptosporidia, M. avium*, and CMV, among the most common organisms infecting the gastrointestinal tract in AIDS patients, can cause severe diarrhea. The CNS is susceptible to infection by *Cryptococcus, Toxoplasma*, and CMV.

The multiple infections cause continuous cell necrosis (death), a major feature of AIDS. The organisms and cell debris provide chronic antigenic stimulation to a deficient immune system. The B cells show evidence of responding to that stimulation; patients have polyclonal hypergammaglobulinemia (elevated serum Ig), circulating immune complexes, and markedly increased plasma cell production. In spite of this B-cell activity, patients are unable to mount an effective antibody response to newly encountered antigens, perhaps due to the T-cell defect; however, they also have particular difficulty with T-cell-independent responses to encapsulated organisms. In addition, B cells infected with EBV (normally eliminated by T cells) are susceptible to additional transforming events, resulting in the B-cell malignancies discussed above.

The CNS is infected with HIV, presumably via macrophage transport. The virus infects microglia cells (bone marrow-derived cells in the same lineage as the macrophage), oligodendrocytes, and astrocytes. This may start the process, resulting in AIDS-related dementia and progressive encephalopathy. In total, up to 50% of AIDS patients show CNS symptoms and more than 70% have CNS changes at autopsy.

Finally, these patients suffer from cachexia, or wasting syndrome, to a degree much more severe than can be attributed to their concurrent illnesses. It is thought that HIV alters the cytokine profile of the macrophages to increase TNF production, leading to the development of extreme weight loss and fatigue.

The clinical course of AIDS has changed, at least for individuals in developed countries with access to medication. The first improvement was seen in the early, prophylactic, and aggressive treatment of infections, particularly PCP. Initially, most patients died early from infection. With the aggressive treatments, more began surviving long enough to develop the malignancies, which took prominence among people with AIDS in the 1990s. A second, more recent improvement was the introduction of multiple antiviral therapies, which prolong the chronic phase of HIV infection, thus delaying entry of the individual to full-blown AIDS.

Prevention, Control, Diagnosis, and Therapy of HIV Infection

Prevention and control of HIV are best accomplished by avoiding unprotected contact with blood and body fluids from infected individuals. Education and public awareness of what to avoid and what is safe (casual contact) are required to control the disease and to prevent possible panic.

All blood donations in the United States have been tested for antibodies to HIV since 1985. Because the development of an antibody response after exposure to HIV can take up to 5 weeks, this testing still left a long window of time in which recent infection might not be detected. Viremia following infection precedes the immune response; testing for viral RNA, which requires an amplification step, is very sensitive and has significantly decreased but not eliminated the window period. The HIV NAT (nucleic acid testing) can be set up to detect either proviral cDNA in WBCs or viral RNA in plasma, reducing the window period to several days. The latter also forms the basis for the quantitative viral load test (see below). Because there is still a short period where signs of infection cannot be detected, each blood donor is screened by an interview process and asked direct questions orally and in writing about high-risk behavior.

HIV$^+$ women who are pregnant are placed on antiviral therapy to decrease viral load and thereby diminish risk of transplacental transfer of virus. Cesarean sections are performed to eliminate infection during passage through the birth canal. Finally, exposure through breast milk is avoided.

For individuals accidentally exposed to infected products, therapy is administered as soon as possible after exposure to prevent establishment of infection.

Diagnosis of HIV infection is generally made by detection of antibodies to the viral particles by enzyme-linked immunosorbent assay (ELISA) and confirmed by Western blot analysis, which detects antibodies to individual viral proteins (see Chapter 6). Patients are monitored by following their absolute CD4$^+$ T-cell count and CD4:CD8 T-cell ratio in the peripheral blood and monitoring viral titers by quantitative analysis of viral RNA. CD4 counts above 500/μL are not associated with opportunistic infections. The CDC has designated CD4 counts below 200/μL as an indicator of full-blown AIDS, making it one of the AIDS-defining criteria.

Therapy using azidothymidine (AZT), a nucleoside inhibitor of reverse transcriptase, was the first promising treatment for HIV infection. Protease inhibitors form a second class of therapeutic agents, and non-nucleoside reverse transcriptase inhibitors a third. Drug resistance to single agents develops rapidly, however, because HIV is capable of an amazing rate of spontaneous mutation during the course of infection in a single individual. The mutations arise from the lack of fidelity of the reverse transcriptase and RNA polymerase.

Individuals who are HIV$^+$ but asymptomatic are placed on triple-agent antiviral therapy, referred to as highly active antiretroviral therapy (HAART). HAART combines three drugs from at least two of the inhibitor classes directed against HIV's reverse transcriptase and protease. It is hoped that the triple-agent therapy will delay the appearance of mutant strains. This therapy prevents infection of new cells; however, previously infected cells remain until they are lysed. After initiating therapy, the fall in viral titers is rapid and dramatic, but a small baseline titer almost always remains. As one might expect, discontinuation of the drugs for a prolonged period results in resurgence of virus. Mutations may allow escape from control by these agents, so there is still a great need to develop an extensive arsenal of drugs to treat the disease. However, HAART, especially when initiated early, has changed the landscape of the AIDS epidemic in developed nations. HIV infection in individuals from those countries with access to the medications has gone from being a virtual death sentence to being a chronic disease. This glimmer of hope should not in any way minimize the seriousness of this infection. The therapy is not without side effects, including suppression of hematopoietic cells, nausea, and malaise. Long-term survivors are beginning to struggle with age-related diseases at younger ages, and additional time is needed to evaluate how successful this approach truly is.

Infections and other AIDS-associated diseases must also be treated; it was the successful institution of prophylactic treatment for infection that first led to extension of life span and improved quality of life.

Many infectious diseases have been controlled by vaccines, the most effective way of preventing the spread of infection through a population. Vaccines induce a long-lasting immune response prior to exposure to the infectious agent (Chapter 21). The development of a vaccine for HIV presents serious challenges, however. First, we do not yet know which effector arm of the immune system—humoral, cell-mediated immunity, and so on—needs to be boosted to mount a response that will eliminate the virus on entry into the organism. HIV escapes eradication despite both antibody and cytotoxic T-cell responses in recently infected individuals. Second, the ability of the virus to "hide out" in reservoir cells and its high mutation rate are major problems that need to be overcome for vaccination to be effective. Third, the availability of animal models, in which candidate vaccines for other infectious diseases are tested extensively, is limited due to their lack of susceptibility to infection by HIV. The best model is the simian, which develops a disease similar to AIDS after infection with simian immunodeficiency virus (SIV). Lastly, testing of HIV vaccines in humans presents a host of ethical problems. An understanding of the molecular biology and structure of all components of HIV throughout its life cycle will be essential to development of a safe vaccine. An alternative may be to genetically engineer an HIV-resistant immune system using the lessons learned from resistant individuals and our one cured bone marrow-transplanted patient.

NEOPLASMS OF LYMPHOID SYSTEM

A common theme throughout this chapter has been the idea that dysregulation of the immune system can result in the emergence of neoplasms, particularly neoplasms of lymphoid cells. This is true for patients with primary immunodeficiency diseases and AIDS, as well as immunosuppressed transplant patients (see also Chapter 19). In these circumstances, the malignancies are most often aggressive B-cell lymphomas, frequently associated with EBV infection. Although malignant transformation of any element of the immune system can occur in the absence of clinically apparent immunodeficiency, when tumors are analyzed at the molecular level, dysregulation intrinsic to the malignant cells or imposed upon them by the environment becomes obvious. In this section, we first describe general concepts of lymphoid neoplasms followed by specific examples of important or informative types.

Referring to a malignancy as a *leukemia* implies that the malignant cells are predominantly present in the circulation and/or bone marrow. A lymphoma presents as a solid mass in the lymph nodes, spleen, thymus, or extranodal organs. Sometimes the same malignant cell type can show either presentation (leukemia/lymphoma).

In 1996, the World Health Organization (WHO) recommended a classification system based on cell of origin (B vs. T/NK cell) and stage of differentiation (immature [precursor] vs. mature [peripheral]) (Table 18.4). These tumors are considered outgrowths of a transformed lymphoid cell that appears frozen in development. They have the same surface markers and many of the same properties as the corresponding normal cells at that developmental stage. However, the malignant cells may not continue to mature, they may accumulate in large numbers, and all originate from a single clone (in other words, they are monoclonal). They will occupy the same sites or traffic in the same pattern as their normal counterparts—for example, bone marrow for immature B cells, thymus for immature T cells—until they spill over into additional locations.

Southern blot analysis of DNA extracted from B- or T-cell neoplasms will show a single band for the Ig genes and TCR genes, respectively. This demonstrates that all the tumor cells have the same rearrangement of these genes and establishes the monoclonality of that lymphoid growth. For some lymphoid neoplasms, a unique molecular abnormality has been identified, which may contribute to the transformation of that cell. These molecular changes are also incorporated into the classification scheme. Since the WHO classification is based on cell of origin rather than clinical presentation, leukemias are no longer designated separately from lymphomas if they are derived from the same malignant cell type. The WHO grouping makes practical sense, because the treatment is often based on the malignant cell type.

TABLE 18.4. World Health Organization Classification for Lymphoid Neoplasms[a]

B-Cell Neoplasms
  Precursor B-cell lymphoblastic
    Leukemia/lymphoma
  Mature B-cell neoplasms
    Chronic lymphocytic leukemia/small lymphocytic
      lymphoma/prolymphocytic leukemia
    Follicular lymphoma
    Mantle cell lymphoma
    Marginal zone lymphoma of mucosa-associated lymphoid
      tissue (MALT) type
    Nodal marginal-zone lymphoma
    Splenic marginal-zone lymphoma
    Hairy cell leukemia
    Diffuse large B-cell lymphoma (including subtypes:
      mediastinal, primary effusion, intravascular)
    Burkitt lymphoma
    Plasma cell myeloma
    Lymphoplasmacytic lymphoma
  B-cell proliferations of uncertain malignant potential
    Lymphomatoid granulomatosis
    Post-transplant lymphoproliferative disorders
T/NK cell neoplasms
  Precursor T-cell lymphoblastic leukemia/lymphoma
  Mature T-cell/NK-cell neoplasms (selected)
    T-cell large granular lymphocytic leukemia
    NK-cell leukemia
    Peripheral T-cell lymphoma (unspecified)
    Mycosis fungoides
    Sézary syndrome
    Primary cutaneous anaplastic large-cell lymphoma
    Systemic anaplastic large-cell lymphoma
    Extranodal NK/T-cell lymphoma, nasal type
    Intestinal T-cell lymphoma
    Hepatosplenic $\gamma\delta$ T-cell lymphoma
    Adult T-cell leukemia/lymphoma
Hodgkin lymphoma
  Nodular lymphocyte predominant Hodgkin lymphoma
  Classical Hodgkin lymphoma
    Nodular sclerosis
    Mixed cellularity
    Classical, lymphocyte rich
    Lymphocyte depleted

[a]Selected neoplasms are discussed in the text.

B-Cell Neoplasms

Precursor B-Cell Lymphoblastic Leukemia/Lymphoma. B-cell acute lymphoblastic leukemias/lymphomas (B-ALL/L) correspond to the stages of development of the pro-B cell, the pre-B cell, or immature B cell, as demonstrated by the expression of surface CD markers along with the extent of Ig gene rearrangement and protein expression in the individual patient's leukemia cells (Figure 18.9). The malignant cells may express the blast or stem-cell marker CD34 (particularly pro-B cells) and will express CD10 and CD19, which are early B-cell markers. Similar to the normal pro-B or pre-pre-B cell and pre-B cell, corresponding B-ALLs express terminal deoxynucleotidyl transferase (TdT) in the nucleus. The expression of this enzyme, normally required to rearrange the Ig genes (and TCR genes), reflects the fact that B-ALL cells are in the process of gene rearrangement. These cells do not yet express a complete Ig molecule on their surfaces and have only cytoplasmic μ chains if at the pre-B-cell stage. Chemotherapy has been successful in treating many of these children with B-ALL with prognosis depending on the underlying molecular changes.

Mature B-Cell Neoplasms

Burkitt Lymphoma/Leukemia. Burkitt may present as a leukemia or lymphoma; both forms are characterized by a translocation that places the c-*myc* oncogene next to either the Ig heavy-chain gene or one of the two light-chain genes [t(8;14), t(8;22), or t(2;8)] (Figure 18.10). The c-myc protein is normally involved in activating genes for cell proliferation when a cell receives a signal to divide. Translocation to the Ig genes leads to increased expression of c-myc and increased cell proliferation. Antigenic stimulation of the B cell may initiate overexpression of c-myc, now under the control of the Ig gene but malignant transformation of the cell requires additional mutations.

In equatorial Africa, this lymphoma is endemic in children and is associated with EBV infection of the B cells. Burkitt lymphoma is one of the malignancies seen in patients who are immunosuppressed medically or have AIDS. In these patients, the EBV genome is sometimes but not always found in the lymphoma cells.

Follicular Lymphoma. The normal cell counterpart of follicular lymphomas is the B cell of the germinal center (Figure 18.11). As described in Chapter 8, B cells stimulated by antigen enter a primary follicle, generating a germinal center. The B cells may respond by proliferating and undergoing affinity maturation, by Ig isotype switching, and by differentiating into memory or plasma cells. If their antibody is a poor match for that antigen or of low affinity, the cell undergoes apoptosis or cell death. In follicular lymphomas, the *bcl-2* gene, which produces a protein that interferes with apoptosis, is translocated to the Ig H-chain gene [t(14;18)] (see Figure 18.10). This results in continuous expression of bcl-2 protein, preventing death of the cells. In fact, these B-cell neoplasms have a low rate of proliferation and a long chronic clinical course. They display the phenotype (surface CD markers) of normal follicular center B cells: CD19[+], CD20[+], CD10[+] and surface Ig.

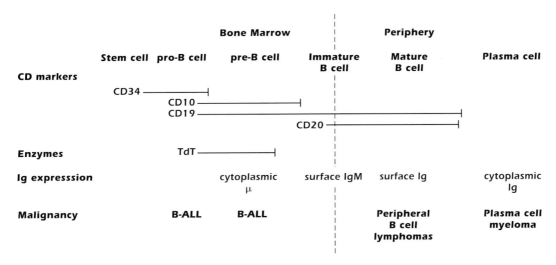

Figure 18.9. Correlation of B-cell development with B-cell malignancies.

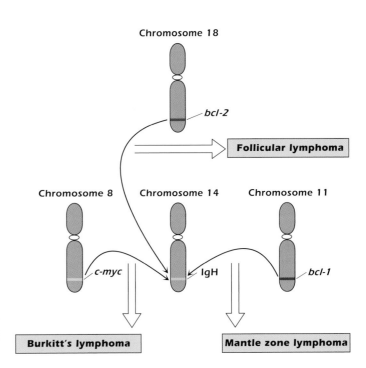

Figure 18.10. Some B-cell neoplasms associated with translocations of genes to chromosomal locus encoding Ig H chain on chromosome 14.

 Read the related case: **Follicular Lymphoma**
In *Immunology: Clinical Case Studies and Disease Pathophysiology*

Mantle Cell Lymphoma. The normal germinal center is surrounded by a collar of small, quiescent B cells that have not responded to antigen (see Figure 18.11). A neoplasm of these mantle zone cells has the same B-cell phenotype as its normal counterpart: CD19+, CD20+, CD5+, and surface IgM. The majority of mantle cell lymphomas demonstrate overexpression of cyclin D1 protein, usually, but not always the result of the translocation of the *bcl-1*

gene to the Ig H-chain gene [t(11;14)] (see Figure 18.10). Cyclin D1 is normally responsible for promoting cell cycle progression from G_1 to S phase, leading to cell division. Mantle cell lymphoma has a higher proliferative rate and a more aggressive course than follicular lymphomas.

Marginal Zone Lymphoma. Marginal zone lymphomas commonly arise in MALT and are often associated with chronic antigenic stimulation or autoimmune disease. The first infectious association recognized was that of chronic *Helicobacter pylori* infection of the stomach leading to the development of gastric lymphoma; it is thus preventable by antibiotic treatment. Recent associations have been reported between *Campylobacter jejuni* and small

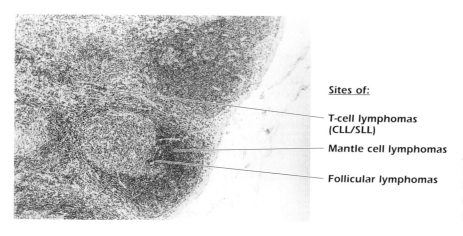

Sites of:

T-cell lymphomas
(CLL/SLL)

Mantle cell lymphomas

Follicular lymphomas

Figure 18.11. Section through normal lymph node showing sites that become involved by T- and B-cell lymphomas. CLL/SLL, mantle cell lymphoma, and follicular lymphoma are all B-cell derived.

intestinal MALT lymphoma, *Borrelia burgdorferi* and primary cutaneous B cell lymphoma, and *Chlamydophila psittaci* and ocular adnexal MALT lymphoma. Patients with autoimmune thyroiditis (Hashimoto's thyroiditis) and autoimmune disease of the salivary glands (Sjögren's syndrome) also have a high incidence of B-cell lymphoma development in the affected organ.

The correlation between autoimmune disease or infection and lymphoma suggests two interesting hypotheses that are not mutually exclusive. First, chronic antigenic stimulation, particularly in response to a limited number of epitopes, provides fertile ground for the development of a B-cell lymphoma. B cells may be particularly vulnerable to developing transforming mutations as they continue to undergo somatic mutation of their Ig genes in response to stimulation. The second hypothesis is that a defect in the regulation of the B cells, whether intrinsic or due to lack of T-cell downregulation, leads to both autoimmune disease and, eventually, lymphoma.

As described earlier in this section, the malignant cells of the immune system follow the trafficking patterns of their normal counterparts. Marginal zone lymphomas of MALT remain localized for a prolonged period and then follow the circulatory pattern for normal MALT cells, traveling to other MALT sites in the body.

Chronic Lymphocytic Leukemia/Small Lymphocytic Lymphoma.
Chronic lymphocytic leukemia (CLL) or small lymphocytic lymphoma (SLL) was originally thought to be a malignant transformation of a subset of B cells known as B-1 cells (see Chapter 8). In some patients, the disease presents first with a leukemic picture, with blood and bone marrow involvement (CLL); in others it presents first in the lymph nodes (SLL) (see Figure 18.11). Similar to B-1 cells, CLL/SLL cells express the mature B-cell markers sIgM, CD19, and CD20, as well as CD5. A subgroup has hypermutated Ig genes, suggesting postgerminal center origin, and therefore the transformation of a different B-cell subset than B-1.

 Read the related case: **Chronic Lymphocytic Leukemia/Small Cell Lymphoma**
In *Immunology: Clinical Case Studies and Disease Pathophysiology*

The majority of CLL cases (over 65%) have a deletion in chromosome 13 at q14.3. This region codes, not for a protein, but for microRNA (miRNA 15 and 16), which normally functions to downregulate the mRNA for *bcl-2*. Therefore, CLL cells often have overexpression of *bcl-2* as the result of posttranscriptional control.

CLL is the most common leukemia in North America and Western Europe and is seen mostly in older individuals. These patients are extremely susceptible to infection, suggesting that their nonmalignant cells are not functioning properly. Autoimmune antibodies are common, particularly against RBCs, resulting in autoimmune hemolytic anemia. The antibodies may be produced by the malignant clone or, more often, by nontransformed B cells. The association of this autoimmune condition with a leukemia/lymphoma again suggests that a lymphoid neoplasm arises in the setting of immune dysregulation or causes it. CLL has a long clinical course, but eventually there is massive involvement of every organ, peripheral blood, and bone marrow.

Diffuse Large B-Cell Lymphoma.
Diffuse large B-cell lymphomas are a heterogeneous group of lymphomas that may arise *de novo* at a single site, may be the progression from one of the above-described slow-growing lymphomas (such as follicular lymphoma or CLL), or may be a consequence of a poorly controlled transforming viral infection (EBV or HHV8) in immunosuppressed individuals. In all cases, the cells generally express the B-cell markers CD19 and CD20 and surface Ig.

Historically, the behavior of the *de novo* diffuse large B-cell lymphomas has been unpredictable. Gene expression microarray analysis (see Chapter 6) has divided the lymphomas into two major groups based on their gene activation patterns and has demonstrated a correlation between these two groups and response to therapy. Those lymphomas with gene expression profiles similar to germinal center B cells have a much better response and prognosis than those with gene expression profiles resembling that of activated or immunoblastic B cells. Similarly, two subgroups could be distinguished based on having a translocation or mutation of the *bcl-6* gene. These genetic alterations result in this protein's continued expression. The *BCL-6* gene is normally expressed in germinal center B cells. It codes for a transcriptional regulator that represses the genes required for plasma cell differentiation and maintains the transcription of genes that allow the B cell to continue as a B cell in the germinal center (i.e., undergo further affinity maturation and isotype switching). Lymphoma patients showing mutations or translocations of *bcl-6* have a better prognosis as compared with those with other large B-cell lymphomas. It is believed that the promiscuity of activation-induced cytidine deaminase (AID), the molecule necessary for somatic hypermutation and isotype class switching, plays a role in mutating *BCL-6* and in lymphogenesis.

The association of EBV infection with diffuse large B-cell lymphomas and Burkitt lymphoma in immunosuppressed patients illustrates the consequences of a breakdown in the immune system's ability to regulate aberrant cell growth. EBV infection of B cells (via the EBV receptor CD21) leads to polyclonal B-cell proliferation. In healthy individuals, these expanded EBV-infected B cells are removed by the body's cytotoxic T lymphocytes (see Chapter 10). In situations in which T cells are lacking, the infected B cells continue to expand; some may acquire mutations, such as c-*myc* translocation, that lead to transformation, independent growth, and the accumulation of additional mutations. For patients on immunosuppressive therapy with an atypical B-cell proliferation, it is still possible to prevent the development of lymphoma by withdrawing the immunosuppressive treatment and allowing the body's immune system to handle the abnormal proliferation. For people with AIDS, control of their HIV infection with antivirals increases their CD4$^+$ T cells and significantly improves their outcome.

Plasma Cell Neoplasms

Neoplastic growths of plasma cells may occur at a single site, resulting in a plasmacytoma. If they occur at multiple sites, predominantly throughout the bone, they are called *multiple myeloma* or *plasma cell myeloma*. Similar to normal plasma cells, malignant plasma cells home to the bone marrow. IL-6 functions as an autocrine growth factor for myeloma cells.

 Read the related case: **Plasma Cell Neoplasms**
In *Immunology: Clinical Case Studies and Disease Pathophysiology*

The neoplastic plasma cells may continue to synthesize and secrete their Ig product. This secreted monoclonal protein causes many difficulties for the patient over and above the malignant cells themselves. Light-chain deposits called amyloid can cause organ failure, especially in the kidneys. As described in Chapter 5, isolation of free light chains excreted in the urine of multiple myeloma patients—Bence Jones proteins—led to an early understanding of Ig light-chain structure.

The monoclonal product of myeloma cells is detected in the serum and sometimes in the urine as a spike, known as an M spike in the γ region of an electrophoretic evaluation (see Figure 5.1). A spike, rather than a broad band, forms because all the immunoglobulins are identical and migrate to the same place by size and charge (see Chapter 5). Most myeloma cases produce monoclonal IgG; IgA is the next most frequent Ig isotype found. The levels of all other normal immunoglobulins are severely decreased in these patients, who are immunosuppressed with respect to antibody production and therefore susceptible to infection. Before the appearance of full-blown myeloma, patients may have a small amount of monoclonal Ig in their serum for many years. Many individuals remain at this stage, never progressing to disease. Small M spikes may also be found in association with other lymphoid neoplasms, such as CLL, or even with nonmalignant conditions.

Lymphoplasmacytic Lymphoma (Waldenström Macroglobulinemia).
Lymphoplasmacytic lymphoma/Waldenström macroglobulinemia is a neoplasm of a single clone of B cells; the microscopic appearance of the clone is a mixture of lymphocytes, plasma cells, and something in between—lymphoplasmacytoid cells. The neoplastic cells involve the lymph nodes, bone marrow, and spleen. Although uncommon, these lymphomas are of interest to immunologists because they overproduce and secrete monoclonal IgM, thus making it accessible for study. The large size and high concentration of the IgM in the blood may combine to slow blood flow and clog vessels (hyperviscosity syndrome). In some patients, the IgM has an abnormal structure, causing it to precipitate in the cold (cryoglobulin); this results in circulatory problems in the patient's extremities (fingers and toes).

T-Cell Neoplasms

Precursor T-Cell Acute Lymphoblastic Leukemia/Lymphoma.
Precursor T-cell acute lymphoblastic leukemia/lymphoma (T-ALL) is a neoplasm of immature T cells with characteristics identical to those of thymocytes frozen in their immature state. As Figure 18.12 shows, T-ALLs express the pan-T markers CD2, CD5, and CD7, which appear early in T-cell development in the thymus. Some T-ALLs have the characteristics of immature or early thymocytes and do not express CD4 or CD8 (they are double

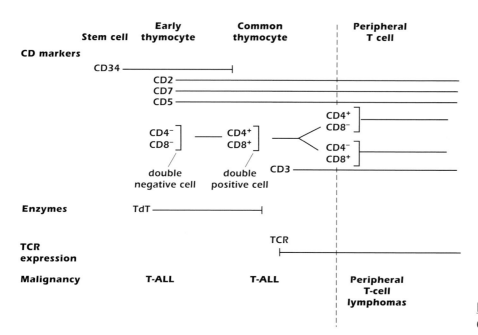

Figure 18.12. Correlation of T-cell development with T-cell malignancies.

negative). Most T-ALLs are slightly more mature and may express both CD4 and CD8 (double positive) but little or no CD3 on their surface, similar to common thymocytes. These cells have not yet completed rearrangement of their TCR genes and still express TdT. T-ALL presents as a leukemia or as a thymic mass. Treatment has not been as successful as for B-ALL.

Mature T-Cell Neoplasms

Peripheral T-cell lymphomas have varied presentations. They are found wherever T cells normally migrate, namely, skin, lung, vessel wall, gastrointestinal tract, and lymph nodes. They also retain some of the functions of normal mature T cells; consequently, cytokine production by the neoplastic cells results in a background of inflammatory cells, including eosinophils, plasma cells, and macrophages. Peripheral T-cell lymphomas usually have a more aggressive course than B-cell lymphomas. Two will be highlighted here: cutaneous T-cell lymphoma and adult T-cell leukemia/lymphoma.

Cutaneous T-Cell Lymphoma. When confined to the skin, this cutaneous T-cell lymphoma is still known by its historical name, mycosis fungoides, because patients were originally believed to have a chronic fungal infection of the skin that waxed and waned over many years. We now understand that the skin disease is due to infiltration of the epidermis by malignant CD4$^+$ T cells with homing receptors for skin. Eventually, the cells may spread to the lymph nodes and even into the blood. When these malignant T cells are present in the circulation they are called Sézary cells, and the patient is said to have Sézary syndrome.

Adult T-Cell Leukemia/Lymphoma. Adult T-cell leukemia/lymphoma (ATLL) is an aggressive T-cell neoplasm that was described in the 1970s in a region of Japan, where it is endemic. It is also found in the Caribbean, parts of central Africa, and a small region of the southeast United States. ATLL is a neoplasm of mature, usually CD4$^+$ T cells. IL-2 is an autocrine growth factor for these cells. In early attempts at treatment, the neoplasm was found to respond temporarily (for a few months) to administration of an antibody (known as anti-Tac) specific for the α chain of the IL-2 receptor (CD25).

ATLL is caused by the retrovirus human T lymphotropic virus 1 (HTLV-1), which was described and isolated before recognition of AIDS and HIV. The proviral genomic structure is similar to HIV, containing an LTR and coding for structural and regulatory proteins as well as viral enzymes, reverse transcriptase, integrase, and protease. Tax, the viral protein that transactivates HTLV-1 transcription by binding to the LTR region, also activates host genes, including those coding for IL-2, IL-2R α chain, and a parathyroid-like hormone (not normally expressed by T cells). Therefore, activation of proviral transcription is associated with activation and proliferation of host T cells. Patients with ATLL frequently have extreme elevations in serum calcium levels as a result of the increased synthesis of the parathyroid-like hormone.

Transmission of HTLV-1 is similar to that of HIV; it is acquired through contact with blood and body fluids, with more efficient transfer through breast milk. Thus, many patients are infected with HTLV-1 during infancy. The incubation period of this virus is long, typically 20–40 years. The virus primarily infects the CD4$^+$ T-cell subset and also infects the nervous system. A subset of patients presents with neurologic disease.

Fortunately, only a very low proportion (approximately 1%) of infected patients develops ATLL. The trigger for the development of disease after so many years is unknown. The CD4$^+$ T cells harbor the virus in a quiescent state. Unlike HIV, the virus is not cytolytic for these cells once activated. To the contrary, HTLV-1 leads to transformation and continuous proliferation of the T cells. Once a patient is diagnosed with ATLL, survival is generally 6–12 months. Blood supplies in the United States and the United Kingdom are screened for this virus.

Hodgkin Lymphoma. Classical Hodgkin lymphoma is characterized by the presence of relatively small numbers of large, binucleate malignant cells called Reed–Sternberg cells in a reactive background of small T cells, eosinophils, plasma cells, macrophages, and fibroblasts. This reactive milieu is the result of abundant cytokine production, particularly IL-5, by the tumor cells and/or background cells. Patients show clinical signs of increased cytokine production: fever, night sweats, and weight loss. Characteristically, these patients demonstrate evidence of depressed cell-mediated immune responses (T$_H$1 type) with no DTH reaction to common test antigens and increased susceptibility to viral and parasitic infections.

The origin of the Reed–Sternberg cell, which expresses no lineage-specific markers and is characterized by the expression of only CD15 and CD30, was the subject of much debate. Microdissection of the malignant cells and analysis by molecular techniques demonstrated rearrangements in the Ig genes, supporting a B-cell origin. The finding of hypermutation in those Ig genes suggests that the Reed–Sternberg cell derives from a post-germinal center B cell. Although the malignant cell has been identified as a B cell (and is large), this lymphoma behaves differently from large

B-cell lymphomas and is therefore classified separately. Lymphomas overall are grouped as Hodgkin versus non-Hodgkin lymphomas.

Immunotherapy

The expanding knowledge of lymphoma biology combined with the technical advances in monoclonal antibody and protein production has led to the development of a new generation of treatment options. Currently, chimeric and humanized monoclonal antibodies directed against CD20, in particular, are widely used for the treatment of B-cell lymphomas. These antibodies are generally used alone ("cold"), causing tumor cell elimination by opsonization of antibody-coated cells. Additional agents to block cytokines or cytokine receptors, which stimulate the proliferation of malignant cells, are being combined with conventional chemotherapy. Conventional chemotherapies, which are largely nonspecific agents, kill all dividing cells. The technology used in developing new specific therapies is also widely applicable to drug development for the treatment of autoimmune diseases and nonlymphoid cancers such as breast cancer.

The immune system normally works as a finely tuned network, responding to foreign invaders, causing no harm to itself, and returning to a more quiescent state (but with memory) once the threat is over. Eliminating, chronically stimulating, or allowing uncontrolled growth of any single component perturbs the remaining elements. Thus, without proper regulation of the network, the occurrence of any one of the major categories of disorders—immunodeficiency, autoimmune disease, or lymphoid neoplasm—allows the emergence of one or both of the other two disease types.

SUMMARY

1. Immunodeficiency disorders are referred to as *primary* when the deficiency is the cause of disease and *secondary* when the deficiency is a result of other diseases or the effects of treatment regimens.

2. Immunodeficiency diseases may be due to disorders in the development or function of B cells, T cells, phagocytic cells, or components of complement.

3. Immunodeficiency disorders predispose patients to recurrent infections. The type of infection that develops is sometimes characteristic of the particular arm of the immune system that is deficient. Defects in humoral immunity lead to increased susceptibility to bacterial infections; in cell-mediated immunity, to viral and fungal infections; in phagocytic cells, to pyogenic organisms; and in complement components, to bacterial infections and autoimmunity.

4. Immune deficiencies constitute one type of defect or disorder of the immune system. Other aspects of such disorders are the unregulated proliferation of B or T lymphocytes, the overproduction of lymphocyte or phagocytic cell products, and the unregulated activation of complement components. This may account for the association of immune deficiencies with autoimmune disease and malignancies.

5. HIV causes a massive immunosuppressive illness known as AIDS by infecting and killing CD4$^+$ T lymphocytes.

6. Lymphoid neoplasms are uncontrolled monoclonal proliferations that can be related to their normal cell counterparts by surface markers and stage of differ-entiation. Many lymphoid neoplasms have specific chromosomal translocations, causing dysregulation of cell proliferation and death. Some are associated with viral infections such as EBV and HTLV-1, acting as either growth promoters or oncogenic viruses, respectively.

REFERENCES AND BIBLIOGRAPHY

Ammann AJ. (1994) Mechanisms of immunodeficiency. In: Stites DP, Terr Al, Parslow TG (eds). *Basic and Clinical Immunology, 8th Ed.* East Norwalk, CT: Appleton & Lange.

Anderson DC, Springer TA. (1987) Leukocyte adhesion defi-ciency: An inherited defect in Mac-1, LFA-1, and p150, 95 glycoproteins. *Annu Rev Med* 38: 175.

Bacchelli C, Buckridge S, Thrasher A, Gaspar HB. (2007) Trans-lational minireview series on immunodeficiency: Molecular defects in common variable immunodeficiency. *Clin Exp Immun* 149: 401.

Baltimore D, Feinberg MB. (1989) HIV revealed: Towards a natural history of the infection. *N Engl J Med* 132: 1673.

Berger EA, Murphy PM, Farber JM. (1999) Chemokine receptors as HIV-1 coreceptors: Roles in viral entry, tropism and disease. *Annu Rev Immunol* 17: 657.

Buckley RH. (2004) Molecular defects in human severe combined immunodeficiency and approaches to immune reconstitution. *Ann Rev Immunol* 22: 625.

Cavazzana-Calvo M, Hacein-Bay S, de Saint Basile G, De Coene F, Selz F, Le Deist F, Fischer A. (1996) Role of interleukin-2 (IL-2), IL-7, and IL-15 in natural killer cell differentiation from cord blood hematopoietic progenitor cells and from γc trans-duced severe combined immunodeficiency X1 bone marrow cells. *Blood* 88: 3901.

Chiorazzi N, Ferrarini M. (2003) B cell chronic lymphocytic leuke-mia: Lessons learned from studies of the B cell antigen receptor. *Annu Rev Immunol* 21: 841.

Cicardi M, Zingale L, Zanichelli A, Deliliers DL. (2007) Estab-lished and new treatments for hereditary angioedema: An update. *Mol Immunol* 44: 3858.

Cimmino A, Calin GA, Fabbri M, Iorio MV, Ferracin M, Shimizu M, Wojcik SE, Aqeilan RI, Zupo S, Dono M, Rassenti L, Alder H, Volinia S, Liu CG, Kipps TJ, Negrini M, Croce CM. (2005) miR-15 and miR-16 induce apoptosis by targeting BCL2. *Proc Natl Acad Sci USA* 102: 13944.

Clerici M, Shearer GM. (1994) The Th1–Th2 hypothesis of HIV infection: New insights. *Immunol Today* 14: 107.

Cunningham-Rundles C, Ponda PP. (2005) Molecular defects in T- and B-cell primary immunodeficiency diseases. *Nature Rev Immunol* 5: 880.

Espeli M, Rossi B, Mancini SJC, Roche P, Gaunthier L, Schiff C. (2006) Initiation of pre-B cell receptor signaling: Common and distinctive features in human and mouse. *Sem Immunol* 18: 56.

Fahey JL. (1993) Update on AIDS. *Immunologist* 1: 131.

Fauci AS. (1993) Multifactorial nature of human immunodeficiency virus disease: Implications for therapy. *Science* 262: 1011.

Geier JK, Schlissel MS. (2006) Pre-BCR signals and the control of Ig gene rearrangements. *Sem Immunol* 18: 31.

Green WC. (1993) AIDS and the immune system. *Sci Am* Sept: 99.

Hazenberg MD, Hamann D, Schuitemaker H, Miedema F. (2000) T-cell depletion in HIV-1 infection: How CD4$^+$ T cells go out of stock. *Nature Immunol* 1: 285.

Helbert MR, Lage-Stehr J, Mitchison NA. (1993) Antigen presen-tation, loss of immunologic memory and AIDS. *Immunol Today* 14: 340.

Jaffe ES, Harris NL, Stein H, Vardiman JW (eds). (2001) *World Health Organization Classification of Tumours. Pathology and Genetics of Tumours of Haematopoietic and Lymphoid Tissues.* Lyon, France: IARC Press.

Jain A, Ma CA, Liu S, Brown M, Cohen J, Strober W. (2001) Specific missense mutations in NEMO result in hyper-IgM syn-drome with hypohydrotic ectodermal dysplasia. *Nature Immunol* 2: 223.

June C, Levine B. (2012) Blocking HIV's attack. *Sci Am* 306: 54.

Kawakami Y, Kitaura J, Hata D, Yao L, Kawakami, T. (1999) Func-tions of Bruton's tyrosine kinase in mast and B cells. *J Leukocyte Biol* 65: 286.

Kohler H, Muller S, Nara P. (1994) Deceptive imprinting in the immune response against HIV-1. *Immunol Today* 15: 475.

Lusso P, Gallo RC. (1995) Human herpes virus 6 in AIDS. *Immunol Today* 16: 67.

McLean-Tooke A, Spickett GP, Gennery AR. (2007) Immunodefi-ciency and autoimmunity in 22q11.2 deletion syndrome. *Scand J Immunol* 66: 1.

Nomura K, Kanegane H, Karasuyama H, Tsukada S, Agematsu K, Murakami G, Sakazume S, Sako M, Tanaka R, Kuniya Y, Komeno T, Ishihara S, Hayashi K, Kishimoto T, Miyawaki T. (2000) Genetic defect in human X-linked agammaglobulinemia impedes a maturational evolution of pro-B cells into a later stage of pre-B cells in the B-cell differentiation pathway. *Blood* 96: 610.

Ochs HD, Smith CIE, Puck JM. (2007) *Primary Immunodeficiency Diseases.* New York: Oxford University Press.

Orkin SH. (1989) Molecular genetics of chronic granulomatous disease. *Annu Rev Immunol* 7: 277.

Quartier P, Bustamamente J, Sanai O, Plebani A, Debre M, Deville A, Litzman J, Levy J, Fermand JP, Lane P, Horneff G, Aksu G, Yakin I, Davies G, Texcan I, Ersoy F, Catalan N, Imai K, Fischer A, Durandy A. (2004) Clinical immunologic and genetic analysis of 29 patients with autosomal recessive hyper-

IgM syndrome due to activation-induced cytidine deaminase deficiency. *Clin Immunol* 110: 22.

Rosenberg ZF, Fauci AS. (1990) Immunopathogenic mechanisms of HIV infection: Cytokine induction of HIV expression. *Immunol Today* 11: 176.

Snapper SB, Rosen FS. (1999) The Wiskott–Aldrich Syndrome Protein (WASP): Roles in signalling and cytoskeletal organization. *Annu Rev Immunol* 17: 905.

Straus SE, Sneller M, Lenardo MJ, Puck JM, Strober W. (1999) An inherited disorder of lymphocyte apoptosis: The autoimmune lymphoproliferative syndrome. *Ann Intern Med* 130: 591.

Wamatz K, Denz A, Dräger R, Braun M, Groth C, Wolff-Vorbeck G, Eibel H, Schlesier M, Peter HH. (2002) Severe deficiency of switched memory B cells (CD27$^+$IIgM$^-$IgD$^-$) in subgroups of patients with common variable immunodeficiency: A new approach to classify a heterogeneous disease. *Blood* 99: 1544.

Zhu Y, Nonoyama S, Morio T, Muramatsu M, Honjo T, Mizutani S. (2003) Type two hyper-IgM syndrome caused by mutation in activation-induced cytidine deaminase. *J Med Dent Sci* 50: 41.

REVIEW QUESTIONS

For each question, choose the ONE BEST answer or completion.

1. An 8-month-old baby has a history of repeated Gram-positive bacterial infections. The most probable cause for this condition is:
   A) the mother did not confer sufficient immunity to the baby *in utero*
   B) the baby suffers from erythroblastosis fetalis (hemolytic disease of the newborn)
   C) the baby has a defect in the alternative complement pathway
   D) the baby is allergic to the mother's milk
   E) none of the above

2. A 50-year-old worker at an atomic plant who previously had a sample of his own bone marrow cryopreserved was accidentally exposed to a minimal lethal dose of radiation. He was subsequently transplanted with his own bone marrow. This individual can expect to:
   A) have recurrent bacterial infections
   B) have serious fungal infections due to deficiency in cell-mediated immunity
   C) make antibody responses to thymus-independent antigens only
   D) all of the above
   E) none of the above

3. Which of the following immune deficiency disorders is associated exclusively with an abnormality of the humoral immune response?
   A) X-linked agammaglobulinemia (Bruton's agammaglobulinemia)
   B) DiGeorge syndrome
   C) Wiskott–Aldrich syndrome
   D) chronic mucocutaneous candidiasis
   E) ataxia telangiectasia

4. A sharp increase in levels of IgG with a spike in the IgG region seen in the electrophoretic pattern of serum proteins is an indication of:
   A) IgA or IgM deficiency
   B) plasma cell myeloma
   C) macroglobulinemia
   D) hypogammaglobulinemia
   E) severe fungal infections

5. Patients with DiGeorge syndrome may fail to produce IgG in response to immunization with T-dependent antigens because:
   A) they have a decreased number of B cells that produce IgG
   B) they have increased numbers of suppressor T cells
   C) they have a decreased number of T helper cells
   D) they have abnormal antigen-presenting cells
   E) They cannot produce IgM during primary responses

6. A 2-year-old child has had three episodes of pneumonia and two episodes of otitis media. All the infections were demonstrated to be pneumococcal. Which of the following disorders is most likely to be the cause?
   A) an isolated transient T-cell deficiency
   B) a combined T- and B-cell deficiency
   C) a B-cell deficiency
   D) transient anemia
   E) AIDS

7. A healthy woman gave birth to a baby. The newborn infant was found to be HIV-seropositive. This finding is most likely the result of:
   A) the virus being transferred across the placenta to the baby
   B) the baby's making anti-HIV antibodies
   C) the baby's erythrocyte antigens cross-reacting with the virus
   D) the mother's erythrocyte antigens cross-reacting with the virus
   E) maternal HIV-specific IgG being transferred across the placenta to the baby

8. Immunodeficiency disease can result from a:
   A) developmental defect of T lymphocytes
   B) developmental defect of bone marrow stem cells

C) defect in phagocyte function
D) defect in complement function
E) all of the above

9. A 9-month-old baby was vaccinated against smallpox with attenuated smallpox virus. He developed a progressive necrotic lesion of the skin, muscles, and subcutaneous tissue at the site of inoculation. The vaccination reaction probably resulted from:
A) B-lymphocyte deficiency
B) reaction to the adjuvant

C) complement deficiency
D) T-cell deficiency
E) B- and T-lymphocyte deficiency

10. The most common clinical consequence(s) of C3 deficiency is (are):
A) increased incidence of tumors
B) increased susceptibility to viral infections
C) increased susceptibility to fungal infections
D) increased susceptibility to bacterial infections
E) all of the above

ANSWERS TO REVIEW QUESTIONS

1. E. None of these is likely to be the underlying cause for the history. The baby is probably hypogammaglobulinemic. Hypogammaglobulinemia leads to recurrent bacterial infections. Viral and fungal infections are controlled by cell-mediated immunity, which is normal in hypogammaglobulinemic individuals. Answer **A** is incorrect because the mother's IgG, which passed through the placenta, would have a half-life of 23 days, and would therefore not be expected to remain in the baby's circulation for 8 months. At this age, any Ig present in the baby's circulation is synthesized by the baby. Answer **B** is irrelevant, since erythroblastosis fetalis is caused by the destruction of the newborn's Rh$^+$ erythrocytes by the Rh$^-$ mother's antibodies to Rh antigen. Answer **C** is unlikely since the classical complement pathway would still be protective; a defect in the alternative pathway would not result in the selective inability to protect from only Gram-positive bacterial infections. Answer **D** is incorrect because, even if allergic to the mother's milk, the baby should not suffer from increased frequency of bacterial infections.

2. E. The autologous bone marrow cells, which contain stem cells, will replicate, differentiate, and repopulate the hematopoietic-reticuloendothelial system, rendering the individual immunologically normal. Thus the individual is not expected to have bacterial, viral, or fungal infections or to respond to antigens differently from a normal individual.

3. A. The only immunodeficiency disorder that is associated with an abnormality exclusively of the humoral response is X-linked (Bruton's) agammaglobulinemia. DiGeorge syndrome results from thymic aplasia, in which there is a deficiency in T cells that influence IgG responses, which require T helper cells. Wiskott–Aldrich syndrome is associated with several abnormalities. Ataxia telangiectasia is a disease with defects in both cellular and humoral immune responses, with T-cell-dependent areas of lymphoid tissues the most severely affected. Chronic mucocutaneous candidiasis is a poorly defined collection of syndromes associated with a selective defect in the functioning of T cells.

4. B. This pattern is characteristic of plasma cell myeloma (IgG myeloma). Plasma cell myeloma may be recognized by the synthesis of large amounts of homogeneous antibody of any one isotype. Although patients with plasma cell myeloma may suffer from a decreased synthesis of other Ig isotypes, the electro-

phoretic pattern is not necessarily an indication of IgA or IgM deficiency.

5. C. Patients with DiGeorge syndrome have a decreased number of T cells, in particular, T helper cells, which are essential for the IgG response to T-dependent antigens. These patients have normally functioning B cells and are capable of responding to T-independent antigens or with only IgM responses (primary responses) to T-dependent antigens.

6. C. The cause of the 2-year-old's infections is very likely B-cell deficiency, which is characterized by recurrent bacterial infections leading to otitis media and pneumonia. T-cell deficiency would usually result in viral, fungal, and protozoal infections. The same is true for combined T- and B-cell deficiency. Answer **D** (transient anemia) is irrelevant in this case; anemia is not generally associated with increased infections. It is unlikely that with a history of only pneumococcal infections the child would have AIDS. The latter syndrome is associated more with characteristic infections such as *Pneumocystis carinii* and various viral infections.

7. E. The most likely explanation is that the "healthy" mother has been infected with HIV-1 and is making anti-HIV IgG, which is transferred to the fetus and newborn transplacentally. While it is possible that the HIV was transferred to the infant across the placenta, this would not cause the newborn to make antibodies to the virus at this young age. Thus answers **A** and **B** are incorrect. Answers **C** and **D** are false because this unlikely situation would result in the recognition of the viral antigen as "self" and the individual would not make anti-self antibodies.

8. E. All are correct. Immunodeficiency disorders may result from defects in the development of bone marrow stem cells into lymphocytes and other cells that participate in the immune response. They can also result from defects in phagocyte functions, which are important in phagocytosis and presentation of antigen. Immunodeficiency disorders may also result from defects in complement function and absence or malfunction of one or more of the complement components, activators, or regulators.

9. D. T-cell deficiency would result in the absence of the crucial immunologic defenses against viral infection, that is, cell-mediated immunity. Cell-mediated immunity plays the major role in immunity to viral infections, much greater than the role of either antibody or complement. In fact, individuals with impaired T-cell-mediated immunity should not be vaccinated with live virus, which, even if attenuated, may cause a serious infection.

10. *D.* Deficiency in C3 is associated with increased susceptibility to bacterial infections, because C3 plays an important role in the opsonization and destruction of bacteria. C3 is a component of all the complement activation pathways: alternative, classical, and mannose-binding lectin pathways. Cell-mediated immunity is generally more important in the resistance of the host to viral and fungal infections. In general, cell-mediated immunity is also considered to be more important than complement in the resistance of the host to tumors.

19

TRANSPLANTATION

INTRODUCTION

The immune system has evolved as a way of discriminating between self and nonself. Once foreignness has been established, the immune system proceeds toward its ultimate goal of destroying the foreign material, be it a microorganism or its product, a substance present in the environment, or a tumor cell. Chapter 20 will describe immune mechanisms associated with the latter.

The same self/nonself discriminating power of the immune system is undesirable in therapeutic settings such as the transplantation of cells, tissues, or organs from one individual to another. Prior to the advent of effective immunosuppressive therapies, organ transplants uniformly culminated in the phenomenon of *graft rejection*, with one notable exception, namely, blood transfusions. Blood transfusions represent the earliest and most successful cell-based "transplants," and they continue to be the most common of all transplants. The reason for this success is due to the fact that red blood cells (RBCs) do not express major histocompatibility complex (MHC) antigens, and they express only a limited number of different types of the major RBC antigens, most importantly, the ABO and Rh blood group antigens. Therefore, it is relatively easy to match the RBCs of the donor and recipient. Matching prevents rapid antibody-mediated destruction of donor RBC. By contrast, the MHC antigens expressed on other cells, tissues, and organs are highly *polymorphic* in the population, so matching donor and recipient is extremely difficult.

Our current understanding of cellular and molecular mechanisms associated with graft rejection and, as noted above, effective immunosuppressive therapies, have made transplantation of various cells, tissues, and organs for therapeutic purposes very commonplace (Table 19.1). For example, over 10,000 kidneys are transplanted annually worldwide with a high degree of success. Transplantations of heart, lungs, corneas, liver, and bone marrow that were considered spectacular and were widely publicized as recently as 25 years ago, have now become commonplace. Although rejection episodes have been significantly reduced due to the use of immunosuppressive therapies, they have not been eliminated. Thus, transplantation immunology continues to be a major area of research.

RELATIONSHIP BETWEEN DONOR AND RECIPIENT

Before we discuss the immunologic mechanisms associated with graft rejection, it is important to understand the various gradations in relationships of transplantation from donor to recipient. These are shown in Figure 19.1 and are described below.

1. An *autograft* is a graft or transplant from one area to another on the same individual such as would occur in the transplantation of normal skin from one area of an individual to a burned area of the same

Immunology: A Short Course, Seventh Edition. Richard Coico and Geoffrey Sunshine.
© 2015 John Wiley & Sons, Ltd. Published 2015 by John Wiley & Sons, Ltd.
Companion Website: www.wileyimmunology.com/coico

individual. The graft is recognized as autochthonous or **autologous** (self), and no immune response is induced against it. Barring technical difficulties in the transplantation process, the graft will survive or take in its new location.

2. An **isograft** or **syngraft** is a graft or transplant of cells, tissue, or an organ from one individual to another individual who is **syngeneic** (genetically identical) to the donor. An example of an isograft is the transplantation of a kidney from one identical (homozygotic) twin to the other. As in the case of an autograft, the recipient who is genetically identical with regard to the donor MHC and all other loci, recognizes the donor's tissue as "self" and does not mount an immune response against it. The two individuals (i.e., donor and recipient) are described as **histocompatible**.

3. An **allograft** is a graft, or transplant, from one individual to an MHC-disparate individual of the same species. Because of the high degree of MHC polymorphism within a given outbred species, this **allogeneic** transplant will result in rejection of the grafted foreign tissue. The donor and recipient, in this case, are **nonhistocompatible** or **histoincompatible**.

4. A **xenograft** is a graft between a donor and a recipient from different species. The transplant is recognized as foreign, and the immune response mounted against it will destroy or reject the graft. Donor and recipient are again histoincompatible.

TABLE 19.1. Transplantation of Specific Organs and Tissues

Organ/Tissue	Clinical Uses	Comments
Skin	Burns, chronic wounds, diabetic ulcers, venous ulcers	Commonly autologous grafts; increasing use of artificial skin consisting of stromal elements and cultured cells of allogeneic or xenogeneic origin
Kidney	End-stage renal failure	Graft survival now exceeds 85% at 1 year even with organs from unrelated donors
Liver	Hepatoma and biliary atresia	Successful in about two thirds of recipients at 1 year
Heart	Cardiac failure	Survival rates in excess of 80% at 1 year
Lung	Advanced pulmonary or cardiopulmonary diseases	Sometimes performed together with heart transplantation
Bone marrow	Incurable leukemias and lymphomas, congenital immunodeficiency diseases	Risk of graft-versus-host disease is a unique feature of bone marrow transplantation; increasingly, transplantation of hematopoietic stem cells being used
Cornea	Blindness	HLA matching is not advantageous because this is a "privileged" site that normally lacks lymphatic drainage
Pancreas	Diabetes mellitus	Pancreas and kidney transplantation are sometimes performed together; success rates are approaching that seen with kidney transplants

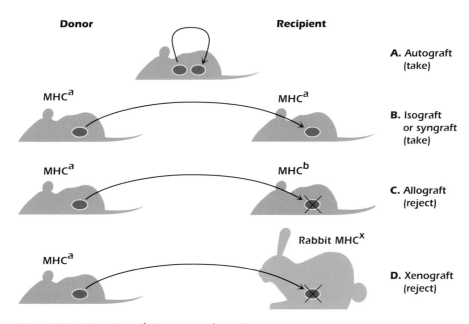

Figure 19.1. Situations of tissue transplantation.

IMMUNE MECHANISMS ARE RESPONSIBLE FOR ALLOGRAFT REJECTION

The most direct evidence that the immune response is involved in graft rejection is provided by experiments in which skin is transplanted from one individual to a genetically different individual of the same species, namely, between allogeneic donor and recipient. Skin from a mouse with black hair transplanted onto the back of an MHC-disparate white-haired mouse appears normal for 1 or 2 weeks. However, after approximately 2 weeks, the skin allograft begins to be rejected, and is completely sloughed off within a few days. This process is called *first-set rejection*. If, after this rejection, the recipient is transplanted with another piece of skin from the same initial donor, the graft is rejected within 6–8 days. This accelerated rejection is termed a *second-set rejection*. By contrast, grafting skin from a different MHC-disparate mouse strain will result in rejection at a rate similar to that of the initial graft, with so-called *first-set kinetics*. Thus, second-set rejection is an expression of specific immunologic memory for antigens expressed by the graft. The participation of CD4$^+$ and CD8$^+$ T cells in the rejection response can be shown by transferring these cells from an individual sensitized to an allograft into a normal syngeneic recipient. If the second recipient is transplanted with the same allograft that was used on the original T-cell donor, a second-set rejection ensues. This establishes that T cells primed in the initial grafting mediate the accelerated rejection in the second host. However, antibodies can also contribute to the destruction of grafted tissue in second-set rejection.

Many other lines of evidence establish the immunologic nature of graft rejection as follows: (1) histologic examination of the site of the rejection reveals lymphocytic and monocytic cellular infiltration reminiscent of the delayed-type hypersensitivity reaction (see Chapter 17); both CD4$^+$ and CD8$^+$ cells are present at the site (and, as we shall see later, both play a crucial role in graft rejection); (2) animals that lack T lymphocytes (such as athymic mice, or humans with DiGeorge syndrome; see Chapter 18) do not reject allografts; and (3) the process of rejection slows down considerably or does not occur at all in individuals treated with immunosuppressive drugs. Direct evidence for the immunologic basis of graft rejection comes from the observation that in the absence of immunosuppressive therapy, animals transplanted with foreign tissues or cells generate alloreactive T cells and alloantigen-specific antibodies that ultimately destroy the graft.

CATEGORIES OF ALLOGRAFT REJECTION

Clinically, allograft rejections fall into three major categories: (1) hyperacute rejection, (2) acute rejection, and (3) chronic rejection. The following are descriptions of the rejection reactions as might be observed, for example, after transplantation of a kidney; they also apply for rejection of other tissues.

Hyperacute Rejection

Hyperacute rejection occurs within a few minutes to a few hours of transplantation. It is a result of destruction of the transplant by so-called *preformed antibodies* to incompatible MHC antigens and, in some cases, to carbohydrates expressed on transplanted tissues (e.g., on endothelial cells). Such antibodies have been produced in the recipient prior to transplant. In some cases, these preformed antibodies are generated as a result of previous transplantations, blood transfusions, or pregnancies. These cytotoxic antibodies activate the complement system, followed by platelet activation and deposition, causing swelling and interstitial hemorrhage in the transplanted tissue, thereby decreasing the flow of blood through the tissue. Thrombosis with endothelial injury and fibrinoid necrosis is often seen in cases of hyperacute rejection. The recipient may have fever, leukocytosis, and will produce little or no urine. The urine may contain various cellular elements, such as erythrocytes. Cell-mediated immunity is not involved at all in hyperacute rejection.

Acute Rejection

Acute rejection is seen in a recipient who has not previously been sensitized to the transplant. There are two types of acute rejection for solid organs. One type is *antibody-mediated* or *humoral acute rejection*, and the other is *acute cellular rejection* (sometimes abbreviated as *acute rejection*). Humoral acute rejection usually occurs within the first 3 months following transplantation. In the case of kidney transplants, this manifests as a sudden decline in kidney function. Donor-specific antibody (DSA) is detected and C4d is deposited on the endothelium of the kidney due to activation of complement. Enlargement and tenderness of the grafted kidney, a rise in serum creatinine level, a fall in urine output, decreased renal blood flow, and presence of blood cells and proteins in the urine are characteristic. Acute cellular rejection usually occurs 1–6 weeks to several years following transplantation when doses of immunosuppressive drugs are lowered. Histologically, cell-mediated immunity, manifested by intense infiltration of lymphocytes and macrophages, is taking place at the rejection site. The distinction between humoral acute rejection and acute cellular rejection is important because treatments may differ. If the acute rejection is antibody mediated, patients are treated with B-cell-directed drugs such as Rituxan and/or plasmaphoresis. Acute rejection may be reduced by immunosuppressive therapy, for example, with cyclosporine and other drugs, as we shall see later in this chapter. Treatment with corticosteroids is used for both types of acute rejection.

Chronic Rejection

Chronic rejection caused by both antibody and cell-mediated immunity occurs in allograft transplantation months or years after the transplanted tissue has assumed its normal function. Subclinical (insidious) microvascular inflammation, associated with antibody-mediated rejection, which can be with or without complement activation, predicts progression to chronic rejection, transplant dysfunction, and failure. It is noteworthy that humoral responses beyond major histocompatibility antigens continue to receive the attention of the transplantation community and these may contribute to such microvascular inflammatory responses. Clinical relevance of antibodies targeting angiotensin type 1 receptor is broadly confirmed in renal and cardiac transplantation, where, in addition, antibodies against endothelin type A receptor have been found. Finally, antibodies directed against K-α 1 tubulin, and collagen-V have been implicated as non-HLA (human leukocyte antigen) targets of antibodies formed following allografts, and more recently anti-perlecan antibodies have been identified as accelerators of obliterative vascular lesions. Clearly, a better understanding of intersections of HLA-related and non-HLA-related mechanisms, and identification of common effector mechanisms would represent an important step towards targeted therapies.

In cases of kidney transplantation, chronic rejection is characterized by slow, progressive renal failure. Histologically, the chronic reaction is accompanied by proliferative inflammatory lesions of the small arteries, thickening of the glomerular basement membrane, and interstitial fibrosis. Because the damage caused by immune injury has already taken place, immunosuppressive therapy at this point is useless, and little can be done to save the graft.

While the preceding example is for kidney transplantation, it is important to point out that the rate, extent, and underlying mechanisms of rejection may vary, depending on the transplanted tissue and site of the transplanted graft. The recipient's circulation, lymphatic drainage, expression of MHC antigens on the graft, and several other factors determine the rejection rate. For example, bone marrow and skin grafts are very sensitive to rejection as compared to heart, kidney, and liver grafts.

ROLE OF MHC MOLECULES IN ALLOGRAFT REJECTION

Antigens that evoke an immune response associated with graft rejection are referred to as *transplantation antigens*, or *histocompatibility antigens*. Indeed, the major histocompatibility complex was so named because of its central role in graft rejection. Why do these molecules serve as the major antigenic targets for the T cells that are ultimately responsible for graft rejection? There are at least two reasons

for this: As discussed in Chapter 9, gene products of the MHC are cell-surface proteins. All nucleated cells express class I MHC molecules whereas class II molecules are normally expressed only on a subset of hematopoietic cells and by thymic stromal cells. Other cell types may also be induced to express class II MHC following their exposure to the proinflammatory cytokine, IFN-γ. In an organ transplantation scenario, when a donor and recipient are MHC disparate (allogeneic), the immune response will be directed predominantly against foreign MHC class I antigens expressed on the cells in the grafted tissue. Furthermore, foreign MHC molecules activate an enormous number of T-cell clones in the recipient. It is estimated that up to 5% of all T-cell clones in the body may be activated in response to alloantigen activation, orders of magnitude higher than the response to other antigens. The combination of nonself MHC molecules plus bound peptides cross-reacts with T-cell receptors (TCRs) expressed on many different T-cell clones. Other mechanisms, discussed below, also contribute to how alloantigens on the transplant are presented to the recipient's T cells.

Mechanisms of Alloantigen Recognition by T Cells

As we discussed in Chapters 9 and 10, the specificity of T cells is normally restricted by self-MHC, the allelic specificity seen in the thymus during T-cell differentiation. Thus, the exposure of an individual to nonself-MHC molecules expressed on the graft represents an artificial but clinically relevant situation.

There are two mechanisms of alloantigen recognition by T cells: direct and indirect. When T cells are exposed to foreign cells expressing nonself MHC (class I or class II), many clones are "tricked" into activation because their TCRs bind to (ligate) the foreign MHC–peptide complex being presented. This *direct mechanism* is presumably due to the recognition of foreign MHC bound to donor-derived peptides. It is important to recall that physiologically, MHC molecules can, and do, normally bind self-peptides. Self-proteins are routinely digested within cytosolic organelles called *proteosomes*, and peptides are delivered to the endoplasmic reticulum where they can bind to MHC class I molecules. Such MHC–self-peptide complexes are believed to stabilize the structure of the MHC molecules and are of no consequence when expressed on the surface of cells in a normal individual because there is tolerance to self-peptides. When foreign peptides are bound to donor MHC molecules expressed by grafted cells, the donor MHC–peptide complex has functional cross-reactivity with the self-MHC–peptide combination and thus activates peptide-specific T cells. Hence, when donor-derived peptides are presented to T cells by antigen presenting cells (APCs) that are "passengers" in the transplanted tissue (donor dendritic cells, in particular), they are recognized as foreign. These passenger APCs

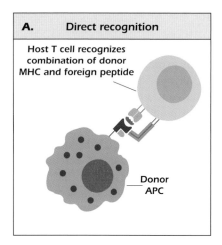
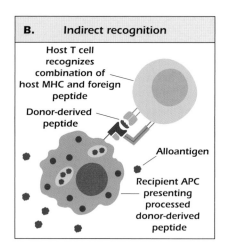

Figure 19.2. Direct and indirect recognition of alloantigens in grafted organs and tissues.

become activated due to the "danger signals" they encounter —unavoidable injurious consequences of organ transplantation. The donor APCs therefore become activated as evidenced by their increased expression of MHC class II molecules, increased expression of T-cell co-stimulatory molecules, and use of chemokine receptors to facilitate their trafficking to host secondary organs. In short, these activated APCs mature to become potent stimulators of host T cells.

The *indirect mechanism* of T-cell alloantigen recognition involves the APCs of the recipient. Host APCs process alloantigenic proteins and present the resulting peptides on self-MHC molecules to T cells expressing TCRs that bind to these foreign epitopes. This is essentially the same process by which epitopes derived from any other foreign protein activate peptide-specific T cells. It is now known that a major source of the donor-derived peptides presented in this direct fashion are the *minor H antigens* encoded by genes outside the MHC. Responses to minor H antigens are generally mediated by CD8⁺ T cells because they are presented by class I MHC molecules. As we will discuss later in this chapter, minor H antigens appear to be important in bone marrow transplantation and have been implicated in graft-versus-host (GVH) disease in cases of HLA-matched bone marrow transplantations.

In short, direct activation of T cells by alloantigens is due to recognition of donor-derived MHC antigens expressed by donor cells serving as APCs. Indirect activation of T cells occurs via recognition of donor-derived cellular peptides (mostly minor H antigens) bound to MHC antigens expressed by host APCs (Figure 19.2). The relative contribution of these two mechanisms to graft rejection is not known. The direct mechanism of alloantigen recognition is believed to be of importance in acute rejection of grafts as discussed earlier in this chapter. The destruction of donor cells, in this case, is therefore directly mediated by T cells. By contrast, indirect alloantigen recognition by T cells also involves activation of host macrophages that cause tissue damage and

fibrosis. Moreover, such activation leads to the development of cytotoxic alloantibody responses, which may also play a role in the destruction of the graft.

ROLE OF T CELL LINEAGES AND CYTOKINES IN ALLOGRAFT REJECTION

Alloactivation of T cells generates both allospecific CD4⁺ and CD8⁺ cells. The cytokines produced are synthesized mainly by activated CD4⁺ T cell clones. The most important cytokines generated are during these responses are IL-2, IFN-α, IFN-β, and IFN-γ, TNF-α, and TNF-β. IL-2 is important for T-cell proliferation, and for differentiation of cytotoxic T lymphocytes (CTLs) and T_H1 cells participating in the delayed-type hypersensitivity reactions associated with allograft rejection. IFN-γ is important for the activation of macrophages, which migrate to the graft area causing tissue damage, and TNF-β is cytotoxic to the cells present in graft. IFN-α, IFN-β, TNF-β, and TNF-α increase the expression of class I molecules, while IFN-γ increases the expression of class II molecules on cells (host and allograft cells), thus increasing the effectiveness of antigen recognition and enhancing graft rejection.

It is now clear that in addition to the roles played by the T_H1 cells, other CD4⁺ T cell lineages also participate in graft rejection (Figure 19.3). As we have discussed in preceding chapters, depending on the microenvironment in peripheral lymphoid organs, helper CD4⁺ T cells differentiate into different types of effector cells that mediate different types of responses. In the presence of IL-12, T_H1 cells dominate and mediate IFN-γ-dependent macrophage activation and delayed-type hypersensitivity; in the presence of IL-4, T_H2 cells mediate IL-5-dependent eosinophilic rejection; in the presence of TGF-β, IL-6, and IL-23, T_H17 cells emerge and are thought to mediate neutrophilic rejection; in the presence of TGF-β alone, Treg cells dominate and promote

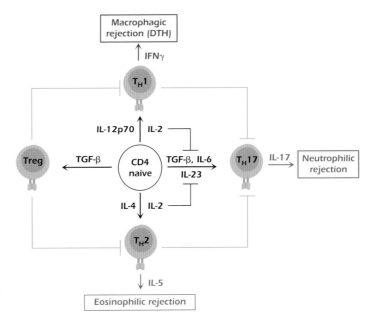

Figure 19.3. Allograft activation of multiple CD4⁺ T cell leading to graft rejection.

allograft acceptance by multiple mechanisms including IL-9-dependent mast-cell recruitment.

LABORATORY TESTS USED IN TISSUE TYPING

In order to minimize the risks of graft rejection, laboratory tests are performed prior to transplantation to determine the MHC phenotypes of both the donor and recipient. These tests are often referred to as *tissue typing*. Tissue typing in humans involves assays that determine HLA allele expression on donor and host cells (usually peripheral blood lymphocytes for convenience). This information is then used to assess the magnitude of MHC parity/disparity between the two individuals. It also serves as a predictive measure for the potential outcome of a transplant procedure. With the advent of highly effective immunosuppressive drugs, attempts to match donor and recipient by the similarity of their HLA antigens is becoming less essential in certain organ transplant settings (e.g., kidney). Nevertheless in many instances—bone marrow transplantation in particular—HLA analyses are critical in order to minimize the occurrence of graft versus host disease.

Historically, HLA typing was conducted using serologic methods. Panels of HLA-specific monoclonal antibodies were used to phenotype the MHC antigens expressed on cells using immunofluorescence methods (Chapter 6). With the advent of the polymerase chain reaction (PCR) in the 1980s, it became possible to perform *molecular typing of donor and recipient*. Genetic variation in the PCR-amplified DNA can then be detected in a number of ways including restriction fragment length polymorphism (RFLP), PCR fingerprinting, sequence analysis, allele specific oligonucleotide typing, and PCR sequence specific primer typing. These highly sensitive methods are far more accurate than serologic typing because they can detect differences on the level of a single amino acid. Indeed, typing at the genomic level has shown differences in instances where complete match has been shown by serologic means.

Assessment of donor and recipient tissue type provides a theoretical evaluation of the suitability of a potential donor. Compatibility is also evaluated in a more direct and immediate manner. The recipient may have a preexisting immune response to donor HLA antigens due to sensitization as a result of pregnancy, blood transfusion, or prior transplantation.

In the case of kidney transplantation, complement-dependent cytotoxicity (CDC) cross-match tests are always carried out to determine whether anti-HLA class I antibodies are present in the serum of the recipient. Lymphocytes from potential donor are used as targets. These cells can be peripheral blood lymphocytes, splenocytes, or lymphocytes from lymph nodes (the latter two in the case of a deceased donor). Cells are mixed with recipient serum at various dilutions in the presence of complement and a vital dye is used to assess cell viability. Cell lysis occurs if specific antibodies are present. The test predominantly measures antibodies against HLA class I. If the test is positive, the transplant is not performed using tissue from the panel of potential donors. If the test is negative, further analysis takes place to determine whether weaker donor-specific class I antibodies or any class II antibodies are present in the serum of the recipient. A so-called cross-match test is used to measure

TABLE 19.2. Cases of Mixed-Lymphocyte Reaction (MLR) Associated with Different Transplantation Situations

Transplantation Situation	HLA Relationship	Treatment of Reacting Leukocytes	MLR
Tissue between identical twins	HLA identical (syngeneic)	No treatment	(−) No reaction
Tissue between nonrelated donor and recipient	HLA different (allogeneic)	No treatment	(+) Reaction intensity depends on the degree of HLA difference between donor and recipient
Tissue between nonrelated donor and recipient	HLA different (allogeneic)	Donor's cells are treated with a mitotic inhibitor, thus testing reactivity of only the recipient cells (performed to test for donor–recipient match)	(+) This is a one-way MLR; reaction intensity depends on the degree of HLA difference between donor and recipient
Bone marrow transplantation, or tissue grafting to an immunoincompetent recipient	HLA different (allogeneic)	Recipient's cells are treated with a mitotic inhibitor, thus testing reactivity of only the donor's cells (performed to avoid GVH reaction)	(+) This is a one-way MLR; reaction intensity depends on the degree of HLA difference between donor and recipient

the presence of donor anti-HLA class I antibodies (reacting against recipient B and T cells) versus the presence of anti-HLA class II antibodies (reacting only against recipient B cells). This is commonly performed using flow cytometric analysis (see Chapter 6). If the cross-match test is positive, the transplant is not performed.

Read the related case: **IgA Nephropathy and Kidney Transplantation**
In *Immunology: Clinical Case Studies and Disease Pathophysiology*

Molecular genotyping of donor and recipient HLA antigens has also eliminated the need to carry out functional assays for tissue typing. In the case of allogeneic stem hematopoietic stem cell transplantation (discussed later in this chapter), the classic approach to functional assessment of HLA compatibility between donor and host cells is the **mixed leukocyte reaction** (MLR). This method is still used in some experimental settings and involves the coculturing of leukocytes from donor and recipient leukocytes for several days. Donor T cells respond to allo-MHC antigens expressed on the recipient cells and are stimulated to produce cytokines and proliferate in the presence of these antigens (see Table 19.2). The same is true for recipient leukocytes, which will proliferate in the presence of alloantigens on the donor cells. The proliferation is usually measured by introducing a radioactively labeled precursor to DNA (e.g., radiolabeled thymidine) into the culture. The greater the extent of proliferation, the more DNA is synthesized by the proliferating cells, and the more radioactivity is incorporated into the cells' DNA.

In most cases, it is essential to ascertain whether the recipient lymphocytes will react against the donor histocompatibility antigen (rather than whether the donor lymphocytes will react against the recipient alloantigens). For this purpose, an MLR is set up as a "one-way MLR" in which the donor cells have been treated with mitomycin C or X-irradiation to prevent their proliferation. In this way, the only cells with the ability to proliferate are the recipient T cells. Under these conditions, recipient CD4+ T cells will proliferate when stimulated with foreign MHC class II molecules. This response will lead to the production of cytokines, which help activate alloreactive cytotoxic CD8+ T. The functional activity of such cells can subsequently be measured in CTL assays cells (see Chapters 6 and 11).

PROLONGATION OF ALLOGRAFT SURVIVAL: IMMUNOSUPPRESIVE THERAPY

A major clinical issue in transplantation immunology is to determine how the components and regulatory interactions involved in graft rejection might be manipulated to allow allograft (or xenograft) acceptance. Nonspecific approaches using immunosuppressive drugs that reduce the overall immunocompence of the recipient to all foreign antigens have been used with success to achieve this goal. However, given the need to treat patients chronically with these drugs to maintain the immunosuppressed state, such individuals are predisposed to opportunistic infections as well as malignancies. Accordingly, chemoprophylaxis using antimicrobial drugs is used in patients undergoing nonspecific, generalized immune suppression to help reduce the incidence of infections. The potential malignancy problem is one that cannot be addressed prophylactically.

More recently, experimental strategies that seek to prevent responses only to the antigens of a particular donor have been investigated. The ultimate goal of this approach is to achieve tolerance, which is lasting and ensures donor-specific nonresponsiveness. As discussed in Chapter 13, there are several mechanisms by which T-cell and B-cell tolerance to self-antigens is achieved. These include clonal deletion, anergy, and suppression. Although clinical trials have begun in which tolerance-inducing strategies are combined with conventional immunosuppressive therapies, none of these strategies have been used to replace such chronic therapy in clinical transplantation.

Currently, immunosuppressive drugs are used for three purposes:

1. *Induction therapy*. Induction therapy is used to suppress the immune system. In circumstances of a scheduled transplant, this may be started before the transplant. For transplant of deceased organs, induction therapy is begun at the time of transplant and continues approximately 2 weeks after transplantation to reduce the incidence of immediate rejection of the graft.

2. *Maintenance therapy*. In order to ensure, over time, that the immune system is kept at bay to facilitate graft survival, combinations of synergistic immunosuppressive drugs are used to interfere with specific immune mechanisms (e.g., T-cell activation). Typically, doses of immunosuppressive drugs used in maintenance therapy are lower than induction therapy to allow the immune system to function (albeit suboptimally) and to minimize the incidence of opportunistic infections.

3. *Specific treatments*. In some cases, episodes of acute rejection may occur months or years after transplantation. Treatment with immunosuppressive drugs are used in these situations and typically at dose levels similar to those used in induction therapy regimens.

Several of the standard and experimental immunosuppressive agents used in transplantation are listed in Table 19.3 and discussed below. Commonly, they are used in various combinations with each other to prevent graft rejection in transplantation of heart, kidney, lungs, pancreatic islet cells, liver, and other organs and tissues.

Anti-Inflammatory Agents

Corticosteroids, such as **prednisone**, **prednisolone**, and **methylprednisolone**, are powerful anti-inflammatory agents. As pharmacologic derivatives of the glucocorticoid family of steroid hormones, their physiologic effects result from their binding to intracellular steroid receptors that are expressed on almost every cell of the body. The immunosuppressive action of corticosteroids is due to several effects, most of which are a consequence of corticosteroid-induced regulation of gene transcription. Corticosteroids downregulate the expression of several genes that code for inflammatory cytokines. These include IL-1, IL-2, IL-3, IL-4, IL-5, IL-8, TNF-α, and GM-CSF. Cortocosteroids also inhibit expression of adhesion molecules causing inhibition of leukocyte migration to sites of inflammation. They therefore inhibit the activity of inflammatory cells. In addition, they promote the release of cellular endonucleases leading to the induction of apoptosis in lymphocytes and eosinophils. Moreover, they reduce phagocytosis and killing by neutrophils and macrophages and reduce expression of MHC class II molecules. In this way, cortocosteroids inhibit T-cell activation and T-cell function.

It is important to acknowledge that despite these beneficial anti-inflammatory effects, corticosteroids also have potent toxic effects including fluid retention, hypertension, weight gain, diabetes mellitus, thinning of the skin, and bone loss. Therefore, the efficacy of corticosteroids in the control of disease involves the judicious use of these agents to strike a careful balance between their beneficial and toxic effects. Given the growing arsenal of immunosuppressive therapies, corticosteroids are often used in combination with other pan-immunosuppressive agents in an effort to keep the dose and toxic side effects to a minimum.

TABLE 19.3. Immunosuppressive Drugs Used in Transplantation

Inhibitors of lymphocyte gene expression	Corticosteroids
	Cyclosporine (Neoral)
	FK-506
Inhibitors of cytokine signal transduction	Anti-CD25
	Rapamycin
	Leflunomide
Inhibitors of nucleotide synthesis	Azathioprine (Imuran)
	Mercaptopurine
	Chlorambucil
	Cyclophosphamide

Cytotoxic Drugs

Antimetabolites that suppress the immune response include the purine antagonists **azathioprine**, **mercaptopurine**, and **mycophenolate mofetil**, which interfere with the synthesis of RNA and DNA by inhibiting inosinic acid, the precursor for the purines adenylic and guandylic acids. **Chlorambucil** and **cyclophosphamide**, compounds that alkylate DNA, also interfere with the metabolism of DNA. These agents were originally developed to treat cancer. The observation that they are also cytotoxic to lymphocytes led to their use as immunosuppressive therapeutic agents. As expected, however, they have a range of toxic effects since they interfere with DNA synthesis in many tissues in the body. Consequently, in addition to their immunosuppressive activity, they can also cause anemia, leukopenia, thrombocytopenia, intestinal damage, and hair loss. Indeed, fatal reactions to these cytotoxic drugs have also been reported. As noted above, the availability of other immunosuppressive agents allows them to be used in combination therapies at lower, less toxic doses.

Agents That Interfere with Cytokine Production and Signaling

A highly effective immunosuppressive therapy strategy involves the use of drugs that interfere with calcineurin—a phosphatase crucial for intracellular events leading to cytokine gene transcription, IL-2 in particular (see Chapter 12). They are commonly used as supplements to immunosuppressive antimetabolite and cytotoxic drugs and include *cyclosporine* and *FK-506* (*tacrolimus*). They exert their pharmacologic effects by binding to immunophilins, a family of intracellular proteins involved with lymphocyte signaling pathways. Upon binding to immunophilins, these agents interfere with signal transduction pathways needed for clonal expansion of lymphocytes.

Cyclosporine is a cyclic peptide derived from a soil fungus (*Tolypocladium inflatum*). When it forms a complex with cytoplasmic receptor, cyclophilin binds to and blocks the phosphatase activity of calcineurin, which is an intracellular signaling protein that is essential for transcriptional activation of the IL-2 gene. It also suppresses production of IL-4 and IFN-γ, as well as the synthesis of IL-2 receptors (CD25). In addition, it is known to induce the synthesis of TGF-β, a cytokine that has immunosuppressive activity. Cyclosporine is effective when administered before transplantation but is ineffective in suppressing ongoing rejection. Evidence indicates cyclosporine is nephrotoxic and is also associated with an increased risk of cancer in patients who take this drug long term. It has been suggested that these and other side effects are largely due to the TGF-β-inducing property of cyclosporine.

FK-506 (tacrolimus) is a macrolide compound obtained from the filamentous bacterium *Streptomyces tsukabaenis*. Macrolides have a multimembered lactone ring to which is attached one or more deoxy sugars. Although its structure is considerably different from that of cyclosporine, its biologic and immunosuppressive activities are similar. FK506 binds to a different cytoplasmic immunophilin (FK506 binding protein). Like cyclosporine, it interferes with T-cell activation by blocking calcineurin activity and the accompanying cytokine production.

Another drug that interferes with cytokine production by T cells is rapamycin (sirolimus). Like FK506, rapamycin is a macrolide compound and is derived from the bacterium *Streptomyces hygroscopicus*. Like cyclosporin and FK-506, it inhibits T-cell activation, but it does so using a different pharmacologic mechanism. Unlike cyclosporin and FK-506, which block calcineurin activity, rapamycin inhibits T-cell activation by blocking signal transduction mediated by IL-2 and other cytokines, not by inhibiting IL-2 production.

Immunosuppressive Antibody Therapy

Antilymphocyte antibody preparations, such as horse antilymphocyte and rabbit anti-thymocyte globulin (ATG), have been used as adjuncts to standard immunosuppressive therapy for many years. While this therapeutic approach can effectively remove unwanted lymphocytes, treatment of humans with large amounts of foreign protein has the disadvantage of inducing a serum sickness caused by the formation of immune complexes (see Chapter 16). Nevertheless, ATG is still used today to prevent acute graft rejection. Clearly, the challenge for those attempting to develop new antibody-based therapies for transplant patients is to develop less immunogenic antibodies while maintaining their targeted effects. To this end, monoclonal antibodies, and engineered mouse–human chimeric antibodies or humanized antibodies are being used (see Chapter 6 for a discussion about these antibodies). The first mouse monoclonal antibody to be used as an immunosuppressive agent in humans was OKT3, which is directed against CD3 expressed on T cells. More recently, two chimeric antibodies (daclizumab and basiliximab) with specificity for the IL-2 receptor α-chain (CD25) have been used. Their molecular effect downregulates expression of the IL-2 receptor on activated T cells—a phenomenon that interferes with the ability of T cells to proliferate in response to IL-2. The advent of engineered antibodies holds great promise in reducing the limitations of alloantibody therapy by minimizing the antigenicity of these proteins.

New Immunosuppressive Strategies and Frontiers

The use of antibodies to several other molecules important for T-cell adhesion (e.g., anti-ICAM-1) and T-cell activation is currently under investigation. Among the latter category of T-cell determinants, a humanized mouse antibody against human CD154 (also known as CD40 ligand) has recently been shown to prevent acute renal allograft rejection in nonhuman primates. Other target pathways include co-stimulatory signaling pathways involving CD28:CD80 (B7.1)/86 (B7.2), CD40:CD154 (CD40L), CD2:LFA-3 and ICAM:LFA-1. As discussed in Chapter 11, binding of CD80/86 to CD28 initiates a cascade of T-cell activation events. As predicted, blocking CD28 ligation interferes with the transmission of signals needed for gene expression and T-cell activation. Thus, antibodies that interfere with co-stimulatory molecule-mediated T-cell activation may have efficacy in transplant patients. It should be noted that a related experimental approach uses the inhibitory ligand, CTLA-4, to suppress the function of these co-stimulatory molecules. Among the newest immunosuppressive biologicals is a *fusion protein* composed of the Fc fragment of a human IgG1 immunoglobulin linked to the extracellular domain of *CTLA-4* (belatacept). Belatacept is now approved by the U.S. Food and Drug Administration (USFDA) to selectively block the process of T-cell activation.

The development of co-stimulation blockers for clinical application in the field of organ transplantation had several setbacks. However, belatacept has recently been approved as first in class for renal transplantation. Several additional co-stimulation blockers are under development with some having already entered into clinical trials. Co-stimulation blockers are a new, emerging class of rationally designed immunosuppressive drugs with considerable potential for improving the outcome of organ transplantation. Additional co-stimulation blockers are under development; some have already entered into clinical trials.

Our knowledge of CD4$^+$ T cell lineages and the cytokines they produce has grown considerably in recent years. The discovery of T$_H$17 T cells that produce a family of IL-17 cytokines (Chapter 12) and the resurgence of interest and investigation of T cells with suppressive activity (Treg cells) have given rise to new hypotheses regarding immune mechanisms for transplant rejections and, by extension, new approaches to prevent rejection (Figure 19.2). For example, it has been suggested that skewing of responses towards T$_H$17 or T$_H$1 and away from Treg cells may be responsible for acute rejection of organ transplants. Blocking key cytokines *in vivo*, most notably IL-6, may result in a shift from T$_H$17 toward a regulatory phenotype (Treg) to help prevent transplant rejection.

It should be clear from the above that several experimental approaches are being taken with the hope of finding immunosuppressive agents that will be less toxic and will not leave the recipient helpless to opportunistic infections in the absence of a fully competent immune response. However, it should be stated that in spite of all the experimental approaches mentioned above, the main agents that are most commonly used for clinical immunosuppression are corticosteroids, cyclosporin, FK506, and azathioprine.

HEMATOPOIETIC STEM CELL TRANSPLANTATION

Transplantation of hematopoietic stem cells constitutes a special transplantation situation because it is performed mostly between an immunocompetent donor and an immunocompromised recipient. Historically, the procedure involved the use of bone marrow as a source of hematopoietic stem cells, but today, a peripheral blood is a more common source of these cells for use in hematopoietic stem-cell transplantation (HCT).

HCT is used to treat a variety of conditions including severe combined immunodeficiency disease (SCID), Wiskott–Aldrich syndrome (see Chapter 18), or some acute leukemias. It is also used to treat blood cell diseases such as thalassemia and sickle cell diseases, in which a mutant gene is inherited. The mutant gene expresses itself only in the blood-forming hematopoietic cells. In these patients, transplantation of hematopoietic stem cells is a form of genetic therapy: the genetically abnormal blood-forming stem cells are replaced with normally functioning cells.

The ultimate goal of HCT is to restore or reconstitute normal hematopoiesis of the recipient. Hematopoietic stem cells give rise to all blood cell lineages (Chapter 2). Small numbers of these pluripotent cells also circulate in the blood. This finding, together with our knowledge regarding the cytokines that control the proliferation and differentiation of hematopoietic stem cells (granulocyte-colony-stimulating factors [G-CSF]), has given rise to the clinical use of G-CSF to increase the numbers of hematopoietic stem cells both in the marrow and blood. The quantitation of these cells is facilitated by their unique expression of CD34. When G-CSF is administered to individuals, it induces myeloid precursor cells to differentiate into mature neutrophils. Neutrophils produce proteases that are able to cleave the proteins that, under normal circumstances, anchor CD34$^+$ cells to the bone marrow microenvironment. Thus, CD34$^+$ hematopoietic stem cells are mobilized to enter the periphery where sufficiently large quantities of cells can be recovered for use in HCT. Given the efficacy and convenience of this procedure, peripheral blood from G-CSF–treated individuals is therefore increasingly used as a source of hematopoietic stem cells.

The two most common types of HCT are *allogeneic* and *autologous* HCT. In rare cases, transplantation is performed between identical twins (syngeneic transplantation). Syngeneic stem cell transplantation is associated with a relatively low immunologic risk because of the genetic similarity between donor and recipient. Autologous HCT is an important therapy, although, strictly speaking, it is not transplantation; rather, it is a technique of obtaining stem cells from blood or marrow and returning them to the same individual. Therefore, immunologic transplantation barriers do not exist. This procedure is commonly used to treat patients with hematological malignancies such as leukemia, lymphoma, or myeloma. The stem cells are recovered from the bone marrow or blood and stored frozen (cryopreserved) while the patient is intensively treated with chemotherapy and/or irradiation to control the malignancy and to markedly decrease the malignant cells in marrow and blood. Finally, the autologous stem cells are infused into the patient so that blood cell production can be restored.

Allogeneic HCT has most commonly been used to treat hematologic malignancies, where it is often the only potentially curative option available. The success of HCT has been limited by transplant-associated toxicities related to the conditioning regimens used and to the common immunologic consequence of donor T-cell recognition of recipient alloantigens, graft-versus-host disease (GVHD), discussed below. The frequency and severity of GVHD observed when extensive HLA barriers are transgressed have essentially precluded the routine use of extensively HLA-mismatched HCTs. Allogeneic HCT also has potential as an approach to organ allograft tolerance induction, but this potential has not been previously realized because of the toxicity associated with traditional conditioning.

Allogeneic HCT involves the use of donor cells obtained from blood, bone marrow, or umbilical cord and placental blood sources where the concentration and growth of blood-cell-forming stem cells is even greater than in the blood of adults. Unlike autologous HCT where there is no risk of immune reactivity to the infused cells, in allogeneic HCT, two potential immune rejection outcomes may result: The donor stem cells and the hematopoietic cells to which they give rise may be rejected by the recipient (host-versus-graft effect) or an immune reaction to host MHC antigens may occur (GVHD). When immunocompetent recipients are used, immune rejection by host T cells is usually prevented by intensive immunosuppressive therapy of the recipient before the transplant is performed. This approach is also used in patients with malignancies to destroy the rapidly dividing cancer cells (induction therapy) followed by HCT. Patients with immunodeficiency diseases (e.g., SCID) do not require such induction therapy since there is no risk of rejection by the host. To reduce this risk of GVHD, T cells are rigorously eliminated from the donor-cell population. This removal, which can be achieved by a number of methods (e.g., treatment with monoclonal anti-T-cell antibodies and complement), widens the choice of bone marrow donors.

GRAFT-VERSUS-HOST DISEASE

HCT from a donor to an HLA-disparate recipient results in a reaction mounted by the grafted T cells against the recipient's MHC (and/or minor H) antigens. This response manifests as *graft-versus-host disease* (GVHD). GVHD occurs when immunocompetent lymphoid cells are transplanted into individuals who are immunologically compromised (e.g., following high-dose radiation therapy or chemotherapy). GVHD can be either acute or chronic. Acute GVHD is responsible for 15–40% of mortality and is the major cause of morbidity after allogeneic HCT, whereas chronic GVHD occurs in up to 50% of patients who survive 3 months after HCT.

Two important principles help to explain the pathophysiology of acute GVHD. First, it represents an exaggerated but "normal" inflammatory response against foreign antigens (the ubiquitous host alloantigens, in this case). Second, donor lymphocytes encounter tissues in the recipient that have often been profoundly damaged due to the underlying disease of the host or pre-HCT therapy regimens such as radiation or chemotherapy.

In humans, GVHD may produce splenomegaly (enlarged spleen), hepatomegaly (enlarged liver), lymphadenopathy (enlarged lymph nodes), diarrhea, anemia, weight loss, and other disorders in which the underlying causes are inflammation and destruction of tissue. GVHD is initiated by donor-derived T cells that recognize the recipient's MHC antigens (and minor H antigens) as foreign. Standard procedures are used to eliminate virtually all mature T cells from the donor hematopoietic stem sell source, but over time, the pluripotent stem cells will give rise to donor-derived T cells. Interestingly, most of the innate inflammatory cells that participate in the destruction of host cells in GVHD are host cells recruited to the site of the reaction by cytokines (mainly TNF-α and IL-1) released by activated donor participating in the GVH reaction. Unless the reaction is controlled, GVHD activates destructive immune defense mechanisms carried out by donor- and host-derived cells that may lead to the death of the recipient. GVHD can be modulated and controlled using a variety of immunosuppressive agents. Calcineurin inhibitors such as cyclosporine or tacrolimus, with short-course methotrexate, have become the standard immunosuppressive regimen for allogeneic HCT.

On the other hand, efforts have been made to harness some of the graft anti-host activity for an antileukemic effect. This requires a balance between the beneficial versus detrimental effects of donor T cells.

XENOGENEIC TRANSPLANTATION

It is estimated that more than 50,000 people who need organ transplants die each year while waiting for a compatible donor. To address the critical shortage of donated human organs for transplantation, studies are under way in the use of nonhuman organs. For ethical and practical reasons, species closely related to the human, such as the chimpanzee, have not been widely used. Attention has focused on the pig; some of the pig's organs are anatomically similar to those of humans. Interestingly, the human T-cell response to xenogeneic MHC antigens is not as strong as to allogeneic MHC molecules.

The major problem with using pig organs, and organs from other species, in human recipients, however, is the existence of natural or preformed antibodies to carbohydrate moieties expressed on the graft's endothelial cells. As a consequence, the activation of the complement cascade occurs rapidly, and hyperacute rejection ensues. Finally, another concern that has stimulated debate about the safe use of xenografts concerns the possibility that animal organs and tissues may harbor viruses that might infect humans. This fear is underscored by the possibility that the HIV pandemic may have been caused by the transmission of a virus from monkeys to humans. In the United States, the Centers for Disease Control and Prevention and other public health agencies have drafted guidelines to monitor patients who receive xenografts using sensitive assays to detect viruses that may be present.

THE FETUS: A TOLERATED ALLOGRAFT

A puzzling phenomenon associated with allograft rejection is that the fetus, which expresses paternal histocompatibility antigens that are not expressed by the mother, is not rejected by the mother as an allograft. It is clear that the mother can mount an antibody response against fetal antigen, as exemplified by anti-Rh antibodies produced by Rh⁻ mothers. More importantly, women who experienced multiple births have antibodies to the father's MHC antigens. It appears, however, that in most cases the antibodies are harmless to the fetus, and what is important is the mother's ability or, rather, inability, to respond with the production of cytotoxic T cells against the fetus. There is evidence that fetal trophoblast cells that constitute the outer layer of the placenta that come in contact with maternal tissue do not express polymorphic MHC class I or class II molecules but express only the nonpolymorphic class Ib MHC molecule, HLA-G. Thus, the fetal trophoblast does not prime for a cellular immune response associated with allograft rejection.

It has been suggested that the major function of HLA-G is to provide a ligand for the killer-cell inhibitory receptors (KIRs) on maternal natural killer (NK) cells, thus preventing them from killing the fetal cells (see Chapter 2). HLA-G is also expressed in thymic medullary epithelium, where it might ensure T-cell tolerance to this molecule. Finally, no cells expressing large amounts of MHC class II molecules (e.g., dendritic cells) have been found in the placenta.

Other factors that affect the immune response and may be involved in the fetal–maternal relationship include cytokines, complement inhibitory proteins, and other as yet unknown factors. Another factor that appears to operate in the survival of the fetus, is α-fetoprotein, a protein synthesized in the yolk sac and fetal liver. α-Fetoprotein has been demonstrated to have immunosuppressive properties. All in all, the fetus and several other tissues in the body that do not initiate an immune response or are not affected by immune components are termed *immunologically privileged sites*. Overall, it appears that multiple factors are responsible for one of the most spectacular immunologically privileged sites: the fetus. Increased knowledge of the immunologic mechanisms responsible for tolerance to the fetus might provide new insights for how we might induce tolerance to grafted cells, tissues, and organs.

SUMMARY

1. Alloreactive T cells are principally responsible for allograft rejection. Alloantigen-specific antibodies are responsible for hyperacute rejection and acute humoral rejection. They can also participate in other types of rejection.

2. The most important transplantation antigens, which cause rapid rejection of the allograft, are derived from the donor major histocompatibility complex (MHC), which is called HLA in humans and H-2 in mice. Genetic differences between donor and host can also result in allogeneic cellular peptides (minor H antigens) being presented by host MHC molecules to T cells. Reactions to these allogeneic proteins can also lead to graft rejection.

3. Two mechanisms for host T-cell alloantigen recognition are known to exist: (1) direct activation of T cells by alloantigens is due to recognition of donor-derived MHC antigens expressed by donor cells serving as APCs; (2) indirect activation of T cells occurs via recognition of donor-derived cellular peptides (mostly minor H antigens) bound to MHC antigens expressed by host APCs.

4. The degree of histocompatibility between donor and recipient can be determined by serologic or, more commonly, molecular tissue typing. MLR assays are also used to assess the MHC compatibility of donor and recipient for hematopoietic stem-cell transplantation.

5. Survival of allografts is prolonged using a cocktail of immunosuppressive agents including anti-inflammatory agents, cytotoxic agents, antimetabolites, and using agents that interfere with IL-2 production and cytokine-mediated signaling. Newer modalities include the use of biologic agents that target co-stimulatory molecules associated with T-cell activation.

6. The fetus is a natural allograft that is tolerated. Multiple factors appear to be involved in this form of tolerance including the absence of MHC class I and II molecules on fetal trophoblast cells, and the "absence" of MHC class II expression on placental cells.

REFERENCES AND BIBLIOGRAPHY

Afzali B, Lombardi G, Lechter RI, Lord GM. (2007) The role of T helper 17 (Th17) and regulatory T cells (Treg) in human organ transplantation and autoimmune disease. *Clinical Exp Immunol* 148: 32.

Alegre ML, Florquin S, Goldman M. (2007) Cellular mechanisms underlying acute graft rejection: time for reassessment. *Curr Opin Immunol* 19: 563.

Auchincloss H Jr, Sachs D. (1998) Xenogeneic transplantation. *Annu Rev Immunol* 16: 433.

Auchincloss H Jr, Sykes M, Sachs D. (1998) Transplantation immunology. In: Paul WE (ed.) *Fundamental Immunology, 4th Ed*. New York: Lippincott-Raven.

Beniaminovitz A, Itescu S, Lietz K, Donovan M, Burk EM, Groff BD, Edward N, Mancini DM. (2000) Prevention of rejection in cardiac transplantation by blockade of the interleukin-2 receptor with a monoclonal antibody. *N Engl J Med* 342: 613.

Charlton B, Auchincloss H Jr, Fathman CG. (1994) Mechanisms of transplantation tolerance. *Annu Rev Immunol* 12: 707.

Devetten M, Armitage JO. (2007) Hematopoietic cell transplantation: progress and obstacles. *Ann Oncol* 18: 1450.

Dragun D, Catar R, Philippe A. (2013) Non-HLA antibodies in solid organ transplantation: recent concepts and clinical relevance. *Curr Opin Organ Transplant* 18(4): 430.

Ferrara JLM, Deeq HJ. (1991) Graft versus host disease. *N Engl J Med* 324: 667.

Hunt JS. (1992) Immunobiology of pregnancy. *Curr Opin Immunol* 4: 591.

Joudeh A, Saliba KA, Topping KA, Sis B. (2013) Pathologic basis of antibody-mediated organ transplant rejection: from pathogenesis to diagnosis. *Curr Opin Organ Transplant* 18(4): 478.

Kirk, AD. (1999) Treatment with humanized monoclonal antibody against CD154 prevents acute renal allograft rejection in nonhuman primates. *Nat Med* 5: 686.

LaRosa DF, Rahman AH, Turka L. (2007) The innate immune system in allograft rejection and tolerance. *J Immunology* 178: 7503.

Nash RA, Antin JH, Karanes C. (2000) Phase 3 study comparing methotrexate and tacrolimus with methotrexate and cyclosporine for prophylaxis of acute graft-versus-host disease after marrow transplantation from unrelated donors. *Blood* 96: 2062.

Pilat N, Schwarz C, Wekerle T. (2012) Modulating T-cell costimulation as new immunosuppressive concept in organ transplantation. *Curr Opin Organ Transplant* 17(4): 368.

Schreiber SL, Crabtree GR. (1992) The mechanism of action of cyclosporin A and FK-506. *Immunol Today* 13: 136.

Strober S, Spitzer TR, Lowsky R, Sykes M. (2011) Translational studies in hematopoietic cell transplantation: treatment of hematologic malignancies as a stepping stone to tolerance induction. *Semin Immunol* 23(4): 273.

Sun Y, Tawara, I, Toubai, T. (2007) Pathophysiology of acute graft-versus-host disease: recent advances. *Transl Res* 150: 197.

REVIEW QUESTIONS

For each question, choose the ONE BEST answer or completion.

1. In clinical transplantation, preformed cytotoxic antibodies reactive against MHC antigens expressed on the grafted tissue cause:
   A) chronic rejection
   B) hyperacute rejection
   C) acute rejection
   D) delayed-type hypersensitivity
   E) no serious problems

2. Following transplantation of a solid organ, skewing an immune response in a direction that promotes activation of T_H1 and T_H17 T cells would be expected to:
   A) help prevent rejection of allografts
   B) minimize progression of autoimmune diseases
   C) promote allograft rejection
   D) promote antibody responses
   E) induce regulatory T cells

3. Which of the following is a pathophysiologic mechanism for activation of donor APCs in individuals who have received organ transplants?

A) their exposure to damaged cells in the recipient
B) generation of antibodies against donor MHC antigens by host B cells
C) failure of regulatory T cells in the recipient to suppress APC activation
D) polyclonal activation of recipient T cells
E) production of IL-4 by T_H2 cells

4. Transplant rejection may involve
   A) cell-mediated immunity
   B) activation of T_H17 cells
   C) complement-dependent cytotoxicity
   D) the release of IFN-γ by alloreactive T_H1 cells
   E) all of the statements are correct

5. Molecular HLA genotyping of peripheral blood lymphocytes from an individual in need of a kidney transplant donor confirms the expression of the following alleles: HLA-A1, -A3; HLA-B7, -B8; HLA-DR3 -DR4. What would be the most likely outcome of a renal transplant performed in this individual using a donor with the following HLA genotype: HLA-A1, A1; HLA-B8, -B22; HLA-DR3, -DR4?

A) The graft would be accepted with no need for immunosuppressive therapy.

B) The graft would undergo hyperacute rejection.

C) The graft would be rejected even if immunosuppressive therapy were used.

D) The graft would be accepted if maintenance immunosuppressive therapy were used.

6. A clinical trial investigating the efficacy of a humanized anti-CD28 monoclonal antibody in prolonging kidney allograft survival shows that patients treated with this biologic reagent have significantly fewer episodes of chronic rejection. The probable mechanism responsible for this effect is best explained by

A) the binding of anti-CD28 to B cells, which blocks their interaction with CD80 (B7.1) and CD86 (B7.2) expressed on T cells

B) the formation of circulating CD28–anti-CD28 immune complexes

C) the binding of anti-CD28 to T cells, which interferes with signal transduction needed for T-cell activation

D) the binding of anti-CD28 to suppressor T cells, which then become activated

E) the binding of anti-CD28 to B and T cells, which interferes with signal transduction and activation of both populations

ANSWERS TO REVIEW QUESTIONS

1. _B._ Hyperacute rejection is caused by preformed cytotoxic, complement-fixing antibodies that cause platelet activation and deposition causing swelling and hemorrhage in the transplanted tissue. This occurs minutes to hours following transplantation and quickly leads to a decrease in the flow of blood through the tissue and ultimate rejection of the graft. Choices **A**, **C**, and **D** are T-cell mediated; therefore they are incorrect. Choice **E** is wrong for obvious reasons.

2. _C._ T_H1 and T_H17 cells produce proinflammatory cytokines. Therefore, skewing immune responses to activate these cells would promote allograft rejection. Skewing the response in the Treg direction would be expected to promote allograft survival.

3. _A._ Activation of donor APCs present in the allograft tissue as "passenger APCs" is mediated, in large part, by their exposure to disease-related or radiation- or chemotherapy-induced damaged host cells.

4. _E._ All are correct. The important process in the rejection of an allotransplant is cell-mediated immunity. Here, T cells, which recognize the alloantigens, become activated; the T cells release

cytokines, one of which is IFN-γ, which recruits and activates phagocytic cells that, together with cytotoxic T cells, destroy the graft. However, the reaction to the allotransplant may also involve antibodies (IgM and IgG), which can cause damage to tissue via activation of complement and the recruitment of polymorphonuclear cells to the site of the reaction. The polymorphonuclear cells would damage the graft by the release of their lysosomal enzymes.

5. _D._ The only mismatched HLA allele between the donor and recipient is seen with regard to HLA-B22 expressed by the donor. All other HLA alleles are matched. Thus, with appropriate maintenance immunosuppressive therapy, the engrafted kidney would most likely survive long term.

6. _C._ Experimental models have demonstrated that injection of allografted mice with anti-CD28 monoclonal antibody does, indeed, prolong survival of the allograft. Blocking CD28 ligation interferes with the transmission of signals needed for gene expression (e.g., IL-2 synthesis) and T-cell activation. B7.1 and B7.2 are co-stimulatory molecules expressed on antigen-presenting cells that ligate CD28 leading to T-cell activation.

20

TUMOR IMMUNOLOGY

INTRODUCTION

Immune responses against tumor cells occur, in large part, because of expression of cell-surface components on malignant cells that do not occur with their normal counterparts and that are recognized as antigenic molecules. Experimental evidence for this phenomenon came from studies in mice, which showed that when tumor cells were injected subcutaneously into syngeneic (major histocompatibility complex [MHC]-matched) mice, the cells formed nodules that grew for a few days and then regressed. When identical tumor cells were reinjected into the mice, they did not produce nodules or grow. These findings were interpreted to mean that the mice that rejected the tumor did so because they had generated an immune response to the tumor. Subsequently, ***tumor-specific transplantation antigens*** (TSTAs), or as they are more commonly called, ***tumor antigens***, have been demonstrated for many tumors in a variety of animal species, including humans.

The major focus of this chapter concerns the role of the immune system in tumor-cell destruction. It is believed that throughout life, tumor cells are generated in normal individuals and then destroyed by normal immune effector mechanisms, without notice or consequence. Obviously, these immunological mechanisms are not always successful. The hope is that our growing knowledge of host defense mechanisms and the phenomenon of ***immunosurveillance*** will provide new insights into how we might prevent and better treat cancer. The two major goals of tumor immunology are (1) to elucidate the immunologic relationship

between the host and the tumor, and (2) to utilize the immune response to tumors for the purpose of diagnosis, prophylaxis, and therapy. We discuss various approaches to meeting these goals in this chapter.

TUMOR ANTIGENS

Advances in immunologic and molecular biologic methodology have greatly facilitated the identification of tumor antigens capable of eliciting immune reactions. Before defining the different categories of tumor antigens, it is important to underscore the principal biologic mechanisms that may lead to the appearance of immunogenic tumor antigens including ***mutation***, ***gene activation***, and ***clonal amplification***. Like normal immune responses to foreign antigens, the immunogenic potential of tumor antigens is manifested when their expression stimulates immune effector mechanisms. The antigenic prerequisites that apply to foreign immunogens also apply to tumor antigens. As discussed in Chapter 4, a substance must possess the following characteristics in order to be immunogenic: (a) foreignness, (b) high molecular weight, (c) chemical complexity, and (d) degradability with the ability to interact with host MHC antigens. Immunogenic tumor antigens fulfill these criteria and thus have the potential to induce immune responses. Nonimmunogenic tumor antigens, on the other hand, are in many cases self-antigens to which some degree of tolerance exists. This poses major barriers to both *de novo* and vaccine-induced tumor immunity. Efforts to overcome these barriers

Immunology: A Short Course, Seventh Edition. Richard Coico and Geoffrey Sunshine.
© 2015 John Wiley & Sons, Ltd. Published 2015 by John Wiley & Sons, Ltd.
Companion Website: www.wileyimmunology.com/coico

include the use of peptides derived from self-antigens expressed on tumor cells that are engineered to contain altered amino acids in order to increase the immunogenicity of the tumor antigen.

Some tumor antigens consist of structures that are unique to the cancerous cells and are not present on their normal counterparts. Other tumor antigens may represent structures that are common to both malignant and normal cells but are masked on the normal cells and become unmasked on malignant cells. Still other antigens on malignant cells represent structures that are present on fetal or embryonic cells but disappear from normal adult cells. These latter antigens are referred to as *oncofetal antigens*. Some tumor antigens expressed on tumor cells represent structures that are qualitatively not different from those found on normal cells, but that are overexpressed and thus present at significantly higher levels on the cancer cell. These are typically products of *oncogenes*. An example of the latter is the high level of *human epidermal growth factor receptor* (HER) expression in certain breast and ovarian cancers due to overexpression of the *HER-2/neu-1* oncogene. Another example is the elevated *ras* oncogene products present on some human prostate cancer cells. In each of these different cases, the structural features of the tumor antigens arising by these various mechanisms are often similar from individual to individual. This similarity has sometimes translated to therapeutic advances in the treatment of cancer since commonly expressed tumor antigens can serve as targets for immune-based therapy (e.g., monoclonal antibodies against HER-2 to treat individuals with breast and ovarian cancer). Finally, oncogenic retroviruses (e.g., human T-cell leukemia virus) that can transform normal cells into cancer cells also induce tumor cell antigens that exhibit extensive structural similarity.

Normal genes that were previously silent may also be activated by *carcinogens*. It is generally assumed that unique tumor antigens on tumors induced by carcinogens are products of mutated genes with hot spots for mutations. There is little or no cross-reactivity between carcinogen-induced tumors. This absence of cross-reactivity is probably due to the random mutations induced by the chemical or physical carcinogens, leading to a large array of different antigens. For example, if the chemical carcinogen methylcholanthrene is applied in an identical manner to the skin of two genetically identical animals, or on two similar sites on the same individual, the cells of the developing tumors (sarcomas, in this case) will exhibit antigens unique to each tumor, with no immunologic cross-reactivity between the tumors. As with chemically induced tumors, there is little or no cross-reactivity among physically induced tumors, such as those induced by ultraviolet light or by X-irradiation. Carcinogens can also be responsible for conversion of an otherwise nonimmunogenic molecule to an immunogenic antigen together with clonal amplification of cells expressing these molecules. The carcinogen-induced

transformation event(s) that cause the emergence of such expanded clones most likely affect the genes that possess mutation-sensitive hot spots while sparing the genes responsible for other normal proteins. When these normal proteins are clonotypic (i.e., only expressed by single clones of cells), their expression is dramatically amplified, therefore making them immunogenic, assuming tolerance can be broken. As an example, the idiotypes of antigen-specific receptors expressed by B or T cells may not be on sufficiently numerous cells to elicit a response in the normal host but may serve as target antigens on lymphoid tumor cells bearing the same idiotype.

The following two sections provide overviews of the various categories and examples of tumor antigens and the immune effector mechanisms that play a role in preventing tumor cell development. Our expanding knowledge of these areas of tumor immunology continues to facilitate the development of clinically useful tumor-specific immonotherapies.

CATEGORIES OF TUMOR ANTIGENS

Tumor antigens may be classified into several major categories (Table 20.1). The categories differ in both the factors that induce the malignancy and the immunochemical properties of the tumor antigens.

Normal Cellular Gene Products

Some tumor antigens are derived from normal genes that, under normal circumstances, are programmed to be expressed only during embryogenesis, namely, *oncofetal antigens*. Examples of these tumor antigens include the *melanoma-associated antigen* (MAGE) family of proteins that is not expressed in any normal adult tissues except for the testes (an immunologically privileged site). MAGE proteins are candidate tumor vaccine antigens because their expression is shared by many melanomas. Another category of oncofetal antigens is the group of cancer testes (CT) antigens. These are encoded by genes that are normally expressed only in the human germline but are also expressed in various tumor types, including melanoma, and carcinomas of the bladder, lung, and liver. Indeed, like many other tumor-associated antigens, the MHC restriction elements of the antigenic epitopes have been identified for both MAGE-1 and CT antigens. This information is being exploited in experiments aimed at developing immunogenic tumor peptide vaccines that can be presented by class I MHC antigens on antigen-presenting cells (APCs) to activate cytotoxic (CD8$^+$) T cell responses.

Other examples of oncofetal antigens include the *carcinoembryonic antigen* (CEA) and *α-fetoprotein* (AFP). CEA is found primarily in serum of patients with cancers of the gastrointestinal tract, especially cancer of the colon.

TABLE 20.1. Categories of Tumor Antigens

Category		Type of Antigen	Name of Antigen	Types of Cancer
Normal cellular gene products	Embryonic	Oncofetal antigens	MAGE-1	Several
			MAGE-2	Several
			CEA	Lung, pancreas, breast, colon, stomach
			AFP	Liver; melanoma; carcinoma of bladder, lung, liver, and testes
	Differentiation	Normal intracellular enzymes	Prostate-specific antigen	Prostate
			Tyrosinase	Melanoma
		Oncoprotein	HER-2/neu	Breast, ovary
		Carbohydrate	T-cell leukemia/ lymphoma 1 oncoprotein	B-cell malignancies
	Clonal amplification	Immunoglobulin idiotype	Specific antibody of B-cell clone	Lymphoma
Mutant cellular gene products	Point mutations	Oncogene product	Mutant Ras proteins	Several
		Suppressor gene product	Mutant p53	Several
		CDK	Mutant CDK-4	Melanoma
Viral gene products	Transforming viral gene	Nuclear proteins	E6 and E7 proteins of HPV	Cervical

Elevated levels of CEA have also been detected in the circulation of patients with some types of lung cancer, pancreatic cancer, and some types of breast and stomach cancer. However, it should be noted that elevated levels of CEA have also been detected in the circulation of patients with nonneoplastic diseases, such as emphysema, ulcerative colitis, and pancreatitis, as well as in the sera of alcoholics and heavy smokers. AFP, which is normally present at high concentrations in fetal and maternal serum but absent from serum of normal individuals, is rapidly secreted by cells of a variety of cancers and is found particularly in patients with hepatomas and testicular teratocarcinomas.

Finally, amplified clones of malignant B or T cells that express antigen-specific receptors represent yet another example of how normal cellular gene products can be characterized as tumor antigens. The idiotype of the particular immunoglobulin or T-cell receptor (TCR) expressed by the transformed B or T cell, respectively, effectively identifies that clone as a unique population of malignant cells.

Mutant Cellular Gene Products

The genetic origins of several tumor antigens that are products of mutated genes have been identified. In every case, these antigens were the result of a somatic mutation (i.e., by a genetic change absent from autologous normal DNA). Often, these mutations occur in genes that encode functionally important parts of the expressed protein. There are

several well-characterized examples of tumor antigens that are derived from mutant cellular gene products. **Chronic myelogenous leukemia** (CML) is characterized by the **Philadelphia chromosome**, a shortened chromosome 22 resulting from a reciprocal translocation between the *bcr* gene on chromosome 22 and the *abl* gene on chromosome 9 [t(9;22)]. The molecular equivalent of t(9;22) can be detected in virtually all cases of CML. It manifests with the expression of a *bcr/abl* fusion gene that encodes chimeric RNAs that produces copious amounts of the *abl* gene tyrosine kinase activity. This chimeric gene product, appears, at least in part, to be responsible for uncontrolled cell proliferation. In 2001, the U.S. Food and Drug Administration approved the use of the first Bcr-Abl tyrosine kinase inhibitor (TKI), namely, imatinib. Bcr-Abl tyrosine kinase TKIs are now the first-line therapy for most patients with CML.

Another example of a mutant cellular gene product is seen in many cases of familial melanoma. This disease is associated with a mutation in **cyclin-dependent kinase-4** (CDK-4) that reduces binding to its inhibitor (p16INK-4), which happens to be a tumor-suppressor protein. Yet another example of a tumor antigen that is generated as a result of a mutant cellular gene is the mutant **p53 protein**. The p53 mutation generates common conformational changes in p53 protein that normally acts as a suppressor of cellular growth. Mutations in *p53* are among the most common seen in tumors of human and experimental animals. They typically occur in evolutionarily conserved regions of the *p53* gene and result in overexpression of the protein, which then

TABLE 20.2. Activation of Cellular Proto-Oncogenes in Human Cancers

Proto-Oncogene	Activation Mechanism	Chromosomal Change	Associated Cancer
c-*myc*	Genetic rearrangement	Translocation: 8:14, 8:2, or 8:22	Burkitt lymphoma
c-*abl*	Genetic rearrangement	Translocation: 9–22	CML
c-*H-ras*	Point mutation		Bladder carcinoma
c-*K-ras*	Point mutation		Lung and colon carcinoma
N-*myc*	Gene amplification		Neuroblastoma

serves as an immunogenic antigen for autologous B and T cells. Antibody and T-cell responses are also seen when mutations occur in *ras* oncogene-encoded proteins. Mutant ras proteins, resulting from a glycine substitution at position 12 of *ras*, represent one of the most common mutations in human cancers.

The potential use of mutated gene products as immunologic targets for immune-based therapies is best illustrated by experimental evidence showing that tumor immunity *in vivo* can be induced against normal p53 by mutant p53 peptides if administered to animals together with IL-12 to promote T-cell responses toward a T_H1 phenotype. Because p53 is commonly overexpressed in cancer cells, the cytotoxic T-cell responses generated can destroy tumor cells. Furthermore, p53 knockout mice can be induced to generate cytotoxic T cells specific for normal p53 that, on adoptive transfer into p53 wild-type mice, can eradicate tumors overexpressing p53 without causing autoimmunity in the host.

Tumor Antigens Encoded by Oncogenes

Although a full discussion of carcinogenesis is beyond the scope of this chapter, it is important to summarize the **oncogene theory** in order to better understand the properties of certain oncogene-derived proteins that can be tumor antigens. All retroviral oncogenes are known to have close relatives in the genomes of virtually all normal vertebrate cells called *c-onc* genes or **proto-oncogenes**. The gene products of proto-oncogenes have been identified as proteins with known functions in normal cells, including growth factor receptors and signal transducers, to name a few. The oncogene theory postulates that when such proto-oncogenes are mutated or activated by other aberrant mechanisms, they overexpress or inappropriately express the mutated forms of their gene products, thereby contributing to neoplastic transformation and the development of cancer. Oncogenes are aberrantly activated in somatic cells in many forms of human cancer, including carcinoma and sarcomas, which include leukemias and lymphomas. The chief mechanisms of activation are chromosomal translocation, point mutation, and gene amplification. Table 20.2 gives a partial list of the known proto-oncogenes and their associated cancers.

Animal studies have shown that tumors induced by oncogenic viruses exhibit extensive immunologic cross-reactivity. This is because any particular oncogenic virus induces the expression of the same antigens in a tumor, regardless of the tissue of origin or the animal species. For example, in animals, DNA viruses such as polyoma, SV40, and Shope papilloma virus induce tumors that exhibit extensive cross-reactivity within each virus group. Many leukemogenic viruses, such as Rauscher leukemia virus, induce the formation of tumors that exhibit cross-reactivity not only within each virus group but also between some groups. There is considerable evidence to suggest that several human cancers, such as Burkitt lymphoma, hepatocellular carcinoma, and nasopharyngeal carcinoma are caused by viruses. Adult T-cell leukemia is known to be caused by infection with human T-cell lymphotropic virus type 1 (HTLV-1).

As might be expected, the viral proteins, which ultimately serve as tumor antigens, are expressed intracellularly as predominantly nuclear proteins. In order for cytotoxic T lymphocytes (CTLs) to recognize these antigens, they must be processed and presented as class I MHC-associated peptides. Studies using SV40-specific CTL have confirmed that these cells can recognize processed fragments of proteins that are primarily located intracellularly. The unique tumor antigens of cells transformed by SV40 and several other viruses, including polyoma virus, adenovirus, and human papilloma virus (HPV) have been studied extensively and, in many cases, shown to be clearly related to the transformed phenotype and the establishment of malignancy. Such viruses have so-called **early region genes** designated *E1A/E1B* and *E6/E7*, which are transcribed during early stages of viral replication and in transformed cells by adenovirus and human papilloma virus, respectively. Like other categories of tumor antigens, these proteins are candidate targets for therapy.

IMMUNOLOGIC FACTORS INFLUENCING THE INCIDENCE OF CANCER

In the late 1950s, a hypothesis emerged to help explain the primary reason for development of T-cell–mediated immunity during the evolution of vertebrates. It was proposed that the main function of this arm of the immune system was to provide specific defense against altered self or neoplastic cells. The term *immunosurveillance* was coined to describe the concept of immunologic resistance against the development of cancer. However, there is growing recognition that immunosurveillance represents only one dimension of the complex relationship between the immune system and cancer. The concept of immunosurveillance is well supported by immunocompromised animal studies and epidemiologic studies of patients with various immunodeficiencies (primary, secondary, or acquired) that correlate an increased incidence of cancer but only with regard to cancers associated with viruses or, in some cases, UV exposure. By contrast, most common forms of cancer are not increased in immunocompromised individuals. However, patients with immunodeficiency diseases are usually susceptible to viral infections and certain malignant neoplasms (Table 20.3).

The absence of immunosurveillance of spontaneous cancers or those induced by carcinogens does not imply that such tumors do not express immunogenic tumor antigens. Indeed, there is sufficient evidence to support the conclusion that these tumor cells, like those induced by viruses, are sensitive to immunologic destruction. Nevertheless, the natural development of tumor-specific immune responses sometimes fails to prevent cancer from developing. Indeed, recent work has shown that the immune system may also promote the emergence of primary tumors with reduced immunogenicity that are capable of escaping immune recognition and destruction. This finding prompted the development of the cancer *immunoediting hypothesis* to more broadly encompass the potential host-protective and tumor-sculpting functions of the immune system throughout tumor development. Cancer immunoediting is a dynamic process composed of three phases: (1) elimination, (2) equilibrium, and (3) escape (Figure 20.1). In the first phase of elimination, cells and molecules of the innate and adaptive immune systems, which comprise the cancer immunosurveillance network, may eradicate the developing tumor and protect the host from tumor formation. However, if this process is not successful, the tumor cells may either enter the equilibrium phase where they may be maintained chronically or immunologically sculpted by immune "editors" to produce new populations of tumor-cell variants. These variants may eventually evade the immune system by a variety of mechanisms and become clinically detectable in the escape phase.

Elimination represents the classical concept of cancer immunosurveillance; equilibrium is the period of immune-mediated latency after incomplete tumor destruction in the elimination phase, and escape refers to the final outgrowth of tumors that have outstripped immunological restraints of the equilibrium phase.

Even at early stages of tumorigenesis, these cells may express distinct tumor-specific markers and generate proinflammatory "danger" signals that initiate the cancer immunoediting process (Figure 20.1). In the first phase of elimination, cells and molecules of innate and adaptive immunity, which comprise the cancer immunosurveillance network, may eradicate the developing tumor and protect the host from tumor formation. However, if this process is not successful, the tumor cells may enter the equilibrium phase where they may be either maintained chronically or immunologically sculpted by immune "editors" to produce new populations of tumor variants. These variants may eventually evade the immune system by a variety of mechanisms and become clinically detectable in the escape phase.

EFFECTOR MECHANISMS IN TUMOR IMMUNITY

Until recently, most of the information concerning tumor antigen-specific immune effector mechanisms and their capacity to destroy tumor cells has been derived from experiments with transplantable tumors in animals or from *in vitro* experiments. There is now ample evidence to suggest that adaptive and innate immune responses play important roles in the relationship between the host and the tumor in humans as well.

Immune effector mechanisms that are potentially capable of destroying tumors *in vitro* are summarized in Table 20.4. In general, destruction of tumor cells by these mechanisms is more efficient in the case of dispersed tumors (i.e., when the target tumor cells exist as single cells) than in the case of solid tumors, probably because dispersed cells are more accessible to immune action.

The character and magnitude of an immune response to tumor antigens depend on the context of antigen

TABLE 20.3. Malignant Neoplasms with an Increased Incidence in Immunodeficiency Patients

Type of Immunodeficiency	Cancer	Associated Virus[a]
Primary (congenital)	Hepatocellular carcinoma	HBV
	B-cell lymphoma	EBV
Secondary (e.g., drug-induced)	B-cell lymphoma	EBV
	Squamous cell carcinoma (skin)	HPV
	Hepatocellular carcinoma	HBV
	Cervical carcinoma	HPV
AIDS	Hepatocellular carcinoma	HBV
	Cloagenic or oral carcinoma	HPV
	B-cell lymphoma	EBV

[a]HBV, hepatitis B virus; EBV, Epstein–Barr virus; HPV, human papilloma virus

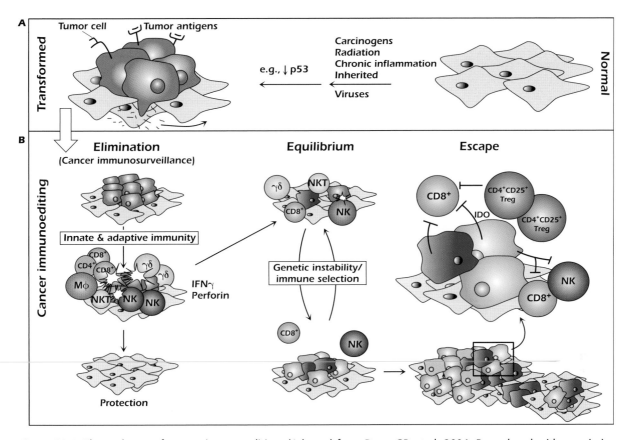

Figure 20.1. Three phases of cancer immunoediting. (Adapted from Dunn GP et al. 2004. Reproduced with permission of Elsevier.)

TABLE 20.4. Effector Mechanisms in Cancer Immunity

Effector Mechanism	Comments
Antibodies and B cells (complement-mediated lysis, opsonization)	Role in tumor immunity poorly understood
T cells (cytolysis, apoptosis)	Critical for rejection of virally and chemically induced tumors
NK cells (cytolysis, ADCC, apoptosis)	Tumor cells not expressing one of the MHC class I alleles are effectively rejected by NK cells
LAK cells (cytolysis, apoptosis)	Antitumor responses seen in certain human cancers following adoptive transfer of LAK cells
Macrophages and neutrophils (cytostasis, cytolysis, phagocytosis)	Can be activated by bacterial products to destroy or inhibit tumor cell growth
Cytokines (apoptosis, recruitment of inflammatory cells)	Growth inhibition can occur using adoptively transferred tumor cells transfected with certain cytokines (e.g., GM-CSF)

presentation. In normal immune responses, when dendritic cells (DCs) acting as APCs encounter certain "danger signals" resulting from cellular damage or invasion by a pathogen (e.g., double-stranded RNA), they are activated and mature to produce cytokines that promote differentiation of $CD4^+$ T_H0 cells to T_H1 cells (Chapter 12). Such DC activation therefore promotes cell-mediated immune responses. Alternatively, when DCs are activated such that they polarize T_H0 cells toward a T_H2 phenotype, antibody responses are facilitated. Both types of immune responses can theoretically participate in the destruction of tumor cells. However, many therapeutic immune-based strategies are aimed at promoting cell-mediated responses since tumor cell destruction by CTLs is the major goal.

B-Cell Responses to Tumors

Both IgM and IgG antibodies have been shown to destroy tumor cells *in vitro* in the presence of complement. Several studies conducted with mice indicate that antitumor antibodies are effective *in vivo* in destroying some leukemia and lymphoma cells and in reducing metastases in several other tumor systems. Other studies *in vivo* and *in vitro*, however, show that the same antibodies, in the presence of complement, are ineffective in destroying the cells of the same tumor in a solid form.

Destruction of Tumor Cells by Opsonization and Phagocytosis

Destruction of tumor cells by phagocytic cells has been demonstrated *in vitro*, but only in the presence of antitumor immune serum and complement. The relevance of this finding *in vivo* is unknown.

Antibody-Mediated Loss of Adhesive Properties of Tumor Cells

Metastatic activity of certain kinds of tumors requires the adhesion of the tumor cells to each other and to the surrounding tissue. Antibodies directed against tumor-cell surfaces may interfere with the adhesive properties of the tumor cells. The relevance of this mechanism *in vivo* is also unknown.

CELL-MEDIATED RESPONSES TO TUMOR CELLS

Destruction of Tumor Cells by T Lymphocytes

Destruction of tumor cells *in vitro* by tumor antigen-specific T cells has been demonstrated numerous times for a variety of tumors, both dispersed and solid. Moreover, from many studies with experimental animals (primarily but not exclusively mice), there is good evidence that tumor-specific, cytotoxic T cells are responsible for destruction of virally induced tumors *in vivo*. As discussed below, certain cytokines are essential players in antitumor responses mediated by CTLs including IFN-γ and TNF-α. CD4⁺ helper T cells also play a major role in the induction, regulation, and maintenance of such CTLs.

Antibody-Dependent Cell-Mediated Cytotoxicity

Antibody-dependent cell-mediated cytotoxicity (ADCC) involves (1) the binding of tumor-specific antibodies to the surface of the tumor cells; (2) the interaction of various cells, such as granulocytes and macrophages, which possess surface receptors for the Fc portion of the antibody attached to the tumor cell; and (3) the destruction of the tumor cells by substances that are released from these cells that carry receptors for the Fc portion of the antibody. The importance of this mechanism in the destruction of tumor cells *in vivo* is still not clear.

Destruction of Tumor by NK Cells, NK/T Cells, and Cytokine-Activated Killer Cells

As we have discussed in earlier chapters, natural killer (NK) cells are a lymphoid population representing the 10–20% of peripheral blood mononuclear cells, able to lyse MHC class

I-negative tumor and virus-infected cells. The majority of NK cells is localized in peripheral blood, lymph nodes, spleen, and bone marrow but can be induced to migrate toward sites of inflammation by different chemoattractants including chemokines.

NK cells have receptors for the Fc region of IgG (CD16) and, as we have seen in Chapters 5 and 16, can participate in ADCC. Like activated macrophages, NK cells secrete TNF-α that induces hemorrhage and tumor necrosis; however, the exact mechanism by which NK cells recognize and kill the tumor cells is still not clear. More recently, evidence has been obtained indicating that NK/T cells are another innate immune cell population that is essential for tumor elimination *in vivo* (see Chapter 11).

Cytokine-activated killer cells (historically and currently called **lymphokine-activated killer** [LAK] cells) are tumor-specific killer cells obtained from the patient. They have been used with minimal success to treat patients with solid tumors; newer strategies using T cells isolated from the tumor called **tumor-infiltrating lymphocytes** (TILs) and then adoptively transferred to patients are showing some therapeutic promise.

Destruction of Tumor Cells by Activated Macrophages and Neutrophils

Macrophages and neutrophils are generally not cytotoxic to tumor cells *in vitro*. They can be activated by bacterial products *in vitro* to cause selective cytostasis or cytolysis of malignant cells. Macrophages may also become highly cytotoxic (Figures 20.2 and 20.3) when they are activated by cytokines, most notably IFN-γ produced by an activated population of T lymphocytes, which, by themselves, are not cytotoxic.

These CD4⁺ T cells are tumor specific: they release IFN-γ after activation by tumor antigen. Other cytokines released by these antigen-activated T lymphocytes attract macrophages to the area of the antigen. IFN-γ also prevents migration of macrophages away from the antigen. The mechanism of activation of macrophages by T cells specific for tumor antigen, leading to destruction of tumor cells, is similar to mechanisms involved in delayed-type hypersensitivity reactions in allograft rejection or in the killing of microorganisms: Antigen-specific T cells become activated by antigen, and they release cytokines, which attract and activate macrophages. These activated macrophages are cytotoxic to the microorganism, to tumor cells, and even to "self" cells in the vicinity of the activated macrophages. The damaging and killing activity of activated macrophages is due to several products that they release, notably lysosomal enzymes and TNF-α. Mounting evidence indicates that destruction of tumor cells by activated macrophages occurs *in vivo*. For example, resistance to a tumor can be abolished by specific depletion of macrophages. In addition, increased resistance to tumors accompanies an increase in the number of activated macrophages. Finally, activated macrophages are frequently found at the site of regression of a tumor. However, the relationship between the tumor and the tumor-associated macrophages is quite complex. On one hand, macrophages can and indeed do kill tumor cells. In addition, macrophages and tumor cells have been shown to produce reciprocal growth factors, leading to an almost symbiotic relationship. Thus, changes in the delicate balance between macrophages and tumor cells may drastically affect the fate of the tumor.

CYTOKINES

As discussed above, cytokines can have a variety of ancillary functions that facilitate immune effector mechanisms in cancer immunity. It is important to note that depending on the cytokines produced, immune effector mechanisms may be stimulated or inhibited. Consequently, the result may either be stimulation or inhibition of the growth of premalignant or malignant cells by acquired and/or innate immunity. The growth-promoting effect of cytokines is seen in the case of certain tumor cells that produce and respond to cytokines in an autocrine fashion. Similarly, production of TGF-β by some tumor cells promotes tumor growth due to the angiogenic and immunosuppressive properties of this cytokine.

Cytokines such as TNF-α and IFN-γ have antitumor effects because, among other functions, they upregulate MHC class I and class II antigens on some tumor cells. Decreased expression of these antigens allows tumor cells to evade the actions of cytotoxic T cells. Cytokine upregulation of MHC antigens thereby facilitates important cell-mediated effector mechanisms. The effects of sustained high levels of certain cytokines have been studied using tumor cells transfected with cytokine genes. Transfection with genes coding for cytokines IL-1, IL-2, IL-7, IL-12, GM-CSF, or IFN-γ followed by adoptive transfer of such cells into tumor-bearing mice has been shown to significantly inhibit the growth of tumors. GM-CSF and IL-12 are commonly used as preclinical and clinical tumor vaccines.

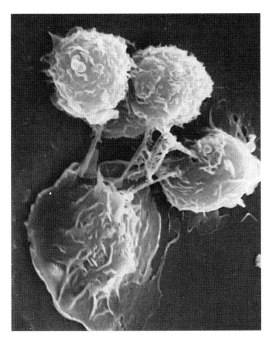

Figure 20.2. A scanning electron micrograph showing an activated macrophage with filopodia extending to the surface of three melanoma cells (×4,500). (Photograph courtesy of Dr. K.L. Erickson, School of Medicine, University of California, Davis.)

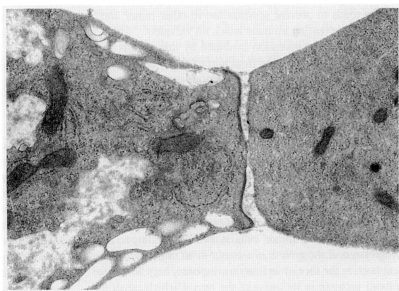

Figure 20.3. The kiss of death. An electron micrograph showing a contact point between an activated macrophage (left) and a melanoma cell after 18 hours of coculture leading to cytolysis of the melanoma target cell. Flocculent material is found between the cells; a dense plate is associated with the cell membranes of the macrophage process; microtubules also appear in these projections (×26,000). (Photograph courtesy of Dr. K.L. Erickson, School of Medicine, University of California, Davis.)

occur preexposure to the virus. Second-generation vaccines are under development and focus on future immunization strategies that may offer protection post-HPV exposure.

Other tumor antigens that have been molecularly characterized have also been used in concert with viral vectors (e.g., vaccinia) to actively vaccinate the host. Active immunization has also been studied by injection of naked DNA plasmid constructs (**DNA vaccines**) with the goal of having the unique tumor antigen encoded and expressed by muscle cells. In some studies, the genes encoding cytokines (e.g., GM-CSF) or immune-enhancing cytokines such as IL-2 and IL-12 are also introduced to improve the presentation of the tumor antigen by DCs at the site of injection.

Immunization strategies focused on oncogenic virus is also expected to provide prophylaxis against other virus-associated cancers. Experimentally, this approach has been successful in the protection of chickens against Marek's disease, and a significant degree of protection against feline leukemia and feline sarcoma has been achieved by immunizing cats with the respective oncogenic viruses. Immunization against the tumor itself requires that the tumor possess specific antigens and that these antigens cross-react immunologically with any prepared vaccine. There are literally thousands of reports of effective immunization against transplantable animal tumors, using as immunogens: (1) sublethal doses of live tumor cells, (2) tumor cells in which replication has been blocked, (3) tumor cells with enzymatically or chemically modified surface membranes, and (4) extracts of antigens from the surface of tumor cells, either unmodified or chemically modified. Despite these reported successes in the protection of experimental animals against transplantable tumors, the efficacy of immunoprophylaxis for protection of humans and animals against spontaneous tumors has not been sufficiently evaluated. This lack of complete study relates to the need for appropriate immunogens and the danger of inducing the production of immunologic elements that may, in fact, enhance metastasis, and thus be detrimental to the host.

IMMUNOTHERAPY

Immunotherapy encompasses a variety of interventions and techniques with the common goal of eliciting tumor-cell destructive immune responses. Numerous attempts have been made to treat cancers in animals and humans by immunologic means. Currently, a wide range of immunotherapeutic strategies are in use (see Figure 20.4). **Tumor-specific monoclonal antibodies** can mediate cytolysis either by engaging NK cells via Fc receptors (ADCC), or by complement activation. Rituximab (anti-CD20) is the first monoclonal antibody approved by the U.S. FDA for the treatment of B-cell lymphomas. Randomized studies have demonstrated its activity when combined with chemotherapy in follicular lymphoma, mantle cell lymphoma, and diffuse large B-cell lymphoma in untreated or relapsing patients. Because of its high activity and low toxicity ratio, rituximab has transformed the prognosis of patients with B-cell lymphoma who are treated with this biological drug.

Xenogeneic chimeric antibodies (e.g., mouse anti-human monoclonal antibodies) that have been molecularly engineered using recombinant DNA technology to humanize their constant regions (see Chapter 6) are now being used as antibody therapeutics in cancer. A growing number of antibodies have been approved by the U.S. FDA for various oncology indications (Table 20.6), and many more are being evaluated in clinical trials. Antibodies for the treatment of hematologic cancers such as chronic lymphocytic leukemia and non-Hodgkin lymphoma, and antibodies to B-cell associated target molecules (e.g., CD52, CD20, CD30) are

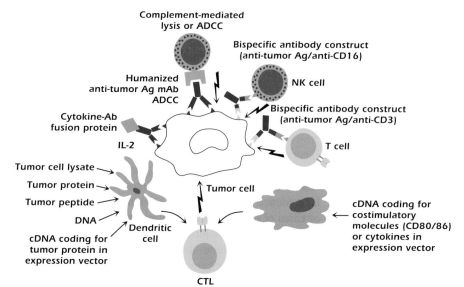

Figure 20.4. Current strategies in experimental immunotherapy.

effective, in part, because of their ability to induce apoptosis after binding to B-cell tumors. ***Bispecific antibody*** constructs designed to bring immune effector cells into contact with tumor cells and to simultaneously stimulate the cytotoxic activity of effector cells are also under investigation. Examples include antibodies that recognize unique tumor antigens and IgG Fc receptors (CD16) to activate NK cells. Similarly, bispecific antibody constructs containing Fabs specific for tumor antigens and CD3 have also been studied. A relatively new approach involves the creation of recombinant fusion proteins consisting of antitumor antibodies and cytokines (***immunocytokines***). Such fusion proteins are designed to concentrate cytokine-mediated immune effector functions at the tumor site. Several approaches are designed to stimulate or bolster the function of tumor-specific CTLs. CTLs can be activated against tumor antigens by tumor cells rendered immunologic by expression of either co-stimulatory molecules such as CD80/CD86 or cytokines. A highly effective method for stimulating tumor-specific CTLs involves the presentation of MHC class I tumor antigen peptides by ***dendritic cells***. These extremely efficient APCs normally express high levels of cell surface co-stimulatory molecules, therefore enhancing their ability to present tumor antigens to effector T cells (see Chapters 9 and 10). Dendritic cells are either directly loaded with peptides or exposed to tumor cell lysates, tumor proteins, or transfection of tumor-derived cDNA in an expression vector. They are then adoptively transferred to the tumor-bearing host in hope of activating cytotoxic T cells to kill the tumor cells.

Antibody–drug conjugates are those joined to a chemotherapy drug, radioactive particle, or a toxin. These antibodies work, at least in part, by acting as homing devices to take these substances directly to the cancer cells. Several antibody–drug conjugates have been approved for clinical use. For example, a modified version of a monoclonal antibody that targets HER2 (trastuzumab; see Table 20.6), which is overexpressed on certain breast and gastric tumors, enables a form of targeted chemotherapy.

Immunostimulatory monoclonal antibodies, and in particular anti-CTLA-4, have also been used together with tumor vaccines to potentiate antitumor responses. CTLA-4 (CD152) is a negative regulator of T-cell responses (see Chapter 11) and therefore can restrict antitumor immune responses. Monoclonal anti-CTLA-4 (ipilimumab) is a fully human, monoclonal anti-CTLA-4 antibody that overcomes CTLA-4-mediated T-cell suppression to enhance the immune response against tumors. Another immunostimulant that acts similarly to monoclonal anti-CTLA-4 antibody is a monoclonal antibody that recognizes programmed death receptor 1 (PD-1; CD279, see Chapter 11). PD-1 is produced by dying T cells. PD-1 interaction with its ligands, PD-L1 (CD274) and PD-L2 (CD273), is one of the many strategies that tumors employ to escape immune surveillance. Upon the binding of PD-Ls to PD-1, TCR signaling is dampened, causing inhibition of proliferation, decreased cytokine production, anergy, and/or apoptosis. Thus PD-L expression by tumor cells serves as a protective mechanism, leading to suppression of tumor-infiltrating lymphocytes in the tumor microenvironment. Anti-PD-1 antibody therapy results in significant increase of antigen-specific immune responses in the periphery and CD8 T-cell infiltration into the tumor.

Given the successful utility of monoclonal antibodies to treat cancer, these biologic therapeutics have a promising future. The use of antibody therapeutics in combination with each other is also emerging. Such combinations may reduce or eliminate the amount of cytotoxic chemotherapy, which is still the mainstay of most oncology treatments. New delivery platforms, new approaches to antibody–drug conjugates and strategies to manipulate the immune response (discussed below) are on the horizon and have the potential for transforming the way cancer patients are effectively treated in the future.

Other Immunotherapeutic Strategies in Cancer

In addition to the growing arsenal of antibody therapeutics in cancer, immunotherapy of human malignancies has also been aimed at the augmentation of specific anticancer immunity, utilizing nonspecific enhancement of the immune response. In particular, stimulation of macrophages, using ***BCG*** (bacille Calmette–Guerin) or *Corynebacterium parvum* has been successfully used in some cases. One example is the use of BCG for treating patients with residual superficial urinary bladder cancer. Repeated instillation of live mycobacteria into the bladder by way of catheter after surgery has become the treatment of choice for superficial bladder cancer.

Trials are also in progress on the effects of ***various cytokines***, such as IFN-α, β, and γ; IL-1, IL-2, IL-4, IL-5, IL-12; tumor necrosis factor; and others either singly or in combination on tumor regression. To date, these trials are mostly inconclusive. The clinical use of LAK cells and TILs has also been applied to the treatment of cancer with variable results. LAK cells are produced *in vitro* by cultivation of the patient's own peripheral lymphocytes with IL-2. Upon reinfusion into the patient, dramatic improvement has been recorded in a number of cases. In the latter case, a documented success has been reported using TIL adoptively transferred to patients with melanoma. These lymphocytes— removed from a tumor biopsy, expanded *in vitro* with IL-2 and returned to the tumor-bearing individual—have an antitumor activity many times higher than LAK cells; thus less is needed for therapy.

Finally, encouraging results using genetically engineered T cells in so-called ***chimeric antigen receptor therapy*** (CAR therapy) are emerging. This personalized treatment involves genetically modifying a patient's T cells to make them target tumor cells. CAR therapy is now the focus of numerous clinical trials.

TABLE 20.6. Antibodies Therapies and Their Indications

Antibody Type	Target	Tumor Types	Dx test	Indication
Cetuximab (Erbitux; Bristol-Myers Squibb): chimeric human-murine IgG1	EGFR	Colon, head, and neck	Yes	Indicated for the treatment of KRAS wild type, EGFR-expressing, metastatic colorectal cancer (mCRC) in combination with FOLFIRI [irinotecan, 5-fluorouracil (5-FU)] In combination with radiation therapy for the initial treatment of locally or regionally advanced squamous cell carcinoma of the head and neck and in combination with platinum-based therapy 5-FU As a single agent, is indicated for the treatment of patients with recurrent or metastatic squamous cell carcinoma of the head and neck for whom prior platinum-based therapy has failed.
Panitumumab (Vectibix; Amgen): human IgG1	EGFR	Colon	Yes	Indicated for the treatment of mCRC with disease progression after fluoropyrimidine-, oxaliplatin-, and iriotecan-containing regimens.
Trastuzumab (Herceptin; Genentech): humanized IgG1	HER2	Breast, gastric	Yes	Indicated for the adjuvant treatment of HER-2 overexpressing node-positive or node-negative breast cancer. In combination with cisplation and capecitabine or 5-FU, for the treatment of patients with HER-2 overexpressing metastatic gastric or gastroesophageal junction adenocarcinoma, who have not received prior treatment for metastatic disease.
Bevacizumab (Avastin; Genentech/Roche): humanized IgG1	VEGF	Colon, non-small cell lung, glioblastoma, kidney	No	mCRC for first- or second-line treatment in combination with intravenous 5-FU-based chemotherapy. Advanced nonsquamous non-small cell lung cancer combination with carboplatin and paclitaxel in people who have not received chemotherapy for their advanced disease. Metastatic kidney cancer when used with IFN-α. Glioblastoma when taken alone in adult patients whose cancer has progressed after prior treatment.
Ipilimumab (Yervoy; Bristol-Myers Squibb): IgG1	CTLA4	Melanoma	Yes	
Rituximab (Rituxan/ Mabthera; Roche): chimeric human-murine IgG1	CD20	Non-Hodgkin lymphoma, chronic lymphocytic leukemia	No	As a single agent, in patients with relapsed or refractory, low grade or follicular, CD20-positive, B-cell non-Hodgkin lymphoma (NHL). Previously untreated and previously treated CD20-positive chronic lymphocytic leukemia in combination with fludarabine and cyclophosphamide.
Ofatumumab (Arzea; Genmab): human IgG1	CD20	Chronic lymphocytic leukemia	No	As a single agent for the treatment of patients with chronic lymphocytic leukemia refractory to fludarabine and alemtuzumab.
Y-labeled ibritumomab tiuxetan (Zevalin; IDEC Pharmaceuticals): murine IgG1, linker-chelator; tiuxetan (N-(2 Bis(carboxymethyl)amino)-3(Pisothio-cyanatophenyl)-propyl)- N-(2 Bis(car-boxymethyl)-amino-2-(Methyl) ethyl)glycine	CD20	Low-grade or follicular B-cell NHL	Yes	Treatment of B-cell NHL (relapsed or refractory, low-grade, follicular, transformed or rituximab-refractory). Patients with previously untreated follicular NHL who achieve a partial or complete response to first-line chemotherapy.

TABLE 20.6. *Continued*

Antibody Type	Target	Tumor Types	Dx test	Indication
l-labeled tositumomab (Bexxar; GlaxoSmithKline): murine lgG2, direct covalent linkage to tositumomab	CD20	Low-grade or follicular B-cell NHL	Yes	Treatment of patients with CD20-positive relapsed or refractory, low-grade, follicular or transformed NHL who have progressed during or after rituximab therapy, including patients with rituximab-refractory NHL.
Alemtuzumab (Campath; Genzyme): humanized lgG1	CD52	Chronic lymphocytic leukemia	No	As a single agent for the treatment of B-cell chronic lymphocytic leukemia.
Brentuximab vedotin (Adcetris; Seattle Genetics): chimeric lgG1, MMAE, maleimidocaproyl valine-citruline-PAB linker	CD30	Hodgkin lymphoma	No	For the treatment of patients with Hodgkin's lymphoma after failure or autologous stem-cell transplant (ASCT) or after failure of at least two prior multiagent chemotherapy regimes in patients who are not ASCT candidates.

Our growing understanding of cancer and of the immune system continues to fuel the development of new immunotherapeutic strategies. In all cases, such strategies must be evaluated in preclinical models for their potential usefulness. The great promise that the immune system can be exploited for the treatment and prevention of cancer must be tempered by the few examples of documented efficacy that have emerged. Nevertheless, given the rapid advances in biotechnology and the molecular identification of human tumor antigens, we are entering a new era of cancer immunotherapy. At the present time, we can say with certainty that tumor immunology has clearly yielded significant improvements in the diagnosis of cancer, and it is likely that immune-based diagnostic methods will continue to offer useful new ways to detect tumor cells and monitor their growth.

SUMMARY

1. Tumor immunology deals with (a) the immunologic aspects of the host–tumor relationship and (b) the utilization of the immune response for diagnosis, prophylaxis, and treatment of cancer.

2. Tumor antigens induced by carcinogens do not cross-react immunologically. On the other hand, extensive cross-reactivity is exhibited with virally induced tumor antigens. Several types of tumors produce oncofetal substances, which are normally present during embryonic development.

3. The immune response to tumors involves both humoral and cellular responses. Destruction of tumor cells may be achieved by (a) antibodies and complement; (b) phagocytes; (c) loss of the adhesive properties of tumor cells caused by antibodies; (d) cytotoxic and helper T lymphocytes; (e) antibody-dependent cell-mediated cytotoxicity (ADCC); and (f) activated macrophages, neutrophils, NK cells, NK/T cells, and LAK cells.

4. The role of the immune response to tumors appears to be important in the host–tumor relationship, as indicated by increased incidence of tumors in immunosuppressed hosts and by the presence of immune components at sites of tumor regression. However, the immune response to a tumor may not be effective in eliminating the tumor because of a variety of tumor- and host-related mechanisms.

5. Immunodiagnosis may be directed toward the detection of tumor antigens or the host's immune response to the tumor.

6. Immunoprophylaxis may be directed against oncogenic viruses or against the tumor itself.

7. Immunotherapy of malignancy employs various preparations for the augmentation of tumor-specific as well as nonspecific immune responses. Approaches include (a) active immunization; (b) passive therapy with antibodies; (c) antibody–drug conjugates, which is antibody joined to a chemotherapy drug, radioactive particle, or a toxin; (d) local application of live bacterial vaccines (BCG); (e) use of cytokines; and (f) adoptive transfer of effector cells.

REFERENCES AND BIBLIOGRAPHY

Bui JD, Schreiober RD. (2007) Cancer immunosurveillance, immunoediting and inflammation: independent or interdependent processes? *Curr Opin Immunol* 19: 203.

Coiffier B. (2007) Rituximab therapy in malignant lymphoma. *Oncogene* 26: 3603.

Dunn GP, Old, LJ, Schreiber RD. (2004) The immunobiology of cancer immunosurveillance and immunoediting. *Immunity* 21: 137.

Haupt K, Roggendorf M, Mann K. (2002) The potential of DNA vaccination against tumor-associated antigens for antitumor therapy. *Exp Biol Med* 227: 227.

Herrera L, Stanciu-Herrera C, Morgan C, Ghetie V, Vitetta ES. (2006) Anti-CD19 immunotoxin enhances the activity of chemotherapy in severe combined immunodeficient mice with human pre-B acute lymphoblastic leukemia. *Leuk Lymphoma* 47: 2380.

Jager E, Chen YT, Drifhout JW. (1998) Simultaneous humoral and cellular immune response against cancer-testis antigen NY-ESO-1: definition of human histocompatibility leukocyte antigen (HLA)-A2-binding peptide epitopes. *J Exp Med* 187: 265.

June C, Rosenberg SA, Sadelain M, Weber JS. (2012) T-cell therapy at the threshold. *Nat Biotechnol* 30: 611.

Ljunggren HG, Malmberg KJ. (2007) Prospects for the use of NK cells in immunotherapy of human cancer. *Nat Rev Immunol* 7: 329.

Meklat F, Li W, Wang Z, Zhang Y, Zhang J, Jewell A, Lim SH. (2007) Cancer-testis antigens in haematological malignancies. *Br J Haematol* 136: 769.

Melief CJ, Offringa R, Toes RE, Kast WM. (1996) Peptide-based cancer vaccines. *Curr Opin Immunol* 8: 651.

Mkrtichyan M, Chong N, Abu Eid R, Wallecha A, Singh R, Rothman J, Khleif SN. (2013) Anti-PD-1 antibody significantly increases therapeutic efficacy of *Listeria monocytogenes (Lm)*-LLO immunotherapy. *J Immunother Cancer* 1: 15.

Noguchi Y, Richards EC, Chen YT, Old LJ. (1995) Influence of interleukin-12 on p53 peptide vaccination against established Meth A sarcoma. *Proc Natl Acad Sci USA* 92: 2219.

Ottmann OG, Druker BJ, Sawers CL, Goldman JM, et al. (2002) A phase two study of imatinib in patients with relapsed or refractory Philadelphia chromosome-positive acute lymphoid leukemias. *Blood* 15: 1965.

Rosenberg SA. (1999) A new era for cancer immunotherapy based on the genes that encode cancer antigens. *Immunity* 10: 281.

Schmitt A, Hus I, Schmitt M. (2007) Dendritic cell vaccines for leukemia patients. *Expert Rev Anticancer Ther* 7: 275.

Sliwkowski MX, Mellman I. (2013) Antibody therapeutics in cancer. *Science* 341: 1192.

Tan TT, Coussens LM. (2007) Humoral immunity, inflammation and cancer. *Curr Opin Immunol* 19: 209.

Weng J, Rawal S, Chu F, Park HJ, Sharma R, Delgado DA, Fayad L, Fanale M, Romaguera J, Luong A, Kwak LW, Neelapu SS. (2012) TCL1: a shared tumor- associated antigen for immunotherapy against B-cell lymphomas. *Blood* 120: 1613.

Wever, J. (2002) Peptide vaccines for cancer. *Cancer Invest* 20: 208.

REVIEW QUESTIONS

For each question, choose the ONE BEST answer or completion.

1. Impairments in which of the following immune mechanisms is associated with the appearance of many primary lymphoreticular tumors in humans?
   A) humoral immunity
   B) NK cell activity
   C) NK/T cell activity
   D) neutrophil function
   E) cell-mediated immunity

2. Tumor antigens have been shown to cross-react immunologically in cases of
   A) tumors induced by chemical carcinogens
   B) tumors induced by RNA viruses
   C) all tumors
   D) tumors induced by irradiation with ultraviolet light
   E) tumors induced by the same chemical carcinogen on two separate sites on the same individual

3. Which of the following is not considered a mechanism by which cytokines mediate antitumor effects?

   A) They enhance the expression of MHC class I molecules.
   B) They activate tumor-infiltrating lymphocytes (TILs).
   C) They have direct antitumor activity.
   D) They induce complement-mediated cytolysis.
   E) They increase activity of cytotoxic T cells, macrophages, and NK cells.

4. Rejection of a tumor may involve which of the following?
   A) T-cell–mediated cytotoxicity
   B) ADCC
   C) complement-dependent cytotoxicity
   D) destruction of tumor cells by phagocytic cells
   E) all are correct

5. Which of the following best defines immunotoxins?
   A) toxic substances released by macrophages
   B) cytokines
   C) toxins completed with the corresponding antitoxins
   D) toxins coupled to antigen-specific immunoglobulins
   E) toxins released by cytotoxic T cells

6. It has been shown that a B-cell lymphoma could be eliminated with anti-idiotypic antibodies. The use of this approach to treat a plasma cell tumor would not be warranted because
   A) plasma cell tumors have no tumor-specific antigens
   B) plasma cell tumors are not expected to be susceptible to ADCC
   C) plasma cell tumors can be killed *in vivo* only by cytotoxic T lymphocytes that bear the same A, B, and C transplantation antigens
   D) the plasma cells do not have surface Ig
   E) the idiotype on the plasma-cell surface is different from that on the B-cell surface

7. Monoclonal antibodies used in hematologic malignancies such as chronic lymphocytic leukemia act, in part, because of their ability to
   A) directly lyse tumor target cells
   B) activate Treg cells
   C) induce apoptosis after binding B-cell tumors
   D) promote antibody-dependent cell-mediated cytotoxicity
   E) reduce microenvironment vascularization

ANSWERS TO REVIEW QUESTIONS

1. *E.* There is a nearly a hundred-fold increase in the incidence of lymphoproliferative tumors in individuals with impaired immunity, in particular with impaired cell-mediated immunity.

2. *B.* Immunologic cross-reactivity has been demonstrated only in cases of virally induced tumors (caused by either RNA or DNA viruses). Tumors induced by chemical or physical carcinogens do not exhibit cross-reactivity, even if induced by the same carcinogen on separate sites on the same individual.

3. *D.* Interferon-α, β, and γ enhance the expression of class I MHC molecules on tumor cells, which makes them more vulnerable to killing by CTLs. IL-2 activates LAK and TIL cells. TNF-α and β both have direct antitumor activity. IFN-γ increases the activity of CTLs, macrophages, and NK cells, each of which plays an important role in tumor cell destruction. Cytokines play no role in the activation of complement, therefore **D** is incorrect.

4. *E.* All are correct. Destruction of tumor cells may be mediated by T-cell–mediated cytotoxicity, by antibody-dependent cell-mediated cytotoxicity (ADCC), by complement-mediated cytotox-

icity, and by phagocytic cells, which are attracted to the tumor by T-cell lymphokines and/or complement components, and become activated by the lymphokines or perform enhanced phagocytosis as a result of the present of opsonins on the target cells.

5. *D.* Immunotoxins consist of toxic substances (or radioactive atoms) conjugated to immunoglobulin molecules specific for tumor cells or other target cells.

6. *D.* The only relevant statement is that plasma cells do not have surface immunoglobulins and would therefore not be susceptible to treatment with anti-idiotypic antibodies. Plasma cell tumors do have tumor-specific antigens and would be susceptible to ADCC with antibodies to these antigens. Statement **C** is not correct.

7. *C.* Antibodies that target B-cell associated targets (CD20 and CD52) have been shown to induce apoptosis of tumor cells. They are not capable of directly lysing targets and have not been shown to activate Treg cells or ADCC. Finally, they have no effects on the tumor microenvironment; therefore choice **E** is incorrect.

21

RESISTANCE AND IMMUNIZATION TO INFECTIOUS DISEASES

INTRODUCTION

By now, the reader should fully appreciate that the primary function of the immune system is to defend the body against diseases caused by pathogens. Historically, infectious diseases have been the leading cause of death for human populations, with most deaths occurring in infancy and childhood. There have been many catastrophic epidemics of infectious diseases in history. For example, the bubonic plague caused by the bacterium *Yersinia pestis* killed one quarter of the European population in the mid-1300s. Hence infectious diseases have provided tremendous selective pressures for the evolution of the immune system. As we have discussed in the early chapters of this book, host defenses are characterized by a considerable amount of layering and redundancy. Layering refers to defense in depth and includes physical barriers, such as the skin and mucosal membranes, and innate and adaptive immune mechanisms. Redundancy is exemplified by the fact that there are several types of phagocytic cells, antigen-presenting cells (APCs), cytokine-producing cells, opsonins, and so on, such that for many immune functions, multiple mechanisms are in place to achieve the desired end. The redundancy of the immune system allows the host to survive for prolonged times, despite severe immune impairment. For example, some individuals with deficiencies in some immunoglobulin isotypes (e.g., IgA deficiency, the most common Ig deficiency) are thought to live a normal existence because other immunoglobulin classes compensate for the immune deficit.

Microbes differ in their pathogenicity and virulence. Only a small minority of all microorganisms on earth are pathogens for humans. Pathogens are defined as microbes capable of causing host damage. Host damage can occur at the cellular, tissue, or organ level. When host damage reaches a certain threshold, it can manifest itself as disease. If sufficient damage occurs, the death of the host can be the outcome. Host damage can result from a variety of mechanisms and can be mediated by the microbe, the host, or both. Examples of mechanisms of microbe-mediated damage include the production of toxins, cellular apoptosis resulting in depletion of immune cells, and the elaboration of enzymes that cause tissue necrosis. Examples of mechanisms of host-mediated damage include destructive inflammation, fibrosis, and autoimmunity. The realization that host damage is the relevant parameter by which to characterize the outcome of the host–pathogen interaction is the basis of the recently proposed ***damage-response framework*** of microbial pathogenesis. According to this conceptual framework, the term ***pathogenicity*** is defined as the capacity of a microbe to cause damage in a host, and ***virulence*** is defined by the relative capacity of a microbe to cause damage in a host. Virulence and pathogenicity are not singular microbial properties, because they can be expressed in only susceptible hosts and reflect complex interactions among hosts; microbes; and myriad environmental, social, and human factors. The damage-response framework is illustrated in Figure 21.1. The host response is represented by a continuum from weak to strong. Weak responses are those that are insufficient,

Immunology: A Short Course, Seventh Edition. Richard Coico and Geoffrey Sunshine.
© 2015 John Wiley & Sons, Ltd. Published 2015 by John Wiley & Sons, Ltd.
Companion Website: www.wileyimmunology.com/coico

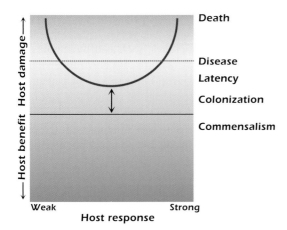

Figure 21.1. Parabolic curve of the damage-response frame-work. The y axis denotes host damage as a function of the host response. Green, yellow, and purple represent health, disease, and severe disease, respectively. (Casadevall and Pirofski 2003. Reproduced with permission of Nature Publishing Group.)

poor, or inappropriate. In other words, they are not strong enough to benefit the host. Strong responses are those that are excessive, overly robust, or inappropriate, and therefore have the ability to cause damage to the host. When a threshold amount of damage is reached, the host will show symptoms of disease. If damage is severe, death can ensue.

Humans harbor many species of microbes. When a human host encounters a microbe, the interaction can result in one of two outcomes: elimination or infection. Elimination can occur when the host–microbe encounter does not result in the establishment of the microbe in the host. Infection is the acquisition of a microbe by a host. Note that although the term *infection* is often used synonymously with the word *disease*, the two are not the same. Infection is followed by one of five outcomes: (1) *elimination*, (2) *commensalism*, (3) *colonization*, (4) *persistence* (or latency), or (5) *disease*. In the latter four outcomes, the relationship between the host and microbe is maintained, but the amount of damage sustained by the host differs (Figure 21.2). Elimination can follow infection as a result of action by host defense mechanisms or therapeutic intervention. Neither commensalism nor colonization rarely, if ever, results in symptomatic or clinically evident host

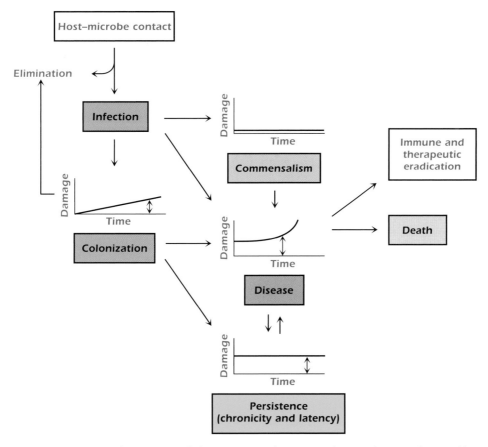

Figure 21.2. Potential outcomes of the interaction between a host and a microbe. Double-headed arrows are situations in which the amount of damage may be variable, depending on the specific host–microbe interaction. (Adapted from Casadevall and Pirofski 2000. *Infect Immun* 68: 6511.)

damage, but these states can differ in the amount of host damage and in their ability to progress to disease. When there is no host damage, commensalism and colonization are essentially indistinguishable states.

Colonization is a term that is usually used for microbes with significant pathogenic potential that establish themselves in the host without causing symptoms. Colonization can lead to elimination, persistence, or disease, depending on the competency of host defenses, the virulence of the microbe, and the effectiveness of the immune response. Many colonizing events stimulate immune responses and prevent future infection and/or disease caused by the relevant microbe. For example, a microbe with high pathogenic potential may establish itself on a mucous membrane, cause a small amount of damage that is insufficient to cause clinical symptoms, and elicit an immune response that eradicates it. In that situation, colonization immunized the host against reacquisition of the microbe.

Persistence (or latency) is a state whereby microbes take up residence in the host and cannot be eradicated, despite causing host damage. For example, in many humans, *Mycobacterium tuberculosis* infection is not symptomatic, even when the microbe has established itself in the host and is able to survive for long periods of time in a granuloma (see Chapter 17). In this state of persistence, local tissue damage and alterations in normal tissue occur due to granuloma formation, but the damage is not sufficient to produce clinical disease. However, unlike colonization, the host defense mechanisms cannot eradicate the mycobacteria, and the infection becomes persistent. In most individuals, this state is maintained with the infection confined to a granuloma. However, in some individuals, this state progresses to tuberculosis, the disease caused by *M. tuberculosis*. In the damage-response framework, disease occurs when the presence of the microbe in the host results in sufficient damage to manifest clinical symptoms.

In individuals with intact immune systems, microbes must be sufficiently virulent to establish themselves and cause infection. However, in individuals with compromised immune systems, low-virulence microbes can cause serious infections. Microbes that are pathogenic only in individuals with weakened immune systems are often referred to as *opportunistic pathogens*. Hence the microbial properties of pathogenicity and virulence are associated with, and partially depend upon, the immune status of the host. In circumstances of normal immune function, commensal microorganisms are not harmful, and some serve important roles for the host, such as the production of vitamin K by gut bacteria. However, commensals can become pathogens in circumstances in which the normal host defenses are breached. For example, both *Staphylococcus epidermitis* and *Candida albicans* are part of the normal skin flora but can cause life-threatening infections in patients with intravenous catheters that provide inappropriate access of these organisms to the circulatory system because of a break in the skin. Some therapies for cancer produce immune suppression, which leaves patients at risk for serious infections with low-virulence microbes, such as commensals.

In this chapter, we will discuss how mammalian hosts protect themselves against various types of pathogens and how the immune system can be primed for antimicrobial defense through active and passive immunization. It is assumed that the reader is now familiar with the principal concepts underlying innate and adaptive immune defenses.

HOST DEFENSE AGAINST THE VARIOUS CLASSES OF MICROBIAL PATHOGENS

The most effective immune response to a particular microbe varies with the type of pathogen and the microbial strategy for pathogenesis. Viruses, bacteria, parasites, and fungi each use different strategies to establish themselves in the host, and, consequently, the effective immune response for each of these classes of microbial pathogens is different. Although each pathogen is different, certain themes emerge when one considers immune responses to the various classes of pathogens.

Immunity to Viruses

All viruses are *obligate intracellular pathogens*, and many have evolved to have highly sophisticated mechanisms for cellular invasion, replication, and evasion of the immune system. Host defenses against viral infections aim to first slow viral replication and then to eradicate infection. The antiviral response can be complex, with several factors affecting the outcome of the host–pathogen interaction, such as the route of entry, site of attachment, aspects of pathogenesis by the infecting virus, induction of cytokines, antibody response, and cell-mediated immunity. An important early defense mechanism consists of the production of various types of interferons (IFNs) including IFN-α by leukocytes, IFN-β by fibroblasts, and INF-γ by T and natural killer (NK) cells. Interferons are antiviral proteins, or glycoproteins, produced by several different types of cell in the mammalian host in response to viral infection (or other inducers, such as double-stranded RNA). Interferons serve as an early protective mechanism. IFN-α and IFN-β produced by virally infected cells diffuse to adjoining cells and activate genes that interfere with viral replication. These interferons also stimulate production of MHC class I molecules and proteasome proteins that enhance the ability of virally infected cells to present viral peptides to T cells. Furthermore, IFN-α and IFN-β activate NK cells that recognize and kill host cells infected with viruses, thus limiting viral production.

NK cells are characterized by their ability to kill certain tumor cells *in vitro* without prior sensitization and constitute an early cellular defense against viruses. Later in the course of infection, when *antibodies* to viral antigens are available, NK cells can eliminate host cells infected with virus through *antibody-dependent cell-mediated cytotoxicity* (ADCC). NK cells also produce INF-γ, a potent activator of macrophage function that helps prime the immune system for producing an adaptive immune response. *Complement* system proteins damage the envelope of some viruses, which may provide some measure of protection against certain viral infections.

While the innate immune mechanisms that include IFNs, NK cells, and possibly complement, function to slow and partially contain many viral infections, the infection may progress, with viral replication and damage triggering an adaptive immune response. The humoral response results in the production of antibodies to viral proteins. Some antibodies can prevent viruses from invading other cells, and these are called *neutralizing antibodies*. IgG appears to be the most active isotype against viruses. Opsonization represents a convergence of humoral and cellular immune mechanisms. IgG, which has combined with viral antigens on the surface of infected host cells through its Fab region, also links to Fc receptors on several cell populations, including NK cells, macrophages, and polymorphonuclear (PMN) cells. These cells then can phagocytose and/or damage the virus-infected cell through ADCC.

Antibodies to viral proteins can prevent infection by interfering with the binding of virus to host cells. The production of secretory IgA can protect the host by preventing infection of epithelial cells in mucosal surfaces. Antibodies can also interfere with the progression of viral infection by agglutinating viral particles, activating complement on viral surfaces, and promoting phagocytosis of viral particles by macrophages. The production of an antibody response serves to limit viral spread and facilitates the destruction of infected host cells by ADCC. Hence the effective antibody response to viruses include the production of antibodies that

- Neutralize (or impede) the infectivity of viruses for susceptible host cells
- Fix complement and promote complement damage to virions
- Inhibit viral enzymes
- Promote opsonization of viral particles
- Promote ADCC of virus-infected cells

Different types of antibodies may be necessary for the control of specific types of viral infections. Consider the case of influenza and measles virus infections. Infection of the epithelium of the respiratory tract by influenza virus leads to production of virus in epithelial cells and spread of the virus to adjacent epithelial cells. An appropriate and sufficient immune response would involve the action of antibody at the epithelial surface. This action might be effected through locally secreted IgA or local extravasation of IgG or IgM. On the other hand, some viral diseases, such

as measles and poliomyelitis, begin by infection at a mucosal epithelium (respiratory and intestinal, respectively) but exhibit their major pathogenic effects after being spread hematogenously to other target tissues. Antibody at the epithelial surface could protect against the virus, but circulating antibody could do likewise.

However, once a virus has attached to a host cell, it is usually not displaced by antibody. Hence an effective antibody response is usually not sufficient to eliminate a viral infection, particularly when the virus has established itself inside host cells. The eradication of an established viral infection usually requires an effective cell-mediated response. The adaptive cellular response results in the production of specific CD4$^+$ and CD8$^+$ T cells that are essential for clearance of viral infections. CD4$^+$ T cells are believed to be intimately involved in the generation of effective antibody responses by facilitating isotype class switching and affinity maturation (see Chapter 11). CD4$^+$ T cells also produce important cytokines to stimulate inflammatory responses at sites of viral infection and activate macrophage function. Cytotoxic lymphocytes CD8$^+$ T cells (CTLs) are the principal effector T cells against viruses. They are generated early in viral infection and usually appear before neutralizing antibody. CD8$^+$ T cells can recognize viral antigens in the context of major histocompatibility complex (MHC) class I molecules and can kill host cells harboring viruses. Since MHC class I molecules are expressed by most cell types in the host, CD8$^+$ T cells can recognize many types of infected cells and thus represent a critically important component of the host adaptive response against viral infections. However, for certain noncytopathic viruses, such as hepatitis B, CD8$^+$ T cells can be responsible for tissue injury. Hence, chronic hepatitis B infection results in persistent inflammation and damage to liver cells, resulting in fibrosis that can progress to organ failure.

In summary, innate immune mechanisms initially interfere with viral infection through the production of IFNs and the killing of infected cells by NK cells. These early defenses buy time until powerful, pathogen-specific adaptive immune responses are generated. The adaptive immune responses produce neutralizing antibodies that reduce the number of viral particles and CTLs that kill infected cells. The presence of neutralizing antibody would then protect against subsequent exposure to the same virus.

Immunity to Bacteria

Host protection against bacterial pathogens is achieved through a variety of mechanisms that include both *humoral* and *cellular-mediated immunity*. Antibacterial defenses include bacterial lysis, via *antibody* and *complement*, *opsonization*, and *phagocytosis*, with elimination of phagocytosed bacteria by the liver, spleen, and other components of the reticuloendothelial system. Bacteria and their products are internalized by APCs such as macrophages and dendritic cells, and processed for antigen presentation to T cells. Peptides resulting from such processing are presented to CD4$^+$ T cells in the context of MHC class II molecules (see Chapter 10). This process amplifies the host response as T cells produce cytokines that activate macrophages and facilitate recruitment of additional inflammatory cells. The relative efficacy of the various immune mechanisms depends on the type of bacteria and, in particular, the cell-surface properties of the bacteria. Bacterial pathogens can be roughly divided into four classes: (1) *Gram-positive*, (2) *Gram-negative*, (3) *mycobacteria*, and (4) *spirochetes*, depending on their cell wall and membrane composition. Some Gram-positive and Gram-negative bacteria have polysaccharide capsules. Another crucial distinction between bacterial pathogens is whether they are *intracellular* or *extracellular* pathogens. Intracellular bacterial pathogens reside in cells and are partially shielded from the full array of host immune defenses, whereas extracellular bacterial pathogens are found outside cells. In general, humoral immunity is very important for protection against extracellular bacteria, whereas cellular immunity is the primary immune mechanism for the control and eradication of intracellular bacteria. T$_H$17 cells are believed to play a crucial role in this host defense mechanism.

Gram-Positive Bacteria. Gram-positive bacteria have thick electron-dense cell walls composed of complex cross-linked *peptidoglycan* that allow them to retain the stain crystal violet (hence Gram-positive). In addition to a thick layer of peptidoglycan, the cell wall of Gram-positive bacteria contains teichoic acids, carbohydrates, and proteins. *Teichoic acids* are immunogenic and constitute major antigenic determinants of Gram-positive bacteria. This type of cell wall provides the Gram-positive bacteria with a thick layer of protection that makes them resistant to lysis by the complement system. Defenses against Gram-positive bacteria include specific antibody responses to provide opsonins and phagocytic cells, such as neutrophils and macrophages, to ingest and kill them. *Opsonization* and *phagocytosis* involve the action of IgG alone or in concert with C3b. The alternative complement pathway may be triggered directly by the Gram-positive bacterial cell wall, resulting in the deposition of complement opsonins in the cell surface and the production of mediators of the inflammatory response. Although the complement system does not lyse Gram-positive bacteria directly, it provides opsonins and mediators of inflammation that are critical for host defense.

Gram-Negative Bacteria. Gram-negative bacteria do not retain crystal violet stain and have a layered cell-wall structure composed of outer and inner membranes separated by a thin layer of peptidoglycan in the periplasmic space. Hence Gram-positive and Gram-negative bacteria have major differences in their cell-wall structure. The outer membrane of Gram-negative bacteria contains *lipopolysaccharide* (LPS), which is also known as *endotoxin*. The polysaccharide portion of LPS has antigenic determinants that confer antigenic specificity. Many Gram-negative bacterial species include variants with different LPS structures that can be identified serologically as serotypes. LPS is highly toxic to humans and can produce cardiovascular collapse, hypotension, and shock during infection with Gram-negative bacteria. The alternative complement pathway may be activated directly by the LPS found in the walls of Gram-negative bacteria or by the polysaccharide capsule of Gram-negative bacteria acting on C3. Activation of the alternative pathway leads to the generation of the chemotactic molecules C3a and C5a and the opsonin C3b and can result in bacteriolytic action by the C5C9 membrane attack complex (see Chapter 14). The ability of the complement system to lyse some Gram-negative bacteria directly is an important distinction from Gram-positive bacteria, which are impervious to complement-mediated lysis because of the thick peptidoglycan layer. Defenses against Gram-negative bacteria include the *complement system*, *specific antibody*, and *phagocytic cells*.

Mycobacteria. Mycobacteria have cell walls distinct from Gram-positive and Gram-negative bacteria. Mycobacterial cell walls are characterized by a high lipid content, which makes the bacteria difficult to stain. A useful diagnostic microbiological property of the mycobacterial cell wall is *acid fastness*, which allows the cell wall to retain certain dyes after being treated with acid. Mycobacteria grow slowly and have hydrophobic surfaces that make them clump. Mycobacterial cell wall components elicit strong immune responses during infection, including *delayed-type hypersensitivity* (DTH) reactions that form the basis for the *tuberculin test* (see Chapter 17). Hypersensitivity reactions to mycobacterial proteins may be involved in the pathogenesis of mycobacterial infections. Mycobacteria elicit strong antibody responses but the protective role of humoral immunity is uncertain. The primary defense mechanisms against mycobacteria are *macrophages* and *cell-mediated immunity*.

Spirochetes. Spirochetes are thin helical microorganisms and include the etiologic agents of syphilis (*Treponema pallidum*) and Lyme disease (*Borrelia burgdorferi*). Spirochetes lack cell walls such as those found in Gram-positive bacteria, Gram-negative bacteria, and mycobacteria. Instead they have a thin outer membrane that contains few proteins. Spirochetes are thin, fragile, and require special techniques for visualization in the microscope, such as dark-field microscopy and immunofluorescence. Important host defenses against spirochetes include *complement*, *specific antibody*, and *cell-mediated immunity*.

Immunity to Parasites

The parasites are a diverse group of complex pathogens that include the multicellular *helminths* and single-celled *protozoa*. Nearly half of the world's population harbors helminth infections. Many parasites have a variety of tissue stages that may differ in cellular location and antigenic composition, thus providing a difficult problem for the immune system. The diversity of parasites is such that it is difficult to make generalizations about effective host mechanisms that protect against parasitic diseases. However, it is clear that both innate and adaptive defense mechanisms are critically important for protection against parasitic infections. So-called *type-2 immune responses* dominate the adaptive immune mechanisms that confer protection to helminths as well as other parasites. The term "type-2 responses" is derived from the fact that these responses are characterized by the induction of T_H2 responses. T_H2 cells secrete cytokines such as IL-4, IL-5, IL-9, and IL-13 and display distinct transcription factor profiles (GATA-3, STAT-5, and STAT-6). It is noteworthy that although type-2 immune responses have been explored largely in the context of helminth infections and allergies (see Chapter 15), they are also induced by venoms, vaccine adjuvants such as alum, and some bacterial and viral infections. How such diverse stimuli trigger prototypic type-2 responses and the nature of the cellular and molecular networks that orchestrate these responses are still unclear.

Protozoa. Protozoa may exist in either a metabolically active form called a *trophozoite* or a dormant tissue form known as a *cyst*. The protozoal diseases include amebiasis, malaria, leishmaniasis, trypanosomiasis, and toxoplasmosis. Host defenses against protozoa include both innate and adaptive humoral and cellular mechanisms, but their relative importance may vary with the individual pathogen. Some protozoal parasites, such as trypanosomes, are able to activate the complement system through the alternative pathway.

Complement activation combined with *phagocytosis* by neutrophils and macrophages of the innate immune system provide an important line of defense against many parasitic pathogens. For some protozoal infections such as amebiasis, malaria, and trypanosomiasis, humoral immunity in the form of antibody has been shown to mediate protection against infection. Vaccines capable of inducing protective antibody responses to each of these parasitic pathogens have not yet been developed. For other protozoal infections such as leishmaniasis and toxoplasmosis, cellular immunity is more important; again, there are currently no vaccines available.

Helminths. Unlike the pathogenic protozoan microorganisms, the multicellular worms called *helminths* are large macroscopic pathogens that can range from 1 cm to 10 m. Their large size poses particular problems for host defenses, and the control of helminth infections requires a complex interplay between tissue and immune responses. The helminths are notorious for causing chronic infections that can elicit intense immune responses to worm antigens.

There is general agreement that components of the innate immune system such as *eosinophils* and *mast cells* are important effector cells against helminths, but many aspects of the host response to worms remain obscure. *IgE* specific for helminth antigens is believed to be important for host defense by priming eosinophils for *ADCC* (see Figure 15.8). Worm infections are often accompanied by an increase in blood eosinophils and serum IgE levels.

Immunity to Fungi

Fungal pathogens are eukaryotes that tend to cause serious infections primarily in individuals with impaired immunity. Fungi cause tissue damage by the elaboration of proteolytic enzymes, inducing inflammatory responses. The most common fungal pathogen is *Candida albicans*. This organism is usually a harmless commensal, but it can cause disease in situations in which the normal defense mechanisms are compromised, such as breaks in skin resulting from intravenous catheters or surgery. Another group at risk for serious *C. albicans*-related diseases comprises individuals who have transient depletion of neutrophils as a result of chemotherapy. The fact that most cases of serious *Candida* infection require a break in the skin or a depletion in neutrophils suggests that *innate defense mechanisms* are largely responsible for preventing systemic diseases. However, patients with advanced human immunodeficiency virus (HIV) infection suffer from mucosal candidiasis, highlighting the importance of cell-mediated immunity in protection against this organism at the mucosal surfaces.

Other fungi, such as *Histoplasma capsulatum* and *Cryptococcus neoformans*, are acquired from the environment by inhalation in regions where the organism is found in soils. *C. neoformans* has a polysaccharide capsule that is required for virulence. Prevalence studies of asymptomatic individuals in such regions have shown a high incidence of infection with a very low incidence of disease, as evidenced by antibody responses or positive skin testing. Hence, for these organisms, it is likely that initial acquisition of the microbe results in an adaptive immune response that controls the infection. Some fungi, such as *H. capsulatum*, survive inside macrophages and are intracellular pathogens. The T_H17 lineage of CD4+ T cells is believed to play an important role in host defenses against intracellular fungal infections.

Fungi differ from bacteria in that they have a different type of cell wall, composed of cross-linked polysaccharides. Fungal cells are generally impervious to lysis by the complement system. The host response to fungal infections includes both humoral and cellular responses. The primary form of host defense against fungal pathogens is widely acknowledged to be cell-mediated immunity. The need for intact T-cell function in resistance to fungi is particularly evident in the predisposition of patients with acquired immunodeficiency syndrome (AIDS) to life-threatening infections with such fungi as *H. capsulatum* and *C. neoformans*. Historically, antibody-mediated immunity was not thought to be very important against fungi, but several protective monoclonal antibodies have been described in recent years against *C. albicans* and *C. neoformans*. Hence it is likely that both cellular and humoral immune mechanisms contribute to protection against fungi.

MECHANISMS BY WHICH PATHOGENS EVADE THE IMMUNE RESPONSE

Despite the formidable defense mechanisms of the intact immune system, some microorganisms manage to establish themselves in the host and cause life-threatening infections. These pathogenic microbes have special adaptations that allow them to evade the immune system or overcome immune responses. Learning about the mechanisms by which microbial pathogens evade the host immune response is important because it can teach us about the efficacy and limitations of host defense mechanisms. Furthermore, a better understanding of the strategies used by microbes to survive immune attack can be used to design new therapies and vaccines to fight infection.

Encapsulated Bacteria

Polysaccharide capsules are important *virulence factors* for several human pathogens, including *Streptococcus pneumoniae* (pneumococcus), *Haemophilus influenzae*, *Neisseria meningitidis* (meningococcus), and *Cryptococcus neoformans*. These capsules are antiphagocytic and thus protect the pathogen from ingestion and killing by host phagocytic cells. Some capsules also interfere with the action of the complement system. Polysaccharide molecules are often weakly immunogenic, and infection by encapsulated pathogens may not necessarily elicit high titer antibody responses. Infants and young children (1–2 years of age) are particularly vulnerable to life-threatening infections with encapsulated bacteria because their immature immune systems do not mount adequate antibody responses. This is attributable, in part, to their lack of marginal B cells in the spleen. Other individuals at high risk are those with inherited or acquired deficiencies in antibody production and those who lack normal spleen function. Because the bacteria are cleared by the reticuloendothelial system in the spleen and liver, these organs are critical for protection against encapsulated pathogens. Individuals with compromised reticuloendothelial function as a result of disease (e.g., sickle cell anemia) or surgical removal of the spleen are particularly vulnerable to encapsulated bacteria. The mechanism of antibody action against encapsulated pathogens involves opsonins for phagocytosis and killing by neutrophils and macrophages. Antibodies to capsular polysaccharide function by promoting phagocytosis directly through Fc receptors or indirectly

by activating complement. The generation of C3b following complement activation also facilitates opsonization for phagocytosis, which is another example of the redundancy of host defenses.

Toxins

For some bacterial infections, the manifestations of disease are caused by virulence factors called *toxins*. Bacterial toxins are proteins that produce their physiologic effects at minute concentrations. Examples of toxin-producing bacteria are *Corynebacterium diphtheriae*, *Vibrio cholerae*, and *Clostridium tetani*, the causes of diphtheria, cholera, and tetanus, respectively. Diphtheria is a condition in which *C. diphtheriae* replication and toxin production in the nasopharynx results in the formation of a tenacious membrane in the throat that can asphyxiate the patient. Cholera is a diarrheal illness caused by *V. cholerae*, resulting from toxin-mediated alteration of water resorption in the cells of the intestinal mucosa. Tetanus is a condition in which toxin produced by *C. tetani* produces unchecked excitation of peripheral muscles, resulting in titanic spasms. The relationship of the toxin function to bacterial invasion and evasion of the immune response is variable and may differ for each pathogen. Some toxins, such as tetanus and botulinum toxin, do not appear to injure the immune system directly. Diphtheria toxin may promote bacterial infection by damaging the mucosa. *Bacillus anthracis*, the causative agent of anthrax, produces pathogenic toxins that cause apoptosis in macrophages. The principle mechanism for this immune evasion involves a toxin called *lethal toxin* (LT). LT inhibits a macrophage protein kinase that is required for the transcription of antiapoptotic genes following cell activation.

Most toxins are highly immunogenic and elicit strong humoral and cellular immune responses. Specific antibodies can bind to and neutralize bacterial toxins. Protection against toxins is predominantly associated with IgG, although IgA may also be important in neutralization of certain exotoxins (e.g., secreted toxins) such as cholera enterotoxin. Because the exotoxins bind firmly to their target tissue, they generally cannot be displaced by subsequent administration of *antitoxin* (passive immunization using toxin-specific antibody and discussed later in this chapter). Hence in toxin-mediated diseases (e.g., diphtheria) prompt administration of antitoxin is necessary to prevent attachment of (additional) exotoxin and the damage caused by the toxin. This can be illustrated by the effectiveness of antitoxin given at varying times as protection against the lethal effects of diphtheria toxin in humans (Table 21.1). As the infection progresses, the effectiveness of administration of diphtheria antitoxin is significantly reduced. Some bacterial toxins are enzymes, such as the lecithinase of the bacterium *Clostridium perfringens* and snake venom. However, antibodies that bind the toxin may not necessarily inhibit the enzymatically active sites of toxin.

TABLE 21.1. Protection of Humans by Diphtheria Antitoxin Given on Indicated Day of Disease

TABLE 21.1. Protection of Humans by Diphtheria Antitoxin Given on Indicated Day of Disease

Day	Number of Cases	Fatality Rate
1	225	9.0
2	1,445	4.2
3	1,600	11.1
4	1,276	17.3
5 (or later)	1,645	18.7

Superantigens

The interaction of certain toxins with the immune system can have major immunologic consequences when they are able to bind the T-cell receptor (TCR) of large numbers of T cells. These toxins are known as **superantigens** and include the staphylococcal **toxic shock syndrome**. In the early 1980s, many cases of staphylococcal toxic shock syndrome were associated with tampon use in menstruating women. Since then, the frequency of the disease has decreased significantly in response to changes to the manufacture of tampons. Superantigens stimulate large numbers of T cells to proliferate, synthesize cytokines, and then die by apoptosis, resulting in the loss of important immune cells. The release of massive amounts of cytokines by the T cells (cytokine storm) is associated with **hypotension, hypolemia**, and **organ failure**, which can lead to death. B-cell superantigens that bind to and alter the expression of certain immunoglobulin gene families have also been described.

Antigenic Variation

Pathogens can escape the immune system by generating variants with different antigenic composition. This mechanism for evasion of host defenses is known as **antigenic variation**. Classical examples of pathogens that evade the host response by antigenic variation are influenza virus, HIV, *Streptococcus pneumonia*, trypanosomes, and Group A streptococcus. Each of these pathogens provides an illustrative example of a mechanism for antigenic variation. In the case of Group A streptococcus, the M protein is required for virulence and functions by preventing phagocytosis through a mechanism that involves deposition of fibrinogen on the bacterial surface. M proteins elicit protective antibody but are antigenically variable, so that streptococcal infection with one strain does not elicit resistance to other strains.

Influenza virus generates antigenic variation because it has a segmented RNA genome that can be resorted to yield virions expressing new combinations of the two main surface antigens: the hemagglutinin and neuraminidase surface proteins. Antigenic variation for influenza virus occurs through both antigenic drift and antigenic shift. **Antigenic drift** is the result of point mutations in the influenza virus genome; these mutations produce antigenic changes in the hemagglutinin and neuraminidase. **Antigenic shift** occurs when influenza virus expresses a new allele of hemagglutinin or neuraminidase protein that results in a major antigenic change and the emergence of a new viral strain. The result of antigenic drift and shift for the influenza virus is that the virus changes rapidly, and one influenza infection does not confer protection against subsequent infection. Furthermore, since each epidemic is antigenically different, a new vaccine against influenza must be reformulated every year.

HIV undergoes rapid antigenic variation *in vivo* because it has an error-prone reverse transcriptase that produces mutations that translates into antigenic changes in surface proteins. The problem of antigenic variation in HIV has been a major hurdle preventing the development of an effective vaccine. Other pathogens, such as *Streptococcus pneumoniae* (pneumococcus), present the host with antigenic variation because they exist in multiple serotypes, each of which has a different antigenic composition. There are 80 known pneumococcal serotypes, and infection with one serotype does not confer protection against infection with a different serotype. Hence the host must deal with infection by each pneumococcal serotype as if it were an infection by a different microbe. However, these have been identified and an effective vaccine exists that covers most serotypes.

Pathogens may also encode for antigenic variation in their genomes. **Trypanosomes** cause chronic infections by the emergence of new antigenic types during infection that express different variant surface glycoproteins (VSGs). In a trypanosome infection, the host mounts an antibody response to the VSG being expressed by the majority of parasites, which clears most of them. However, in every trypanosome infection there are small numbers of organisms that express a different VSG antigen that is not recognized by the antibody response. As the antibody response helps clear the original trypanosome population, the remaining organisms expressing a different VSG then proliferate, while also generating a new subpopulation of antigenic variants that can survive the new antibody response. The cycle then repeats itself. Since there are many VSG genes, trypanosomes are able to cause persistent infections by producing escape variants that differ in antigenic composition in every generation.

Intracellular Survival

Some microorganisms are taken up by **phagocytic cells** but manage to survive in the intracellular environment. These pathogens include the bacteria *Mycobacterium tuberculosis* and *Listeria monocytogenes*, the fungus *Histoplasma capsulatum*, and the protozoa *Toxoplasma gondii*. *M. tuberculosis* is the cause of tuberculosis, a pulmonary infection. *L. monocytogenes* is a food-borne microbe that can cause meningitis in individuals with immune suppression.

H. capsulatum is a fungus common in the soil of the Ohio and Mississippi River valleys of the United States that usually causes a self-limited pneumonia in normal individuals. However, in individuals with impaired immunity, *H. capsulatum* can cause disseminated infections that are life threatening. *T. gondii* is a parasite that is acquired from eating undercooked meat, which usually causes asymptomatic infections. However, in pregnant women, *T. gondii* can infect the fetus, causing severe birth defects. Patients with advanced HIV infection are particularly vulnerable to toxoplasmosis. These organisms cause very different types of diseases, but each has in common the ability to survive inside host cells.

Intracellular residence of pathogens provides an advantageous environment for the microorganism that is nutrient-rich yet outside the reach of humoral factors and neutrophils. In general, protection against intracellular microorganisms is the domain of cell-mediated immunity, although for several pathogens antibody responses also contribute to host defense. This concept is illustrated by the fact *M. tuberculosis*, *L. monocytogenes*, *H. capsulatum*, and *T. gondii* cause serious diseases in individuals with impaired T-cell function, such as patients with AIDS. Furthermore, NK cells may play an important role during early stages of infection by destroying infected cells before the development of specific resistance. Granulomatous inflammation is a tissue manifestation of cell-mediated immunity associated with containment of several intracellular pathogens.

Although phagocytic cells are generally efficient antimicrobial cells, microbes capable of intracellular survival use any of several strategies to avoid being killed after phagocytosis. *M. tuberculosis* blocks the fusion of lysosomes with the phagocytic vacuole, thus preventing delivery of antimicrobial substances to the phagosome (see Chapter 2). *H. capsulatum* interferes with acidification of the phagolysosomal vacuole, a phenomenon that is believed to interfere with killing of yeast cells inside macrophages. *L. monocytogenes* produces bacterial products that allow it to escape from the phagolysosomal vacuole to the cell cytoplasm, a mechanism that presumably provides a more nutritionally favorable niche and defeats intracellular antimicrobial mechanisms. *T. gondii* generates its own vacuole in which it remains insulated from host lysosomes; this avoids triggering recognition of infected cells by the immune system. Other bacteria—such as *Shigella flexneri*, a microbe that causes a diarrheal illness—may promote their survival inside phagocytic cells by triggering apoptosis and death of the phagocytic cell.

Suppression of the Immune System

Some pathogens ensure their survival in a mammalian host by actively suppressing the immune response. Many viruses include genes capable of modulating the immune response. For example, Epstein–Barr virus (EBV), which infects B cells, encodes a gene that produces a protein that is a homolog of IL-10 that downregulates the immune response. Other viruses such as herpes simplex have virally encoded proteins that resemble Ig Fc regions and complement receptors that interfere with the function of antibody and complement, respectively. Herpes simplex virus can also interfere with recognition of infected cells by the immune system through a mechanism that inhibits MHC class I expression on the infected cell thereby thwarting its ability to present virally derived peptides. Adenoviruses encode genes that downregulate the host inflammatory response. The fungus *Cryptococcus neoformans* sheds large amounts of capsular polysaccharide, which interferes with the formation of inflammatory responses in tissue. HIV infects a variety of cells, including CD4$^+$ T cells and hence is able to directly interfere with the cells necessary for an effective immune response. HIV-induced CD4$^+$ T-cell depletion produces a spiraling deterioration of immune function that culminates in AIDS and leaves the patient vulnerable to many opportunistic infections.

Extracellular Enzymes

Some bacteria produce enzymes that degrade immune molecules. For example, *Neisseria meningitidis* and *N. gonorrhoeae*, the causes of meningococcal meningitis and gonorrhea, respectively, produce ***IgA proteases*** that destroy IgA in mucosal surfaces. Streptococci, such as Group A streptococcus (which causes **strep throat**), produce ***hemolysins***, which are believed to aid the organism in dissemination; some elaborate ***a peptidase*** that cleaves the C5a complement protein.

Expression of Antibody-Binding Proteins

Some bacteria, such as *Staphylococcus aureus*, express cell-surface proteins that can bind immunoglobulins through their Fc region. Examples of these ***Fc-binding proteins*** are ***protein A*** and ***protein G***. The ability of these proteins to bind immunoglobulin molecules is exploited in immunologic research by using them in affinity chromatography to purify IgG (see Chapter 6).

PRINCIPLES OF IMMUNIZATION

Protection against infectious diseases by the use of vaccines represents an immense, if not the greatest, accomplishment of biomedical science. One disease, smallpox, has been totally eliminated by the use of vaccination, and the incidence of other diseases has been significantly reduced, at least in areas of the world where vaccines are available and administered properly.

If a large enough number of individuals can be immunized, ***herd immunity*** is achieved, and the transmission of

TABLE 21.2. Examples of Active and Passive Immunization

Type of Immunity	How Acquired
Active	
Natural (unintended)	Infection
Artificial (deliberate)	Vaccination
Passive	
Natural	Transfer of antibody from mother to infant in placental circulation or colostrum
Artificial	Passive antibody therapy (serum therapy, administration of immune human globulin)

communicable diseases among individuals is interrupted. Although deliberate immunization alone can sometimes reduce the incidence of a disease to a very low level, successful immunization programs require the intelligent practice of other measures, both hygienic and sanitary, which contribute to general improvements in public health.

Immunization can be either active or passive. ***Active immunization*** generally refers to the administration of a vaccine that can elicit a protective immune response. ***Passive immunization*** refers to the administration of antibodies or lymphocytes, which then provide temporary protection in the recipient host (Table 21.2).

OBJECTIVES OF IMMUNIZATION

The objective of active immunization is to provide the individual with long-lasting immunologic protection against infectious agents. Many vaccines are given in childhood to protect against infections that are usually acquired early in life. The objective of passive immunization is to provide transient protection against a particular infection. For example, an individual bitten by a rabid animal may be given an injection of immune globulin to rabies virus to protect against infection with this virus. Protection against the development of disease can also be conferred by postexposure immunization. For example, an individual exposed to the rabies virus can be protected against this lethal infection by administration of both rabies vaccine and immune globulin against rabies virus. Other examples of postexposure immunization include the use of toxoid and antitoxin against diphtheria, vaccination with tetanus toxoid after trauma, and administration of immune serum globulins against hepatitis A virus (HAV) and hepatitis B virus (HBV) after exposure. Great effort is currently aimed at the development of therapeutic vaccines that will forestall the relentless progression of AIDS in HIV-infected individuals.

The potential for use of vaccines to prevent certain cancers in humans was discussed in Chapter 20. Some cancers may be prevented by vaccines that prevent infections associated with the subsequent development of carcinoma. For example, there is a strong association between primary carcinoma of the liver and infection by HBV. Hence the use of the recombinant HBV vaccine in high-risk groups may provide protection against both hepatitis and the subsequent development of hepatocellular carcinoma.

ACTIVE IMMUNIZATIONS

As discussed in Chapter 1, the terms *vaccination* and *vaccine* derive from the work of Edward Jenner. More than 200 years ago, Jenner showed that inoculating a young boy with pus from a lesion of a dairy maid who had contracted cowpox (a relatively benign disease that is related to smallpox) from working with cows protected the boy from the highly contagious and frequently fatal smallpox. Jenner coined the word *vaccine* from the Latin *vacca* for cow, and the process came to be called *vaccination*. Cowpox (vaccinia virus) induces protective immune responses to smallpox virus because the two viruses share antigenic epitopes, thus inducing a protective immune response. Table 21.3 lists some of the different kinds of vaccines currently in use. Later in this chapter, we discuss more recent approaches to vaccine development.

Recommended Immunizations

The usual recommended schedule in the United States for active immunization at various ages is given in Table 21.4. It is important to note that in other parts of the world, the immunization schedule may be different. In recent years, a *Haemophilus influenzae* type b polysaccharide diphtheria toxoid conjugate was added to the vaccination schedule of young children (first dose at 2 months of age). *H. influenzae* type b is a major cause of meningitis in nonimmunized young children. The use of this vaccine has resulted in a dramatic reduction in *H. influenzae* type b infections in vaccinated children. Recently, a heptavalent pneumococcal conjugate vaccine was approved for use in children for the prevention of invasive disease, including pneumonia and otitis media.

Recombinant DNA technology has contributed significantly to the development of safe, effective vaccines. These include vaccines to prevent infections with hepatitis B virus and oncogenic forms of human papillomaviruses (HPVs). The HPV vaccine is also known as the ***cervical cancer vaccine***.

Use of Vaccines in Selected Populations

In addition to the usual schedule of immunizations given in Table 21.4, some individuals receive additional vaccinations (listed in Table 21.5). Influenza virus (inactivated) is given

TABLE 21.3. Vaccines Used in Active Immunization

Vaccine Type	Vaccine Composition	Examples
Killed whole organisms	Made from the entire organism, killed to make it harmless	Typhoid
Attenuated bacteria	Organism cultured to reduce its pathogenicity but still retains some of the antigens of the virulent form	Bacille Calmette–Guérin, vaccine against *M. tuberculosis* used in Western European countries, India, and Russia, but rarely used in the United States
Toxoids	Bacterial toxins treated (e.g., with formaldehyde) to denature the protein so that it is no longer dangerous but still retains some epitopes that will elicit protective antibodies	Diphtheria, tetanus
Surface molecules	Purified surface molecules isolated from various pathogens (e.g., hemagglutinins from influenza virus)	Influenza, hepatitis B surface antigen, *S. pneumoniae* capsular polysaccharides, and *H. influenzae* type b capsular oligosaccharides (the latter are formulated as protein conjugates)
Inactivated virus	Whole virus particles treated (e.g., with formaldehyde) so that they cannot infect the host's cells but still retain some unaltered epitopes	Salk vaccine for polio
Attenuated virus	Live viruses that are weakened and nonpathogenic	Sabin oral polio vaccine, measles, mumps, rubella vaccines
Recombinant viral proteins	Major capsid proteins	Hepatitis B, human papilloma virus (HPV)

TABLE 21.4. Schedule for Active Immunization in Children[a]

Age	Vaccine
Birth	Hepatitis B (Hep B), first dose
2 months	Diphtheria, tetanus toxoids, acellular pertussis vaccine (DTP); *H. influenzae* type b (Hib); inactivated polio vaccine (IPV); and pneumococcal conjugate vaccine (PCV), first doses
4 months	DTP, Hib, IPV, and PCV, second doses
6 months	DTP, Hib, and PCV, third doses
6–18 months	Hep B and IPV, third doses
12–15 months	Measles, mumps, rubella (MMR), first doses varicella vaccine
14 months	Hep B, second dose
15–18 months	DTP, fourth dose
4–6 years	DTP, fifth dose; IPV, fourth dose; MMR, second dose
11–12 years	Tetanus toxoid booster
11–12 years	Human papillomavirus (HPV)

[a]Adapted from the Centers for Disease Control and Prevention (www.cdc.gov/vaccines).

to individuals older than 60 years of age and to children and adults with cardiorespiratory ailments. Hepatitis B vaccine (viral protein produced by recombinant DNA technology) is given to health care and emergency workers who are exposed to human blood. Hepatitis A (inactivated virus) has been approved for use in children and adults. Adenovirus vaccines are used to prevent outbreaks of respiratory infections in military recruits. Anthrax vaccine is used in military personnel, given the threat posed by the use of *Bacillus anthracis* spores in biological warfare. Vaccination against smallpox is no longer recommended for civilians but is still given to selected military personnel. However, there is currently a great debate on whether to make greater use of this vaccine given heightened concerns about the use of smallpox as a biological weapon.

Several vaccines against bacterial infections are also used in specific populations. A polyvalent vaccine consisting of several antigenic types of capsular polysaccharides from *Streptococcus pneumoniae* is given to individuals with cardiorespiratory ailments, to anatomically or functionally asplenic individuals, and to patients with sickle cell anemia, renal failure, alcoholic cirrhosis, or diabetes mellitus. These individuals have limited capability to mount the antibody/complement/phagocytic activity required against the encapsulated bacteria such as *S. pneumoniae*. Unfortunately, this vaccine may not be as effective in persons at high risk for pneumococcal pneumonia as in normal individuals because the immune defects preclude the generation of strong antibody responses. *Neisseria meningitidis* vaccine (several serogroups of capsular polysaccharide) is given to military recruits and to children in high-risk regions. This vaccine is also recommended for young adults who live in close quarters such as college dormitories who are at high risk for meningococcal meningitis. Both live attenuated and polysaccharide vaccines are available for protection against

TABLE 21.5. Additional Vaccinations[a]

Vaccine	Population(s)
Anthrax	Military personnel; handlers of animal hides, furs, bone meal, wool, and animal bristles; researchers who work with *B. anthracis*; veterinarians likely to be exposed
Hepatitis A	Children and adults in high-risk areas
Hepatitis B	All children, susceptible health care workers, male homosexuals, intravenous drug users, individuals exposed to blood products
Japanese B encephalitis	Travelers to high-risk areas
Haemophilus Influenzae Type b (Hib)	Children starting at 2 months of age
Measles, mumps, influenza, varicella, rubella	Susceptible health care personnel
Meningococcus	Military personnel, young adults living in college dormitories, sleep-away camp
Plague	Persons in regular contact with rodents, investigators working with *Yersinia pestis*
Rabies	Veterinarians, animal handlers, animal bite victims
Typhoid	Travelers to high-risk areas
Yellow fever	Travelers to high-risk areas

[a]Adapted from the Centers for Disease Control and Prevention (www.cdc.gov/vaccines).

Salmonella typhi, the cause of typhoid fever. Because of unique needs or limited efficacy, some vaccines are recommended under only limited circumstances. These vaccines and appropriate circumstances are listed in Table 21.5.

BASIC MECHANISMS OF PROTECTION

Significance of the Primary and Secondary Responses

The rapidity of the ***anamnestic response*** to a reencounter with antigen provides the host with potential protection on repeated exposures to an infectious agent. This anamnestic response is relevant in at least two significant ways in the application of ***immunoprophylaxis***. First, it may be of particular importance in infections with a relatively long incubation period (greater than 7 days), as shown in Figure 21.3. Thus an individual infected by agent A, which causes disease after a 3-day incubation period, would produce a primary immune response some time (e.g., 7–14 days) after onset of the infection. On a second encounter with agent A, the individual may again develop disease, because an anamnestic response may not be sufficiently rapid to inhibit agent A. The individual infected with agent B, which causes disease after a 14-day incubation period, would produce a primary response (e.g., 7–14 days after infection). On a second encounter with agent B, the anamnestic response occurring within 7 days would be sufficient to reduce the severity or prevent the disease with the 14-day incubation period.

The second influence of the anamnestic response concerns the level to which the immune response has been raised. In the example cited above, agent A, which causes disease in 3 days, may be prevented from causing disease

after a reexposure if there is a persisting high enough level of antibody. Such a level can be achieved deliberately by a series of immunizations (especially applicable with nonviable antigens). Thus, it is customary to give several injections of tetanus toxoid (as the combined diphtheria, tetanus, and pertussis [DTP] vaccine) over a period of 6 months in childhood immunizations. Such a primary series of injections generates anamnestic secondary responses that successively raise the concentration of antitoxin antibodies to protective levels, which are sustained in the serum for 10–20 years.

Age and Timing of Immunizations

The various mechanisms involved in protection can be affected by several factors, including nutritional status, presence of underlying disease (which affects levels of globulin and cell-mediated immunity), and age. The timing of childhood immunization is driven largely by the fact that the efficacy of certain vaccines depends on the age of the child.

In utero, the human fetus normally appears well insulated from antigens and most infectious agents, although certain pathogens (e.g., rubella virus, *Toxoplasma gondii*) can infect the mother and seriously injure the fetus. The immunity of the mother protects the fetus by permitting interception and removal of infectious agents before they can enter the uterus, or it protects the newborn by virtue of transplacental or mammary gland antibody.

The fetus and neonate have poorly developed lymphoid organs, with the exception of the thymus, which at the time of birth is largest in size relative to the body size at any age. The fetus appears capable of synthesizing mainly IgM, which becomes apparent after 6 months of gestation. Levels

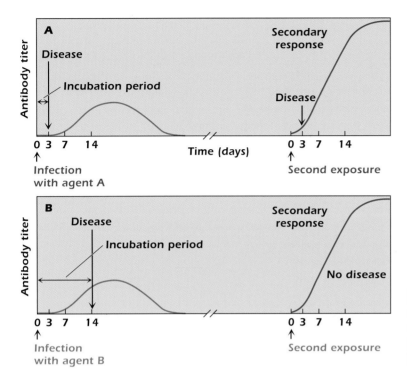

Figure 21.3. The relationship between the primary and secondary immune responses and disease produced by infection with agent A or B. Infection caused by agent A has a shorter incubation period than infection caused by agent B.

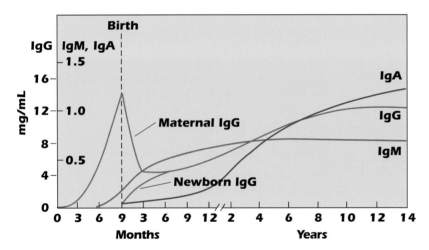

Figure 21.4. Concentration of immunoglobulin in the serum during human development.

of IgM gradually increase to about 10% of the adult level at the time of birth.

IgG becomes detectable in the fetus at about the second month of gestation, but it is IgG of maternal origin. Figure 21.4 shows the concentration of immunoglobulin in serum during human development.

The level of IgG increases significantly at about 4 months of gestation and markedly in the last trimester. At the time of birth, the concentration of IgG slightly exceeds the maternal concentration of IgG. Thus the fetus is provided with maternally synthesized IgG antibodies, which can provide antitoxic, antiviral, and some kinds of antibacte-

rial protection. The levels of these maternal antibodies gradually decline according to the half-life of the immunoglobulin, but the infant begins to synthesize its own antibodies so that total IgG at 23 months of age is less than 50% of the level at birth. Nursing helps maintain levels of certain maternal antibodies and provides maternal derived IgA. The serum concentrations of immunoglobulins during human development are shown in Figure 21.3.

Some aspects of the immune response of the newborn—for example, against some infectious agents (*Toxoplasma gondii*, *Listeria monocytogenes*, herpes simplex virus)—in which cell-mediated immunity is critical are not well developed. But the newborn can produce antibody to various antigens, such as parenterally administered toxoid, inactivated poliomyelitis virus, hepatitis B antigens, and others. However, administration of pertussis vaccine very soon after birth not only fails to induce a protective response but also creates an impaired response (tolerance) to the vaccine when it is given again later in infancy. Therefore, with the exception of the hepatitis B vaccine that is given shortly after birth, in most industrialized countries the initial administration of vaccines is deferred until the child is 2 months old. However, the World Health Organization (WHO) recommends earlier commencement of immunization (at 6 weeks) in developing countries.

Maternal antibody, while capable of providing protection to the neonate against a variety of infectious agents or their toxins, may also reduce the response to antigen. For example, a sufficient quantity of maternal measles antibody persists in the 1-year-old infant to interfere with the active response of the infant to the vaccine, so that vaccination is usually delayed until the child is at least 1 year of age.

Children younger than 2 years of age have a general inability to produce adequate levels of antibody in response to injection of bacterial capsular polysaccharides such as those of *Haemophilus influenzae* type b, various serogroups of *Neisseria meningitidis*, and *Streptococcus pneumoniae* serotypes. It has been suggested that this inability arises because infants do not respond to T-independent antigens, despite their early (*in utero*) capacity to generate IgM. Chemical linkage of polysaccharide to T-dependent antigens (e.g., diphtheria toxoid) or to the *N. meningitidis* outer membrane protein has improved the immunogenicity so that children younger than 2 years of age respond to polysaccharides. An effective conjugate vaccine is already available against *H. influenzae*, which has virtually eliminated this infection in vaccinated children. For *S. pneumoniae*, a heptavalent vaccine containing polysaccharides of pneumococcal serotypes common in childhood infections is now in routine use.

At the other end of the age spectrum, in individuals older than 60 years of age there also appears to be a reduced capability to mount a primary response to some antigens, such as influenza virus vaccine. However, older adults retain the ability to mount a secondary response to antigens to which they have been previously exposed. Healthy older adults also respond well to bacterial polysaccharides, so that administration of pneumococcal polysaccharide vaccine can usually induce protective levels of antibody. Other groups that are especially susceptible to pneumococcal pneumonia (see earlier in this chapter) should also be immunized. Groups that have enhanced susceptibility to the encapsulated respiratory pathogen *Streptococcus pneumoniae* and those at high risk of exposure (e.g., residents of nursing homes and medical personnel) should also receive influenza virus vaccines.

VACCINE PRECAUTIONS

Site of Administration of Antigen

The usual site of parenteral (intradermal, subcutaneous, intramuscular) administration of vaccines in adults is the arm, in particular the deltoid muscle. In children, the thigh is routinely used. Studies have shown a suboptimal response to hepatitis B vaccine when given by intragluteal injection than by injection in the arm. The parenteral administration of inactivated polio vaccine may induce a higher antibody response in the serum than the attenuated oral polio vaccine, but the response to the latter, which includes secretory IgA, affords adequate protection. However, use of the attenuated oral polio vaccine has been discontinued because the live virus can, in exceptionally rare circumstances, cause disease.

Some vaccines may provide a greater antibody response when given by the respiratory route than when given by injection (e.g., attenuated measles vaccine), but administration via the respiratory route remains an investigational method.

Hazards

There are potential hazards associated with the use of some vaccines. Vaccines made from attenuated agents (e.g., measles, mumps, rubella, oral polio, bacille Calmette–Guérin) have the potential for causing progressive disease in the ***immunocompromised patient*** or in the patient on ***immunosuppressive therapy***. In rare cases, reversion of attenuated poliovirus type III to virulence in the intestine of the vaccinated individual has caused paralytic polio. Concern about vaccine-associated paralytic polio has resulted in a change in recommendations for vaccination against polio virus; the inactivated poliovirus vaccine is now the recommended vaccine in the United States. This illustrates the need for constant vigilance in monitoring the prevalence of a given infectious disease in a given population and weighing the risks of disease versus the risks of vaccination. Although vaccines are generally associated with very low toxicity, they are administered to large numbers of individuals, and it must be recognized that as the prevalence of an infectious disease is reduced, the risks of vaccination may be magnified. Hence, the paradoxical situation can occur whereby an effective vaccine reduces the prevalence of an infectious disease to such a low level that rare vaccine-related complications are more frequent than the disease in the population. When that happens, public anxiety about vaccination can result in concerns about vaccine use in general and may reduce its acceptance.

Live attenuated organisms should ordinarily not be given to pregnant women because of potential damage to the fetus. The virions in rubella vaccine have been transmitted to the fetus, although without any recognized injurious effect. Live attenuated vaccines are generally contraindicated for patients with severe immune disorders who may not be able to control the weakened pathogen in the vaccine preparation. Vaccination against smallpox is no longer carried out (except in some military personnel) since the disease has been eradicated. However, as noted above, concerns about the potential of variola virus as a biological weapon have led to debate as to whether universal vaccination should be reintroduced. At this time, the plan is to vaccinate only individuals who are likely to respond or be exposed to a potential biological attack and reserve the vaccine for use in postexposure prophylaxis. One argument against universal vaccination is that vaccinia virus inoculation carries significant risks, not only in immunocompromised individuals but also in individuals with certain cutaneous lesions. Contact between vaccinated and vulnerable individuals must be avoided until the vaccinia lesions have healed.

Arthritis, arthralgia, and rashes are common but transient complications following vaccination with attenuated rubella virus, particularly in adult women. Of the inactivated vaccines, the killed *Bordetella pertussis* bacterial vaccine in DTP was associated with some serious side effects, including encephalopathy in the infant. Although serious side effects were relatively rare and the benefits of the pertussis vaccine outweighed any of alleged risks of immunization, the killed bacteria vaccine was replaced by an acellular vaccine containing inactivated pertussis toxin and one or more antigenic components (e.g., filamentous hemagglutinin and fimbriae). The acellular pertussis vaccine has significantly fewer side effects than the earlier vaccine while retaining efficacy.

Tetanus and diphtheria toxoids may provoke local hypersensitivity reactions. Because an adequate initial series of immunizations in childhood appears to give immunity that lasts about 10 years, the use of booster injections of tetanus toxoid should be guided by the nature of an injury and the history of immunization. The increased hypersensitivity to diphtheria toxoid of adolescents and adults necessitates use of a smaller dose of diphtheria toxoid than is used for children. Because influenza virus is cultivated in chick embryos, allergy to egg protein is a contraindication to vaccination against this virus. Whole influenza virus vaccine is used in adults but gives side effects in children, so a split-virus component vaccine is recommended for children younger than 13 years of age. Some vaccines contain preservatives, such as the organomercurial compound thimerosal (Merthiolate), or antibiotics, such as neomycin or streptomycin, to which the vaccinated individual may be allergic.

RECENT APPROACHES TO PRODUCTION OF VACCINES

Advances in recombinant DNA technology and in the technology of rapid, automated synthesis of peptides and other areas of bioengineering (e.g., monoclonal antibodies) hold promise for improvements in available vaccines and new approaches to the production of vaccines.

Vaccines Produced by Recombinant DNA

Recombinant DNA technology provides the means for expressing protein antigens in large amounts for vaccine use. As noted earlier, one example of the successful application of recombinant DNA technology to vaccine production is provided by the experience with the hepatitis B vaccine. Hepatitis B is a major cause of liver infection and is associated with a long-term risk of hepatocellular carcinoma. An effective vaccine against hepatitis B was developed in the 1970s by purifying viral antigen from the blood of chronically infected donors. In the 1980s, the HIV epidemic heightened awareness about transmission of blood-borne pathogens, and there were concerns that this vaccine could transmit disease. Although several studies showed the plasma-derived vaccine was safe, an alternative was developed by expressing the hepatitis B antigen in yeast using recombinant DNA technology. This recombinant vaccine simplified the production of antigen by avoiding reliance on human blood plasma and eliminated any potential hazard arising from inadvertent contamination of vaccine antigen with blood-borne pathogens.

In 2006, the first recombinant vaccine against HPV was approved for use in girls aged 11–12 years old. HPV vaccination is now recommended for preteen girls and boys in the same age group. This marked the first vaccine developed to prevent cancer, specifically cervical cancer and other diseases in women that are caused by HPV. Other vaccines produced by recombinant DNA technology are in various stages of clinical testing. Some of these molecular approaches may provide practical, safer, and more effective means of immunization than are currently available.

Conjugated Polysaccharides

Conjugated polysaccharide vaccines have revolutionized the approach to vaccination against encapsulated bacterial pathogens. Humoral immunity is critical for protection against encapsulated pathogens, but most microbial polysaccharides are T-independent antigens, which are usually poorly immunogenic. Another problem with polysaccharide vaccines is that young children tend not to mount antibody responses to polysaccharide antigens. Children are at high risk for infection with encapsulated bacteria such as *Streptococcus pneumoniae* and *Haemophilus influenzae*. Conjugation of polysaccharide to a protein (e.g., **tetanus** or **diphtheria toxoid**) results in a molecule that behaves as a T-dependent antigen and elicits strong antibody responses to the polysaccharide moiety. Conjugation of such (bacterial) polysaccharides or oligosaccharides (e.g., of *H. influenzae*), to proteins such as diphtheria toxoid has provided vaccines that are effective in this age group. Conjugated polysaccharide vaccines are currently available against *H. influenzae* type B and certain serotypes of *S. pneumoniae*. Conjugated polysaccharide vaccines are under development for other pathogens, including meningococci, group B streptococci, *Salmonella typhi* and *Shigella* spp. Conjugated polysaccharide vaccines are protective by eliciting strong antibody responses to the polysaccharide portion of the conjugate.

Synthetic Peptide Vaccines

The premise underlying synthetic peptide vaccine development is to use immunogenic peptides to elicit a protective immune response. Synthetic peptide vaccines are designed using the knowledge of the amino acid sequence of the protein antigen that elicits a protective immune response. In theory, synthetic peptide vaccines have the advantage that highly purified peptides may be made in large quantities and their simpler antigenic composition may afford protection with fewer side effects. The general approach is to identify potential epitopes in a protective protein antigen using various algorithms, synthesize a series of peptides corresponding to the amino acid sequence, and test these for immunologic activity. One problem with peptide vaccines is that peptides are poorly immunogenic due to their small size, and they require conjugation to carrier proteins. Several synthetic peptide vaccines are currently in clinical testing. Peptide vaccines have shown promise against viruses that cause hand-foot-and-mouth disease (Coxsackie virus A16 or enterovirus 71), and malaria.

Virus-Carrier Vaccine

It is possible to introduce into a live virus, such as vaccinia, adenovirus, or poliovirus, by means of a vector, a gene from another organism that codes for a desired antigen. The vaccinia virus construct replicates in the host, expresses the foreign gene, and then serves as a vaccine for that particular antigen. This approach is useful provided that the vaccinia virus is not hazardous to the host (as it may be to an immunocompromised individual). This virus-carrier vaccine has the additional advantage in that it can potentially induce both cell-mediated and antibody-mediated immunity to the incorporated antigen.

Bacterium-Carrier Vaccine

Attenuated bacteria such as strains of *Salmonella typhimurium*, *Escherichia coli*, and bacillus Calmette–Guérin can also serve as carriers for pathogen genes in an effort to elicit pathogen-specific responses. These bacteria are altered by recombinant techniques, which introduce a foreign gene that can express the antigens of pathogenic microbes and induce immune responses. In the future, *Salmonella typhimurium*, an intestinal pathogen, could be used to induce mucosal immunity to the foreign antigens.

DNA Vaccines

Vaccination with a plasmid encoding the DNA sequence for an antigenic epitope that elicits protective immunity and that is linked to a strong mammalian promoter can elicit an immune response to the protein. DNA vaccines are thought to work by allowing the expression of the microbial antigen inside host cells that take up the plasmid. DNA vaccines function by generating the desired antigen inside cells, thereby facilitating MHC presentation. Other advantages of DNA vaccines are the absence of infection risk, greater stability relative to protein vaccines, and the possibility for better modulation of the immune response by delivering the antigen to cells that are not usually infected by the pathogen. DNA vaccines could be useful for immunizing young children who still have maternal antibody. The feasibility of DNA immunization has now been demonstrated against several viral, bacterial, and protozoal infections in laboratory animals. Several DNA vaccines are undergoing testing in humans to determine their usefulness in prevention or treatment of malaria and hepatitis B infection. However, no DNA vaccines are currently in use in humans. A recent clinical trial to examine the efficacy of a DNA-based HIV vaccine comprising a non-replicating adenovirus vector and the HIV *gag*, *pol*, and *nef* genes was, unfortunately, abruptly terminated. It was found that administration of the vaccine to uninfected people was associated with significantly increased incidences of HIV infection as compared with individuals given a placebo control vaccine. The apparent explanation for this disappointing outcome was that an earlier infection with adenovirus (common cold virus) activated memory CD4$^+$ T cells, which are the ideal targets of HIV. Another, unrelated concern with DNA vaccines has been possibility that they could be mutagenic by integrating in host DNA. At this time, DNA vaccines continue to be the subject of intense experimental study.

Toxoids

Toxins can be inactivated to produce nonpathogenic toxoids used for vaccination. Toxoids are among the earliest and most successful vaccines. Administration of toxoids prepared from inactivated tetanus, botulism, or diphtheria toxin elicit antibody responses that prevent disease. Toxoids are effective despite the fact that natural infection does not always confer long-lasting immunity, presumably because the amount of toxin produced in infection may not be sufficient to elicit a strong immune response. Hence a bout of tetanus or diphtheria does not confer immunity to recurrent infection, but vaccination with a toxoid provides full protection.

PASSIVE IMMUNIZATION

Passive immunization results from the transfer of antibody or immune cells to an individual from another individual who has already responded to direct stimulation by antigen. Passive immunization differs from active immunization in that it does not rely on the ability of the host's immune system to make the appropriate response. Hence passive immunization with antibodies results in the immediate availability of antibodies that can mediate protection against pathogens. Passive immunization can occur naturally as is the case during transfer of antibodies through the placenta or colostrum, or therapeutically when preformed antibody is administered for the prophylaxis or therapy of infectious diseases.

Passive Immunization through Placental Antibody Transfer

The developing fetus is passively immunized with maternal IgG as a result of placental transfer of antibody. Such antibodies are present at birth and protect the infant against infections for which IgG is sufficient and for which the mother had immunity. For example, transfer of antibody to toxins (tetanus, diphtheria), viruses (measles, poliovirus, mumps, etc.), and certain bacteria (*Haemophilus influenzae* or *Streptococcus agalactiae* group B) can provide protection to the child in the first months of life. Hence adequate active immunization of the mother is a simple and effective means of providing passive protection to the fetus and infant. (However, some premature infants may not acquire the maternal antibodies to the extent that full-term infants do.) Toxoid vaccination can elicit IgG responses that cross the placenta to provide protection to the fetus and newborn. This protection is extremely important in areas of the world where an unclean obstetric environment can lead to *tetanus neonatorum* (of the newborn).

Passive Immunization via Colostrum

Human milk contains a variety of factors that may influence the response of the nursing infant to infectious agents. Some of these factors are natural selective factors that can affect the intestinal microflora by the enhancement of growth of desirable bacteria, and by nonspecific inhibitors of some microbes, through the action of lysozyme, lactoferrin, interferon, and leukocytes (macrophages, T cells, B cells, and granulocytes). Antibodies (IgA) are found in breast milk, with the concentration being higher in the colostrum (first milk) immediately postpartum (Table 21.6). The production of antibody is the result of B cells that are stimulated by intestinal antigens and migrate to the breast where they produce immunoglobulin (the enteromammary system). Thus organisms colonizing or infecting the alimentary tract of the mother may lead to production of colostral antibody,

TABLE 21.6. Levels of Immunoglobulin in Colostrum[a]

	Day Postpartum				
Class	1	2	3	4	Approximate Normal Adult
IgA[b]	600	260	200	80	200
IgG[c]	80	45	30	16	1,000
IgM	125	65	58	30	120

[a]After Michael, Ringenbaek, and Hottenstein, 1971; values given are mg/100 mL.
[b]Approximately 80% is secretory IgA.
[c]IgG$_4$ represents 15% of colostral IgG and 3.5% of serum IgG.

which affords mucosal protection to the nursing infant against pathogens that enter via the intestinal tract. Antibody to the enteropathogens *Escherichia coli*, *Salmonella typhi*, *Shigella* spp., poliomyelitis virus, coxsackievirus, and echovirus have been demonstrated. Feeding a mixture of IgA (73%) and IgG (26%) derived from human serum to low birth weight infants who did not have access to mothers' breast milk protected them against necrotizing enterocolitis. Antibodies to non-alimentary pathogens have also been demonstrated in colostrums—for example, tetanus and diphtheria antitoxins and antistreptococcal hemolysin.

Tuberculin-sensitive T lymphocytes are also transmitted to the infant through the colostrum, but the role of such cells in passive transfer of cell-mediated immunity is uncertain.

Passive Antibody Therapy and Serum Therapy

The administration of specific antibody preparations was one of the first effective antimicrobial therapies. Antibody against particular pathogens could be raised in animals, such as horses and rabbits (heterologous antibody), and administered to humans for treatment of various infections as serum therapy. Serum from individuals recovering from infection is rich in antibodies and can also be used for passive antibody therapy (homologous antibody). In recent years, some monoclonal antibodies made in the laboratory have been used for passive antibody therapy of infectious diseases. This is an area of intense research activity, and it is likely that more antimicrobial therapies based on antibody administration will be developed in the future.

The active agent in serum therapy is specific antibody. In the pre-antibiotic era (before 1935), serum therapy was often the only therapy available for the treatment of infection. Serum therapy was used for the treatment of diphtheria, tetanus, pneumococcal pneumonia, meningococcal meningitis, scarlet fever, and other serious infections. For example, in World War I, tetanus antitoxin produced in horses injected with tetanus toxoid was used to treat the wounded British troops and resulted in prompt reduction in cases of tetanus. This experience allowed the determination of the minimum

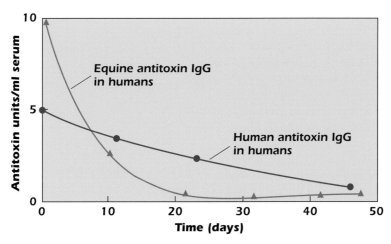

<u>Figure 21.5.</u> Serum concentration of human and equine IgG antitoxin following administration into humans.

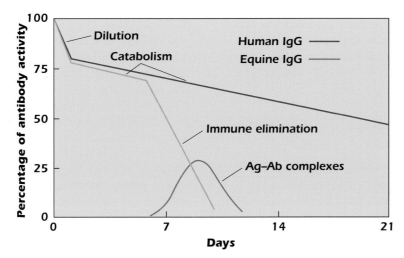

<u>Figure 21.6.</u> The fate of human and equine IgG following administration into humans. The lighter red line illustrates the rate of elimination of equine IgG caused by the host's antibody response to non-human IgG.

concentration of antitoxin needed to provide protection and showed that the period of protection in the human was brief. The basis for the latter is shown in Figures 21.5 and 21.6. The heterologous equine antibody in the human undergoes dilution, catabolism, immune complex formation, and immune elimination. By contrast, the homologous human antibody, which reaches a peak level in the serum about 2 days after subcutaneous injection, undergoes dilution and catabolism with a reduction to half the maximal concentration in about 23 days (the half-life of human IgG_1, IgG_2, and IgG_4 is 23 days; that of IgG_3 is 7 days). The protective level of the human antibody is thus sustained considerably longer than that of the equine antibody. Heterologous antibody, such as that from the horse, can cause at least two kinds of hypersensitivity reaction: type I (immediate, anaphylaxis [see Chapter 15]) or type III (serum sickness from immune complexes [see Chapter 16]). If no other treatment is avail-

able, it is possible to use the heterologous antiserum in an individual with type I sensitivity by administration of gradually increasing but minute amounts of the foreign serum, given repeatedly over several hours. Some preparations of heterologous antibody (e.g., equine diphtheria antitoxin and antilymphocyte serum [ALS]) are still used in humans. In recent years, advances in hybridoma and recombinant DNA technology provided the means to synthesize human immunoglobulins for therapy, and we no longer depend on animal sources for therapeutic antibodies. Human antibodies have significantly longer half-life and reduced toxicity in humans.

Monoclonal and Polyclonal Preparations

Hybridoma technology that allows the production of monoclonal antibodies was discovered in 1975 (see Chapter 6). Polyclonal preparations result from the antibody response to immunization or recovery from infection in a host. In general, antibody to a specific agent is only a small fraction of the total antibody in a polyclonal preparation. Furthermore, polyclonal preparations usually contain antibodies to multiple antigens and include antibodies of various isotypes. Monoclonal antibody preparations differ from polyclonal antibody preparations in that a monoclonal antibody has one specificity and one isotype. As a result, the activity of monoclonal antibody preparations is considerably greater for the amount of protein present than polyclonal preparations. Another advantage of monoclonal preparations is that they are invariant and do not have the lot-to-lot variability associated with polyclonal preparations that depend on quantitative and qualitative aspects of the immune response for their potency. However, polyclonal preparations have the advantage, by including antibodies with multiple specificities and isotypes, of encompassing a higher biologic diversity. In the past 5 years at least a dozen monoclonal antibodies have been licensed for clinical use. Most of them have been developed for therapy of cancer, although one is now licensed for the prevention of respiratory syncytial virus infections in young children. Several monoclonal and polyclonal antibody preparations are currently used for human therapy.

Preparation and Properties of Human Immune Serum Globulin

The use of immune globulin from human serum began in the early 1900s, when serum of patients convalescing from measles was given to children who had been exposed to measles but had not yet developed symptoms. Additional attempts in 1916 and later showed that early administration of serum obtained from individuals who had recovered from infection with measles virus could protect against the emergence of clinically apparent measles. In 1933, human placentas were also recognized as a source of measles antibody. A problem with using serum for passive therapy is that it contains relatively little antibody in a large volume. In the early 1940s, Cohn and co-workers devised a method for the separation of the *gammaglobulin* (γ-globulin) fraction from human serum by precipitation with cold ethanol. This so-called **Cohn fractionation** represented a practical and safe method for production of homologous human antibody for clinical use.

Plasma is collected from healthy donors or placentas. The plasma or sera from hundreds of donors are pooled, and the preparation is then processed for clinical use. If the plasma or serum is from donors who are specially selected after an immunizing or booster dose of antigen or after convalescence from a specific infection, the specific immune globulin preparation is designated accordingly: tetanus immune globulin (TIG), hepatitis B immune globulin (HBIG), varicella-zoster immune globulin (VZIG), and rabies immune globulin (RIG). Large quantities can be

TABLE 21.7. Comparison of Human Immune Serum Globulin

Source	Immunoglobulin (mg/100 mL)		
	IgG	IgA	IgM
Whole serum	1,200	180	200
Immune serum globulin	16,500	100–500	25–200
Intravenous immunoglobulin	3,000–5,000	trace	trace
Placental immune serum globulin	16,500	200–700	150–400

obtained by plasmapheresis removal of the plasma while returning the blood cells to the donor. The fraction containing antibody globulin(s) is precipitated by cold ethanol. The resultant preparation (1) is theoretically free of viruses such as hepatitis virus and HIV, (2) concentrates many of the IgG antibodies about 25-fold, (3) is stable for years, and (4) can provide peak levels in blood approximately 2 days after intramuscular injection. Preparations that are safe when administered intravenously (called IVIG or IVGG) involve cold alcohol precipitation followed by various other treatments, including fractionation using polyethylene glycol or ion exchangers; acidification to pH 4.5; exposure to pepsin or trypsin; and stabilization with maltose, sucrose, glucose, or glycine. Such stabilization reduces aggregation of the globulins that can trigger anaphylactoid reactions (see below). In these intravenous preparations, IgG is present in one third to one fourth its concentration in the intramuscular immune globulin preparations, and there is only a trace of IgA and IgM (Table 21.7).

Indications for the Use of Immune Globulin

Antibody to RhD antigen (**Rhogam**) is given to Rh⁻ mothers at 28 weeks' gestation and a second dose after birth within 72 hours to prevent their immunization by fetal Rh⁺ erythrocytes that could affect future pregnancies. As discussed in Chapter 16, Rhogam administration protects by promoting the removal of Rh⁺ fetal cells to which the mother is exposed during pregnancy and parturition, and thus avoids the sensitizing of the Rh⁻ mother by Rh⁺ antigens. TIG (antitoxin) is used to provide passive protection after certain wounds and in the absence of adequate active immunization with tetanus toxoid. Varicella-zoster globulin (VZIG) is given to patients with leukemia who are highly vulnerable to the varicella-zoster (chickenpox) virus and to pregnant women and their infants exposed to or infected with varicella virus. Cytomegalovirus human immune globulin (CMV-IVIG) is used prophylactically for recipients of bone marrow transplants. RIG is given together with active immunization with human diploid cell rabies vaccine to individuals bitten by potentially rabid animals (human RIG is not universally available, so equine antibody may be necessary in some areas). HBIG may be given to a newborn child of a mother who has evidence of hepatitis B infection, to medical personnel after an accidental stick with a hypodermic needle, or after sexual contact with an individual with hepatitis B. (Immune serum globulin [ISG] may also be used against hepatitis B.) Vaccinia immune globulin is given to eczematous or immunocompromised individuals with intimate exposure to others who have been vaccinated against smallpox by live attenuated vaccinia vaccine. Such compromised individuals can develop destructive progressive disease from the attenuated vaccine.

IVIG has also been used in certain circumstances for its antimicrobial properties and has had significant success against group B streptococcal infections in premature neonates, echovirus-induced chronic meningoencephalitis, and Kawasaki disease (a condition of unknown cause). Intravenous administration of immune globulin can reduce bacterial infections in patients with hematopoietic malignancies, such as chronic B-cell lymphocytic leukemia and multiple myeloma. Chronic IVIG administration has been useful in children who have immunosuppressive conditions and in premature infants; in hypogammaglobulinemia and primary immune deficiency disease, repeated injections of ISG are required. IVIG also has therapeutic value in a variety of autoimmune conditions. For example, in immune thrombocytopenic purpura (ITP), IVIG presumably blocks the Fc receptors on phagocytic cells and prevents them from phagocytosing and destroying platelets coated with autoantibodies. IVIG has also been used with varying success in other immune cytopenias.

Precautions on the Uses of Human Immune Serum Globulin Therapy

The preparations of globulin other than IVIG have to be given by the intramuscular route; intravenous administration is contraindicated because of possible anaphylactoid reactions. These are probably due to aggregates of immunoglobulin formed during the fractionation by ethanol precipitation. These aggregates activate complement to yield anaphylatoxins (IgG_1, IgG_2, IgG_3, and IgM by the classical pathway; IgG_4 and IgA, by the alternative pathway) or cross-link Fc receptors directly, leading to the release of inflamma-

tory mediators. The IVIG that is safe for intravenous administration has been increasingly used, particularly when repeated administration is required, as in patients with agammaglobulinemia.

One unique contraindication to the use of the usual immune globulin preparations is in cases of congenital deficiency of IgA. Since these patients lack IgA, they recognize it as a foreign protein and respond by making antibodies against it, including IgE antibodies, which can lead to a subsequent anaphylactic reaction. The IVIG preparations with only a trace of IgA may pose less of a problem. IVIG preps do not have IgA.

Colony-Stimulating Factors

Colony-stimulating factors (CSFs), as discussed in Chapter 12, are cytokines that stimulate the development and maturation of white blood cells. Granulocyte colony-stimulating factor (G-CSF), granulocyte-macrophage colony-stimulating factor (GM-CSF), and macrophage colony-stimulating factor (M-CSF) have been cloned by recombinant DNA technology and are now available for clinical use. CSFs have proven to be useful in accelerating the recovery of bone marrow cells in patients who have undergone myelosuppressive therapy for cancer or organ transplantation. In these patients, neutrophil depletion (neutropenia) is a major predisposing factor for severe infection. By shortening the period of neutropenia, CSFs can reduce the incidence of serious infections in patients receiving myelosuppressive therapy. CSFs also enhance leukocyte function, and there is encouraging preliminary information suggesting that these proteins may be useful as immunotherapy for enhancing host defenses against various pathogens.

Several other cytokines are powerful activators of the immune system, and there is great interest in learning how to use them as adjunctive therapy against infectious diseases. IFN-γ is a powerful activator of macrophage function, which has been shown to reduce the incidence of severe infections in patients with chronic granulomatous disease. IFN-γ has shown encouraging results as adjunctive therapy for some infections, including drug-resistant *Mycobacterium tuberculosis* infection, hepatitis B and hepatitis C infections, and several unusual fungal infections.

SUMMARY

1. To cause disease, microbes must cause damage to the host.

2. The effective host defenses against individual pathogens depend on the type of pathogen. In general, successful protection against most pathogens

involves both humoral and cellular components of the innate and adaptive immune systems.

3. Pathogens use a variety of strategies to escape host defenses, including polysaccharide capsules, antigenic variation, intracellular survival, proteolytic

enzymes, and active suppression of the immune response.

4. In general, an effective host response to a pathogen uses components of both humoral and cellular immunity. However, for some pathogens, one arm of the immune system may provide the primary protection.

5. Protection against infectious diseases may be achieved by active as well as passive immunization.

6. Active immunization may result from previous infection or from vaccination, while passive immunization may occur by natural means (such as the transfer of antibodies from mother to fetus via the placenta or to an infant via the colostrum) or by artificial means (such as by the administration of immune globulins).

7. Active immunization may be achieved by administration of one immunogen or a combination of immunogens.

8. The incubation period of a disease and the rapidity with which protective antibody titers develop influence both the efficacy of vaccination and the anamnestic effect of a booster injection.

9. The site of administration of a vaccine may be of great importance; many routes of immunization lead to the synthesis predominantly of serum IgM and IgG; oral administration of some vaccines leads to the induction of secretory IgA in the digestive tract.

10. Immunoprophylaxis has had striking success against subsequent infection; immunotherapy has had limited success in infectious diseases.

REFERENCES AND BIBLIOGRAPHY

Barr E, Tamms G. (2007) Quadrivalent human papillomavirus vaccine. *Clin Infect Dis* 45: 609.

Bijker MS, Melief CJ, Offringa R, van der Burg SH. (2007) Design and development of synthetic peptide vaccines: past, present and future. *Expert Rev Vaccines* 6: 591.

Carruthers VB, Cotter PA, Kumamoto CA. (2007) Microbial pathogenesis: mechanisms of infectious disease. *Cell Host Microbe* 2: 214.

Casadevall A, Pirofski L. (2000) Host-pathogen interactions: basic concepts of microbial commensalism, colonization, infection, and disease. *Infect Immun* 68: 6511.

Casadevall A, Pirofski L. (2003) The damage-response framework of microbial pathogenesis. *Nat Rev Micro* 1: 17.

Casadevall A, Scharff MD. (1994) "Serum therapy" revisited: animal models of infection and the development of passive antibody therapy. *Antimicrob Agents Chemother* 38: 1695.

Centers of Disease Control and Prevention. (2006) Recommended childhood immunization schedule—United States. *Ann Pharmacother* 40: 369.

Deitsch KW, Moxon ER, Wellems TE. (1997) Shared themes of antigenic variation and virulence in bacterial, protozoal, and fungal infections. *Microbiol Molec Biol Rev* 61: 283.

Doherty PC, Turner SJ. (2007) The challenge of viral immunity. *Immunity* 27: 363.

Hanke T. (2006) On DNA vaccines and prolonged expression of immunogens. *Eur J Immunol* 36: 806.

Hemming VG. (2001) Use of intravenous immunoglobulins for prophylaxis and treatment of infectious diseases. *Clin Diagn Lab Immunol* 8: 85963.

Hubel K, Dale DC, Liles WC. (2002) Therapeutic uses of cytokines to modulate cytokine function for the treatment of infectious diseases: current status of granulocyte colony-stimulating factor, granulocyte-macrophage colony-stimulating factor, macrophage colony-stimulating factor, and interferon-gamma. *J Infect Dis* 185: 1490.

Letvin NL. (2007) Correlates of immune protection and the development of a human immunodeficiency virus vaccine. *Immunity* 27: 366.

Mirza A, Rathore MH. (2007) Immunization update. *Adv Pediatr* 54: 135.

Park JM, Greten FR, Li ZW, Karin M. (2002) Macrophage apoptosis by anthrax lethal factor through p38 MAP kinase inhibition. *Science* 297: 2048.

Pulendran B, Artis D. (2012) New paradigms in type 2 immunity. *Science* 337: 431.

Reichert JM. (2001) Monoclonal antibodies and the clinic. *Nat Biotech* 19: 819.

Robinson HL. (2007) HIV/AIDS vaccines. *Clin Pharmacol Ther* 82: 686.

Schiffman M, Castle PE, Jeronimo J, Rodriguez AC, Wacholder S. (2007) Human papillomavirus and cervical cancer. *Lancet* 370: 890.

REVIEW QUESTIONS

For each question, choose the ONE BEST answer or completion.

1. The usual sequence of events in the development of an effective immune response to a viral infection is
   A) interferon secretion, antibody synthesis, cellular immune response, NK cell ADCC
   B) antibody synthesis, interferon secretion, NK cell ADCC, cellular immune response
   C) NK cell ADCC, interferon secretion, antibody synthesis, cellular immune response
   D) interferon secretion, cellular immune response, antibody synthesis, NK cell ADCC
   E) cellular immune response, interferon secretion, antibody synthesis, NK cell ADCC

2. Differences between Gram-positive and Gram-negative bacteria include
   A) staining with crystal violet
   B) ability of complement to lyse cells
   C) thickness of the peptidoglycan layer
   D) endotoxin in the cell walls of Gram-negative bacteria
   E) all of the above

3. Antigenic variation is a mechanism of immune evasion that results in
   A) interference with attachment to host receptors
   B) induction of immune suppression
   C) alterations in important surface antigens so that escape variants arise as a result of immune selection
   D) changes in the nature of expression of surface antigens
   E) destruction of antigens by proteolytic enzymes

4. The best way to provide immunologic protection against tetanus neonatorum (of the newborn) is to
   A) inject the infant with human tetanus antitoxin
   B) inject the newborn with tetanus toxoid
   C) inject the mother with toxoid within 72 hours of the birth of her child
   D) immunize the mother with tetanus toxoid before or early in pregnancy
   E) give the child antitoxin and toxoid for both passive and active immunization

5. Active, durable immunization against poliomyelitis can be accomplished by oral administration of attenuated vaccine (Sabin) or by parenteral injection of inactivated (Salk) vaccine. These vaccines are equally effective in preventing disease because
   A) both induce adequate IgA at the intestinal mucosa, the site of entry of the virus
   B) antibody in the serum protects against the viremia that leads to disease
   C) viral antigen attaches to the anterior horn cells in the spinal cord, preventing attachment of virulent virus
   D) both vaccines induce formation of interferon
   E) both vaccines establish a mild infection that can lead to formation of antibody

6. The administration of vaccines is not without hazard. Of the following, which is least likely to adversely affect an immunocompromised host?
   A) measles vaccine
   B) pneumococcal vaccine
   C) bacille Calmette–Guérin
   D) mumps vaccine
   E) Sabin poliomyelitis vaccine

7. The administration of foreign (e.g., equine) antitoxin for passive protection in humans can lead to serum sickness, which is characterized by all of the following except which?
   A) production by host of antibody to foreign antibody
   B) onset in 24–48 hours
   C) use of homologous antitoxin
   D) deposition of antigen–antibody complexes at various sites in the host
   E) although delayed, the reaction is not a type IV hypersensitivity response

8. The pneumococcal polysaccharide vaccine should be administered to all except which group?
   A) individuals with chronic cardiorespiratory disease
   B) older adults (>60 years of age)
   C) children (<2 years of age)
   D) persons with chronic renal failure
   E) individuals with sickle cell disease

9. The following statements about human immune serum globulin are true except which one?
   A) The source is human placenta.
   B) The globulins are obtained by precipitation with cold ethanol.
   C) The concentration of IgG is more than tenfold greater than in plasma.
   D) IgA and IgM are present in concentrations slightly lower than in plasma.
   E) The ethanol precipitation does not render preparation of globulin free of hepatitis virus.

10. A common feature of helminth infections is that the host response immune mechanisms involved are dominated by:
    A) T_H1 responses
    B) T_H2 responses
    C) T_H17 responses
    D) antibody responses
    E) NK responses

ANSWERS TO REVIEW QUESTIONS

1. D. The usual sequence of events in the host immune response to a viral infection is interferon secretion, cellular immune response, antibody synthesis, NK cell ADCC. Interferon is produced early in the course of viral infection and serves to slow the infection of adjoining cells. Cellular immune responses in the form of cytotoxic CD8⁺ T cells occur early in viral infection and usually precede the appearance of serum-neutralizing antibody or NK cell-mediated ADCC (which requires specific antibody).

2. E. Differences between Gram-positive and Gram-negative bacteria include staining with crystal violet. Gram-negative cells can be lysed by complement, but Gram-positive cells are complement resistant because of a thick peptidoglycan layer. Gram-negative bacteria have endotoxin in their cell walls that can cause hemodynamic compromise and septic shock in patients with Gram-negative sepsis. Gram-positive bacteria lack endotoxin but have teichoic acids that are immunogenic.

3. C. Antigenic variation is common to many pathogens and is a mechanism by which they are able to escape the immune system. Antigenic variation can be the result of various mechanisms including mutation, changes in surface protein expression, and natural variation among strains such as occurs in the pneumococci. The potential of a microorganism for antigenic variation is a major consideration in vaccine design.

4. D. The simplest and most effective way to protect the newborn infant against exotoxic disease, such as tetanus and diphtheria, is to induce antibody in the mother. The antitoxic IgG passing through the placenta will provide the necessary protection. While tetanus antitoxin could be used to provide short-term passive protection, it would be more costly and require an otherwise unnecessary and painful injection. Injection of toxoid in the mother within 72 hours of delivery of the child would not allow time for induction of antibody. While antitoxin and toxoid could provide immediate passive and future active protection, the latter would have to be accompanied by future injections of toxoid, and the former is expensive; both would require undesirable injections.

5. B. Both attenuated and inactivated vaccines lead to formation of circulating antibody, which would provide protection by intercepting the infecting virus before it reaches the target tissue in the central nervous system. While the Sabin vaccine induces mucosal gut IgA that may intercept virus at the portal of entry, the parenterally injected Salk vaccine is not effective in inducing mucosal IgA.

Viral antigen in the vaccine might attach to the anterior horn cells in the nervous system, but it probably would not provide durable immunity. Induction of interferon would represent potentially only brief protection. Only the Sabin vaccine, being attenuated and live, would induce a mild infection.

6. B. The pneumococcal vaccine consists of capsular polysaccharides from *Streptococcus pneumoniae* and represents a nonviable vaccine that cannot lead to infection. Measles, mumps, and Sabin polio vaccines contain attenuated viruses, and bacille Calmette–Guérin is an attenuated bacterium. These attenuated organisms are capable of proliferating in the human host. The normal host limits their replication, but the immunocompromised host may not be able to do so, and progressive infection may occur.

7. B. The reactions that constitute serum sickness follow administration of the foreign substance within 6–12 days. During this time, the host produces antibody that reacts with the foreign substance(s), which persists in the host and leads to antigen–antibody complexes that can be deposited in joints, lymph nodes, skin, and elsewhere. The manifestation of the immune reaction, although appearing later, nevertheless is classified as type III rather than cell-mediated delayed (type IV) hypersensitivity because it involves antibodies rather than T cells.

8. C. Children younger than 2 years of age do not respond adequately to immunization with pure bacterial capsule polysaccharide vaccine due to the absence of marginal zone B cells that can respond to T-independent antigens. Therefore, vaccinating them may be useless. The various other individuals listed are particularly vulnerable to infection with *Streptococcus pneumoniae*. While some of them may mount a suboptimal response to the vaccine, they should nevertheless be vaccinated.

9. E. The potential hazard of hepatitis viruses in human plasma is overcome by the separation of ethanol-precipitated globulins. The concentration of IgG is about 16,500 mg/dL, compared to 1,200 mg/dL in plasma. Whereas the IgG thus becomes highly concentrated in immune serum globulin, IgA and IgM are relatively depleted, and their concentration in the ethanol-precipitated immune serum globulin is close to their original concentration in the plasma.

10. B. A common feature of individuals that harbor helminth infections is the so-called type 2 immune response mediated by T_H2 cells.

GLOSSARY

ABO blood group system Antigens expressed on red blood cells used for typing human blood for transfusion. Individuals who do not express A or B antigens on their red blood cells naturally form antibodies that interact with these antigens.

accessory cell Cell required to initiate immune responses, often used to describe an antigen-presenting cell. See also **antigen-presenting cell**.

accessory molecules Molecules other than the antigen receptor and the major histocompatibility complex (MHC) that participate in activation and effector functions of T-lymphocytes.

acquired immune response Response of antigen-specific lymphocytes to antigen, including the development of immunologic memory; also known as the adaptive immune response.

acquired immunodeficiency syndrome (AIDS) Disease caused by human immunodeficiency virus (HIV) infection, characterized by depletion of CD4$^+$ T cells, leading to a profound defect in cell-mediated immunity. Clinically, AIDS manifests with opportunistic infections, malignant tumors, encephalopathy, and wasting.

activation-induced cytidine deaminase (AID) Enzyme induced in activated B cells that plays a key role in initiating the three major pathways that generate diversity of antibodies: class switch recombination, somatic hypermutation, and gene conversion. It removes cytidine groups from DNA to form uridine.

activation protein 1 (AP-1) Family of DNA-binding transcription factors that bind to one another through a shared structural motif called a leucine zipper. Important members of the AP-1 family include Fos and Jun.

acute-phase proteins Found in the blood after the onset of an infection, they participate in the early phases of host defense. Include cytokines such as IL-1, IL-6, TNF and interferons as well as C-reactive protein.

acute-phase response (APR) Early phase (within hours) of systemic response to infection. See also **acute-phase proteins**.

acute rejection Form of graft rejection involving injury mediated by T cells, macrophages, and antibodies that usually begins the first week following transplantation.

adaptive immune response See **acquired immune response**.

adaptor proteins Key linkers between antigen-specific receptors and downstream components of signaling pathways.

ADCC See **antibody-dependent cell-mediated cytotoxicity**.

addressins Glycoproteins expressed on high endothelial venules of the vascular endothelium at the boundary of

Immunology: A Short Course, Seventh Edition. Richard Coico and Geoffrey Sunshine.
© 2015 John Wiley & Sons, Ltd. Published 2015 by John Wiley & Sons, Ltd.
Companion Website: www.wileyimmunology.com/coico

the nodes that bind adhesion molecules expressed on leukocytes.

adenosine deaminase (ADA) deficiency Form of severe combined immunodeficiency (SCID) in which B and T cells fail to develop. Affected individuals lack the enzyme adenosine deaminase (ADA), which catalyzes the deamination of adenosine as well as deoxyadenosine to produce inosine and deoxyinosine, respectively.

adhesion molecules Molecules that mediate the binding of one cell to another or to extracellular matrix proteins. They include integrins, selectins, and members of the immunoglobulin gene superfamily.

adjuvant Substance given with antigen that enhances the response to the antigen.

adoptive transfer Transfer of the capacity to make an immune response by transplantation of immunocompetent cells.

affinity Measure of the binding constant of a single antigen-combining site with a monovalent antigenic determinant.

affinity chromatography Purification of a substance by means of its affinity for another substance immobilized on a solid support; for example, an antigen purified by affinity chromatography on a column of antigen-specific antibody molecules covalently linked to beads.

affinity maturation Sustained increase in affinity of antibodies for an antigen with time following immunization. The genes encoding the antibody variable regions undergo somatic hypermutation with concomitant selection of B lymphocytes whose receptors express high affinity for the antigen.

agammaglobulinemia See **X-linked agammaglobulinemia**.

agglutination Aggregation of particulate antigen by antibodies.

agonist peptides Peptide antigens that activate T cells with specific TCRs, inducing them to make cytokines and to proliferate.

AIRE See **autoimmune regulator**.

alleles Two or more alternate forms of a gene that occupy the same position or locus on a specific chromosome.

allelic exclusion Ability of heterozygous lymphoid cells to produce only one allelic form of antigen-specific receptor (Ig or TCR) when they have the genetic endowment to produce both. Genes other than those for the antigen-specific receptors are usually expressed codominantly.

allergen Antigen responsible for producing allergic reactions by inducing IgE synthesis.

allergic asthma Clinical phenomenon caused by constriction of the bronchial tree due to allergic reaction to inhaled antigen.

allergic reaction Response to environmental antigens or allergens, which most commonly involves responses mediated by IgE and CD4$^+$ T$_H$2 cells.

allergic rhinitis Allergic reaction in the nasal mucosa, also known as hay fever, that causes runny nose, sneezing, and tears.

allergy Reaction to nonpathogenic antigens in the environment. See **allergic reaction**.

alloantigens MHC antigens expressed on the cells of one individual that differ from the MHC antigens expressed by the cells of a genetically distinct individual. Differences in alloantigen expression stimulate powerful T-cell responses when a tissue is transplanted from one individual to a genetically distinct individual (an **allograft**).

allogeneic Describes genetic variations or differences among members or strains of the same species. Refers to organ or tissue grafts between genetically dissimilar humans or between unrelated members of the same species.

allograft Tissue transplant (graft) between two genetically nonidentical members of a species.

allotypes Antigenic determinants present in allelic (alternate) forms. When used in association with immunoglobulin, describes allelic variants of immunoglobulins detected by antibodies raised between members of the same species.

alternative complement pathway Complement activation initiated by deposition of C3b on cell surface. Occurs in the absence of antibody and part of the innate immune response. Many foreign substances activate this pathway.

alveolar macrophage Macrophage found in the lung alveoli; ingests inhaled material.

anamnestic Term used to describe immunologic memory, which leads to a rapid increase in response after reexposure to antigen.

anaphylatoxin Molecules including C3a and C5a synthesized during complement activation that are potent inducers of inflammatory responses. Trigger histamine release from mast cells, smooth muscle contraction, and enhance vascular permeability.

anaphylaxis Rapid, life-threatening allergic reaction (e.g., after insect bite or sting), resulting in throat swelling and low blood pressure. Caused by immediate hypersensitivity response mediated by IgE binding to mast cells, followed by release of pharmacologically active agents.

anchor residues Amino acid residues of peptide whose side chains fit into pockets in the peptide-binding cleft of an

MHC molecule, thus "anchoring" the peptide in the cleft of the MHC molecule. Each MHC molecule binds preferentially to peptides with specific anchor residues.

anergy State of antigen-specific nonresponsiveness in which a T and/or B cell is present but functionally unable to respond to antigen.

ankylosing spondylitis Chronic inflammatory disease affecting the spine, sacroiliac joints, and/or large peripheral joints, leading to stiffening. Has major genetic predisposition—approximately 90% of patients are HLA-B27$^+$; however, only 1–2% of HLA-B27$^+$ individuals develop the disease.

antibody Serum protein formed in response to an immunogen; binds specifically to an antigen.

antibody-dependent cell-mediated cytotoxicity (ADCC) Mechanism by which target cells coated with IgG antibody are destroyed by specialized killer cells (NK cells and/or macrophages) that express receptors for the Fc portion of coating antibody (Fc receptors). These Fc receptors allow killer cells to bind to the antibody-coated target.

antigen Any foreign material specifically bound by antibody or lymphocytes; also used loosely to describe materials used for immunization (contrast with **immunogen**).

antigen-binding site Site on an antibody or TCR molecule where an antigenic determinant (epitope) is bound. In an Ig molecule, it is located in a cleft bordered by N-terminal variable regions of heavy- and light-chain parts of the Fab region.

antigen capture assay Antigen that binds to a specific antibody; presence is detected using a second antibody that binds to a different epitope.

antigen presentation Display of antigen as peptide fragments bound to MHC molecules on the surface of a cell. T cells recognize antigen only when it is presented in this way.

antigen-presenting cell (APC) Cells such as dendritic cells, macrophages, and B cells that express MHC class II molecules and are involved in presentation of antigen to T cells.

antigen processing Catabolism of proteins into peptides, some of which bind to MHC molecules for presentation to T cells.

antigen receptor The specific antigen-binding receptor expressed on T (=TCR) or B (=BCR) lymphocytes. The receptor is coded for by Variable and Constant region genes.

antigenic determinant Single antigenic site on a complex antigenic molecule or particle. See also **epitope**.

antigenic drift Variations in antigenicity of microorganisms (e.g., viruses, parasites) resulting from point mutations of genes, causing small differences in surface antigen expression.

antigenic shift Reassortment of segmented influenza virus genome with another influenza virus, causing surface antigens to change radically.

anti-immunoglobulin antibodies Antibodies specific for immunoglobulin constant domains useful for detecting bound antibody molecules in immunoassays and other applications.

antiserum (plural: *antisera*) Fluid component of clotted blood from an immune individual containing a heterogeneous collection of antibodies made in response to the immunizing molecule. This heterogeneity makes each antiserum unique. Antibodies in the antiserum bind the antigen used for immunization.

antitoxin Antibody specific for exotoxins produced by certain microorganisms, such as the causative agents of diphtheria and tetanus.

APC See **antigen-presenting cell**.

APECED See **autoimmune polyendocrinopathy-candidiasis–ectodermal dystrophy**.

apoptosis Form of programmed cell death caused by activation of endogenous molecules leading to the fragmentation of DNA.

appendix Gut-associated lymphoid tissue located at the beginning of the colon.

Arthus reaction Type of hypersensitivity reaction produced by local formation of antigen–antibody aggregates that activate the complement cascade and cause thrombosis, hemorrhage, and acute inflammation.

asthma Disease of the lungs characterized (in most cases) by reversible airway obstruction, airway inflammation with prominent eosinophil participation, and increased airway responsiveness to various stimuli. Some cases of asthma are allergic (see **allergic asthma**) and are mediated, in part, by IgE antibody to environmental allergens. Other cases are provoked by nonallergic factors.

ataxia telangiectasia Disorder characterized by cerebellar ataxia, oculocutaneous telangiectasis, variable immunodeficiency affecting function of both T and B lymphocytes, development of lymphoid malignancies, and recurrent sinopulmonary infections.

atopic allergy or atopy Term used to describe IgE-mediated allergic responses in humans, usually showing a genetic predisposition.

autoantibody Antibody produced in an individual that is specific for a self-antigen; can cause damage to cells and tissues.

autochthonous Pertaining to self.

autograft Tissue transplant from one area to another in single individual.

autoimmune disease Disease caused by breakdown of self-tolerance, such that the adaptive immune system responds to self-antigens and mediates cell and tissue damage. Autoimmune diseases can be classified as systemic (e.g., systemic lupus erythematosus) versus organ specific (e.g., thyroiditis or diabetes); alternatively defined by predominant mechanism: either T-cell or B-cell and antibody mediated.

autoimmune polyendocrinopathy candidiasis ectodermal dystrophy Multiorgan autoimmune disease resulting from defects in the AIRE gene product and lack of negative selection in the thymus.

autoimmune regulator (AIRE) AIRE gene product codes for a protein that at least partly controls the expression of self-molecules in thymic medullary epithelial cells. When the AIRE gene product is lacking, deletion of autoreactive lymphocytes (negative selection) is impaired, resulting in autoimmune responses in several tissues. See **autoimmune polyendocrinopathy candidiasis ectodermal dystrophy**.

autoimmunity Immune response to self-tissues or components. Such immune responses may have pathologic consequences leading to autoimmune disease.

autologous Derived from the same individual, or self.

autophagy Pathway that transports proteins from cytoplasm into lysosomes for degradation and possible association with MHC class II molecules.

avidity Summation of multiple affinities; for example, when a polyvalent antibody binds to a polyvalent antigen.

azathioprine Potent immunosuppressive drug converted to its active form *in vivo*, then kills rapidly proliferating cells, including lymphocytes responding to grafted tissues.

$\alpha\beta$ T cell receptor ($\alpha\beta$TCR) Form of TCR expressed by the majority of T cells. Each chain contains highly variable (V) regions which form the antigen-binding site, and constant (C) regions that insert in the cell membrane.

B cell See **B lymphocyte**.

B-cell receptor (BCR) B-cell antigen-specific receptor expressed at the surface and composed of a transmembrane immunoglobulin molecule associated in a noncovalent complex with the invariant Igα and Igβ chains.

B-cell tyrosine kinase (Btk) A Src family tyrosine kinase involved in B-cell activation. Mutations in the gene expressing Btk cause X-linked agammaglobulinemia, in which B cells fail to develop beyond the pre-B-cell stage.

B lymphocyte Lymphocyte that expresses immunoglobulin on its surface. It is the precursor of the plasma cell that synthesizes and secretes antibodies and is thus the central cellular component of humoral immune responses. B lymphocytes develop in the bone marrow, and mature B cells are found mainly in lymphoid follicles in secondary lymphoid tissues, in bone marrow, and in low numbers in the circulation.

B7 Family of co-stimulator proteins (B7.1 and B7.2) in the immunoglobulin superfamily; expression restricted to the surface of APC (e.g., dendritic cells, B cells, macrophages) that activate T lymphocytes. B7 binds to CD28 and CTLA-4 expressed on T cells.

BALT See **bronchus-associated lymphoid tissue**.

bare lymphocyte syndrome Immunodeficiency condition characterized by failure to express either HLA class I or class II gene products.

basophils White blood cells containing granules that stain with basic dyes. Thought to have a function similar to mast cells.

BCG (bacille Calmette–Guerin) *Mycobacterium bovis* strain long used outside the United States as a vaccine against tuberculosis.

BCR See **B-cell receptor**.

Bence Jones protein Dimers of immunoglobulin light chains in the urine of patients with multiple myeloma.

Blk See **tyrosine kinases**.

blocking antibody An antibody capable of blocking the interaction of antigen with cells or with other antibodies.

Bloom's syndrome Disease caused by mutations in DNA helicase and characterized by low T-cell numbers, reduced antibody levels, and increased susceptibility to respiratory infections, cancer, and radiation damage.

bone marrow Site of hematopoiesis, in which stem cells give rise to the cellular elements of blood, including red blood cells, monocytes, polymorphonuclear leukocytes, platelets, and lymphocytes.

bone marrow transplantation Procedure used to treat a variety of conditions, including neoplasia, that are not amenable to other forms of therapy. It has been especially used in cases of aplastic anemia, acute lymphocytic leukemia, and acute nonlymphocytic leukemia.

bradykinin Vasoactive peptide produced as a result of tissue damage and acts as an inflammatory mediator.

bronchus-associated lymphoid tissue (BALT) Secondary lymphoid organs connected to the bronchial tree.

Bruton's agammaglobulinemia See **X-linked agammaglobulinemia**.

bursa of Fabricius Site of development of B cells in birds; an outpouching of the cloaca.

β_2 microglobulin Invariant molecule that associates with the transmembrane α chain of MHC class I to form a four-domain molecule; coded for outside the MHC.

C (constant region) DNA sequence in an immunoglobulin or T-cell receptor gene that encodes the nonvariable portion of an Ig light or heavy chain or TCR chain.

C1 Complement component that initiates the classical complement pathway by attaching to the Fc regions of IgG or IgM.

C1 deficiencies Patients with C1 defects may manifest systemic lupus erythematosus, glomerulonephritis, or pyogenic infections as well as increased incidence of type III (immune complex) hypersensitivity diseases. (Only a few cases of C1q, C1r, or C1r and C1s deficiencies have been reported.)

C1 esterase inhibitor See **C1 inhibitor**. A serum protein that counteracts activated C1. This diminishes the generation of C2b, which facilitates development of edema.

C1 inhibitor or C1 esterase inhibitor (C1INH) Serum protein that binds to C1r and C1s, causing them to dissociate from C1q and preventing the first step in the activation of the classical complement pathway. C1INH also regulates the alternative pathway by inhibiting the function of C3bBb, and the lectin pathway by inhibiting MASP1 and MASP2. In addition, C1INH inhibits the function of enzymes in other serum cascades, particularly those involved in clotting and in the formation of kinins, potent mediators of vascular effects.

C1 inhibitor (C1 INH) deficiency Absence of C1 INH is the most frequently found deficiency of the classic complement pathway; seen in patients with hereditary angioedema.

C1q An 18-polypeptide-chain subcomponent of C1, the first component of the classical complement pathway.

C1q deficiency Deficiency of C1q may be found in association with lupus-like syndromes.

C1r Subcomponent of C1, the first component of complement in the classical activation pathway. Also, a serine esterase.

C1s Serine esterase that is a subcomponent of C1. Ca^{2+} binds two C1s molecules to the C1q stalk.

C2 Third complement protein in the classical complement pathway activation; a single polypeptide chain that binds to C4b molecules on the cell surface in the presence of magnesium.

C2 deficiency Rare deficiency with autosomal recessive mode of inheritance, characterized by pyogenic infections and systemic lupus erythematosus–like symptoms.

C3 Pivotal component of complement activation. All three activation pathways—the classical, alternative, and lectin—converge at C3. Cleavage of C3 results in the formation of C3a and C3b, described below.

C3a Low-molecular-weight (9-kDa) peptide fragment of complement component C3; it is an **anaphylatoxin**.

C3b Key opsonin and the principal fragment produced when complement component C3 is split by either the classical or alternative pathway convertases, i.e., C4b2a or C3bBb, respectively. It results from C3 convertase digestion of C3.

C3 convertase Enzyme that splits C3 into C3b and C3a. There are two types: one in the classical pathway designated C4b2a and one in the alternative pathway of complement activation termed *C3bBb*.

C3 tickover Continual generation of C3b from C3 in the alternative pathway. Hydrolysis of the C3 internal thioester bond is the initiating event.

C4 Cleaved immediately following C1 in the classical pathway of complement activation.

C5 Component in the complement cascade that binds to the C5 convertase in the classical and alternative pathways.

C5a An anaphylatoxin, a small peptide fragment released into the fluid after cleavage of C5.

C5b The larger molecular species that remains after C5 convertase splits C5. It has a binding site for complement component C6 and complexes with it on the cell surface to begin generation of the membrane attack complex (MAC).

C5 convertase Molecular complex that splits C5 into C5a and C5b in both the classical and the alternative pathways of complement activation.

C5 deficiency Very uncommon genetic disorder that has an autosomal recessive mode of inheritance. Individuals with this deficiency have a defective ability to form the membrane attack complex (MAC), which is necessary for the efficient lysis of some clinically relevant microorganisms. They have an increased susceptibility to disseminated infections by *Neisseria*.

C6 Complement component that participates in the membrane attack complex (MAC).

C6 deficiency Very uncommon genetic defect with autosomal recessive mode of inheritance. Affected individuals have only trace amounts of C6 in their plasma and have defective ability to form a membrane attack complex (MAC), with increased susceptibility to disseminated infections by *Neisseria* microorganisms.

C7 Complement component that binds to C5b and C6 to form C5b67 on the surface of a cell as part of the MAC. The complex has the appearance of a stalk with a leaf type of structure.

C7 deficiency Rare genetic disorder, with an autosomal recessive mode of inheritance, associated with a defective ability to form a membrane attack complex (MAC) and increased incidence of disseminated infections caused by *Neisseria* microorganisms.

C8 Complement component that binds to C5bC6C7 and participates in the membrane attack complex (MAC).

C8 deficiency Rare genetic disorder with an autosomal recessive mode of inheritance; associated with a defective ability to form a membrane attack complex (MAC) and an increased propensity to develop disseminated infections caused by *Neisseria* microorganisms such as meningococci.

C9 Complement component that binds to the C5b678 complex on the cell surface. The interaction of 12–15 C9 molecules with one C5b678 complex is the final step in the production of the membrane attack complex (MAC).

C9 deficiency Rare genetic disorder with an autosomal recessive mode of inheritance; defective ability to form the membrane attack complex (MAC).

c-*myc* Cellular proto-oncogene that encodes a nuclear factor involved in cell cycle regulation. Translocations of the c-*myc* gene into Ig loci are associated with B-cell malignant neoplasms.

C-reactive protein Serum protein produced by hepatocytes as part of the acute-phase response. Inflammation induced by bacterial infection, necrosis of tissue, trauma, or malignant tumors may cause an increase in the serum concentration within 48 hours of the inducing condition.

C region See **constant region**.

C-type lectin receptors (CLRs) Type of pattern recognition receptor—large family of membrane-bound receptors that bind to carbohydrates in a calcium-dependent manner (by definition, all lectins bind to carbohydrates). Involved in fungal recognition and modulation of the innate immune response.

calcineurin Cytosolic serine/threonine phosphatase that plays a crucial role in signaling via the TCR. The immunosuppressive drugs cyclosporine A and tracolimus (FK506) form complexes with cellular proteins called *immunophilins* that inactivate calcineurin, thereby suppressing T-cell responses.

calnexin Endoplasmic reticulum (ER) protein that binds partly folded molecules of the Ig superfamily of proteins and returns them to the ER until folding is completed.

calreticulin Molecular chaperone that binds initially to MHC class I, class II, and other proteins containing immunoglobulin-like domains such as the TCR and BCR.

CAM Cell-surface adhesion molecule. See **adhesion molecules**.

carcinoembryonic antigen (CEA) Membrane glycoprotein epitope present in the fetal gastrointestinal tract in normal conditions. CEA levels are elevated in almost one third of patients with colorectal, liver, pancreatic, lung, breast, head and neck, cervical, bladder, medullary thyroid, and prostatic carcinomas.

carrier Large immunogenic molecule or particle to which a hapten or other nonimmunogenic, epitope-bearing molecule may attach, allowing it to become immunogenic.

caspases Family of closely related cysteine proteases that cleave proteins at aspartic acid residues; play important roles in apoptosis.

CD See **cluster of differentiation**.

CDR See **complementarity-determining regions**.

CEA See **carcinoembryonic antigen**.

cell-mediated cytotoxicity Killing (lysis) of a target cell by an effector lymphocyte.

cell-mediated immunity (CMI) Immune reaction mediated by T cells, as opposed to humoral immunity, which is antibody mediated. Also referred to as **delayed-type hypersensitivity**.

central lymphoid organs Sites of lymphocyte development. In humans, B lymphocytes develop in bone marrow, whereas T lymphocytes develop with the thymus from bone marrow-derived progenitors.

central tolerance Self-tolerance induced in primary lymphoid organs as a consequence of immature self-reactive lymphocytes recognizing self-antigens, subsequently leading to their death or inactivation. Central tolerance prevents emergence of lymphocytes with high-affinity receptors for self-antigens present in the bone marrow or thymus.

centroblasts Large, rapidly dividing cells found in germinal centers that undergo somatic hypermutation and give rise to antibody-secreting and memory B cells.

CFU See colony-forming unit.

CH50 unit The amount of complement (serum dilution) that induces lysis of 50% of erythrocytes coated with specific antibody.

chaperone Molecule that binds to a newly synthesized molecule inside a cell and ensures that it traffics to the correct compartment.

Chédiak–Higashi syndrome Disorder with a defect in lysosomal fusion that leads to impaired intracellular killing of microorganisms.

chemokines Cytokines of relatively low molecular weight, released by a variety of cells. They are involved in inflammatory responses, and migration and activation of primarily phagocytic cells and lymphocytes.

chemotaxis Migration of cells along a concentration gradient of an attractant.

chimera Mythical animal possessing the head of a lion, the body of a goat, and the tail of a snake. Refers to an individual containing cellular components derived from another, genetically distinct, individual.

chromosomal translocation Chromosomal abnormality in which a segment of one chromosome is transferred to another chromosome. Malignant diseases of lymphocytes are associated with chromosomal translocations involving an Ig or TCR locus and a chromosomal segment containing a cellular oncogene.

chronic granulomatous disease (CGD) Disorder inherited as an X-linked trait characterized by an enzyme defect associated with NADPH oxidase. This enzyme deficiency causes neutrophils and monocytes to have decreased consumption of oxygen and diminished glucose utilization by the hexose monophosphate shunt.

chronic lymphocytic leukemia (CLL) A B-cell leukemia in which long-lived small lymphocytes continually collect in the spleen, lymph nodes, bone marrow, and blood. Most express CD5.

chronic rejection Form of allograft rejection characterized by fibrosis with loss of normal organ structures occurring during a prolonged period. In many cases, the major pathologic event in chronic rejection is graft arterial occlusion.

class II-associated invariant chain peptide (CLIP) Peptide of variable length cleaved by proteases from the invariant chain when bound to newly synthesized MHC class II molecules. CLIP remains associated with the MHC class II molecule until removed by HLA-DM in endosomes. Once the CLIP is removed, antigenic peptides bind to the MHC class II molecule.

class switch Phenomenon in which B cells initially synthesizing antibodies of class (=isotype) IgM switch to synthesizing antibodies of a different class: IgG, IgA or IgE. Class switch does not change the specificity of the antibody.

class switch recombination Mechanism by which a germinal center B cell interacting with a T follicular helper cell (Tfh) switches from synthesizing IgM to IgG, IgA, or IgE. The enzyme AID induced in germinal center B cells is essential for class switch recombination.

classical complement pathway Mechanism of complement activation initiated by component C1 binding to antigen–antibody aggregates.

clonal deletion Removal of lymphocytes of particular specificity after contact with either self- or foreign antigen.

clonal expansion Increase in the number of lymphocytes specific for antigen that results from antigen stimulation and proliferation of naïve T cells.

clonal ignorance Form of lymphocyte unresponsiveness in which self-antigens are ignored by the immune system even though lymphocytes with receptors specific for those antigens remain viable and functional.

clonal selection theory Prevalent concept that specificity and diversity of an immune response are the result of selection by antigen of specifically reactive clones from a large repertoire of preformed lymphocytes, each with individual specificities.

cluster of differentiation (CD) Antibodies that react with cell-surface molecules; used to name and define specific cell-surface molecule, e.g., CD1, CD8, etc.

cold agglutinin Antibody that agglutinates particulate antigen, such as bacteria or red blood cells, optimally at temperatures less than 37°C. In clinical medicine, the term usually refers to antibodies against red blood cell antigens, as in *cold agglutinin syndrome*.

colony-forming unit (CFU) Hematopoietic stem cell and progeny cells deriving from it. Mature hematopoietic cells in the blood are considered to develop from one CFU.

colony-stimulating factors (CSFs) Glycoproteins that govern the formation, differentiation, and function of hematopoietic progenitor cells. CSFs promote the growth, maturation, and differentiation of stem cells to produce progenitor cell colonies *in vitro*.

combinatorial joining The joining of V, D, and J segments of Ig and TCR genes to generate a genetic information unit that codes for the Variable region of Ig or TCR during development of B and T cells. Combinatorial joining allows multiple opportunities for two sets of genes to combine in different ways.

common lymphoid progenitors Stem cells that give rise to all lymphocytes.

common variable immunodeficiency (CVID) Relatively common congenital or acquired immunodeficiency that may be either familial or sporadic. The familial form may have a variable mode of inheritance. Hypogammaglobulinemia is common to all CVID patients and usually affects all classes of immunoglobulin, but in some cases only IgG is affected.

complement Key effector mechanism in both innate and adaptive immunity for the elimination of microbial pathogens. See also under individual components: **C1**, **C2**, etc.).

complement receptors (CRs) Cell-surface proteins on a variety of cells that recognize and bind complement proteins that have bound pathogens or other antigens. CRs on phagocytes allow them to identify pathogens coated with complement proteins for uptake and destruction. Complement receptors include CR1, the receptor for C1q, CR2, CR3, and CR4.

complementarity-determining regions (CDRs) Hypervariable regions of immunoglobulins and T-cell receptors that determine their specificity and make contact with specific ligand. CDRs are the most variable parts of the molecule. Three such regions (CDR1, CDR2, and CDR3) exist in each V domain.

complete Freund's adjuvant (CFA) See **Freund's complete adjuvant**.

concanavalin A (Con A) A jack bean (*Canavalia ensiformis*) lectin that induces erythrocyte agglutination and is mitogenic for T lymphocytes; that is, activating all T cells to undergo mitosis and proliferate.

conformational epitopes Discontinuous epitopes on a protein antigen that are formed from several separate regions in the primary sequence of a protein brought together by protein folding. Antibodies that bind conformational epitopes bind only native-folded, not denatured, proteins.

congenic (also coisogenic) Describes two individuals who differ only in the genes at a particular locus and are identical at all other loci.

constant (C) region Invariant carboxyl-terminal portion of an Ig or TCR molecule, as distinct from the variable region at the amino terminus of the chain.

contact hypersensitivity Delayed-type (type IV) hypersensitivity mediated by T lymphocytes that develops 48–72 hours after contact with an allergen in contact with the skin. For example, poison ivy hypersensitivity is a contact hypersensitivity reaction resulting from exposure to pentadecacatechol found in poison ivy leaves. Chemicals eliciting contact hypersensitivity typically bind to and modify self-proteins or molecules on the surfaces of APCs, which are then recognized by CD4$^+$ and CD8$^+$ T cells.

convertase Enzymatic activity that converts a complement protein into its reactive form by cleaving it. Generation of the C3/C5 convertase is the pivotal event in complement activation.

Coombs test Named for its originator, R.R.A. Coombs; conducted to detect antibodies by addition of an anti-immunoglobulin antibody.

co-receptor Cell surface protein—Igα/β on B cells and CD4 or CD on T cells—that increases the sensitivity of the antigen-receptor to antigen; i.e., it lowers the threshold for activation by antigen and enhances signaling through the BCR or TCR complex.

cortex Outer region of a gland, such as the adrenal gland or thymus.

corticosteroids Lympholytic steroid hormones derived from the adrenal cortex. Glucocorticoids (e.g. prednisone, dexamethasone) can diminish size and lymphocyte content of lymph nodes and spleen, while sparing proliferating myeloid or erythroid stem cells of the bone marrow.

co-stimulator molecules Membrane-bound molecules expressed by APCs that interact with the T-cell surface and provide a stimulus (second signal) in addition to antigen required for full activation of naïve T cells. The best defined co-stimulators are the B7 molecules expressed on professional APCs that bind to the CD28 and CTLA-4 molecules expressed on T cells. B7 molecules activate signal transduction events in addition to those induced by MHC/TCR interactions. The interaction of CD40 expressed on APCs and CD40 ligand expressed on T cells is another critical co-stimulator interaction.

cowpox The common name for the virus and disease in cows caused by vaccinia virus. Antibodies generated after inoculation with cowpox cross-react with and thus protect against smallpox, a much more serious human disease. This was the principal that underlay Edward Jenner's successful vaccination (*vaccinus* = "of the cow" in Latin) against smallpox in the 1700s.

CpG nucleotides Unmethylated cytidine–guanine sequences found in microbial DNA that stimulate innate immune responses. CpG nucleotides are recognized by TLR-9 and have adjuvant properties in the mammalian immune system.

CR See **complement receptors**.

cromolyn sodium Drug blocking release of pharmacologic mediators from mast cells, diminishing symptoms and tissue reactions of type I hypersensitivity (i.e., anaphylaxis) mediated by IgE.

cross-presentation Pathway in APCs, particularly dendritic cells, for generating peptides derived from exogenous protein antigens and presenting them on MHC class I molecules to CD8$^+$ T cells.

cross-reactivity Ability of an antibody specific for one antigen to react with a second antigen; a measure of relatedness between two different antigenic substances.

CTLA-4 High-affinity receptor for B7 molecules expressed on activated T cells. Interaction with B7 inhibits T-cell activation.

cutaneous lymphocyte antigen (CLA) Cell surface molecule involved in lymphocyte homing to the skin in humans.

cyclophosphamide Alkylating agent used to treat some tumors and autoimmune diseases. Predominantly kills T lymphocytes; may have severe side effects.

cyclosporine (also called cyclosporine A or ciclosporin) Immunosuppressive drug used in organ transplantation that inhibits T-cell signaling, thus preventing T-cell activation and effector function. It acts by binding to cyclophilin to create a complex that binds to and inactivates the serine/threonine phosphatase calcineurin.

cytokine receptors Cellular receptors for cytokines. Binding of the cytokine to the cytokine receptor stimulates signal transduction, resulting in new activities in the cell, such as growth, differentiation, or death.

cytokines Soluble substances secreted by cells that have a variety of effects on other cells.

cytophilic antibody Antibody that attaches via its FcR region to a cell expressing an Fc receptor, for example, IgE molecules binding to the Fcε receptor expressed on the surface of mast cells and basophils.

cytotoxic (or cytolytic) T lymphocyte (CTL) A type of T lymphocyte that expresses CD8 and interacts with cells expressing peptides bound to MHC class I molecules. Its major effector function is to recognize and kill host cells infected with viruses or other intracellular microbes and also kill tumors and transplanted tissues. CTL killing of infected cells involves the release of cytoplasmic granules whose contents include membrane pore-forming proteins and enzymes that initiate apoptosis of the infected cell.

cytotoxins Proteins made by cytotoxic T cells that participate in the destruction of target cells. Perforins and granzymes or fragmentins are the major defined cytotoxins.

D gene A small gene segment used in V(D)J recombination that is found in immunoglobulin heavy-chain and T-cell receptor β and δ loci DNA. It codes for amino acids found in the highly variable part of the V region of IgH and TCR β and δ chains.

death domain Originally defined in proteins encoded by genes involved in programmed cell death but now known to be involved in protein–protein interactions.

decay-accelerating factor (DAF, CD55) Widely distributed cell surface glycoprotein molecule (human erythrocytes, leukocytes, and platelets) that regulates the classical and alternative pathway C3 convertases, C4b2a and C3bBb. Absent from the red blood cell membrane in paroxysmal nocturnal hemoglobulinuria, patients with this disorder experience destruction of their own red blood cells.

degranulation Mechanism whereby cytoplasmic granules in cells fuse with the cell membrane to discharge the contents from the cell. A classic example is degranulation of the mast cell or basophil in immediate (type I) hypersensitivity.

delayed-type hypersensitivity (DTH) Form of type IV, cell-mediated immunity elicited by antigen that appears hours to days after reexposure to antigen. Mediated by CD4$^+$ T$_H$1 cells and involves release of cytokines and recruitment of monocytes and macrophages to the area. See also **granuloma**.

dendritic cells Stellate cells derived from bone marrow precursors and closely related to monocytes/macrophages. Found in many tissues and organs as well as T-cell areas of secondary lymphoid organs. They are the most potent activators of naïve CD4$^+$ and CD8$^+$ T-cell responses. Dendritic cells present in nonlymphoid tissues stimulate T-cell responses once they have been activated by pathogens and after migration to the T-cell areas of draining lymphoid organs.

desensitization Procedure in which an allergic individual is exposed to increasing doses of allergens with the goal of inhibiting his or her allergic reaction. The mechanism involves shifting the response away from CD4$^+$ T$_H$2 responses to T$_H$1 or Treg types, thus changing the pattern of antibody produced from IgE to IgG.

determinant Part of the antigen molecule that binds to an antibody-combining site or to a receptor on T cells; also termed *epitope* (see **hapten** and **epitope**).

diapedesis Movement of blood cells, particularly leukocytes, from the blood across blood vessel walls into tissues.

differentiation antigen Cell-surface antigenic determinant found only on cells of a certain lineage and at a particular developmental stage; used as an immunologic marker.

DiGeorge syndrome Immunodeficiency condition in which the thymus and parathyroid glands do not develop. Heart problems are also found. T-cell development is severely impaired, resulting in chronic viral and fungal infections.

diphtheria toxoid Immunizing preparation generated by formalin inactivation of *Corynebacterium diphtheriae* exotoxins. This toxoid, used in the immunization of children against diphtheria, is usually administered as a triple vaccine along with pertussis microorganisms and tetanus toxoid (DPT).

diversity Existence of a large number of lymphocytes with different antigenic specificities in any individual. A fundamental property of the adaptive immune system and the result of variability in the structures of the antigen-binding sites of lymphocyte receptors for antigens (antibodies and TCRs).

diversity gene segments See **D gene**.

DNA vaccination Vaccination procedure in which plasmid DNA is used to initiate an adaptive immune response to the encoded protein.

domain A compact segment of an immunoglobulin or TCR chain, made up of amino acids around an S–S bond.

double-negative thymocyte Early T-lymphocyte lineage cells in the thymus that do not express either CD4 or CD8.

double-positive thymocyte T lymphocytes in the thymus that express both CD4 and CD8. T cells outside the thymus generally do not express both CD4 and CD8.

DP, DQ, and DR molecules Human MHC class II molecules expressed constitutively on B cells, APCs, and thymic epithelial cells.

draining lymph node Any lymph node downstream of an infection or site of antigen injection that receives microbes and antigens from the site via the lymphatic system. Often enlarges during an immune response and can be palpated (a phenomenon known as "swollen glands").

DTH See **delayed-type hypersensitivity**.

ECAM Endothelial cell adhesion molecule. See **adhesion molecules**.

effector cells Lymphocytes that can mediate the removal of pathogens or antigens from the body without the need for further differentiation. They are distinct from naïve lymphocytes, which need to proliferate and differentiate before they can mediate effector cell functions. Also distinct from memory cells, which must differentiate and sometimes proliferate before they become effector cells.

ELISA See **enzyme-linked immunosorbent assay**.

ELISPOT assay An adaptation of ELISA in which cells are placed over antibodies or antigens attached to a surface. The antigen or antibody traps the cells' secreted products, which can then be detected using an enzyme-coupled antibody that cleaves a substrate to make a localized colored spot.

encapsulated bacteria Bacteria with thick carbohydrate coats that protect them from phagocytosis. They can cause extracellular infections and are effectively engulfed and destroyed by phagocytes only if they are first coated with antibody and/or complement components produced in an adaptive immune response.

endocytosis Mechanism whereby substances are taken into a cell from the extracellular fluid through plasma membrane vesicles; accomplished by either pinocytosis or receptor-facilitated endocytosis.

endogenous antigen Antigen synthesized inside host cells.

endogenous pyrogens Cytokines (e.g., IL-1, TNF-α) that can induce a rise in body temperature. Distinct from exogenous substances such as endotoxin from Gram-negative bacteria that induce fever by triggering endogenous pyrogen synthesis.

endosome Intracellular membrane-bound acidic vesicle into which extracellular proteins are internalized during antigen processing. Contain proteolytic enzymes that degrade proteins into peptides (epitopes), allowing these peptides to bind to MHC class II molecules.

endotoxins Bacterial toxins released when bacterial cells are damaged or destroyed. The most important endotoxin is the lipopolysaccharide of Gram-negative bacteria, which induces cytokine synthesis.

enzyme-linked immunosorbent assay (ELISA) Assay in which an enzyme is linked to an antibody and a colored substrate is used to measure the activity of bound enzyme and hence the amount of bound antibody.

eosinophils Bone marrow-derived granulocytes important in defense against parasitic infections, including helminths. Found in abundance in inflammatory infiltrates of immediate hypersensitivity late-phase reactions, eosinophils contribute to many of the pathologic consequences of allergic diseases.

epitope Specific portion of a macromolecular antigen to which the antibody or TCR binds. An alternative term for **antigenic determinant**.

erythrocyte sedimentation rate (ESR) Test that measures the rate at which red blood cells settle in a tube. It is nonspecific in that it is increased in inflammation, infectious diseases, and some neoplasms (e.g., myeloma). It may also be increased in hypercholesterolemia or anemia. ESR is increased when positively charged proteins in the serum (e.g., myeloma Ig, acute phase proteins) neutralize the negative charges on red blood cells, overcoming the normal repulsion; this causes them to settle faster.

exocytosis Release of intracellular vesicle content to the exterior of the cell. The vesicles traffic to the plasma membrane, with which they fuse to permit the contents to be released to the external environment.

exogenous antigen An antigen taken into a cell, particularly an APC.

exon Region of DNA coding for a protein or a segment of a protein.

experimental allergic encephalomyelitis (EAE) Inflammatory disease of the central nervous system in rodents used as a model of multiple sclerosis. Develops after mice or rats are immunized with antigens of the nervous system together with an adjuvant.

extravasation Escape of the fluid and cellular components of blood from a blood vessel into tissues.

Fab Fragment of antibody containing one antigen-binding site; generated by cleavage of the antibody with the enzyme papain, which cuts at the hinge region N terminally to the inter-heavy-chain disulfide bond. This generates two Fab fragments from one antibody molecule.

F(ab)′₂ Fragment of an antibody containing two antigen-binding sites; generated by cleavage of the antibody molecule with the enzyme pepsin, which cuts at the hinge region C-terminally to the inter-heavy-chain disulfide bond.

FACS See **fluorescence-activated cell sorter**.

factor B Alternative complement pathway component that combines with C3b and is cleaved by factor D to produce alternative pathway C3 convertase.

factor H A key regulator of complement activation: competes with factor B for binding to C3b on a cell surface; binds to C3b when it is part of the C3b convertase, C3bBb; and promotes the dissociation of the convertase.

factor I Regulator of both classical and alternative complement pathways; serine protease that splits C3b and C4b.

factor P (properdin) A key participant in the alternative pathway of complement activation that combines with C3b and stabilizes alternative pathway C3 convertase (C3bB) to produce C3bBbP.

farmer's lung Hypersensitivity disease caused by the interaction of IgG antibodies with large amounts of an inhaled allergen in the alveolar wall of the lung, causing alveolar wall inflammation and compromising gas exchange.

Fas (CD95) Member of the TNF receptor family expressed on many types of cells, making them susceptible to killing by cells expressing Fas ligand. The binding of Fas ligand to Fas triggers apoptosis in the Fas-expressing cells.

Fas ligand (CD178 or CD95 ligand) Cell surface protein and member of the TNF family. Binding of Fas to Fas ligand triggers apoptosis in the Fas-expressing cell.

Fc Fragment of antibody without antigen-binding sites, generated by cleavage with papain. The Fc fragment contains the C-terminal domains of the immunoglobulin heavy chains.

Fc receptor (FcR) Receptor on a cell surface with specific binding affinity for the Fc portion of an antibody molecule. FcRs are found on many types of cells.

ficolin Family of serum lectins that trigger the lectin pathway of complement activation. See **lectin pathway of complement activation**.

FITC See **fluorescein isothiocyanate**.

FK506 See **tacrolimus**. An immunosuppressive polypeptide drug that inactivates T cells by inhibiting signal transduction from the T-cell receptor.

fluorescein isothiocyanate (FITC) Fluorescent dye that emits a yellow-green color and can be conjugated to antibody or other proteins.

fluorescence-activated cell sorter (FACS) Instrument that uses a laser to differentially deflect cells bound to fluorochrome-linked antibodies, thus sorting the cells into fluorescent-positive and fluorescent-negative populations.

fluorescence microscopy Microscope method that uses ultraviolet light to illuminate a tissue or cell stained with a fluorochrome-labeled substance, such as an antibody against an antigen of interest in the tissue.

fluorescent antibody Antibody coupled with a fluorescent dye used to detect antigen on cells, tissues, or microorganisms.

follicles Circular or oval areas of lymphocytes in lymphoid tissue rich in B cells, present in the cortex of lymph nodes and in the splenic white pulp. Primary follicles contain B lymphocytes that are small and medium sized. Antigen stimulation causes development of secondary follicles that contain large B lymphocytes in the germinal centers where tingible body macrophages (those phagocytizing nuclear particles) and follicular dendritic cells are present.

follicular dendritic cells Cells within lymphoid follicles crucial in selecting antigen-binding B cells during antibody responses. They have Fc receptors not internalized by receptor-mediated endocytosis; thus they hold antigen–antibody complexes on their surface for long periods.

Freund's complete adjuvant An oil containing killed mycobacteria and an emulsifier that forms an emulsion when mixed with an immunogen in aqueous solution. Injection of the emulsion enhances the immune response to the immunogen. Called *incomplete Freund's adjuvant* if mycobacteria are not included.

FYN See **tyrosine kinases**.

G proteins Proteins that bind GTP and convert it to GDP in the process of cell signal transduction.

GALT See **gut-associated lymphoid tissue**.

gene knockout Term for gene disruption by homologous recombination.

gene therapy Correction of a genetic defect by the introduction of a normal gene into bone marrow or other cells. Also known as *somatic gene therapy* because it does not affect the germline genes of the individual.

genetic immunization Technique for inducing adaptive immune responses by injecting plasmid DNA encoding a protein of interest, usually into muscle; the protein is then expressed *in vivo* and elicits antibody and T-cell responses.

genotype All the genes possessed by an individual; in practice it refers to the particular alleles present at the loci in question.

germinal centers Structures in secondary lymphoid organs that are sites of B-cell somatic hypermutation and class switch and the development of memory and plasma cells. They also include follicular dendritic cells and T (follicular) helper cells.

germline Refers to genes in germ cells as opposed to somatic cells. In immunology, it refers to immunoglobulin or TCR genes in their unrearranged state.

glomerulonephritis Group of diseases characterized by glomerular injury. Patients usually have glomerular deposits of immunoglobulins frequently associated with complement components.

Goodpasture's syndrome Autoimmune disease in which autoantibodies against basement membrane or type IV collagen are produced and cause extensive vasculitis. Can be rapidly fatal.

graft-versus-host reaction (GVH) Pathologic consequences of a response generally initiated by transplanted immunocompetent T lymphocytes into an allogeneic, immunologically incompetent host. The host is unable to reject the grafted T cells and becomes their target. The emerging graft-versus-host disease (GVHD) most often affects skin, liver, and intestines.

granulocyte See **polymorphonuclear leukocytes**.

granulocyte-macrophage colony-stimulating factor (GM-CSF) Cytokine involved in the growth and differentiation of myeloid and monocytic lineage cells, including dendritic cells, monocytes and tissue macrophages, and cells of the granulocyte lineage.

granuloma Structure in the form of a mass of mononuclear cells at the site of a persisting inflammation; mostly macrophages with some T lymphocytes at the periphery. A common delayed type hypersensitivity reaction associated with continuous presence of a foreign body or infection.

granzyme Serine protease enzyme found in the granules of CTL and NK cells released by exocytosis, enters target cells, and proteolytically cleaves and activates caspases to induce apoptosis.

Graves' disease Autoimmune disease in which antibodies against the thyroid-stimulating hormone receptor cause overproduction of thyroid hormone and thus hyperthyroidism.

Guillain–Barre syndrome Type of idiopathic polyneuritis in which autoimmunity to peripheral nerve myelin leads to a condition characterized by chronic demyelination of the spinal cord and peripheral nerves.

gut-associated lymphoid tissue (GALT) Lymphoid tissue situated in the gastrointestinal mucosa and submucosa that constitutes the gastrointestinal immune system. GALT is present in the Peyer's patches, appendix, and tonsils.

GVH See **graft-versus-host reaction**.

$\gamma\delta$ T cell receptor ($\gamma\delta$ TCR) The form of the TCR expressed by a minority of T cells, found mostly in epithelial barrier tissues. Each chain contains variable (V) regions, which form the antigen-binding site, and constant (C) regions that insert in the cell membrane.

H chain See **heavy chain**.

H-2 The major histocompatibility complex of the mouse, situated on chromosome 17. H-2 contains the subregions K, I, D, and L. (Haplotypes are designated by a lowercase superscript, as in H-2^b.)

haplotype Linked set of genes associated with one haploid genome; used mainly in connection with the linked genes of the major histocompatibility complex (MHC), usually inherited as one haplotype contributed by each parent. Some MHC haplotypes are overrepresented in the population, a phenomenon known as *linkage disequilibrium*.

hapten Compound, usually of low molecular weight, that is not itself immunogenic but becomes immunogenic and induces an antibody response after conjugation to a carrier protein or cells. The hapten alone can bind to the antibody in the absence of carrier.

Hashimoto's thyroiditis Autoimmune disease characterized by persistent high levels of antibody against thyroid-specific antigens, primarily thyroid peroxidase and the hormone thyroglobulin. CD4$^+$ T$_H$1 cells also contribute to the destruction of the thyroid gland.

HAT Hypoxanthine–aminopterin–thymidine, commonly used as a selective media cocktail in cell cultures to generate hybridomas.

heavy (H) chain Larger of the two types of chains that comprise a normal immunoglobulin or antibody molecule.

helper T cells Class of CD4$^+$ T cell that cooperates with B cells to make antibody in response to thymus-dependent antigens.

hemagglutinin Any substance that causes red blood cells to agglutinate. Hemagglutinins in human blood are antibodies that recognize the ABO blood group antigens. Influenza and some other viruses have hemagglutinins that bind to glycoproteins on host cells to initiate the infectious process.

hematopoiesis Generation of cellular elements of blood, including the red blood cells, leukocytes, and platelets.

hematopoietic stem cell (HSC) Bone marrow cell that is undifferentiated and serves as a precursor for multiple hematopoietic cell lineages. Also demonstrable in the yolk sac and later in the liver in the fetus.

hemolytic disease of the newborn (HDN) Also called *erythroblastosis fetalis*, HDN is caused by a maternal IgG antibody response to paternal antigens expressed on fetal red blood cells. The usual target of this response is the Rh blood group antigen. Maternal anti-Rh IgG antibodies cross the placenta, bind to fetal red blood cells, and trigger their destruction.

herd immunity Protection afforded to non-vaccinated individuals in a population when the majority have been successfully vaccinated.

hereditary angioedema Disorder due to decreased or absent C1 inhibitor (C1 INH) in which recurrent attacks of edema occur in the skin and gastrointestinal and respiratory tracts. The most serious consequence is epiglottal swelling leading to suffocation.

heterodimer Molecule comprising two components that are different but closely joined structures, such as a protein comprised of two separate chains. Major examples include the TCR—either α plus β chains or γ plus δ chains—and MHC class I and class II molecules.

heterophile antigen A cross-reacting antigen expressed by widely different species including humans and bacteria.

heterozygous Refers to individuals with two different alleles of a particular gene.

HEV See **high endothelial venules**.

high endothelial venules (HEV) Specialized venules found in lymphoid tissues. Lymphocytes migrate from blood into lymphoid tissues by attaching to and migrating across the high endothelial cells of these vessels.

highly active antiretroviral therapy (HAART) Combination chemotherapy for HIV infection consisting of a viral protease inhibitor and reverse transcriptase inhibitors. Can reduce plasma virus titers to below detectable levels and slow the progression of HIV disease.

hinge region Flexible, open segment of an antibody molecule that allows it to bend. Located between the Fab and Fc regions of an antibody molecule and susceptible to enzymatic cleavage.

histamine Vasoactive amine stored in mast cell granules released by antigen binding to IgE molecules on mast cells, causing dilation of local blood vessels and smooth muscle contraction. Histamine release produces some symptoms of immediate hypersensitivity reactions.

histocompatibility Literally, the ability of tissues to be compatible; in immunology, identity in all transplantation antigens. These antigens, in turn, are collectively referred to as *histocompatibility antigens*.

HIV See **human immunodeficiency virus**.

HLA See **human leukocyte antigen**.

Hodgkin disease and Hodgkin lymphoma Malignant disease of B lymphocytes characterized by the presence of large cells, called *Reed–Sternberg cells*.

homing Directed migration of different types of leukocytes into particular tissue sites and regulated by the selective expression of adhesion molecules and chemokine receptors. See also **lymphocyte homing**.

homodimer A protein comprising two identical peptide chains, for example, CD8.

human immunodeficiency virus (HIV) Retrovirus that infects human CD4$^+$ cells and causes AIDS.

human leukocyte antigen (HLA) The human major histocompatibility complex; contains the genes coding for the polymorphic HLA class I and II molecules and many other important genes.

humanization Describes the genetic engineering of mouse hypervariable loops of a desired specificity into otherwise human antibodies. DNA encoding hypervariable loops of mouse monoclonal antibodies or V regions selected in phage display libraries is inserted into the framework regions of human immunoglobulin genes. This allows the production of antibodies of a desired specificity that do not cause an immune response in humans treated with them.

humoral immunity Refers to immune responses that involve antibody (contrast with cell-mediated immunity: T-cell responses in the absence of antibody). Can be transferred to another individual using antibody-containing serum.

hybridoma Immortalized hybrid cell resulting from the *in vitro* fusion of an antibody-secreting B cell with a myeloma; it secretes antibody without stimulation and proliferates continuously, both *in vivo* and *in vitro*. The term is also used for a hybrid T cell resulting from the fusion of a T lymphocyte with a thymoma (a malignant T cell), in which the T-cell hybridoma proliferates continuously and secretes cytokines upon activation by antigen and APC.

hyperacute rejection Form of graft rejection that begins within minutes to hours after transplantation, particularly of a xenograft, characterized by thrombotic occlusion of the graft vessels. Mediated by preexisting antibodies in the host circulation that bind to donor endothelial antigens, such as blood group antigens or MHC molecules, and activate the complement and blood-clotting cascades, leading to an engorged, ischemic graft and rapid loss of the organ.

hypergammaglobulinemia Elevated serum immunoglobulin levels. A polyclonal increase in immunoglobulins in the serum occurs in any condition where there is continuous stimulation of the immune system, such as chronic infection, autoimmune disease, or systemic lupus erythematosus. Hypergammaglobulinemia may also result from a monoclonal increase in immunoglobulin production, as in multiple myeloma, Waldenström's macroglobulinemia, or other conditions associated with the formation of monoclonal immunoglobulins.

hyper-IgM syndromes Conditions in which high levels of IgM but not other Ig classes are made. They result from defects in class switch recombination, most commonly from defects in CD40 ligand expression (T cells) but also may result from mutations in CD40 (B cells and APCs) or AID (B cells).

hyperimmune A descriptor for an animal with a high level of immunity that is induced by repeated immunization to generate large amounts of functionally effective antibodies, in comparison to animals subjected to routine immunization protocols, generally with fewer boosters.

hypersensitivity State of reactivity to antigen that is greater than normal; denotes a deleterious rather than a protective outcome. Four types are defined. See **types I–IV hypersensitivity**.

hypersensitivity diseases Immune-mediated diseases that include autoimmune diseases, in which immune responses are directed against self-antigens, and diseases resulting from uncontrolled or excessive responses against foreign antigens, such as microbes and allergens. The tissue damage that occurs in hypersensitivity diseases is due to the same effector mechanisms used by the immune system to protect against microbes.

hypervariable regions Portions of the antigen-specific receptors on T cells and B cells, the TCR and BCR, respectively, that are highly variable in amino acid sequence from one molecule to another and constitute the antigen-binding site. See also **complementarity-determining region**.

Ia (I region associated) An older term for mouse MHC class II I-A and I-E genes and molecules.

idiotype Combined antigenic determinants (idiotopes) expressed in the variable region of antibodies of an individual; directed at a particular antigen.

Ig See **immunoglobulin**.

IgA Class of immunoglobulin characterized by α heavy chains. IgA antibodies are secreted mainly by mucosal associated lymphoid tissues.

IgD Class of immunoglobulin characterized by δ heavy chains. IgD is a cell-surface immunoglobulin co-expressed on naïve B cells together with IgM. May function as a co-receptor that binds to IgD receptors expressed on T cells.

IgE Class of immunoglobulin characterized by ε heavy chains; involved in allergic reactions.

IgG Class of immunoglobulin characterized by γ heavy chains. The most abundant class of immunoglobulin found in plasma.

IgM Class of immunoglobulin characterized by μ heavy chains. IgM is the first immunoglobulin to appear on the surface of B cells and to be secreted following B-cell stimulation with antigen.

Igα/β (CD79a/CD79b) Heterodimeric signal transduction molecule expressed at the surface of B lymphocyte lineage cells and associated with Ig heavy chains.

IL See **interleukins**.

immature B cell IgM$^+$ cell in the B-cell lineage; tolerized by exposure to antigen.

immature dendritic cell Antigen-presenting cell in tissue that takes up and processes antigen.

immediate-type hypersensitivity Type I hypersensitivity reaction occurring within minutes after exposure to allergen and interaction with IgE antibody.

immune adherence Adherence of particulate antigen coated with C3b to cells expressing C3b receptors; results in enhanced phagocytosis of bacteria by macrophages.

immune complex Molecules formed by the interaction of a soluble (i.e., nonparticulate) antigen with antibody molecules. Large immune complexes are cleared rapidly, but smaller complexes formed in antigen excess may deposit in tissues resulting in tissue damage (immune complex disease).

immune modulators Substances that control the level of the immune response.

immune surveillance Concept that a physiologic function of the immune system is to recognize and destroy clones of transformed cells before they grow into tumors.

immunity General term for resistance to a pathogen.

immunodeficiency Decrease in immune responses that result from absence or defect of some component of the immune system.

immunodiffusion Identifies antigen or antibody by the formation of antigen–antibody complexes in a gel.

immunogen Substance capable of inducing an immune response (as well as reacting with the products of an immune response). Compare with **antigen**.

immunoglobulin (Ig) General term for all antibody molecules (IgM, IgD, IgG, IgA, and IgE); each Ig unit is made up of two heavy chains and two light chains and has two antigen-binding sites.

immunoglobulin A See **IgA**.

immunoglobulin D See **IgD**.

immunoglobulin domain A three-dimensional globular structure found in many proteins in the immune system, including Igs, TCRs, and MHC molecules. Ig domains are about 110 amino acid residues in length, include an internal disulfide bond, and contain β-pleated sheets.

immunoglobulin E See **IgE**.

immunoglobulin G See **IgG**.

immunoglobulin heavy (H) chain With the light chain, it is one of the two basic structural units of a four-chain antibody molecule. The H chain can be μ, δ, γ, α, or ε, and so gives rise to the different antibody classes (isotypes): IgM, IgD, IgG, IgA, or IgE. The H chain variable (V) region combines with the light chain V region to form the antigen-binding site. The constant (C) region of the H chain mediates the effector function of the antibody molecule, such as binding to receptors on phagocytic cells and the activation of complement.

immunoglobulin light (L) chain With the heavy chain, it is one of the two basic structural units of a four-chain antibody molecule. The L chain can be either κ or λ, which are functionally identical. About 60% of human antibodies have κ light chains and 40% have λ light chains.

immunoglobulin M See **IgM**.

immunoglobulin superfamily Proteins involved in cellular recognition and interactions that are structurally and genetically related to immunoglobulins.

immunologic synapse Area of contact between the surfaces of a T cell and an APC, such as dendritic cells or a B cell.

immunoreceptor tyrosine-based activation motif (ITAM) Pattern of amino acids in the cytoplasmic tail of many transmembrane receptor molecules, including Igα and Igβ and CD3 and ζ (zeta) chains, which are phosphorylated and then associate with intracellular molecules as an early consequence of cell activation.

immunoreceptor tyrosine-based inhibitory motif (ITIM) Pattern of amino acids in the cytoplasmic tail of receptors, such as the B-cell molecules FcγRIIB and CD22, which recruit phosphatases to the receptor site that remove the phosphate groups added by the tyrosine kinases.

immunosuppression Inhibition of one or more components of the adaptive or innate immune system, either as a result of an underlying disease or intentionally induced by drugs for the purpose of preventing or treating graft rejection or autoimmune disease. A commonly used immunosuppressive drug is cyclosporine, which blocks T-cell cytokine production.

immunotherapy Treatment of a disease with therapeutic agents that promote or inhibit immune responses. Cancer immunotherapy, for example, involves either promoting active immune response to tumor antigens (e.g., by pulsing them onto dendritic cells) or by administering antibodies specific for molecules expressed on tumor cells to establish passive immunity.

immunotoxins Antibodies that are chemically coupled to toxic proteins usually derived from plants or microorganisms. They are being tested as anticancer agents and as immunosuppressive drugs.

inducible NO synthase (iNOS) Produced by macrophages and many other cell types. Induced by many stimuli to activate NO synthesis, thereby playing a major role in host resistance to intracellular infection.

inflammasome Multiprotein complex, assembled from NOD-like receptors (NLRs) and expressed in myeloid cells, activating the enzyme caspase-1 that in turn cleaves immature forms of certain cytokines, particularly IL-1, into active, mature cytokines.

inflammation An acute or chronic response to tissue injury or infection involving accumulation of leukocytes, plasma proteins, and fluid.

innate immunity Mechanisms involved in the early response to pathogens and antigens; key components include phagocytic and NK cells, cytokines, and complement. Not expanded by repeat stimulation with the pathogen, so does not induce memory.

integrins Family of two-chain cell surface adhesion molecules found on leukocytes; important in the adhesion of APCs and lymphocytes and in leukocyte migration into tissues.

intercellular adhesion molecule (ICAM) 1, 2, and 3 Adhesion molecules on surface of several cell types, including APCs and T cells, which interact with integrins; members of the immunoglobulin superfamily.

interferons (IFNs) Group of proteins having antiviral activity and capable of enhancing and/or modifying the immune response.

interleukins (ILs) Glycoproteins secreted by a variety of leukocytes that have effects on other leukocytes.

intron Segment of DNA that does not code for protein; the intervening sequence of nucleotides between coding sequences or exons.

invariant chain (Ii) Nonpolymorphic protein that binds to newly synthesized MHC class II molecules in the endoplasmic reticulum; prevents loading of MHC class II peptide-binding cleft with peptides present in the endoplasmic reticulum. also promotes folding and assembly of MHC class II molecules and directs newly formed MHC class II molecules to the specialized endosomal MHC compartment, where peptide loading takes place.

ISCOMs Immune stimulatory complexes of antigen held within a lipid matrix that act as an adjuvant and enable antigen to be taken up into the cytoplasm after fusion with the cytoplasmic membrane.

isoelectric focusing Protein identification technique; proteins migrate in an electric field under a pH gradient to the pH at which their net charge is zero (their isoelectric point).

isograft Tissue transplanted between two genetically identical individuals (same as **syngraft**).

isohemagglutinins Naturally occurring IgM antibodies specific for the red blood cell antigens of the ABO blood groups; thought to result from immunization by bacteria in the gastrointestinal and respiratory tracts.

isotype switch See **class switch**.

isotypes Also known as *antibody classes*, isotypes are antibodies that differ in the heavy-chain constant regions: IgM, IgG, IgD, IgA, and IgE. These differences result in distinct biological activities of the antibodies; distinguishable also on the basis of reaction with antisera raised in another species.

ITAM See **immunoreceptor tyrosine-based activation motif**.

ITIM See **immunoreceptor tyrosine-based inhibition motif**.

J (joining) chain Polypeptide involved in the polymerization of immunoglobulin molecules IgM and IgA, so is associated with the IgM pentamer and IgA dimer.

JAK See **Janus kinases**.

JAK/STAT signaling pathway A signaling pathway initiated by cytokine binding to type I and type II cytokine receptors, sequentially activating receptor-associated Janus kinase (JAK) tyrosine kinases, JAK-mediated tyrosine phosphorylation of the cytoplasmic tails of cytokine receptors, docking of signal transducers and activators of transcription (STATs) to the phosphorylated receptor chains, JAK-mediated tyrosine phosphorylation of the associated STATs, dimerization, nuclear translocation of the STATs, and binding of STAT to regulatory regions of specific target genes, causing transcriptional activation of those genes.

Janus kinases (JAKs) Tyrosine kinases activated by cytokines binding to their cellular receptors.

joining (J) gene segment Short gene segment within Ig and TCR loci that together with V and D segments, codes for the variable region of Ig or the TCR.

junctional diversity The diversity in Ig and TCR repertoires that results from the random addition or removal of nucleotide sequences at junctions between V, D, and J gene segments.

Kaposi sarcoma Malignant tumor of vascular cells; associated with infection by the Kaposi-sarcoma-associated herpes virus 8 that frequently arises in patients with AIDS.

killer activatory receptor (KAR) Receptor expressed on NK or cytotoxic cells that can activate killing by these cells.

killer-cell inhibitory receptor (KIR) Receptor expressed on NK cells that binds to MHC class I molecules on target cells; ligation of MHC class I inhibits the signaling that would otherwise lead to target cell killing.

killer T cell A T cell, also known as a cytotoxic T cell (CTL) that kills a target cell expressing antigen bound to MHC class I molecules on the surface of the target cell.

KIR See **killer-cell inhibitory receptor**.

knockout mouse Mouse with a targeted disruption of one or more genes created by homologous recombination techniques.

L chain See **light chain**.

LAK cells See **lymphokine-activated killer cells**.

Langerhans cell Cell of the monocyte/dendritic cell family that takes up and processes antigens in the epidermal layer of the skin. It migrates through lymphatics to lymph nodes draining the site of exposure to antigen, where it differentiates into a dendritic cell.

late-phase reaction Component of the immediate hypersensitivity reaction that develops 2 to 4 hours after mast-cell and basophil degranulation characterized by an inflammatory infiltrate of neutrophils, eosinophils, basophils, and lymphocytes. Recurring late-phase inflammatory reactions can cause tissue damage.

Lck An Src family nonreceptor tyrosine kinase that noncovalently associates with the cytoplasmic tails of CD4 and CD8 molecules in T cells. Lck is involved in the early signaling events of antigen-induced T-cell activation and mediates tyrosine phosphorylation of the cytoplasmic tails of CD3 and ζ proteins of the TCR complex.

lectin pathway of complement activation Pathway of complement activation triggered, in the absence of antibody, by the binding of microbial polysaccharides to circulating lectins such as mannose-binding lectin (MBL) and ficolin. MBL and ficolin in the circulation associate with proteases, the mannose-associated serine proteases (MASPs). Once bound to a pathogen, one of the proteases, MASP-2, sequentially cleaves C4 and C2 to form C4b2a on the surface of the bacterium. The remaining steps of the lectin pathway, beginning with cleavage of C4, are identical to the classical complement pathway.

Leishmania An obligate intracellular protozoan parasite that infects macrophages and can cause a chronic inflammatory disease involving many tissues. T_H1 responses and associated IFN-γ production control *Leishmania major* infection, whereas T$_H$2 responses with IL-4 production lead to disseminated lethal disease.

leukemia Uncontrolled proliferation of a malignant leukocyte.

leukocyte adhesion deficiency (LAD) One of a rare group of immunodeficiency diseases with infectious complications; caused by defective expression of the leukocyte adhesion molecules required for tissue recruitment of phagocytes and lymphocytes.

leukocyte common antigen (LCA, CD45) Protein tyrosine phosphatase that is expressed by both T and B lymphocytes.

leukocytes White blood cells; they comprise monocytes/macrophages, lymphocytes, and polymorphonuclear cells.

leukotrienes Class of arachidonic-acid-derived lipid inflammatory mediators produced by the lipoxygenase pathway in many cell types. They contribute significantly to the pathologic processes of bronchial asthma.

ligand Molecule or part of molecule that binds to a receptor.

ligation Binding of a molecule or a part of a molecule to a receptor.

light (L) chain The light chain of the immunoglobulin molecule, either κ or λ.

linked recognition The requirement for the T helper and B cell involved in the antibody response to a thymus-dependent antigen to interact with different epitopes physically linked in the same antigen.

lipopolysaccharide (LPS) Component of Gram-negative bacteria cell walls; also known as *endotoxin*.

LPS See **lipopolysaccharide**.

Lyme disease Chronic infection with the spirochete *Borrelia burgdorferi*.

lymph Extracellular fluid that bathes tissues; contains tissue products, antigens, antibodies, and cells (predominantly lymphocytes).

lymph nodes Secondary lymphoid organs in which mature B and T lymphocytes interact with antigen and with each other.

lymphatic system System of vessels through which lymph travels and which includes organized structures, with lymph nodes at the intersection of vessels. It has three major functions: (1) to concentrate antigen from all parts of the body into a few lymphoid organs; (2) to circulate lymphocytes through lymphoid organs so that antigen can interact with rare antigen-specific cells; and (3) to carry products of the immune response (antibody and effector cells) to the bloodstream and tissues.

lymphoblast Lymphocyte with enlarged and increased rate of RNA and protein synthesis.

lymphocyte homing Directed migration of subsets of circulating lymphocytes into particular tissue sites; regulated by the selective expression of adhesion molecules and chemokine receptors.

lymphocyte maturation Process by which bone marrow precursor cells develop into mature, antigen receptor-expressing naïve B or T lymphocytes in primary lymphoid organs—bone marrow (B cells) and thymus (T cells).

lymphocyte migration Movement of lymphocytes around the body. See also **lymphocyte homing**.

lymphocyte recirculation Continuous movement of lymphocytes through the blood and lymphatics, between the lymph nodes or spleen, and, if activated, to peripheral inflammatory sites.

lymphocytes Leukocytes that express antigen-specific receptors; divided into two major sets: B cells (Ig) and T cells (TCR); small cells with virtually no cytoplasm found in blood, tissues, and lymphoid organs such as lymph nodes, spleen, and Peyer's patches. Responsible for specificity, diversity, memory, and self–nonself discrimination.

lymphoid follicle B-cell-rich region of a lymph node or the spleen that is the site of antigen-induced B-cell proliferation and differentiation. In T-cell-dependent B-cell responses to protein antigens, a germinal center forms within the follicles.

lymphokine A cytokine secreted by lymphocytes.

lymphokine-activated killer (LAK) cells The heterogeneous population of lymphocytes, including NK cells, derived from the *in vitro* cytokine-driven activation of peripheral blood lymphocytes from a tumor-bearing patient.

lymphoma Lymphocyte tumors in lymphoid tissues or other sites but not generally found in the blood.

lymphotoxin (LT, TNF-β) Cytokine produced by CD4$^+$ T$_H$1 cells and CTL that kills infected T cells and tumor cells and also has proinflammatory effects, including endothelial and neutrophil activation; also critical for the normal development of lymphoid organs.

lysosome Organelle abundant in phagocytic cells that contains proteolytic enzymes that degrade proteins derived both from the extracellular environment and from within the cell.

M cells Specialized epithelial cells overlaying Peyers's patches in the gut that deliver antigens to Peyer's patches.

macrophages Large phagocytic leukocytes found in tissues; derived from blood monocytes.

major histocompatibility complex (MHC) Cluster of genes encoding polymorphic cell surface molecules (MHC class I and class II) that are involved in interactions with T cells. These molecules also play a major role in transplantation rejection. Several nonpolymorphic proteins are also encoded in this region.

MALT See **mucosa-associated lymphoid tissue**.

mannose-binding lectin (MBL) Plasma protein that binds to mannose residues on bacterial cell walls and activates complement in the absence of antibody.

mannose receptor Carbohydrate-binding receptor (lectin) expressed by macrophages that binds mannose and fucose residues on microbial cell walls and mediates phagocytosis of the organisms.

marginal zone Peripheral region of splenic lymphoid follicles containing macrophages; associated with the trapping of polysaccharide antigens that may persist locally for prolonged periods of time within macrophages and allow them to be recognized by antigen-specific B cells or to be transported into follicles.

marginal zone B lymphocytes Subset of B lymphocytes, found exclusively in the marginal zone of the spleen, which respond rapidly to blood-borne microbial antigens by producing IgM antibodies with limited diversity.

mast cell Bone marrow-derived granule-containing cell found in connective tissues; releases mediators such as histamine and cytokines following cell activation; plays a major role in allergic responses.

mature B cell B cells that express both IgM and IgD of identical antigenic specificity on their surface.

medulla Inner region of a gland such as the thymus or adrenal.

membrane attack complex Terminal components of the complement cascade (C5b–C9), which form a pore on the surface of a target cell, resulting in cell damage or death.

memory Denotes second interaction of B or T lymphocytes with antigen or antigenic peptides, leading to a more effective and more rapid response than the first interaction (primary response).

memory lymphocytes B or T lymphocytes that mediate rapid and enhanced responses to antigen in a second or subsequent exposure. Memory B and T cells are produced by antigen stimulation of naïve lymphocytes and survive in a functionally quiescent state for long periods of time (years).

MHC See **major histocompatibility complex**.

MHC class I molecule Molecule encoded by highly polymorphic genes of the MHC that binds peptides derived from exogenous antigens in the endoplasmic reticulum and interacts with CD8$^+$ (cytotoxic) T cells.

MHC class II molecule Molecule encoded by highly polymorphic genes of the MHC that binds peptides derived from exogenous antigens in acid compartments of the cell and interacts with CD4$^+$ T cells.

MHC class III molecules Complement components including C2, C4, and factor B that are encoded by genes in the MHC.

MHC restriction Property of T lymphocytes that they respond to antigenic peptides only when presented in association with either self-MHC class I or class II molecules.

minor histocompatibility antigens Antigens encoded outside the MHC that stimulate graft rejection, but not as rapidly as MHC molecules.

mitogen Substance that stimulates the proliferation of many different clones of lymphocytes.

mixed-lymphocyte reaction (MLR) Proliferative response occurring when leukocytes from two individuals are mixed *in vitro*; T cells from one individual (the responder) are activated by MHC antigens expressed by APCs of the other individual (the stimulator).

MLR See **mixed-lymphocyte reaction**.

Mls antigens Non-MHC antigens that provoke strong primary mixed-lymphocyte responses.

molecular mimicry Identity or similarity of epitopes expressed by a pathogen and by a self-molecule. Molecular mimicry may explain how autoimmune responses develop.

monoclonal Derived from a single clone, the progeny of a single cell. Generally refers to a homogeneous population of T cells, or B cells, or an antibody that is reactive to only one antigen epitope.

monoclonal antibody An antibody produced by a B-cell hybridoma (a cell line derived by the fusion of a single normal B cell and an immortal B-cell tumor line) that is specific for one epitope of an antigen. Monoclonal antibodies are widely used in research, clinical diagnosis, and therapy. Contrast with **antiserum**.

monocyte Phagocytic leukocyte found in the blood; precursor to tissue macrophage.

motif Pattern of amino acids in the sequence of a molecule critical for the binding of a ligand.

mucins Highly glycosylated cell surface proteins. Mucin-like molecules are bound by L-selectin in lymphoid organs.

mucosa-associated lymphoid tissue (MALT) System that connects lymphoid structures found in the gastrointestinal and respiratory tracts; includes tonsils, appendix, and Peyer's patches of the small intestine.

mucosal immune system Part of the immune system that responds to and protects against microbes that enter the body through mucosal surfaces within the gastrointestinal and respiratory tracts. The mucosal immune system comprises mucosa-associated lymphoid tissues composed of collections of lymphocytes and accessory cells in the epithelia and lamina propria of mucosal surfaces.

multiple myeloma Malignant tumor of antibody-producing clones of B cells that often secretes immunoglobulins or parts of Ig molecules. The monoclonal antibodies produced by multiple myelomas were critical for early biochemical analyses of antibody structure.

multiple sclerosis Disease of the central nervous system believed to be autoimmune in nature in which an inflammatory response results in demyelination and loss of neurologic function.

myasthenia gravis Autoimmune disease in which antibody specific for the acetylcholine receptor expressed in muscle blocks function at the neuromuscular junction.

myeloma Tumor of plasma cells generally secreting a single monoclonal immunoglobulin.

naïve lymphocytes Lymphocytes that have not yet encountered their specific antigen and therefore have never responded to it. All lymphocytes leaving the central lymphoid organs (bone marrow and thymus) are naïve.

natural killer (NK) cells Large granular lymphocyte-like cells that kill various tumor cells *in vitro* and may play a role in resistance to tumors; they also participate in ADCC.

negative selection A step in the development of B and T cells at which cells with potential reactivity to self-molecules are functionally inactivated.

neonatal immunity Immunity mediated by maternally produced antibodies transported across the placenta into the fetal circulation before birth or derived from ingested maternal milk and transported across the epithelium.

neutralization Ability of an antibody to block or inhibit the effects of a virus or bacterium.

neutropenia A situation in which there are fewer neutrophils in the blood than normal.

neutrophil Phagocytic cell morphologically characterized by a segmented lobular nucleus and cytoplasmic granules filled with degradative enzymes. Short-lived (<1 day) and the most abundant type of circulating white blood cells. It is the major innate immune cell type mediating acute inflammatory responses to bacterial infections.

nitric oxide A vasoactive and microbicidal effector molecule produced by macrophages from L-arginine.

nitric oxide synthase Member of a family of enzymes that synthesize nitric oxide from L-arginine. Macrophages express an inducible form of this enzyme (see **iNOS**) following activation by various microorganisms or cytokines.

NK cells See **natural killer cells**.

NKT cells Small subset of T cells that express the NK1.1 marker normally found on NK cells as well as a TCR of limited diversity. They rapidly produce cytokines in response to pathogens. They are considered to have features of both innate and adaptive immunity, and are thought to play a regulatory role in several diseases and conditions.

NOD-like receptors (NLRs) Family of intracellular pattern recognition receptors (PRRs) whose primary role is to recognize cytoplasmic pathogen-associated molecular patterns (PAMPs) and/or endogenous danger signals, inducing immune responses.

nuclear factor of activated T cells (NFAT) Transcription factor complex of a protein called NFATc that is held in the cytosol by serine/threonine phosphorylation and the Fos/Jun dimer called AP-1. Following cleavage of the phosphate residues of NFAT by calcineurin, it moves from the cytosol to the nucleus.

nuclear factor κB (NF-κB) Family of transcription factors composed of homodimers or heterodimers of proteins important in the transcription of many genes in both innate and adaptive immune responses.

nude mice Mice in which the thymus does not develop, so they lack T cells; also *hairless*.

oncofetal antigens Proteins expressed at high levels on some types of cancer cells and in normal developing fetal tissue but not adult tissues. Antibodies specific for these proteins are used as diagnostic histologic tools to identify tumors or to monitor the progression of tumor growth in patients. Carcinoembroyonic antigen (CEA, CD66) and α-fetoprotein are two oncofetal antigens commonly expressed by some carcinomas.

oncogenes Genes involved in regulating cell growth that, when defective in structure or expression, can cause cells to grow continuously to form a tumor.

opsonin A molecule that becomes attached to the surface of a microbe and increases the efficiency of phagocytosis of the microbe by phagocytic cells (neutrophils and macrophages). Opsonins include IgG antibodies whose Fc regions are recognized by Fcγ receptors on phagocytes, and C3b and other fragments of complement proteins, which are recognized by CR1 (CD35) and by the leukocyte integrin Mac-1.

opsonization The coating of a particle such as a bacterium with antibody and/or a complement component (an opsonin) that leads to enhanced phagocytosis by phagocytic cells.

paracortical area (or paracortex) The T-cell area of the lymph node.

passive cutaneous anaphylaxis (PCA) Transfer of anaphylactic sensitivity by intradermal injection of serum from a sensitized donor.

passive hemagglutination Technique for measuring antibody in which antigen-coated red blood cells are agglutinated by adding antibody specific for the antigen.

passive immunization Immunization of an individual by the transfer of antibody synthesized in another individual.

pathogen An agent that causes disease.

pathogen-associated molecular patterns (PAMPs) Evolutionarily conserved structures such as lipopolysaccharide, teichoic acid, and double-stranded RNA that are expressed by pathogens (viruses, bacteria, fungi) and bind to pattern recognition receptors (PRRs) expressed by cells of the innate immune system.

pattern recognition receptors (PRRs) Germline-encoded membrane or cytoplasmic receptors expressed by cells of the innate immune system that recognize pathogen-associated molecular patterns (PAMPs) expressed by microorganisms. Based on their molecular structure, PRRs can be divided into multiple families, including Toll-like receptors (TLRs), C-type lectin receptors (CLRs), NOD-like receptors (NLRs), and RIG-I-like receptors (RLRs).

PCA See **passive cutaneous anaphylaxis**.

PCR See **polymerase chain reaction**.

peptide-binding cleft The portion of an MHC molecule that binds peptides derived from antigen processing. The cleft or groove is composed of paired α helices resting on an eight-stranded β-pleated sheet. The polymorphic residues that account for differences in sequences among MHC alleles are located in and around the peptide-binding cleft.

perforin A molecule synthesized by cytotoxic T cells (CTLs) and NK cells that polymerizes on the surface of a target cell and creates a pore in the membrane, resulting in target-cell death.

periarteriolar lymphoid sheath (PALS) Part of the inner region of the white pulp of the spleen that mainly contains T cells.

peripheral lymphoid organs Lymphoid organs other than the thymus and bone marrow; they include the spleen, lymph nodes, and mucosa-associated lymphoid tissue.

peripheral tolerance Physiologic unresponsiveness to antigens induced in mature lymphocytes outside the primary lymphoid organs: bone marrow (B cells) and thymus (T cells).

Peyer's patches Clusters of lymphocytes distributed in the lining of the small intestine.

PHA See **phytohemagglutinin**.

phagocytosis The engulfment of a particle or a microorganism by leukocytes such as macrophages and neutrophils.

phagolysosome A phagocytic vacuole formed by the fusion of lysosomes and phagosomes containing foreign particles. Phagolysosomes release powerful enzymes, which digest the particle (e.g., bacteria).

phagosome Membrane-bound intracellular vesicle that contains particulate material, such as microbes, from the extracellular environment. Phagosomes are formed during the process of phagocytosis and fusion with other vesicular structures such as lysosomes, forming the phagolysosome (see above). This leads to enzymatic degradation of the ingested material.

phenotype Physical expression of an individual's genotype.

phosphatase Enzyme that removes phosphate groups from the side chains of specific amino acids.

phospholipase C-γ (PLC-γ) Enzyme involved in T- and B-cell activation pathways; splits phosphatidylinositol bisphosphate into diacylglycerol (DAG) and inositol triphosphate, leading to the activation of two major intracellular signaling pathways.

phytohemagglutinin (PHA) Mitogen that polyclonally activates T cells.

pinocytosis Ingestion of liquid or very small particles by vesicle formation in a cell.

plasma Fluid component of unclotted blood.

plasma cell Antibody-producing cell that is the end stage of B-cell differentiation.

platelets Bone marrow-derived cells crucial in blood clotting.

pluripotency Ability of a cell to differentiate into numerous other types of cells.

PMN See **polymorphonuclear leukocytes**.

poison ivy Plant whose leaves contain pentadecacatechol, a potent contact-sensitizing agent and a frequent cause of contact hypersensitivity.

pokeweed mitogen Mitogen that polyclonally activates T and B cells.

polyclonal activator Substance that induces activation of many individual clones of either T or B cells. See also **mitogen**.

poly-Ig receptor Binds to IgA at one surface of an epithelial cell, transports it through the cell, and releases it at the opposite lumenal surface; IgA can then participate in protecting the outer surface of the mucosal system.

polymerase chain reaction (PCR) Reaction that produces large amounts of DNA from a sequence by repeated cycles of synthesis.

polymorphism Literally, having many shapes; in genetics, the existence of multiple alleles at a particular genetic locus, resulting in variants of the gene and product among different members of the species.

polymorphonuclear (PMN) leukocytes Leukocytes containing cytoplasmic granules with characteristic multilobed nucleus; the three major types are neutrophils, eosinophils, and basophils.

polyvalency The presence of multiple identical copies of an epitope on a single antigen molecule, cell surface, or particle; examples include bacterial capsular polysaccharides. Polyvalent antigens are often capable of activating B lymphocytes independent of helper T cells.

positive selection The process by which the double-positive thymocyte interacts with MHC molecules and peptides expressed on cortical epithelial cells in the thymus, receiving signals both to survive and commit to either the CD4$^+$ or CD8$^+$ lineages. In the absence of this interaction, the double-positive cell dies.

pre-B cell Cell in the B-cell lineage that has rearranged heavy- but not light-chain genes; expresses surrogate light chains and μ heavy chain at its surface in conjunction with Igα and Igβ; all these molecules comprise the pre-B-cell receptor.

pre-B-cell receptor (pre-BCR) Complex expressed in pre-B cells comprising μ and surrogate light chains plus Igα/β. Once expressed, the pre-B cells are ready to rearrange their light chains.

precipitin reaction Mixing of soluble antigen and antibody at different proportions that can result in the precipitation of insoluble antigen–antibody complexes.

prednisone Synthetic steroid with potent anti-inflammatory and immunosuppressive activity used to treat acute graft rejection, autoimmune disease, and lymphoid tumors.

pre-T cell Cell in T-lymphocyte differentiation in the thymus that has rearranged TCR β genes and expresses TCR β polypeptide on its surface in association with pT-α (gp33), and CD3, forming the pre-T-cell receptor.

pre-T-cell receptor (pre-TCR) Expressed on the surface of pre-T cells, consisting of TCR β chains, pT-α, and CD3.

primary follicle Region of a secondary lymphoid organ containing predominantly unstimulated B lymphocytes;

develops into a germinal center following antigen stimulation.

primary immunodeficiency A genetic defect in which an inherited deficiency in some aspect of the innate or adaptive immune system leads to an increased susceptibility to infections. Primary immunodeficiencies are frequently manifested early in infancy and childhood but sometimes are detected clinically later in life.

primary lymphoid organs Organs in which the early stages of T- and B-lymphocyte differentiation take place and antigen-specific receptors are first expressed.

primary response The adaptive immune response resulting from first encounter with antigen; generally small in magnitude with a long induction phase or lag period. In the primary B-cell response, IgM antibodies are made first.

priming Activation of naïve lymphocytes by exposure to antigen.

pro-B cell Earliest stage of B-cell differentiation in which a heavy-chain D gene segment rearranges to a J gene segment.

professional antigen-presenting cells (APCs) Refers to dendritic cells, mononuclear phagocytes, and B lymphocytes. APCs are capable of presenting antigen to T lymphocytes. All are capable of expressing MHC class II molecules and co-stimulators. Dendritic cells are the most important professional APCs for initiating primary T-cell responses.

programmed cell death See **apoptosis**.

promoter DNA sequence immediately 5′ to the transcription start site of a gene where the proteins that initiate transcription bind. The term *promoter* is often used to mean the entire 5′ regulatory region of a gene, including enhancers, which are additional sequences that bind transcription factors and interact with the basal transcription complex to increase the rate of transcriptional initiation. Other enhancers may be located at a significant distance from the promoter, either 5′ of the gene, in introns, or 3′ of the gene.

properdin (factor P) A positive regulator of the alternative pathway of complement activation; stabilizes C3bBb.

prophylaxis Protection.

prostaglandins Lipid products of metabolism of arachidonic acid that, like leukotrienes, have multiple effects (e.g., inflammatory mediators) on a variety of tissues.

protease Enzyme that cleaves peptide bonds and thereby breaks proteins down into peptides. Different kinds of proteases have different specificities for bonds between particular amino acid residues. Proteases within phagocytes are important for killing ingested microbes during innate immune responses. Within APCs, proteases generate peptide fragments of protein antigens that bind to MHC molecules during T-cell–mediated immune responses. Finally, when released from phagocytes at inflammatory sites, proteases can cause tissue damage.

proteasome Multiprotein cytoplasmic complex that catabolizes proteins to peptides.

protein A A membrane component of *Staphylococcus aureus* that binds to the Fc region of IgG and is thought to protect the bacteria from IgG antibodies by inhibiting their interactions with complement and Fc receptors. It is useful in purifying IgG.

protein kinase C Enzyme activated by calcium and diacylglycerol during T- and B-lymphocyte activation.

protein tyrosine kinases (PTKs) Enzymes that mediate the phosphorylation of tyrosine residues in proteins and thereby promote phosphotyrosine-dependent protein–protein interactions. PTKs are involved in many signal transduction pathways in cells of the immune system.

proto-oncogenes Cellular genes regulating growth control; mutation or aberrant expression can lead to malignant transformation of the cell.

protozoa Single-celled eukaryotic organisms, many of which are human parasites and cause disease. Examples of pathogenic protozoa include *Leishmania*, which causes leishmaniasis; *Entamoeba histolytica*, which causes amebic dysentery; and *Plasmodium*, which causes malaria.

provirus DNA form of a retrovirus integrated into the host DNA.

pseudogene Sequence of DNA resembling a gene but containing codons that prevent transcription into full-length RNA species.

pus Mixture of cell debris and dead neutrophils that is present in wounds and abscesses infected with extracellular encapsulated bacteria.

pyogenic Refers to the generation of pus at the sites of response to bacteria with large capsules.

pyrogen Substance that causes fever.

Rac Small guanine-nucleotide-binding protein that is activated by the GDP–GTP exchange factor Vav during the early events of T-cell activation. GTP-activated Rac triggers a three-step protein kinase cascade that culminates in activation of the stress-activated protein (SAP) kinase, c-*jun* N-terminal kinase (JNK), and p38 kinase, which are similar to the MAP kinases.

radioallergosorbent test (RAST) Solid-phase radioimmunoassay for detecting IgE antibody specific for a particular allergen.

radioimmunoassay (RIA) Technique for measuring the level of a biologic substance in a sample, by measuring the binding of antigen to radioactively labeled antibody (or vice versa).

RAG-1* and *RAG-2 Recombination-activating genes; their products are expressed specifically in developing B and T cells and play a key role in V(D)J recombination.

rapamycin Immunosuppressive agent used to prevent transplantation rejection; blocks cytokine production.

Ras Member of a family of nucleotide-binding proteins with intrinsic GTPase activity that are involved in many different signal transduction pathways in diverse cells types. Mutated Ras genes are associated with neoplastic transformation. Physiologically, during T-cell activation, Ras is recruited to the plasma membrane by tyrosine-phosphorylated adaptor proteins, where it is activated by GDP–GTP exchange factors. Activated Ras then initiates the MAP kinase cascade, which leads to *fos* gene expression and assembly of the AP-1 transcription factor.

reactive oxygen intermediates (ROIs) Highly reactive metabolites of oxygen, including superoxide anion, hydrogen peroxide, and hydroxyl radical, that are produced by activated phagocytes. Phagocytes use ROIs to form oxyhalides that damage ingested bacteria. ROIs may also be released from cells and promote inflammatory responses or cause tissue damage.

reagin IgE antibody that mediates an immediate hypersensitivity reaction.

receptor Generally in the immune system, a transmembrane molecule that binds to a ligand on the exterior surface of the cell, leading to biochemical changes inside the cell.

receptor editing Process in which the interaction of an immature B cell with self-antigen induces a secondary rearrangement of immunoglobulin light-chain genes generating a different antigenic specificity.

recombinant vaccine See **synthetic vaccine**.

recombination See **V(D)J recombination**.

recombination-activating genes See ***RAG-1* and *RAG-2***.

red pulp An anatomic and functional compartment of the spleen composed of vascular sinusoids in which large numbers of erythrocytes, macrophages, dendritic cells, sparse lymphocytes, and plasma cells are scattered. Macrophages within red pulp clear the blood of microbes, other foreign particles, and damaged red blood cells.

Reed–Sternberg cells Large malignant B cells that are found in Hodgkin disease.

regulatory T (Treg) cells A population of T cells, most of which are CD4$^+$, that regulate the activation of other T cells and is necessary to maintain peripheral tolerance to self-antigens. Many Treg cells constitutively express CD25, the α chain of the IL-2 receptor, and the transcription factor FoxP3.

repertoire The complete and enormous range of antigenic specificities of either B or T lymphocytes in an individual.

RES See **reticuloendothelial system**.

respiratory burst Process by which reactive oxygen intermediates such as superoxide anion, hydrogen peroxide, and hydroxyl radical are produced in macrophages and polymorphonuclear leukocytes. Mediated by the enzyme phagocyte oxidase and often triggered by inflammatory mediators, such as TNF, LTB$_4$, and platelet-activating factor (PAF), or by products uniquely produced by bacteria, such as N-formylmethionyl peptides.

reticuloendothelial system (RES) A general term for the network of phagocytic cells.

reverse transcriptase Enzyme that transcribes the RNA genome of a retrovirus into DNA; used in molecular biology to convert RNA into complementary DNA (cDNA).

Rh blood group antigens A complex system of protein alloantigens expressed on red blood cell membranes. Differences between maternal and paternal Rh antigens are the cause of transfusion reactions and hemolytic disease of the newborn.

rheumatic fever Caused by antibodies elicited after infection with some *Streptococcus* species. Some of these antibodies cross-react with heart, kidney, and joint antigens.

rheumatoid arthritis Autoimmune, inflammatory disease of the joints.

rheumatoid factor Autoantibody (usually IgM) that reacts with the individual's own IgG; present in rheumatoid arthritis.

ring vaccination Public health strategy for immunizing a select group of individuals, usually within a relatively small geographic location, who have either been exposed to or potentially exposed to an infectious microorganism that poses a public health threat such as a biological weapon.

SCID See **severe combined immunodeficiency disease**.

second set rejection Accelerated rejection of an allograft in a primed recipient.

secondary immune response Adaptive immune response that occurs on second exposure to an antigen; characterized by more rapid kinetics and greater magnitude relative to the primary immune response, which occurs after initial exposure to the antigen.

secondary lymphoid organs Organs such as the spleen and lymph nodes in which antigen-driven proliferation and differentiation of mature B and T lymphocytes take place following antigen recognition.

secretory component Cleaved component of the poly-Ig receptor that attaches to dimeric IgA and protects it from proteolytic cleavage as it is transported through an epithelial cell.

selectins A family of cell-surface adhesion molecules found on leukocytes and endothelial cells; they bind to sugars on glycoproteins.

selective immunoglobulin deficiency Immunodeficiencies characterized by the inability to produce one or more Ig classes or subclasses. Selective IgA deficiency is the most common selective Ig deficiency, followed by IgG$_3$ and IgG$_2$ deficiencies. Patients with these disorders may be at increased risk for bacterial infections, but many are normal.

self-MHC restriction Phenomenon in which an individual's T cells respond only to peptides associated with MHC molecules that were present in the thymus during T-cell maturation (i.e., self-MHC molecules).

self-tolerance Unresponsiveness of B and T lymphocytes to self-antigens, largely as a result of inactivation or death of self-reactive lymphocytes induced by exposure to those self-antigens. Self-tolerance is a cardinal feature of the normal immune system, and failure of self-tolerance leads to autoimmune diseases.

sensitization Immunization by antigen; generally used for first encounter with allergen.

sepsis Infection of the bloodstream.

septic shock Often lethal complication of severe Gram-negative bacterial infection with spread to the bloodstream (sepsis) that is characterized by vascular collapse, disseminated intravascular coagulation, and metabolic disturbances. Typically triggered by bacterial lipopolysaccharides (LPS, or endotoxin) that can induce a cytokine storm characterized by immune cell production of dangerous levels of multiple cytokines, including IL-1, IL-12, and TNF. Septic shock is also called *endotoxin shock*.

seroconversion The production of detectable antibodies in the serum specific for a microorganism during the course of an infection or in response to immunization.

serology Use of antibodies to detect antigens.

serotype Antigenically distinct subset of a species or subspecies of an infectious organism that is distinguished from other subsets by serologic tests (i.e., serum antibody). Antibody responses to one serotype of microbes (e.g., influenza virus) may not be protective against another serotype.

serum Residual fluid derived from clotted blood; contains antibodies.

serum sickness Type III hypersensitivity reaction resulting from deposition of circulating, soluble, antigen–antibody complexes leading to complement and neutrophil activation in tissues such as the kidney; typically induced following therapy with large doses of antibody from a foreign source, such as monoclonal antibodies made in mice (or, originally, by treating patients with horse serum).

severe combined immunodeficiency (SCID) Disease resulting from early block in differentiation pathways of both B and T lymphocytes.

signal transducers and activators of transcription (STATs) Intracellular proteins phosphorylated by Janus kinases as a consequence of cytokine–cytokine receptor engagement.

signal transduction Processes involved in transmitting the signal received on the outer surface of the cell (e.g., by antigen binding to its receptor) into the nucleus of the cell, which leads to altered gene expression.

SLE See **systemic lupus erythematosus**.

slow-reacting substance of anaphylaxis (SRS-A) Group of leukotrienes released by mast cells during anaphylaxis that induce a prolonged contraction of smooth muscle.

smallpox Infectious disease caused by the virus *Variola* that has been eliminated in the world by vaccination.

somatic gene conversion Nonreciprocal exchange of sequences between genes: Part of the donor gene or genes is copied into an acceptor gene, but only the acceptor gene is altered; it is the mechanism for generating diverse Ig repertoire in many nonhuman species.

somatic hypermutation Mutation in the variable-region sequence of an antibody produced by a B cell following antigenic stimulation in the germinal center; results in increased antibody affinity for antigen.

specificity Used in the immune system to indicate that adaptive immune responses are directed toward and able to distinguish between distinct antigens or small parts of antigens. Derives from the ability of BCRs and TCRs on B and T cells, respectively, to bind to one molecule but not to another with only minor structural differences.

spleen Largest of the secondary lymphoid organs; traps and concentrates foreign substances carried in the blood; composed of white pulp, and rich in lymphoid cells and red pulp, which contains many erythrocytes and macrophages.

Src homology 2 (SH2) domain Three-dimensional domain structure of about 100 amino acid residues present in many signaling proteins that permits specific noncovalent interactions with other proteins by binding to phosphotyrosines. Each SH2 domain has a unique binding specificity that is determined by the amino acid residues adjacent to the phos-

photyrosine on the target protein. Several proteins involved in early signaling events in T and B lymphocytes interact with one another through SH2 domains.

Src homology 3 (SH3) domain Structural domain of about 60 amino acid residues present in many signaling proteins that mediates protein–protein binding. SH3 domains bind to proline residues and function cooperatively with the SH2 domains of the same protein.

STATs See **signal transducers and activators of transcription**.

stem cell Precursor cell that can differentiate into multiple lineages; for example, all blood cells arise from a common hematopoietic stem cell.

strain Set of animals (particularly mice and rats) in which every animal is bred to be genetically identical.

superantigen A molecule that activates all T cells with a particular $V\beta$ gene segment, irrespective of their $V\alpha$ expression.

suppression A mechanism for producing a specific state of immunologic unresponsiveness by which one cell or its products inhibit the function of another.

surrogate light chains Non-rearranging chains ($V\lambda 5$ and V pre-B) expressed in conjunction with the μ chain in the pre-B cell; they form part of the pre-BCR.

switch recombination The molecular mechanism underlying Ig isotype switching in which a rearranged VDJ gene segment in an antibody-producing B cell recombines with a downstream C gene and the intervening C genes are deleted. It involves nucleotide sequences called *switch regions* located in the introns at the 5′ end of each C_H locus. Switch recombination is triggered by the binding of CD40 to CD40 ligand, and by interaction of antigen-stimulated B cells with T-cell-derived cytokines.

switch region Region of B-cell heavy-chain DNA at which recombination occurs in an antigen-stimulated cell; allows class (or isotype) switch (e.g., IgM to IgE).

syngeneic Literally, genetically identical; e.g., monozygotic twins or mice of the same strain.

syngraft Same as **isograft**.

synthetic vaccine Vaccine composed of recombinant-DNA-derived antigens; also called *recombinant vaccine*. Synthetic vaccines for hepatitis B virus and herpes simplex virus are now in use.

systemic inflammatory response syndrome (SIRS) The systemic changes observed in patients who have disseminated bacterial infections ranging from mild forms characterized by neutrophilia, fever, and a rise in acute-phase reactants in the plasma to severe cases that include disseminated intravascular coagulation, adult respiratory distress syndrome, and septic shock. SIRS is stimulated by bacterial products such as LPS and mediated by cytokines of the innate immune system.

systemic lupus erythematosus (SLE) Autoimmune disease that affects many organs of the body and causes fever and joint pain. Patients produce high levels of antibodies against the components of cell nuclei, particularly DNA, and form circulating soluble antigen–antibody complexes. These complexes deposit in tissues such as the kidney, activate the complement cascade, and result in tissue damage.

T-bet A T-box family transcription factor that promotes the differentiation of T_H1 cells from naïve T cells.

T cell See **T lymphocyte**.

T-cell receptor (TCR) Two-chain clonally distributed heterodimer on the T cell that recognizes antigen. Each chain contains one Ig-like variable (V) domain, one Ig-like constant (C) domain, a hydrophobic transmembrane region, and a short cytoplasmic region. $\alpha\beta$ is the most common form. It interacts with complexes of foreign peptides bound to self-MHC molecules on the surface of host cells. A smaller population of T cells uses γ and δ chains as their TCR. $\gamma\delta$ T cells are found mostly in epithelial barrier tissues.

T-cell receptor complex Multiprotein plasma membrane complex expressed by T lymphocytes composed of the clonally distributed, antigen-binding TCR heterodimer and the invariant signaling proteins CD3 δ, ε, and γ plus the ζ chain.

T-dependent antigen Immunogen that requires helper $(CD4^+)$ T cells for B cells to synthesize antibody. Helper T cells produce cytokines and express cell surface molecules that stimulate B-cell growth and differentiation into antibody-secreting cells. Antibody responses to T-dependent antigens are characterized by class switching, affinity maturation, and memory.

T-independent (TI) antigen Immunogen that induces B lymphocyte antibody synthesis in the absence of T cells or their products; usually stimulates only IgM responses (no class switching) and no memory response.

T lymphocyte The lymphocytes (also called *T cells*) that require the thymus for differentiation; they expresses an antigen-specific receptor, the TCR, and mediate cell-mediated immune responses in the adaptive immune system. Major subsets are defined by expression of different TCRs such as $\alpha\beta$ or $\gamma\delta$, and surface markers and function: $CD4^+$ (cytokine synthesis), $CD8^+$ (cytotoxic), and NKT.

tacrolimus Immunosuppressive polypeptide drug (also called FK506) that inactivates T cells by inhibiting signal transduction from the T-cell receptor.

TAP-1 and TAP-2 See **transporter associated with antigen processing**.

tapasin TAP-associated protein that is a key molecule for the assembly of MHC class I molecules. Cells deficient in this protein are unable to express MHC class I molecules on their surface.

target A cell killed by one of the body's killer cells, such as a CTL or NK cell.

TCR See **T-cell receptor**.

terminal deoxynucleotidyl transferase (TdT) Enzyme that inserts nontemplated nucleotides at the junctions of V, D, and J gene segments of Ig and TCR locus DNA; these nucleotides increase the diversity of antigen-specific receptors.

T_H1 cells Subset of $CD4^+$ T cells that synthesize the signature cytokines IL-2, IFN-γ, and TNF-β, and are mainly involved in activating cells of cell-mediated immunity and in stimulating B cells to produce IgG_3 antibody.

T_H2 cells Subset of $CD4^+$ T cells that synthesize the signature cytokines IL-4, IL-5, and IL-13, and are mainly involved in activating effector cells involved in responses to parasitic worms and to allergens.

T_H17 cells Subset of $CD4^+$ T cells that secrete the IL-17 family of proinflammatory cytokines as well as IL-22 and other cytokines. They are protective against certain bacterial and fungal infections and also involved in autoinflammatory diseases.

thymic epithelial cells Epithelial cells found in the cortical and medullary stroma of the thymus that play a critical role in T-cell development. Cortical epithelial cells play a key role in positive selection: T cells must recognize self-peptides bound to MHC molecules on the surface to be rescued from programmed cell death. Medullary epithelial cells play a role in negative selection (also see **AIRE gene**).

thymocytes T cells differentiating in the thymus.

thymus The primary lymphoid organ for T-cell differentiation, comprising an outer cortex and inner medulla; developing thymocytes interact with MHC molecules and peptides expressed by thymic epithelial cells and dendritic cells.

TIL See **tumor-infiltrating lymphocyte**.

tingible body macrophages Macrophages in the germinal center that phagocytize apoptotic B cells.

tissue typing A laboratory method to determine the particular MHC alleles expressed by an individual for the purpose of matching allograft donors and recipients. Often called *HLA typing*, it can be performed by testing whether sera known to be reactive with certain MHC gene products mediate complement-dependent lysis of an individual's lymphocytes. More commonly, PCR techniques are used to determine HLA allele expression.

titer Reciprocal of the last dilution of a titration giving a measurable effect; e.g., if the last dilution of an antibody giving significant agglutination is 1:128, the titer is 128. It is used generally as an empirical measure of the avidity of an antibody.

TNF See **tumor necrosis factor**.

tolerance Antigen-specific unresponsiveness of B or T cells.

Toll-like receptors (TLRs) Family of pattern-recognition receptors (PRRs) expressed on cells of the innate immune system that recognize microorganisms and evoke a host defense response and the development of adaptive immunity through production of inflammatory cytokines and expression of co-stimulatory molecules.

Toll pathway Signaling pathway that activates transcription factor NF-κB by degrading its inhibitor I-κB.

toxic-shock syndrome Systemic reaction produced by the toxin derived from the bacterium *Staphylococcus aureus*; the toxin acts as a superantigen, which activates a high proportion of $CD4^+$ cells to produce cytokines.

toxoid Nontoxic derivative of a toxin used as an immunogen in vaccines to induce antibodies capable of cross-reacting with the toxin.

transfusion Transplantation of blood cells, platelets, or plasma from one individual to another. Performed to treat blood loss from hemorrhage or to treat a deficiency in one or more blood cell types resulting from inadequate production or excess destruction.

transfusion reaction Immunologic reaction against transfused blood products, usually mediated by preformed antibodies in the recipient that bind to donor blood cell antigens, such as ABO blood group antigens or histocompatibility antigens. In severe cases, transfusion reactions can cause disseminated intravascular coagulation, kidney damage, fever, and shock.

transgenic mouse A mouse that expresses an exogenous gene that has been introduced into the genome by injection of a specific DNA sequence into the pronuclei of fertilized mouse eggs. Transgenes insert randomly at chromosomal break points and are subsequently inherited as simple Mendelian traits.

transplantation Grafting solid tissue (such as a kidney or heart) or cells (particularly bone marrow) from one individual to another. See **allograft** and **xenograft**.

transporter associated with antigen processing (TAP) Two-chain peptide transporter (TAP-1 and TAP-2) that mediates the active transport of peptides from the cytosol to the site of assembly of MHC class I molecules inside the endoplasmic reticulum.

Treg cells Subset of $CD4^+$ T cells that regulate or inhibit the function of other lymphocyte subsets. Synthesize inhibitory cytokines TGF-β and IL-10. See also **regulatory T cells**.

tuberculin test Subcutaneous injection of antigens derived from the organism causing tuberculosis; individuals who have been exposed to the organism and those who have been previously vaccinated with BCG develop a delayed hypersensitivity response at the injection site 24–48 hours later.

tumor immunity Describes immune responses against tumor cells.

tumor-infiltrating lymphocyte (TIL) Mononuclear cells derived from the inflammatory infiltrate of solid tumors.

tumor necrosis factor-β (TNF-β) See **lymphotoxin**.

tumor necrosis factor (TNF) Proinflammatory cytokine with functions including the selective killing of tumor cells; toxicity may be the result of the production of free radicals following the binding of high-affinity cell-surface receptors.

tumor-specific transplantation antigen (TSTA) Antigens uniquely expressed by certain tumor cells.

TUNEL assay Identifies apoptotic cells *in situ* by the characteristic fragmentation of their DNA.

type I hypersensitivity Immediate hypersensitivity reactions occurring rapidly after reexposure to allergen and involving IgE responses and triggering of mast cells.

type II hypersensitivity Hypersensitivity reactions involving IgG antibodies against cell-surface antigens that result in direct killing of the cell expressing the antigen.

type III hypersensitivity Hypersensitivity reactions that involve antigen–antibody complexes depositing in filtering organs and triggering cytotoxic reactions.

type IV hypersensitivity T-cell–mediated, delayed (24–72 hours after reexposure to antigen) hypersensitivity reactions involving mainly T_H1 cells and monocytes.

tyrosine kinases Family of enzymes that phosphorylates proteins on tyrosine residues, a critical step in lymphocyte activation. The key tyrosine kinases in T-cell activation are Lck, Fyn, and ZAP-70; those in B-cell activation are Blk, Fyn, Lyn, and Syk.

unresponsiveness Inability to respond to antigenic stimulation. Unresponsiveness may be specific for a particular antigen (see **tolerance**) or broadly nonspecific as a result of damage to the entire immune system such as that occurring after whole-body irradiation.

urticaria Swelling and redness of the skin caused by localized and transient leakage of fluid and plasma proteins from small vessels into the dermis during an immediate hypersensitivity reaction.

V region See **variable region**.

vaccination Any protective immunization against a pathogen. Originally referred to immunization against smallpox with the less virulent cowpox (vaccinia) virus.

variable (V) region The N-terminal portion of an Ig or TCR that contains the antigen-binding region of the molecule; V regions are formed by the recombination of V, D, and J gene segments.

V(D)J recombination Mechanism for generating antigen-specific receptors of T and B cells. The process is mediated by the enzyme complex V(D)J recombinase and products of the *RAG-1* and *RAG-2* genes and involves the joining of V, D, and J gene segments.

virion Complete virus particle.

virus Organism comprising a protein coat and DNA or RNA genome; it requires a host cell for replication.

Western blotting Technique to identify a specific protein in a mixture; proteins separated by gel electrophoresis are blotted onto a nitrocellulose membrane, and the protein of interest is detected by adding radiolabeled antibody specific for the protein.

wheal and flare Itchy reaction at skin site where antigen has been injected into an allergic individual; characterized by erythema (redness due to dilation of blood vessels) and edema (swelling produced by release of serum into tissue).

white pulp Part of the spleen composed predominantly of lymphocytes, arranged in periarteriolar lymphoid sheaths and follicles, and other leukocytes. The remainder of the spleen (the red pulp) contains sinusoids lined with phagocytic cells and filled with blood.

Wiskott–Aldrich syndrome An X-linked immunodeficiency disease characterized by eczema and thrombocytopenia (reduced blood platelets). Individuals with this disease are highly susceptible to bacterial infections. The defective gene encodes a cytosolic protein involved in signaling cascades and regulation of the actin cytoskeleton.

xenoantigen Antigen expressed by a graft from another species.

xenogeneic Originating from a foreign species.

xenograft Tissue transplantation between individuals belonging to two different species.

X-linked agammaglobulinemia Disease in boys (also known as *Bruton's agammaglobulinemia*) in which B-cell differentiation does not progress beyond the pre-B-cell stage and so manifests as the absence of mature B cells; a tyrosine kinase btk is mutated in these individuals.

X-linked hyper-IgM syndrome Disease in boys manifesting as the inability to synthesize Ig isotypes other than IgM; it is a result of defect in CD40 ligand.

ZAP-70 Tyrosine kinase expressed normally only in T cells and critical in T-cell activation; defects result in immunodeficiency. Also expressed in chronic lymphocytic leukemia (CLL) cells.

APPENDIX

Partial List of CD Antigens

CD Antigen	Other Name(s)	Cellular Expression	Function/Comments	Ligand
CD1		Langerhans cells, dendritic cells, B cells, thymocytes	MHC class I-like molecule, presents lipids and glycolipids to T cells	Lipids, glycolipids
CD2	T11, LFA-2	T cells, NK cells	T-cell adhesion molecule	CD58
CD3	T3	T cells	TCR signal transduction	
CD4	T4	Thymocytes, major set of mature T cells (MHC class II restricted), monocytes, macrophages	T-cell co-receptor, signal transduction	MHC class II, HIV-1 and HIV-2, gp 120
CD5	T1, Tp67	B-cell subset, T cells	B-cell expression associated with polyreactive IgM production	
CD8	T8	Thymocytes, major set of mature T cells (MHC class I restricted) = cytotoxic T cells	T-cell co-receptor, signal transduction	MHC class I
CD11a	LFA-1 chain	Leukocytes	Subunit of adhesion molecule CD11a/CD18 (LFA-1)	ICAM-1, -2, -3
CD18		Leukocytes	Integrin chain that associates with CD11a, b, c, or d	
CD19		B cells	B-cell signal transduction	
CD20		B cells	Ca^{2+} channel in B-cell activation	
CD21	CR2	B cells, follicular dendritic cells	Involved in B-cell activation	Complement component C3d and EBV
CD25	TAC	Activated T cells, B cells	IL-2 receptor α chain	IL-2
CD28	Tp44	T-cell subsets	T-cell co-stimulator molecule	B7 (CD80 and CD86)

Immunology: A Short Course, Seventh Edition. Richard Coico and Geoffrey Sunshine.
© 2015 John Wiley & Sons, Ltd. Published 2015 by John Wiley & Sons, Ltd.
Companion Website: www.wileyimmunology.com/coico

CD Antigen	Other Name(s)	Cellular Expression	Function/Comments	Ligand
CD32	FcγRII	Monocytes, granulocytes, B cells, eosinophils	Low-affinity receptor for IgG	Aggregated IgG and antigen–antibody complexes
CD34		Endothelial cells, hematopoietic precursors	Marker for early stem cells	L-Selectin (CD62L)
CD40		B cells, macrophages, dendritic cells	Involved in T-cell interactions with APCs and class switching; receptor for co-stimulatory signals	CD154 (CD40L)
CD44	Pgp-1, H-CAM	Leukocytes, erythrocytes	Lymphocyte adhesion to HEV	Hyaluronic acid
CD50	ICAM-3	Broad (not on endothelial cells)	Adhesion molecule	LFA-1
CD54	ICAM-1	Broad	Adhesion molecule	CD11a/CD18, rhinovirus
CD55	DAF	Broad	Dissociates C3 convertases of complement cascades	C3b, C4b, CD97
CD58	LFA-3	Leukocytes, endothelial cells, epithelial cells, fibroblasts	Adhesion molecule	CD2
CD62L	L-Selectin, MEL-14	B cells, T cells, monocytes, NK cells	T-cell adhesion to HEV	CD34
CD74	Invariant chain	B cells, macrophages, monocytes, activated T cells	Associated with MHC class II in endoplasmic reticulum	
CD79a, CD79b	Igα, Igβ	B cells, pre-B cells	Signal transduction molecules associated with Ig in of BCR	
CD80	B7.1	B cells, macrophages, dendritic cells	Co-stimulatory molecule on APCs	CD28, CD152 (CTLA-4)
CD81	Target of antiproliferative antibody (TAPA-1)	Broad	Associates with CD19, CD21, and CD225 on B cells to form B-cell co-receptor	
CD86	B7.2	Activated B cells, macrophages, dendritic cells	Co-stimulatory molecule on APCs	CD28, CD152 (CTLA-4)
CD95	Fas, Apo-1	Activated T and B cells, NK cells	Induces apoptosis following ligation with Fas ligand (CD178, CD95L)	CD178 (Fas ligand, CD95L)
CD97	GR1	Granulocytes, macrophages, activated T and B cells	Counter-receptor for CD55	CD55
CD102	ICAM-2	Endothelial cells, resting lymphocytes, platelets	Adhesion molecule	CD11a (LFA-1)
CD152	CTLA-4	Activated T cells	Negative regulator for T-cell activation	CD80 (B7.1) and CD86 (B7.2)
CD154	CD40L	Activated T cells	Binding to CD40 on B cells induces B-cell proliferation and class switching	CD40
CD178	Fas ligand, CD95 ligand	T cells and NK cells	Induces apoptosis in cells expressing CD95; humans and KO mice with CD178 mutation show severe autoimmune disease	CD95 (Fas)
CD210	IL-10 receptor	T and B cells, NK cells, monocytes, macrophages	Receptor for IL-10; binding to IL-10 inhibits macrophage, monocyte, and dendritic cell cytokine production	IL-10

CD Antigen	Other Name(s)	Cellular Expression	Function/Comments	Ligand
CD212	IL-12 receptor β chain	Majority of T cells, NK cells, some B-cell lines	Dimerizes and associates with an unknown chain to form the IL-12 receptor; IL-12 directs immune responses preferentially toward T_H1-type responses.	IL-12
CD213	IL-13 receptor	Broadly expressed in hematopoietic tissue, nervous system, and other tissues	Binding to IL-13 mediates signals to suppress inflammatory cytokine production by monocytes and macrophages; IL-13 induces B-cell proliferation and Ig production	IL-13
CD217	IL-17 receptor	Broad tissue distribution; cord blood lymphocytes, peripheral blood lymphocytes, thymocytes	Binds IL-17 with low affinity; IL-17 induces proinflammatory cytokine secretion	IL-17
CD220	Insulin receptor	Ubiquitous, including erythrocytes, liver, muscle, adipose tissue	Cellular receptor for insulin; mutation in CD220 leads to insulin-resistant diabetes mellitus	Insulin
CD225	Leu 13	Broad	Associates with CD19, CD21, and CD81 on B cells to form B-cell co-receptor	
CD247	ζ (zeta) chain, also known as CD3 ζ or TCR ζ	All T cells and NK cells	Part of TCR complex; couples antigen recognition to intracellular signal transduction pathways	Not applicable
CD281	Toll-like receptor (TLR) 1, TIL	Monocytes and neutrophils; detectable in breast milk	Plays role in innate immunity; induction of signal cascade leads to proinflammatory cytokine release	Recognizes outer surface protein A lipoprotein of *Borrelia burgdorferi*, mycobacterial lipoprotein, and triacylated lipopeptides
CD282	Toll-like receptor (TLR) 2, TIL4	Peripheral blood leukocytes; high expression in monocytes in bone marrow, lymph nodes, and spleen; detectable in other tissues	Plays role in innate immunity; induction of signal cascade leads to proinflammatory cytokine release	Recognizes molecular patterns of fungi, protozoan pathogens, and bacteria
CD283	Toll-like receptor (TLR) 3, TLR3	Fibroblasts, myeloid dendritic cells, microglia, and astrocytes; mostly intracellular	Response to double-stranded viral RNA; activation leads to initiation of caspase-dependent apoptotic cascade	
CD284	Toll-like receptor (TLR) 4, TLR4	Monocytes, macrophages, granulocytes, dendritic cells, and activated $CD4^+$ T cells	Activation of signaling pathways by binding to LPS ligand results in inflammatory cytokine production favoring a T_H1 response	LPS, taxol, RSV fusion protein, endogenous ligands include fibronectin, hyaluronic acid
CD288	Toll-like receptor (TLR) 8, TLR8	Endosomal compartments of macrophages and subsets of dendritic cells	Part of innate defense against RNA viruses; ligation triggers secretion of inflammatory and regulatory cytokines	Single-stranded GU-rich viral RNA
CD289	Toll-like receptor (TLR) 9, TLR9	High-level expression by plasmacytoid dendritic cells, by primary and secondary lymphoid organs, and at low levels by peripheral blood leukocytes	Receptor for DNA present in endosomes during bacterial and viral infection; triggers adaptive response toward T_H1	Unmethylated CpG DNA motifs

INDEX

Note: Page entries in *italics* refer to figures/photos; tables are noted with a t.

Immunology: A Short Course, Seventh Edition. Richard Coico and Geoffrey Sunshine.
© 2015 John Wiley & Sons, Ltd. Published 2015 by John Wiley & Sons, Ltd.
Companion Website: www.wileyimmunology.com/coico